Oxorn-Foote

HUMAN LABOR & BIRTH

Oxorn-Foote

HUMAN LABOR & BIRTH

Seventh Edition

GLENN D. POSNER, MDCM, MEd, FRCSC
Professor, University of Ottawa
Department of Obstetrics and Gynecology
The Ottawa Hospital
Ottawa, Ontario, Canada

AMANDA Y. BLACK, MD, MPH, FRCSC
Professor, University of Ottawa
Department of Obstetrics and Gynecology
The Ottawa Hospital
Division of Pediatric Gynecology, Children's Hospital of Eastern Ontario
Ottawa, Ontario, Canada

GRIFFITH JONES, MBBS, MRCOG, FRCSC
Assistant Professor, University of Ottawa
Department of Obstetrics and Gynecology
Division of Maternal–Fetal Medicine
The Ottawa Hospital
Ottawa, Ontario, Canada

DARINE EL-CHAÂR, MD, MSc (Epi), FRCSC
Associate Professor, University of Ottawa
Department of Obstetrics and Gynecology
Division of Maternal–Fetal Medicine
The Ottawa Hospital
Ottawa, Ontario, Canada

New York Chicago San Francisco Athens London Madrid Mexico City
Milan New Delhi Singapore Sydney Toronto

2 3 4 5 6 7 8 9   DSS   27 26 25 24

ISBN 978-1-260-01941-4
MHID 1-260-01941-1

This title was set in Minion Pro by KnowledgeWorks Global Ltd.
The editors were Jason Malley and Christina M. Thomas.
The production supervisor was Richard Ruzycka.
Project management was provided by Revathi Viswanathan, KnowledgeWorks Global Ltd.
The cover designer was W2 Design.

Library of Congress Cataloging-in-Publication Data

Names: Posner, Glenn D., editor. | Black, Amanda Y. (Professor of obstetrics and gynecology), editor. | Jones, Griffith editor. | El-Chaar, Darine, editor.
Title: Oxorn-Foote human labor & birth / [edited by] Glenn D. Posner, Amanda Y. Black, Griffith Jones, Darine El-Chaar.
Other titles: Human labor & birth
Description: Seventh edition. | New York : McGraw Hill, [2023] | Preceded by Oxorn-Foote human labor & birth. 6th ed. / edited by Glenn D. Posner ... [et al.]. c2013. | Includes bibliographical references and index. | Summary: "A must-buy for the ob-gyn, ob nurse, and midwife, the book presents vital information in a clearly illustrated manner, making it an essential for any practitioner performing or assisting in childbirth. It includes a review of anatomy and proper examination of the patient; variations of fetal presentation are detailed along with proper management and birthing technique. The seventh edition continues to offer explicit management instruction for a variety of complications and delivery scenarios including hemorrhage, fetal concerns, preterm and prolonged labor, dystocia, and more. The book ends with a chapter on preliminary neonatal care"— Provided by publisher.
Identifiers: LCCN 2022017636 | ISBN 9781260019414 (paperback) | ISBN 1260019411 (paperback) | ISBN 9781260019421 (ebook)
Subjects: MESH: Labor, Obstetric | Delivery, Obstetric | Parturition
Classification: LCC RG525 | NLM WQ 300 | DDC 618.2—dc23/eng/20220615
LC record available at https://lccn.loc.gov/2022017636

To: Dr. Andrée Gruslin, we miss you.

DEDICATION

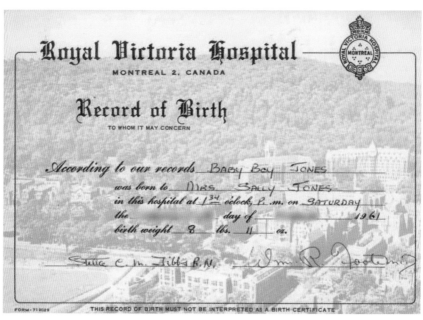

Birth record of Dr. Griffith D. Jones. Dr. Foote played an even more important role in HIS history!

Part I: Clinical Anatomy   1

Part II: First Stage of Labor   87

Part VI: Other Issues   593

Numbers in brackets refer to the chapter(s) written or co-written by the contributor.

Nika Alavi-Tabari, MD, MEd, FRCSC
Assistant Professor, University of Ottawa
Department of Obstetrics and Gynecology
The Ottawa Hospital
Ottawa, Ontario, Canada [23]

Hadeel Alenezi, MD, KBOGyn
Maternal Fetal Medicine Sub-Specialist Affiliate RCSC
Department of Obstetrics and Gynecology
Maternity Hospital
Kuwait [28, 29]

Yaa A. Amankwah, MBChB, FRCSC
Assistant Professor, University of Ottawa
Department of Obstetrics and Gynecology
The Ottawa Hospital
Ottawa, Ontario, Canada [18]

Asma Assiri, MD
Maternal Fetal Medicine and
  Advanced Obstetrics Ultrasound Specialist
Department of Obstetrics and Gynecology
King Faisal Medical City
Abha, Saudi Arabia [37]

Susan L. Aubin, BScH, MD, FRCSC
Assistant Professor, University of Ottawa
Department of Obstetrics and Gynecology
The Ottawa Hospital
Ottawa, Ontario, Canada [11, 12]

Nadya Ben Fadel, MD, FRCPC, FAAP, MMedEd
Assistant Professor, University of Ottawa
Department of Pediatrics, Division of Neonatology
The Children's Hospital of Eastern Ontario
Ottawa, Ontario, Canada [39]

Amanda Y. Black, MD, MPH, FRCSC
Professor, University of Ottawa
Department of Obstetrics, Gynecology, and Newborn Care
The Ottawa Hospital
Division of Pediatric and Adolescent Gynecology
Children's Hospital of Eastern Ontario
Ottawa, Ontario, Canada [13, 16, 17, 23]

Brigitte Bonin, MD, MBA, FRCSC
Associate Professor, University of Ottawa
Department of Obstetrics and Gynecology
The Ottawa Hospital
Ottawa, Ontario, Canada [33]

Innie Chen, MD, MPH, FRCSC
Associate Professor, University of Ottawa
Department of Obstetrics and Gynecology
The Ottawa Hospital
Ottawa, Ontario, Canada [13]

Aisling A. Clancy, MD, MSc, MPH, FRCSC
Assistant Professor, University of Ottawa
Department of Obstetrics and Gynecology
The Ottawa Hospital
Ottawa, Ontario, Canada [21]

Jessica Dy, MD, MPH, FRCSC
Medical Director, Maternal, Newborn, Women's Health Service Line
The Ottawa Hospital
Associate Professor, Department of Obstetrics and Gynecology
University of Ottawa
Ottawa, Ontario, Canada [9, 10]

Wesley J. Edwards, MBBS, MPH, FRCA
Assistant Professor, University of Ottawa
Department of Anesthesia and Pain Medicine
The Ottawa Hospital
Ottawa, Ontario, Canada [34]

Abdalmajed Eisa, MD
Maternal–Fetal Medicine and Advanced Obstetrics and
 Gynecology Ultrasound Specialist
King Khalid University Medical City
Abha, Saudi Arabia [37]

Darine El-Chaâr, MD, MSc (Epi), FRCSC
Associate Professor, University of Ottawa
Department of Obstetrics and Gynecology
Division of Maternal–Fetal Medicine
The Ottawa Hospital
Ottawa, Ontario, Canada [12, 14, 15, 22, 24, 25, 28]

Tamer Elfazari, MD, FRCSC
Assistant Professor, University of Ottawa
Department of Obstetrics and Gynecology
The Ottawa Hospital
Ottawa, Ontario, Canada [25]

Ramadan El Sugy, MD, FRCSC
Department of Obstetrics and Gynecology
William Osler Health System
Brampton, Ontario, Canada [21]

Karen M. Fung-Kee-Fung, MD, FRCSC, MHPE
Professor, University of Ottawa
Department of Obstetrics and Gynecology
The Ottawa Hospital
Ottawa, Ontario, Canada [29]

Catherine Gallant, MD, FRCPC
Assistant Professor, University of Ottawa
Department of Anesthesiology and Pain Medicine
The Ottawa Hospital
Ottawa, Ontario, Canada [36]

Adam Garber, MD, MSc (Ed.), FRCSC
Assistant Professor, University of Ottawa
Department of Obstetrics and Gynecology
The Ottawa Hospital
Ottawa, Ontario, Canada [9, 10, 40]

Laura M. Gaudet, MSc, MD, FRCSC
Associate Professor, Queen's University
Department of Obstetrics and Gynecology
Kingston Health Sciences Centre
Kingston, Ontario, Canada [35]

Megan M. Gomes, MScHQ, FRCSC
Assistant Professor, University of Ottawa
Department of Obstetrics and Gynecology
The Ottawa Hospital
Ottawa, Ontario, Canada [41]

Griffith Jones, MBBS, MRCOG, FRCSC
Assistant Professor, University of Ottawa
Medical Director, Obstetrics & Gynecology Ultrasound
Division of Maternal–Fetal Medicine
Department of Obstetrics and Gynecology
The Ottawa Hospital
Ottawa, Ontario, Canada [30, 34]

Sally Mashally, MD
Neonatal Perinatal Medicine Fellow
University of Ottawa
Ottawa, Ontario, Canada [39]

Roxanna Mohammed, BSc(Pharm), MD, FRCSC
University of Ottawa
Department of Obstetrics and Gynecology
The Ottawa Hospital
Ottawa, Ontario, Canada [14, 15, 26, 27]

Felipe M. Moretti, MD
Associate Professor, University of Ottawa
Department of Obstetrics and Gynecology
The Ottawa Hospital
Ottawa, Ontario, Canada [33, 38]

Lawrence Oppenheimer, MA (Oxon), MB BS, FRCS (Eng), FRCOG, FRCSC
Professor, University of Ottawa
Division of Maternal Fetal Medicine
Department of Obstetrics and Gynecology
The Ottawa Hospital
Ottawa, Ontario, Canada [16, 19]

Dante U. Pascali, MD, FRCSC
Assistant Professor, University of Ottawa
Division of Urogynecology
Department of Obstetrics and Gynecology
The Ottawa Hospital
Ottawa, Ontario, Canada [1, 2, 3, 4]

Glenn D. Posner, MDCM, MEd, FRCSC
Professor, University of Ottawa
Department of Obstetrics and Gynecology
The Ottawa Hospital
Ottawa, Ontario, Canada [5, 6, 7, 8, 20]

Gihad Shabib, MD, MRCOG, FRCSC
Assistant Professor, University of Ottawa
Department of Obstetrics and Gynecology
The Ottawa Hospital
Ottawa, Ontario, Canada [17]

Tammy Shaw, MD, CCFP, FRCPC, MEd
Lecturer, University of Ottawa
Department of General Internal Medicine
The Ottawa Hospital
Ottawa, Ontario, Canada [32]

Sukhbir S. Singh, MD, FRCSC
Professor, University of Ottawa
Department of Obstetrics, Gynecology & Newborn Care
The Ottawa Hospital
Ottawa, Ontario, Canada [19]

Julia Tai, MD, FRCPC
Resident Physician, University of Ottawa
Department of Medicine
The Ottawa Hospital
Ottawa, Ontario, Canada [32]

George Tawagi, BSc, MD, FRCSC
Assistant Professor, University of Ottawa
Department of Obstetrics and Gynecology
The Ottawa Hospital
Ottawa, Ontario, Canada [26, 27]

Ana Werlang, MD, MSc, RCPSC affiliated
Assistant Professor, University of Ottawa
Department of Obstetrics and Gynecology
Division of Maternal–Fetal Medicine
The Ottawa Hospital
Ottawa, Ontario, Canada [31]

It is hard to release a textbook in 2023 without mentioning the global pandemic. We began the process of revising this book in early March of 2020 and our contributors worked on their chapters during one of the most challenging times for health care workers we hope to ever face. Regardless of the wave of the pandemic, we tried to continue providing high-quality maternity care and to work on sharing this knowledge with you. Once again, we are proud that this book represents a tremendous collaboration between obstetricians, pediatricians, internists, and anesthesiologists at The Ottawa Hospital. New chapters on medical education and quality assurance complement the previous content that has all been refreshed for this edition. We hope that Harry Oxorn would continue to be proud.

PART I

Clinical
Anatomy

CHAPTER 1

Pelvis: Bones, Joints, and Ligaments

Dante U. Pascali

PELVIC BONES

The pelvis is the bony basin located at the inferior aspect of the trunk and through which the body weight is transmitted to the lower extremities. In women, it is adapted for childbearing. The pelvis consists of four bones: the two innominate bones, the sacrum, and the coccyx. These are united by four joints.

Innominate Bones

The innominate bones are placed laterally and anteriorly. Each is formed by the fusion of three bones: the ilium, ischium, and pubis located around the acetabulum.

Ilium

The ilium is the superior bone: It has a body (which is fused with the ischial body) and an ala.

Anatomical Landmarks

1. The anterior superior iliac spine gives attachment to the inguinal ligament
2. The posterior superior iliac spine marks the level of the second sacral vertebra. Its presence is indicated by a dimple in the overlying skin
3. The iliac crest extends from the anterior superior iliac spine to the posterior superior iliac spine

Ischium

The ischium consists of a body in which the superior and inferior rami merge.

Anatomical Landmarks

1. The body forms part of the acetabulum
2. The superior ramus is posterior and inferior to the body
3. The inferior ramus fuses with the inferior ramus of the pubis
4. The ischial spine separates the greater sciatic from the lesser sciatic notch. It is an important landmark because this is the attachment for a portion of the levator ani muscle
5. The ischial tuberosity is the inferior part of the ischium and is the bone on which humans sit

Pubis

The pubis consists of the body and two rami.

Anatomical Landmarks

1. The body has a rough surface on its medial aspect. This is joined to the corresponding area on the opposite pubis to form the symphysis pubis. The levator ani muscles are attached to the pelvic aspect of the pubis
2. The pubic crest is the superior border of the body
3. The pubic tubercle, or spine, is the lateral end of the pubic crest. The inguinal ligament and conjoined tendon are attached here
4. The superior ramus meets the body of the pubis at the pubic spine and the body of the ilium at the iliopectineal line, where it forms a part of the acetabulum
5. The inferior ramus merges with the inferior ramus of the ischium

Other Anatomical Relations

1. The iliopectineal line extends from the pubic tubercle back to the sacroiliac joint. It forms the greater part of the boundary of the pelvic inlet
2. The greater sacrosciatic notch is between the posterior inferior iliac spine superiorly and the ischial spine inferiorly
3. The lesser sacrosciatic notch is bounded by the ischial spine superiorly and the ischial tuberosity inferiorly
4. The obturator foramen is delimited by the acetabulum, the ischial rami, and the pubic rami

Sacrum

The sacrum is a triangular bone with the base superiorly and the apex inferiorly. It consists of five vertebrae fused together; rarely, there are four or six. The sacrum lies between the innominate bones and is attached to them by the sacroiliac joints.

The upper surface of the first sacral vertebra articulates with the lower surface of the fifth lumbar vertebra. The anterior (pelvic) surface of the sacrum is concave, and the posterior surface is convex.

The sacral promontory is the anterior superior edge of the first sacral vertebra. It protrudes slightly into the cavity of the pelvis, reducing the anteroposterior diameter of the inlet.

Coccyx

The coccyx (tail bone) is composed of four rudimentary vertebrae. The superior surface of the first coccygeal vertebra articulates with the inferior surface of the fifth sacral vertebra to form the sacrococcygeal joint. Rarely, there is fusion between the sacrum and coccyx, with resultant limitation of movement.

The coccygeus muscle, levator ani muscles, and sphincter ani externus are attached to the anterior aspect of the coccyx. They are important to pelvic floor function.

PELVIC JOINTS AND LIGAMENTS

The sacrum, coccyx, and two innominate bones are linked by four joints: the symphysis pubis, the sacrococcygeal, and the two sacroiliac synchondroses (Fig. 1-1).

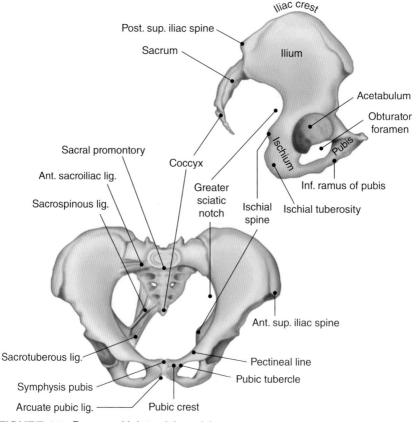

FIGURE 1-1. Bones and joints of the pelvis.

Sacroiliac Joint

The sacroiliac joint lies between the articular surfaces of the sacrum and the ilium. The weight of the body is transmitted through it to the pelvis and then to the lower limbs. It is a synovial joint and permits a small degree of movement. The capsule is weak, and stability is maintained by the muscles around it as well as by four primary and two accessory ligaments.

Primary Ligaments

1. The anterior sacroiliac ligaments are short and transverse, running from the preauricular sulcus on the ilium to the anterior aspect of the ala of the sacrum
2. The interosseus sacroiliac ligaments are short, strong transverse bands that extend from the rough part behind the auricular surface on the ilium to the adjoining area on the sacrum
3. The short posterior sacroiliac ligaments are strong transverse bands that lie behind the interosseus ligaments
4. The long posterior sacroiliac ligaments are each attached to the posterosuperior spine on the ilium and to the tubercles on the third and fourth sacral vertebrae

Accessory Ligaments

1. The sacrotuberous ligaments are attached on one side to the posterior superior iliac spine; posterior inferior iliac spine; tubercles on the third, fourth, and fifth sacral vertebrae; and lateral border of the coccyx. On the other side, the sacrotuberous ligaments are attached to the pelvic aspect of the ischial tuberosity
2. The sacrospinous ligament is triangular. The base is attached to the lateral parts of the fifth sacral and first coccygeal vertebrae, and the apex is attached to the ischial spine

Sacrococcygeal Joint

The sacrococcygeal joint is a synovial hinge joint between the fifth sacral and the first coccygeal vertebrae. It allows both flexion and extension. Extension, by increasing the anteroposterior diameter of the outlet of the pelvis, plays an important role in parturition. Overextension during delivery may break the small cornua by which the coccyx is attached to the sacrum. This joint has a weak capsule, which is reinforced by anterior, posterior, and lateral sacrococcygeal ligaments.

Symphysis Pubis

The symphysis pubis is a cartilaginous joint with no capsule and no synovial membrane. Normally, there is little movement. The posterior and superior ligaments are weak. The strong anterior ligaments are reinforced by the tendons of the rectus abdominis and the external oblique muscles. The strong inferior ligament in the pubic arch is known as the arcuate pubic ligament. It extends between the rami and leaves a small space in the subpubic angle.

MOBILITY OF PELVIS

During normal pregnancy, under the influence of progesterone and relaxin, there is increased flexibility of the sacroiliac joints and the symphysis pubis. Hyperemia and softening of the ligaments around the joints also take place. The pubic bones may separate by 1 to 12 mm. Excessive mobility of the symphysis pubis leads to pain and difficulty in walking. It has been shown that, besides the local changes that may take place in the pelvic ligaments, a generalized change in the laxity of joints occurs in pregnancy.

MALE AND FEMALE PELVISES

At birth, there is no difference between male and female pelvises. Sexual dimorphism does not take place until puberty. A female pelvis develops in offspring born with no gonads. Thus, ovaries and estrogen are not necessary for the formation of the female-type pelvis, but the presence of a testis that is producing androgen is essential for development of the male-type pelvis.

ADOLESCENCE

Adolescent girls' pelvises are smaller than those of mature women. The pattern of growth of the pelvic basin is different from that of bodily stature. Among girls, the growth in stature decelerates rapidly in the first year after menarche and ceases within 1 or 2 years. The pelvic basin, on the other hand, grows more slowly and more steadily during late adolescence. At the same time, it changes from an anthropoid to a gynecoid configuration. Thus, maturation of the reproductive system and attainment of adult size do not indicate that the growth and development of the pelvis are complete. The smaller pelvic capacity in adolescent girls may contribute to the higher incidence of cephalopelvic disproportion and other dystocias in primigravid girls younger than the age of 15 years.

CHAPTER 2

The Pelvic Floor

Dante U. Pascali

THE PELVIC FLOOR

The pelvic floor (Fig. 2-1) is a muscular diaphragm that separates the pelvic cavity above from the perineal space below. It is formed by the levator ani and coccygeus muscles and is covered completely by parietal fascia.

The urogenital hiatus is an anterior gap through which the urethra and vagina pass. The rectal hiatus is posterior, and through which the rectum and anal canal pass.

PELVIC FLOOR FUNCTIONS

1. The pelvic floor supports the pelvic viscera in humans
2. To build up effective intra-abdominal pressure, the muscles of the diaphragm, abdominal wall, and pelvic floor must contract together
3. During parturition, the pelvic floor helps the anterior rotation of the presenting part and directs it downward and forward along the birth passage

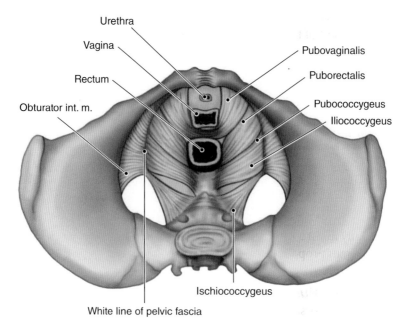

FIGURE 2-1. Pelvic floor.

PELVIC FLOOR MUSCLES

1. Levator ani, each composed of two muscles:
   a. Pubococcygeus, which has three divisions: pubovaginalis, puborectalis, and pubococcygeus proper
   b. Iliococcygeus
   c. Coccygeus (ischiococcygeus)

Levator Ani Muscle

The levator ani muscle has a lateral origin and a central insertion, where it joins with the corresponding muscle from the other side. The direction of the muscle from origin to insertion is inferior and medial. The origin of each levator ani is from the:

1. Posterior side of the pubis
2. Arcuate tendon of the pelvic fascia (the white line of the pelvic fascia)
3. Pelvic aspect of the ischial spine

The insertion, from anterior to posterior, is into:

1. Vaginal walls
2. Central point of the perineum
3. Anal canal
4. Anococcygeal body
5. Lateral border of the coccyx

Pubococcygeus Muscle

The pubococcygeus is the most important, most dynamic, and most specialized part of the pelvic floor. It lies in the midline; is perforated by the urethra, vagina, and rectum; and is often damaged during delivery. It originates from the posterior side of the pubis and from the white line of the pelvic fascia anterior to the obturator canal. The muscle passes posterior and medially in three sections: (1) pubovaginalis, (2) puborectalis, and (3) pubococcygeus proper.

Pubovaginalis Muscle. The most medial section of the pubococcygeus is shaped like a horseshoe and is open anteriorly. The fibers make contact and blend with the muscles of the urethral wall, after which they form a loop around the vagina. They insert into the sides and back of the vagina and into the central point of the perineum.

The principal function of the pubovaginalis is to act as a sling for the vagina. Since the vagina helps to support the uterus and appendages, bladder and urethra, and rectum, this muscle is the main support of the female pelvic organs. Tearing or overstretching predisposes to uterovaginal prolapse. The muscle also functions as the vaginal sphincter, and when it goes into spasm, the condition is called *vaginismus*.

Puborectalis Muscle. The intermediate part of the pubococcygeus forms a loop around the anal canal and rectum. The insertion is into the lateral and posterior walls of the anal canal adjacent to the external anal sphincter. They together form a functional unit contributing to fecal continence and evacuation. The puborectalis also inserts into the anococcygeal body.

The puborectalis suspends the rectum, but since this organ does not support the other pelvic viscera, the puborectalis plays a small role in holding up the pelvic structures. The main work of this muscle is in controlling the descent of feces and in so doing it acts as an auxiliary sphincter for the anal canal. When the anococcygeal junction is pulled forward, the puborectalis increases the anorectal flexure and slows the descent of feces.

Pubococcygeus Proper. This muscle is composed of the most lateral fibers of the pubococcygeus muscle. It has a Y-shaped insertion into the lateral margins of the coccyx. When it contracts, it pulls the coccyx anteriorly, increasing the anorectal juncture. Thus, in combination with the external sphincter ani, it helps control the passage of feces.

Iliococcygeus Muscle

The iliococcygeus muscles arise from the white line of the pelvic fascia posterior to the obturator canal. They join with the pubococcygeus muscle proper and insert into the lateral margins of the coccyx. These are less dynamic than the pubovaginalis and act more like a musculofascial layer.

Ischiococcygeus Muscle

The ischiococcygeus or coccygeus muscles originate from the ischial spines and insert into the lateral borders of the coccyx and the fifth sacral vertebra. These muscles supplement the levator ani and occupy most of the posterior portion of the pelvic floor.

PELVIC FLOOR DURING PARTURITION

When the presenting part has reached the proper level during the second stage of labor, the central point of the perineum becomes thin. The levator ani muscles and the anal sphincter relax, and the muscles of the pelvic floor are drawn over the advancing head. Tearing and overstretching these muscles weaken the pelvic floor and may cause extensive damage.

CLINICAL ANATOMY

Perineum

Dante U. Pascali

The perineum is a diamond-shaped space that lies below the pelvic floor (Fig. 3-1). Its boundaries are as follows:

1. Superiorly: the pelvic floor is made up of the levator ani muscles and the coccygei muscles
2. Laterally: the bones and ligaments that make up the pelvic outlet; anteriorly to posteriorly are the subpubic angle, ischiopubic rami, ischial tuberosities, sacrotuberous ligaments, and coccyx
3. Inferiorly: the skin and fascia

This area is divided into two triangles: anteriorly, the urogenital triangle and posteriorly, the anal triangle. These are separated by a transverse band composed of the transverse perineal muscles and the base of the urogenital diaphragm.

UROGENITAL TRIANGLE

The urogenital triangle is bounded:

1. Anteriorly: by the subpubic angle
2. Laterally: by the ischiopubic rami and the ischial tuberosities

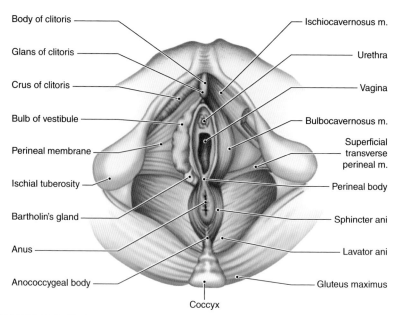

FIGURE 3-1. **Perineum.**

3. Posteriorly: by the transverse perineal muscles and the base of the urogenital diaphragm

The urogenital triangle contains:

1. Opening of the vagina
2. Terminal part of the urethra
3. Crura of the clitoris with the ischiocavernosus muscles
4. Vestibular bulbs (erectile tissue) covered by the bulbocavernosus muscles
5. Bartholin's glands and their ducts
6. Urogenital diaphragm
7. Muscles that constitute the central point of the perineum (perineal body)
8. Perineal pouches, superficial and deep
9. Blood vessels, nerves, and lymphatics

Urogenital Diaphragm

The urogenital diaphragm (triangular ligament) lies in the anterior triangle of the perineum. It is composed of muscle tissue covered by fascia.

1. The two muscles are the deep transverse perineal and the sphincter of the membranous urethra
2. The superior layer of fascia is thin and weak
3. The inferior fascial layer is a strong fibrous membrane. It extends from a short distance beneath the arcuate pubic ligament to the ischial tuberosities. The fascial layers fuse superiorly and form the transverse perineal ligament. Inferiorly, they join in the central point of the perineum

The deep dorsal vein of the clitoris lies in a small space between the apex of the urogenital diaphragm and the arcuate pubic ligament. The urethra, the vagina, blood vessels, lymphatics, and nerves pass through the urogenital diaphragm.

Superficial Perineal Pouch

The superficial perineal pouch is a space that lies between the inferior layer of the urogenital diaphragm and Colles' fascia.

Superficial Transverse Perineal Muscles

The superficial transverse perineal muscles are the superficial parts of the deep muscles and have the same origin and insertion. These are outside the urogenital diaphragm. Sometimes they are entirely lacking.

Ischiocavernosus Muscles

The ischiocavernosus muscles cover the clitoral crura. The origin of each is the inferior ramus of the pubis, and they insert at the lateral aspect of the crus. These muscles compress the crura and by blocking the venous return cause the clitoris to become erect.

Bulbocavernosus Muscle

The bulbocavernosus muscle surrounds the vagina. With the external anal sphincter, it makes a figure eight around the vagina and rectum. It is also called the *bulbospongiosus*. It originates from the central point of the perineum and inserts into the dorsal aspect of the clitoral body. The muscle passes around the orifice of the vagina and surrounds the bulb of the vestibule.

The bulbocavernosus muscle compresses the erectile tissue around the vaginal orifice (bulb of the vestibule) and helps in clitoral erection by closing its dorsal vein. It acts as a weak vaginal sphincter. The real sphincter of the vagina is the pubovaginalis section of the levator ani muscles.

Deep Perineal Pouch

The deep perineal pouch lies between the two fascial layers of the urogenital diaphragm.

Sphincter of the Membranous Urethra

The sphincter of the membranous urethra lies between the fascial layers of the urogenital diaphragm. It is also called the *compressor of the urethra*.

The voluntary fibers have their origin from the inferior rami of the ischium and pubis. They join with the deep transverse perineal muscles. Their action is to expel the last drops of urine.

The involuntary fibers surround the urethra and act as its sphincter.

Deep Transverse Perineal Muscles

The deep transverse perineal muscles lie between the layers of fascia of the urogenital diaphragm. They blend with the sphincter of the membranous urethra. The origin is the ischiopubic ramus on each side, and they insert at the central point of the perineum (perineal body).

ANAL TRIANGLE

The anal triangle is bounded:

1. Anteriorly: by the transverse perineal muscles and the base of the urogenital diaphragm
2. Laterally: by the ischial tuberosities and the sacrotuberous ligaments
3. Posteriorly: by the coccyx

The anal triangle contains the following:

1. Lower end of the anal canal and its sphincters
2. Anococcygeal body
3. Ischiorectal fossa
4. Blood vessels, lymphatics, and nerves

Sphincter Ani Externus

The sphincter ani externus or external anal sphincter has two parts:

1. The superficial portion surrounds the anal orifice. Its fibers are voluntary and act during defecation or in an emergency. The origin is the tip of the coccyx and the anococcygeal body. Insertion is in the central point of the perineum
2. The deep part is an involuntary muscle that surrounds the lower part of the anal canal and acts as a sphincter for the anus. It blends with the levator ani muscles and the internal anal sphincter. When inactive, the deep circular fibers are in a state of tonus, occluding the anal orifice

Anococcygeal Body

The anococcygeal body is composed of muscle tissue (levator ani and external sphincter ani) and fibrous tissue. It is located between the tip of the coccyx and the anus.

PERINEAL BODY

The central point of the perineum or perineal body lies between the posterior angle of the vagina anteriorly and the anus posteriorly. In obstetrics, it is referred to as the *perineum*. It is often torn during delivery. The following muscles meet to form this structure:

1. Sphincter ani externus (external anal sphincter)
2. Two levator ani muscles
3. Superficial and deep transverse perineal muscles
4. Bulbocavernosus muscle

CHAPTER 4

Uterus and Vagina

Dante U. Pascali

UTERUS

The normal uterus is a small muscular organ in the female pelvis. It is composed of three layers:

1. An outer, covering, serous peritoneal layer: the **perimetrium**
2. A thick middle layer made up of muscle fibers: the **myometrium**
3. An inner mucous layer of glands and supporting stroma: the **endometrium**, which is attached directly to the myometrium

   The *myometrium* is made up of three layers of muscle:

1. An outer layer of mainly longitudinal fibers
2. An inner layer whose fibers run, for the most part, in a circular direction
3. A thick middle layer whose fibers are arranged in an interlacing pattern and through which the blood vessels course. When these fibers contract and retract after the products of conception have been expelled, the blood vessels are kinked and constricted. In this way, postpartum bleeding is controlled

Uterine Shape

In the nonpregnant state and at the time of implantation, the uterus is pear-shaped (pyriform). By the third month of gestation, the uterus is globular. From the seventh month to term, the contour is again pyriform.

Uterine Size

The uterus grows from the nonpregnant dimensions of about 7.5 × 5.0 × 2.5 cm to 28 × 24 × 21 cm. The weight rises from 30 to 60 g to 1000 g at the end of pregnancy. The uterus changes from a solid organ in the nullipara to a large sac in pregnancy. The capacity increases from almost nil to 4000 mL.

Uterine Location

Normally, the uterus is entirely in the pelvis. As it enlarges, it gradually rises, and by the fourth month of gestation, it extends into the abdominal region.

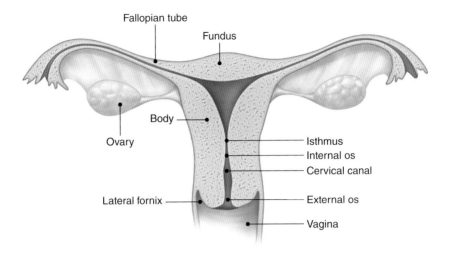

FIGURE 4-1. Uterus, cervix, and vagina.

Uterine Divisions

1. The fundus (Fig. 4-1) is the part superior to the openings of the fallopian tubes
2. The body (corpus) is the main part; it has thick walls, lies between the tubal openings and the isthmus, and is the main contractile portion. During labor, the contractions force the baby downward, distend the lower segment of the uterus, and dilate the cervix
3. The isthmus is a small constricted region of the uterus. It is about 5 to 7 mm in length and lies superior to the internal os of the cervix
4. The cervix (Fig. 4-2) is composed of a canal with an internal os superiorly, separating the cervix from the uterine cavity, and an external os inferiorly, which closes off the cervix from the vagina. The cervix is about 2.5 cm in length. The lower part pierces the anterior wall of the vagina, and its tissue blends with that of the vagina

MYOMETRIUM

Most of the uterine growth takes place in the myometrium of the body and fundus. During the first half of pregnancy, the main factor in uterine growth is hyperplasia (formation of new muscle fibers). In the second half, hypertrophy predominates (enlargement of existing myometrial cells). Individual myometrial fibers increase 10-fold during pregnancy from a

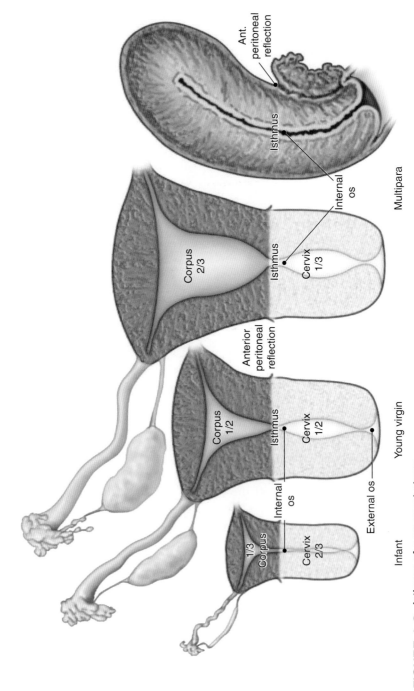

FIGURE 4-2. Isthmus of a pregnant uterus.

nonpregnant length of 50 to 100 μ to 500 to 800 μ during pregnancy. At term, the estimated number of cells is 200 billion. The myometrial fibers are composed of four major proteins: myosin, actin, tropomyosin, and troponin. The main stimulus to growth is provided by 17 β-estradiol, although some myometrial hypertrophy occurs in response to stretch.

There is also an increase in the number and size of the blood vessels and lymphatics, as well as a marked overgrowth of connective tissue.

During early pregnancy, the uterine walls are thicker than in the nonpregnant state. As gestation continues, the lumen becomes larger and the walls thinner. At the end of the fifth month, they are 3 to 5 mm thick and remain so until term. Thus, during late pregnancy, the uterus is a large muscular sac with thin, soft, easily compressible walls. This makes the corpus indentable and enables the fetus to be palpated. The walls of the uterus are so malleable that the uterus changes shape easily and markedly to accommodate changes in fetal size and position.

Isthmus

The isthmus lies between the body of the uterus and the cervix. In humans, its boundaries are not well defined, and it is important as a physiologic rather than as an anatomic entity. In the nonpregnant uterus it is 5 to 7 mm long. It differs from the corpus in that it is free of mucus-secreting glands. The upper limit of the isthmus corresponds to a constriction in the lumen of the uterus, which marks the lower boundary of the body of the uterus (the anatomic internal os of Aschoff). The lower limit is the site of transition from the mucosa of the isthmus to the endocervical mucous membrane (histologic internal os).

Although the isthmus is of little importance in the normal state, in pregnancy it plays an important role. As the uterus grows, the isthmus increases in length (Fig. 4-2) to about 25 mm and becomes soft and compressible. The Hegar sign of early pregnancy depends on palpation of the soft isthmus between the body of the uterus above and the cervix below.

The ovum implants, in the great majority of cases, in the upper part of the uterus. At about the third month, the enlarging embryo grows into the isthmus, which unfolds and expands to make room for it. As this process continues, the isthmus is incorporated gradually into the general uterine cavity, and the shape of the uterus changes from pyriform to globular. The expanded isthmus forms part of the lower uterine segment of the uterus during labor. The histologic internal os becomes the internal os of pregnancy, and the anatomic internal os becomes the physiologic retraction ring of normal labor (and pathologic retraction ring of obstructed labor).

The unfolding of the isthmus continues until it has reached the firm cervix, where it stops. After the seventh month, most of the enlargement takes place in the body and fundus, and the uterus becomes pear-shaped again. At the onset of labor, the lower uterine segment comprises about one-third of the whole uterus. Although this area is not the passive part it was once thought to be, its contractions during normal labor are extremely weak when compared with those of the body.

Cervix

The cervix is composed mostly of connective tissue interspersed with muscle fibers. It feels hard and fibrous in the nonpregnant state. During pregnancy, the cervix becomes progressively softer. This is caused by increased vascularity, general edema, and hyperplasia of the glands. The compound tubular glands become overactive and produce large quantities of mucus. The secretion accumulates in the cervical canal and thickens to form the so-called mucous plug. This inspissated mucus effectively seals off the canal from the vagina and prevents the ascent of bacteria and other substances into the uterine cavity. The plug is expelled early in labor.

At the end of gestation and during labor, the internal os gradually disappears, and the cervical canal also becomes part of the lower uterine segment, leaving only the external os.

VAGINA

The vagina is a fibromuscular membranous tube surrounded by the vulva inferiorly, the uterus superiorly, the bladder anteriorly, and the rectum posteriorly. Its direction is obliquely superior and posterior. The cervix uteri enters the vagina through the anterior wall, and for this reason, the anterior wall of the vagina (6-8 cm) is shorter than the posterior wall (7-10 cm). The protrusion of the cervix into the vagina divides the vaginal vault into four fornices: an anterior, a posterior, and two lateral fornices. The posterior fornix is much deeper than the others.

The wall of the vagina is made up of four layers:

1. The mucosa is the epithelial layer
2. The submucosa is rich in blood vessels
3. The muscularis is the third layer
4. The outer connective tissue layer connects the vagina to the surrounding structures

Even in the normal condition, the vagina is capable of great distention, but in pregnancy, this ability is increased many times. In the pregnant state, there is greater vascularity, thickening and lengthening of the walls, and increased secretion, so that most women have varying quantities of vaginal discharge during the period of gestation.

UTERINE ABNORMALITIES

Prolapse of the Uterus

Prolapse of the uterus during pregnancy is rare but troublesome. As a rule, the uterus rises out of the pelvis by the end of the fourth month. Occasionally, it fails to do so. In most cases, it is only the cervix, with or without an associated hypertrophic elongation, that protrudes through the vagina. Occasionally, the whole uterus is involved. Pregnancy cannot carry to term with the uterus completely out of the vagina.

Complications

Antepartum

1. Abortion and preterm labor
2. Cervical edema, ulceration, and sepsis
3. Urinary retention and infection

Intrapartum

1. Cervical dilatation may begin outside the vagina, resulting in resistance to progress
2. The edema and fibrosis may cause cervical dystocia
3. Lacerations of the cervix are common
4. Obstructed labor may lead to uterine rupture

Postpartum
Puerperal infection is increased.

Treatment

Antepartum

1. Bed rest in the Trendelenburg position to reduce edema and permit repositioning of the uterus
2. Pessary to maintain the position of the uterus

Intrapartum

1. Most patients have a normal vaginal delivery, but arrest of progress may ensue
2. If cervical dystocia develops, several procedures may be considered:
   a. Dührssen incisions of the cervix
   b. Oxytocin augmentation of labor
   c. Cesarean section

Postpartum

A pessary should be inserted to elevate the uterus and support the ligaments.

ANOMALIES OF THE UTERUS

Abnormal fusion of the Müllerian ducts or failure of absorption of the septum leads to a variety of congenital malformations of the uterus. The reported incidence is one in 594 fertile women and one in 29 infertile women. The prevalence of uterine anomalies in the general population is one in 201 women. Most Müllerian anomalies are never detected because of the absence of clinical symptoms. Only about 25 percent of women with uterine anomalies have serious reproductive problems. Concurrent renal abnormalities are common.

Miscarriage occurs in all trimesters, including spontaneous abortion, early or late, and preterm labor and delivery. Malpresentation, especially breech, is common. Women with uterine anomalies are in a high-risk group and have to be followed closely during pregnancy, labor, and delivery.

The theoretical reasons for reproductive failure include:

1. Poor vascularization of the endometrium
2. Distortion of the uterine cavity
3. Incompetent cervix

Diagnosis

During pregnancy, a uterine anomaly may be suspected when the following conditions are present:

1. Notching and broadening of the uterine fundus
2. Abnormal lie
3. Recurring breech
4. Trapped or retained placenta

5. Prolonged third stage of labor
6. Recurrent spontaneous abortion
7. Axial deviation of the uterus
8. Flanking of the fetal limbs
9. Cervix located in the lateral fornix of the vagina
10. Presence of a vaginal septum

In any suspicious case, hysterography should be performed postpartum.

Complications

1. Breech presentation
2. Transverse lie; the fetus often assumes the hammock position with the head in one horn and the feet in the other
3. Incoordinate uterine contractions may result in failure of progress necessitating cesarean section
4. Premature rupture of membranes
5. Placenta previa
6. Obstruction of descent of the fetus by the nonpregnant horn
7. Obstruction by a thick vaginal septum

Labor and Delivery

In many cases, labor progresses without incident and results in a normal delivery. Therefore, a trial of labor is indicated. Failure to progress is treated with a cesarean section. The incidence of the latter is higher than in normal patients.

Postpartum Complications

1. Retained placenta
2. Subinvolution of the placental site
3. Postpartum hemorrhage

Arcuate Uterus

The uterine fundus has a midline curved indentation that projects into the cavity of the uterus (Fig. 4-3A). The external contours of the uterus are not affected and at laparoscopy, the uterus appears normal. Hysteroscopy and hysterosalpingography help in establishing the diagnosis. It is rare for this abnormality to lead to fetal loss from either abortion or preterm delivery. Most pregnancies are normal, and the diagnosis is not made.

Septate Uterus

The longitudinal septum may be complete (Fig. 4-3B), extending down to the internal or external os of the cervix, or incomplete or partial (Fig. 4-3C),

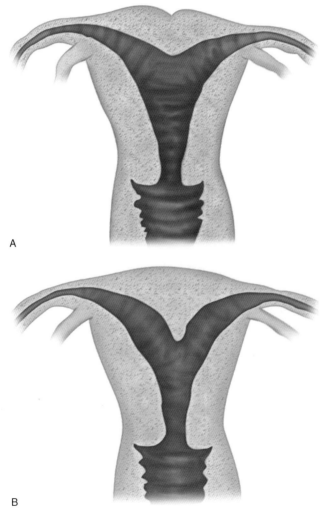

FIGURE 4-3. **A.** Arcuate uterus. **B.** Septate uterus, partial. **C.** Septate uterus, complete.

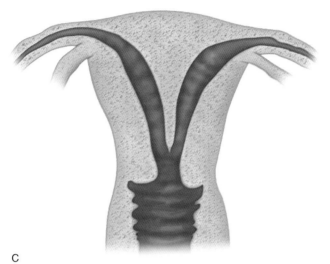

C

FIGURE 4-3. *(Continued)*

when it extends part way from the uterine fundus. Fetal loss in the first half of pregnancy is common. In such cases, the septum should be excised hysteroscopically.

Unicornuate Uterus

This is a uterus with a single horn (Fig. 4-4). A normal vagina and a single normal tube are present in most cases. The other half of the uterus is absent or rudimentary. In many patients, the kidney is absent on the same side as the uterine abnormality.

In this condition, there is an increased incidence of difficulty or inability to conceive, spontaneous abortion, preterm labor, abnormal presentation of the fetus, and intrauterine growth restriction. A possible explanation of the latter is that, with one uterine artery being absent, there is inadequate perfusion of the uterus resulting in reduced fetal nutrition. There may also be insufficient room in the uterus for normal growth. An incompetent cervix is often present.

If there is a rudimentary horn, transmigration of sperm or ova can occur with a resultant pregnancy that cannot progress normally with the possible risk of rupture. In such cases, the rudimentary horn should be

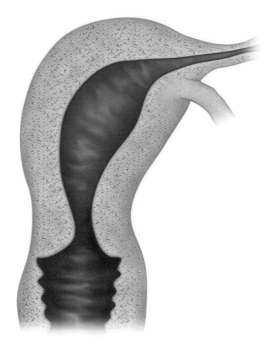

FIGURE 4-4. Unicornuate uterus.

excised. If the patient is unable to conceive, removal of the rudimentary horn may be followed by a successful pregnancy.

Bicornuate Uterus

The division down the middle of the uterus is complete to the internal os (Fig. 4-5). Diagnosis is made by palpation, postpartum exploration of the uterine cavity, during curettage, by hysteroscopy, by hysterography, and by laparoscopy. Abortion, incompetent cervix, premature rupture of membranes, preterm labor, abnormal presentation (especially breech and transverse lie), and cesarean section are all more common than when the uterus is normally shaped. Fetal outcome is good in many cases. When fetal loss recurs, a unification operation can be considered.

Labor proceeds to vaginal delivery in many cases. Cesarean section is indicated only for obstetric reasons. Dystocia may be caused by uterine inertia, obstruction by the nongravid horn, and hypertrophy of a septum. Occasionally, the nonpregnant horn may rupture during labor.

Retained placenta occurs in 20 percent of cases and may lead to postpartum hemorrhage.

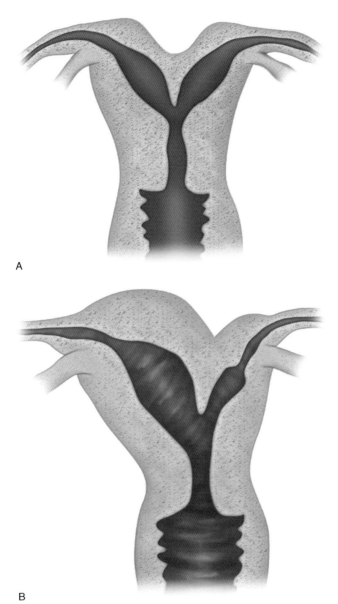

FIGURE 4-5. A. Bicornuate uterus. **B.** Bicornuate uterus with a rudimentary horn.

Double Uterus: Uterus Didelphys

The reported incidence of complete duplication of the female reproductive tract is between one in 1500 and one in 15,000 pregnant women (Fig. 4-6). The cervices are externally united, and the uterine fundi are externally

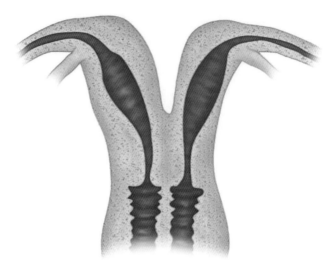

FIGURE 4-6. **Double uterus: uterus didelphys.**

separate. In most cases, there are two vaginas. The halves of the uterus are often of different sizes.

Ineffectual contractions and slowly dilating cervices are common during the first stages of labor. Postpartum atony leading to hemorrhage is observed often. Sloughing of a decidual cast from the nonpregnant uterus can cause excessive bleeding. The cervix of the nongravid uterus may interfere with the descent and rotation of the fetal presenting part and may obstruct progress necessitating a cesarean section. Many women have normal vaginal deliveries; however, preterm labor is common.

TORSION OF THE GRAVID UTERUS

Uterine torsion is defined as rotation of the uterus on its long axis of more than 45°. Torsion of the pregnant uterus is rare; the condition was first reported in animals in 1662 and in the human 200 years later. The exact cause is not known, but some uterine malformation or tumor is present in many instances.

Most pregnant uteri show a slight degree of rotation, to the right in 80 percent and toward the left in 20 percent. In most abnormal situations, the rotation has been 180°, although a case was reported of a 540° torsion associated with uterine necrosis.

In 20 percent of cases, no causative factor is apparent. Predisposing conditions include:

1. Malpresentation, especially transverse lie
2. Uterine myomas
3. Anomalies of the uterus
4. Pelvic adhesions
5. Ovarian cyst
6. Uterine suspension
7. Abnormal pelvis
8. Placenta previa

Preoperative diagnosis is rare. The picture is one of an acute abdominal crisis, including pain, shock, bleeding, obstructed labor, and symptoms referable to the intestinal and urinary tracts. The most serious complication is uterine rupture. Acute torsion results in compromise of the uterine circulation. Treatment at or near term is by cesarean section. Before viability of the fetus has been reached, laparotomy is performed, the uterus is rotated to its normal position, and the pregnancy is allowed to continue to term.

SELECTED READING

Andrews MC, Jones HW Jr: Impaired reproductive performance of the unicornuate uterus: Intrauterine growth retardation, infertility, and recurrent abortion in five cases. Am J Obstet Gynecol 144:173, 1982

Ansbacher R: Uterine anomalies and future pregnancies. Clin Perinatol 10:295, 1983

Heinonen PK, Saarikoski S, Pystynen P: Reproductive performance of women with uterine anomalies. Acta Obstet Gynecol Scand 61:157, 1982

Liang R, Ghandi J, Rahmani B, Ali Khan S: Uterine torsion: A review with critical considerations for the obstetrician gynecologist. Trans Res Anat 21:1000842, 2020

Nahum G: Uterine anomalies. How common are they, and what is their distribution among subtypes? J Reprod Med 43:877-887, 1998

Nielsen TF: Torsion of the pregnant uterus without symptoms. Am J Obstet Gynecol 141:838, 1981

Valle, R, Ekpo, G: Hysteroscopic metroplasty for the septate uterus: Review and meta-analysis. J Minim Invasive Gynecol 20:22-42, 2013

Visser AA, Giesteira MUK, Heyns A, Marais C: Torsion of the pregnant uterus. Case reports. Br J Obstet Gynaecol 90:87, 1983

CHAPTER 5

Obstetric Pelvis

Glenn D. Posner

THE PELVIS

The pelvis is made up of the two innominate bones (which occupy the front and sides) and the sacrum and coccyx (which are behind). The bones articulate through four joints. The sacroiliac joint is the most important, linking the sacrum to the iliac part of the innominate bones. The symphysis of the pubis joins the two pubic bones. The sacrococcygeal joint attaches the sacrum to the coccyx.

The *false pelvis* lies above the true pelvis, superior to the linea terminalis. Its only obstetric function is to support the enlarged uterus during pregnancy. Its boundaries are:

1. Posteriorly: lumbar vertebrae
2. Laterally: iliac fossae
3. Anteriorly: anterior abdominal wall

The *true pelvis* (Fig. 5-1A) lies below the pelvic brim, or linea terminalis, and is the bony canal through which the fetus must pass. It is divided into three parts: (1) the inlet, (2) the pelvic cavity, and (3) the pelvic outlet.

The *inlet* (pelvic brim) is bounded:

1. Anteriorly by the pubic crest and spine
2. Laterally by the iliopectineal lines on the innominate bones
3. Posteriorly by the anterior borders of the ala and promontory of the sacrum

The *pelvic cavity* (Fig. 5-1B) is a curved canal.

1. The anterior wall is straight and shallow. The pubis is approximately 5 cm long
2. The posterior wall is deep and concave. The sacrum is approximately 10 to 15 cm long
3. The ischium and part of the body of the ilium are found laterally

The *pelvic outlet* is diamond shaped. It is bounded:

1. Anteriorly by the arcuate pubic ligament and the pubic arch
2. Laterally by the ischial tuberosity and the sacrotuberous ligament
3. Posteriorly by the tip of the sacrum

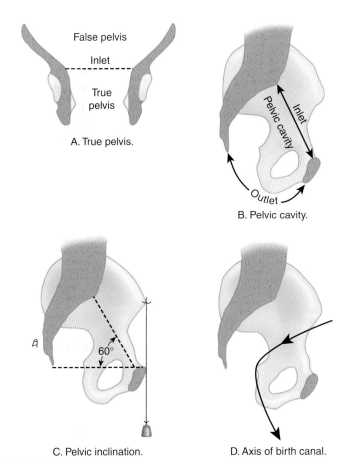

A. True pelvis.

B. Pelvic cavity.

C. Pelvic inclination.

D. Axis of birth canal.

FIGURE 5-1. Pelvic cavity.

The *pelvic inclination* (Fig. 5-1C) is assessed when the woman is in the upright position. The plane of the pelvic brim makes an angle of about 60° with the horizontal. The anterior superior iliac spine is in the same vertical plane as the pubic spine.

The *axis of the birth canal* (Fig. 5-1D) is the course taken by the presenting part as it passes through the pelvis. At first it moves downward and backward to the level of the ischial spines, which is the area of the bony attachment of the pelvic floor muscles. Here the direction changes and the presenting part proceeds downward and forward.

The *pelvic planes* (Fig. 5-2) are imaginary flat surfaces passing across the pelvis at different levels. They are used for the purposes of description. The important ones are as follows:

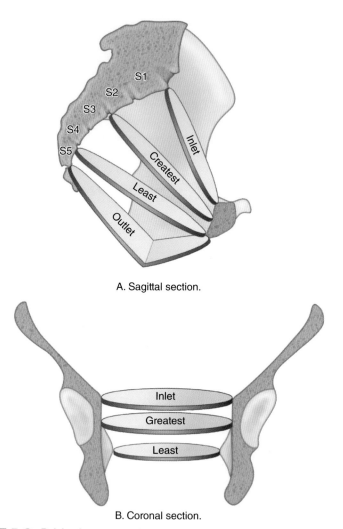

A. Sagittal section.

B. Coronal section.

FIGURE 5-2. Pelvic planes.

1. The plane of the inlet is also called the superior strait
2. The pelvic cavity has many planes, two of which are the plane of greatest dimensions and the plane of least dimensions
3. The plane of the outlet is also called the inferior strait

The *diameters* are distances between given points. Important ones are as follows:

1. Anteroposterior diameters
2. Transverse diameters

3. Left oblique: Oblique diameters are designated left or right according to their posterior terminal
4. Right oblique
5. Posterior sagittal diameter: This is the back part of the anteroposterior diameter, extending from the intersection of the transverse and antero-posterior diameters to the posterior limit of the latter
6. Anterior sagittal diameter: This is the front part of the anteroposterior diameter, extending from the intersection of the transverse and antero-posterior diameter to the anterior limit of the latter

PELVIC INLET

Plane of Obstetric Inlet

The plane of the obstetric inlet is bounded:

1. Anteriorly by the posterior superior margin of the pubic symphysis
2. Laterally by the iliopectineal lines
3. Posteriorly by the promontory and ala of the sacrum

Diameters of Inlet

The diameters of the inlet are as follows:

1. Anteroposterior diameters:
   a. The anatomic conjugate (Fig. 5-3) extends from the middle of the sacral promontory to the middle of the pubic crest (superior surface of the pubis). It measures approximately 11.5 cm. It has no obstetric significance
   b. The obstetric conjugate extends from the middle of the sacral prom-ontory to the posterior superior margin of the pubic symphysis. This point on the pubis, which protrudes back into the cavity of the pel-vis, is about 1.0 cm below the pubic crest. The obstetric conjugate is approximately 11.0 cm in length. This is the important anteroposte-rior diameter, because it is the one through which the fetus must pass
   c. The diagonal conjugate extends from the subpubic angle to the mid-dle of the sacral promontory. It is approximately 12.5 cm in length. This diameter can be measured manually in the patient. It is of clinical significance because by subtracting 1.5 cm, an approximate length of the obstetric conjugate can be obtained

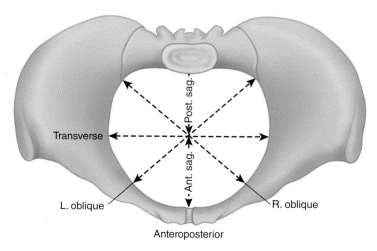

A. Anteroposterior view.

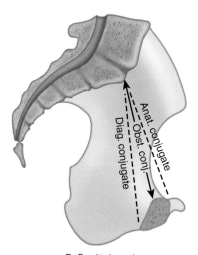

B. Sagittal section.

FIGURE 5-3. Pelvic inlet.

2. Transverse diameter is the widest distance between the iliopectineal lines and is approximately 13.5 cm
3. Left oblique diameter extends from the left sacroiliac joint to the right iliopectineal eminence and is approximately 12.5 cm
4. Right oblique diameter extends from the right sacroiliac joint to the left iliopectineal eminence and is approximately 12.5 cm
5. Posterior sagittal diameter extends from the intersection of the anteroposterior and transverse diameters to the middle of the sacral promontory and is approximately 4.5 cm long

PELVIC CAVITY

The pelvic cavity extends from the inlet to the outlet.

Plane of Greatest Dimensions

This is the roomiest part of the pelvis and is almost circular. Its obstetric significance is small. Its boundaries are:

1. Anteriorly: midpoint of the posterior surface of the pubis
2. Laterally: upper and middle thirds of the obturator foramina
3. Posteriorly: the junction of the second and third sacral vertebrae

The diameters of importance are:

1. The anteroposterior diameter extends from the midpoint of the posterior surface of the pubis to the junction of the second and third sacral vertebrae and measures approximately 12.75 cm
2. The transverse diameter is the widest distance between the lateral aspects of the plane and is approximately 12.5 cm

Plane of Least Dimensions

This is the most important plane of the pelvis (Fig. 5-4). It has the least room, and it is here that most instances of arrest of progress take place. This plane extends from the apex of the subpubic arch, through the ischial spines, to the sacrum, usually at or near the junction of the fourth and fifth sacral vertebrae. The boundaries are, from front to back:

1. Lower border of the pubic symphysis
2. White line on the fascia covering the obturator foramina
3. Ischial spines
4. Sacrospinous ligaments
5. Sacrum

The diameters of importance are:

1. Anteroposterior diameter, extending from the lower border of the pubic symphysis to the junction of the fourth and fifth sacral vertebrae and measuring approximately 12.0 cm

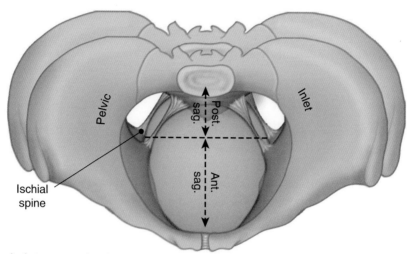

A. Anteroposterior view showing the anteroposterior and transverse diameters.

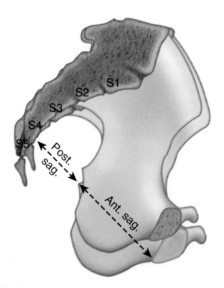

B. Sagittal section showing the anteroposterior diameter.

FIGURE 5-4. Pelvic cavity: the plane of least dimensions.

2. Transverse diameter, lying between the ischial spines and measuring approximately 10.5 cm
3. Posterior sagittal diameter, extending from the bispinous diameter to the junction of the fourth and fifth sacral vertebrae and measuring approximately 4.5 to 5.0 cm

PELVIC OUTLET

The outlet is made up of two triangular planes, having as their common base and most inferior part, the transverse diameter between the ischial tuberosities (Fig. 5-5).

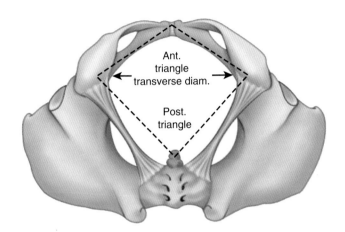

A. Inferior view.

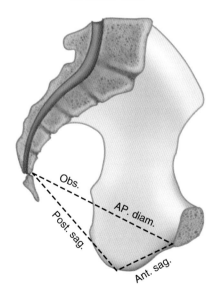

B. Sagittal section.

FIGURE 5-5. Pelvic outlet.

Anterior Triangle

The anterior triangle has the following boundaries:

1. The base is the bituberous diameter (transverse diameter)
2. The apex is the subpubic angle
3. The sides are the pubic rami and ischial tuberosities

Posterior Triangle

The posterior triangle has the following boundaries:

1. The base is the bituberous diameter
2. The obstetric apex is the sacrococcygeal joint
3. The sides are the sacrotuberous ligaments

Diameters of the Outlet

1. The anatomic anteroposterior diameter is from the inferior margin of the pubic symphysis to the tip of the coccyx. It measures approximately 9.5 cm. The obstetric anteroposterior diameter is from the inferior margin of the pubic symphysis to the sacrococcygeal joint. This measures approximately 11.5 cm. Because of the mobility at the sacrococcygeal joint, the coccyx is pushed out of the way by the advancing presenting part, increasing the available space
2. The transverse diameter is the distance between the inner surfaces of the ischial tuberosities and measures approximately 11.0 cm
3. The posterior sagittal diameter extends from the middle of the transverse diameter to the sacrococcygeal junction and is approximately 9.0 cm
4. The anterior sagittal diameter extends from the middle of the transverse diameter to the subpubic angle and measures approximately 6.0 cm

IMPORTANT MEASUREMENTS

In assessing the obstetric capacity of the pelvis, the most important measurements are the following:

1. Obstetric conjugate of the inlet
2. Distance between the ischial spines

3. Subpubic angle and bituberous diameter
4. Posterior sagittal diameters of the three planes
5. Curve and length of the sacrum

CLASSIFICATION OF THE PELVIS

Variations in the female pelvis and in the planes of any single pelvis are so great that a rigid classification is not possible. A pelvis of the female type in one plane may be predominantly male in another. Many pelves are mixed in that the various planes do not conform to a single parent type.

For the purpose of classification, the pelvis is named on the basis of the inlet, and mention is made of nonconforming characteristics. For example, a pelvis may be described as a female type with male features at the outlet.

The classification of Caldwell and Moloy is used commonly (Table 5-1 and Figs. 5-6 through 5-8).

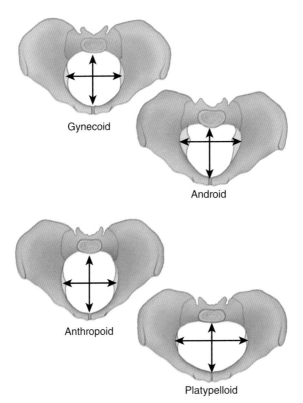

Gynecoid

Android

Anthropoid

Platypelloid

FIGURE 5-6. Pelvic outlet (Caldwell-Moloy classification).

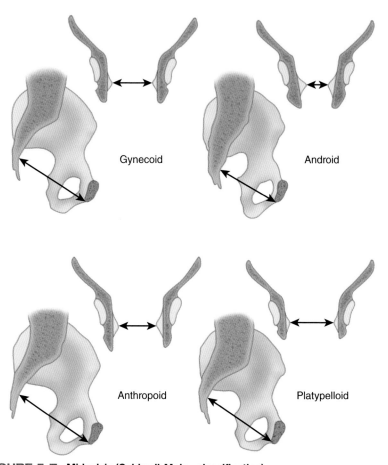

Gynecoid

Android

Anthropoid

Platypelloid

FIGURE 5-7. Midpelvis (Caldwell-Moloy classification).

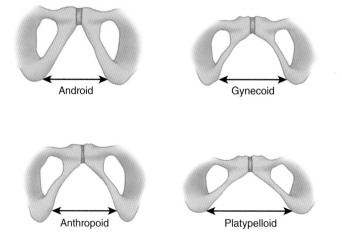

Android

Gynecoid

Anthropoid

Platypelloid

FIGURE 5-8. Pelvic outlet (Caldwell-Moloy classification).

TABLE 5-1: CLASSIFICATION OF PELVIS (CALDWELL AND MOLOY)

	Gynecoid	Android	Anthropoid	Platypelloid
INLET				
Sex type	Normal female	Male	Apelike	Flat female
Incidence	50%	20%	25%	5%
Shape	Round or transverse oval; transverse diameter is a little longer than the anteroposterior	Heart or wedge shaped	Long anteroposterior oval	Transverse oval
Anteroposterior diameter	Adequate	Adequate	Long	Short
Transverse diameter	Adequate	Adequate	Adequate but relatively short	Long
Posterior sagittal diameter	Adequate	Very short and inadequate	Very long	Very short
Anterior sagittal diameter	Adequate	Long	Long	Short
Posterior segment	Broad, deep, roomy	Shallow; sacral promontory indents the inlet and reduces its capacity	Deep	Shallow
Anterior segment	Well rounded forepelvis	Narrow, sharply angulated forepelvis	Deep	Shallow

(Continued)

TABLE 5-1: CLASSIFICATION OF PELVIS (CALDWELL AND MOLOY) *(Continued)*

	Gynecoid	Android	Anthropoid	Platypelloid
PELVIC CAVITY: MIDPELVIS				
Anteroposterior diameter	Adequate	Reduced	Long	Shortened
Transverse diameter	Adequate	Reduced	Adequate	Wide
Posterior sagittal diameter	Adequate	Reduced	Adequate	Shortened
Anterior sagittal diameter	Adequate	Reduced	Adequate	Short
Sacrum	Wide, deep curve; short; slopes backward; light bone	Flat; inclined forward; long; narrow; heavy	Inclined backward; narrow; long	Wide, deep curve; often sharply angulated with enlarged sacral fossa
Sidewalls	Parallel, straight	Convergent; funnel pelvis	Straight	Parallel
Ischial spines	Not prominent	Prominent	Variable	Variable
Sacrosciatic notch	Wide; short	Narrow; long; high arch	Wide	Short
Depth: iliopectineal eminence	Average	Long	Long	Short
capacity	Adequate	Reduced in all diameters	Adequate	Reduced

OUTLET

Anteroposterior diameter	Long	Short	Long	Short
Transverse diameter (bituberous)	Adequate	Narrow	Adequate	Wide
Pubic arch	Wide and round; 90°	Narrow; deep; 70°	Normal or relatively narrow	Very wide
Inferior pubic rami	Short; concave inward	Straight; long	Long; relatively narrow	Straight; short
Capacity	Adequate	Reduced	Adequate	Inadequate

EFFECT ON LABOR

Fetal head	Engages in transverse or oblique diameter in slight asynclitism; good flexion; occiput anterior (OA) position is common	Engages in transverse or posterior diameter in asynclitism; extreme molding	Engages in anteroposterior or oblique; often occiput posterior position	Engages in transverse diameter with marked asynclitism

(Continued)

TABLE 5-1: CLASSIFICATION OF PELVIS (CALDWELL AND MOLOY) *(Continued)*

	Gynecoid	Android	Anthropoid	Platypelloid
Labor	Good uterine function; early and complete internal rotation; spontaneous delivery; wide pubic arch reduces perineal tears	Deep transverse arrest is common; arrest as occiput posterior (OP) position with failure of rotation; delivery is often by difficult forceps application, rotation, and extraction; the narrow pubic arch may lead to major perineal tears	Delivery and labor usually easy; birth face to pubis is common	Delay at inlet
Prognosis	Good	Poor	Good	Poor; disproportion; delay at inlet; labor often terminated by cesarean section

CHAPTER 6

The Passenger:
Fetus

Glenn D. Posner

GENERAL CONSIDERATIONS

1. Resemblance to the adult human form may be perceptible at the end of 8 weeks' gestation and is obvious at the end of 12 weeks' gestation
2. By the end of 12 weeks and sometimes sooner, the sexual differences in the external genitalia may be recognized in abortuses
3. Quickening (the perception by the pregnant woman of fetal movements in utero) occurs between the 16th and 20th weeks of pregnancy. The time of quickening is too variable to be of value in determining the expected date of confinement or when term has been reached. Active intestinal peristalsis is the most common phenomenon mistaken for quickening
4. Depending on maternal body habitus, the fetal heart is audible using a fetal Doppler by the 12th to 13th weeks of gestation
5. The fetal heart is audible using a stethoscope by the 18th or 20th week
6. The average length of the fetus at term is 50 cm
7. Within wide variations, the average boy in Canada (7 pounds, 15 oz or ~3600 g) is a little heavier at birth (based on 40 weeks' gestational age) than the average girl (7 pounds, 10 oz or ~3500 g)
8. In premature babies, the circumference of the head is relatively large compared with the shoulders. This fact is of clinical relevance when contemplating preterm breech delivery. As the fetus matures, the body grows faster than the head, so that at term, the circumferences of the head and the shoulders are nearly the same

FETAL OVOIDS

In its passage through the pelvis, the fetus presents two oval parts, movable on each other at the neck. The oval of the head is longer in its anteroposterior diameter, while that of the shoulders and body is longer transversely. Thus, the two ovoids are perpendicular to each other.

FETAL HEAD

From the obstetric standpoint, the fetal head (Fig. 6-1) is the most important part of the fetus. It is the largest, the least compressible, and the most frequently presenting part of the baby. Once the head has been born, rarely is there delay or difficulty with the remainder of the body.

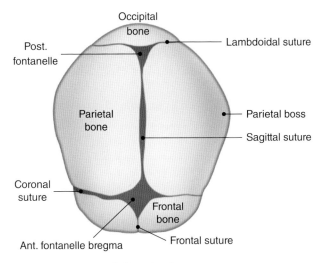

A. Superior view.

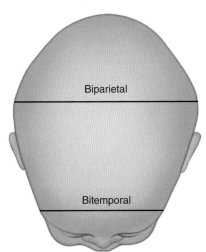

B. Transverse diameters.

FIGURE 6-1. Fetal skull.

Base of Skull

The bones of the base of the skull are large, ossified, firmly united, and not compressible. Their function is to protect the vital centers in the brain stem.

Vault of Skull: Cranium

The cranium is made up of several bones. Important ones are the occipital bone posteriorly, the two parietal bones on the sides, and the two temporal and the two frontal bones anteriorly. The bones of the cranial vault are laid down in membrane. At birth they are thin, poorly ossified, easily compressible, and joined only by membrane. This looseness of union of the bones (actually, there are spaces between them) permits their overlapping under pressure. In this way, the head can change its shape to fit the maternal pelvis, an important function known as *molding*. The top of the skull is wider posteriorly (biparietal diameter) than anteriorly (bitemporal diameter).

Sutures of Skull

Sutures are membrane-occupied spaces between the bones. They are useful in two ways (Fig. 6-1A):

1. Their presence makes molding possible
2. By identifying the sutures on vaginal examination, the position of the baby's head can be diagnosed

The important sutures include the following:

Sagittal Suture
The sagittal suture lies between the parietal bones. It runs in an anteroposterior direction between the fontanelles and divides the head into left and right halves.

Lambdoidal Sutures
The lambdoidal sutures extend transversely from the posterior fontanelle and separate the occipital bone from the two parietals.

Coronal Sutures
The coronal sutures extend transversely from the anterior fontanelle and lie between the parietal and frontal bones (Fig. 6-1).

Frontal Suture
The frontal suture is between the two frontal bones and is an anterior continuation of the sagittal suture. It extends from the glabella to the bregma.

Fontanelles

Where the sutures intersect are the membrane-filled spaces known as fontanelles. Two are important, the anterior and the posterior. These areas are useful clinically in two ways (Fig. 6-1A):

1. Their identification helps in diagnosing the position of the fetal head in the pelvis
2. The large fontanelle is examined in assessing the condition of the child after birth. In dehydrated infants, the fontanelle is depressed below the surface of the bony skull. When the intracranial pressure is elevated, the fontanelle is bulging, tense, and raised above the level of the skull

Anterior Fontanelle

The anterior fontanelle (bregma) is at the junction of the sagittal, frontal, and coronal sutures. It is by far the larger of the two, measuring about 3 × 2 cm, and is diamond shaped. It becomes ossified by 18 months of age. The anterior fontanelle facilitates molding. By remaining patent long after birth, it plays a part in accommodating the remarkable growth of the brain.

Posterior Fontanelle

The posterior fontanelle (lambda) is located where the sagittal suture meets the two lambdoidals. The skull is not truly deficient at this point, and the area is a meeting point of the sutures rather than a true fontanelle. It is much smaller than the anterior one. The intersection of the sutures makes a Y with the sagittal suture as the base and the lambdoidals as the arms. This fontanelle closes at 6 to 8 weeks of age.

Landmarks of Skull

From posterior to anterior, certain areas are identified (Fig. 6-2A).

1. Occiput: the area of the back of the head occupied by the occipital bone. It is behind and inferior to the posterior fontanelle and the lambdoidal sutures
2. Posterior fontanelle
3. Vertex: the area between the two fontanelles. It is the top of the skull and is bounded laterally by the parietal bosses
4. Bregma or large anterior fontanelle
5. Sinciput (or brow): the region bounded superiorly by the bregma and the coronal sutures, inferiorly by the glabella and the orbital ridges
6. Glabella: the elevated area between the orbital ridges
7. Nasion: the root of the nose
8. Parietal bosses: two eminences, one on the side of each parietal bone. The distance between them is the widest transverse diameter of the fetal head

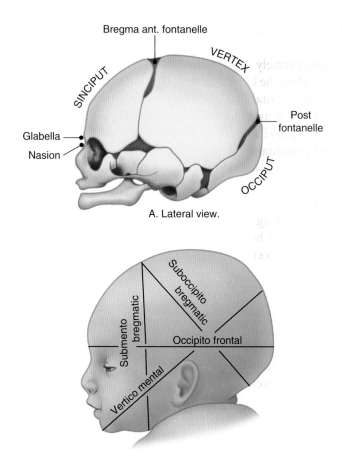

A. Lateral view.

B. Anteroposterior diameters.

FIGURE 6-2. Landmarks and diameters of fetal skull.

Diameters of Fetal Skull

The diameters are distances between given points on the fetal skull (Fig. 6-2B). Their size varies, and the particular anteroposterior diameter that presents to the maternal pelvis depends on the degree of flexion or extension of the fetal head.

1. The biparietal diameter (Fig. 6-1B) is between the parietal bosses. It is the largest transverse diameter and measures approximately 9.5 cm
2. The bitemporal diameter lies between the lateral sides of the temporal bones. It is approximately 8.0 cm in length and is the shortest transverse diameter of the skull

3. The suboccipitobregmatic diameter extends from the undersurface of the occipital bone, where it meets the neck, to the center of the bregma. It is approximately 9.5 cm long. It is the anteroposterior diameter that presents when the head is well flexed
4. The occipitofrontal diameter presents in the military attitude, neither flexion nor extension. It extends from the external occipital protuberance to the glabella and is approximately 11.0 cm long
5. The verticomental diameter is involved in brow presentations (halfway extension of the head). It runs from the vertex to the chin, measures approximately 13.5 cm, and is the longest anteroposterior diameter of the head
6. The submentobregmatic is the diameter in face presentations (complete extension of the head). Reaching from the junction of the neck and lower jaw to the center of the bregma, it is approximately 9.5 cm long

Circumferences of Fetal Skull and Shoulders

1. In the occipitofrontal plane, the circumference of the head is approximately 34.5 cm
2. In the suboccipitobregmatic plane, it is approximately 32 to 34 cm
3. At term, the bisacromial diameter of the shoulders is approximately 33 to 34 cm

Molding

Molding is the ability of the fetal head to change its shape and so adapt itself to the unyielding maternal pelvis (Fig. 6-3). This property is of the greatest value in the progress of labor and descent of the head through the birth canal.

The fetal bones are joined loosely by membranes so that actual spaces exist between the edges of the bones. This permits the bones to alter their relationships to each other as pressure is exerted on the head by the bony pelvis; the bones can come closer to each other or move apart. The side-to-side relationships of the bones are changeable, and one bone is able to override the other. When such overlapping takes place, the frontal and occipital bones pass under the parietal bones. The posterior parietal bone is subjected to greater pressure by the sacral promontory; therefore, it passes beneath the anterior parietal bone. A contributing factor to molding is the softness of the bones.

Compression in one direction is accompanied by expansion in another, and hence the actual volume of the skull is not reduced. Provided that

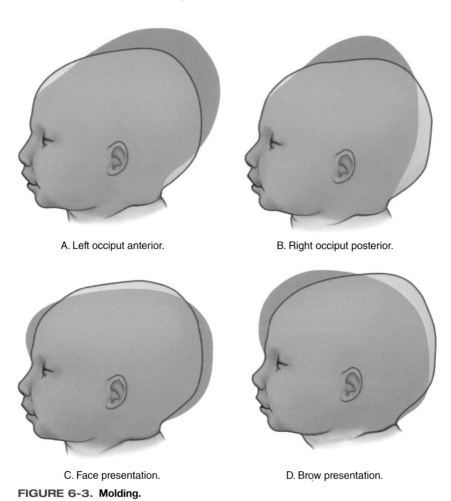

A. Left occiput anterior.   B. Right occiput posterior.

C. Face presentation.   D. Brow presentation.

FIGURE 6-3. Molding.

molding is not excessive and that it takes place slowly, no damage is done to the brain.

Alteration of the shape of the head is produced by compression of the presenting diameter, with resultant bulging of the diameter that is at right angles. For example, in the occipitoanterior (OA) position, the suboccipitobregmatic is the presenting diameter. The head therefore is elongated in the verticomental diameter, with bulging behind and above.

Caput Succedaneum

The caput succedaneum is a localized swelling of the scalp formed by the effusion of serum (Fig. 6-4). Pressure by the cervical ring causes obstruction of the venous return, so that the part of the scalp that lies within the

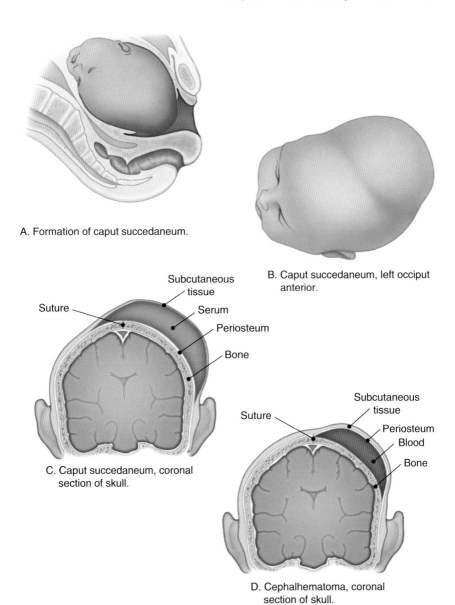

A. Formation of caput succedaneum.

B. Caput succedaneum, left occiput anterior.

Subcutaneous tissue

Suture

Serum

Periosteum

Bone

C. Caput succedaneum, coronal section of skull.

Subcutaneous tissue

Suture

Periosteum

Blood

Bone

D. Cephalhematoma, coronal section of skull.

FIGURE 6-4. Caput succedaneum and cephalohematoma.

cervix becomes edematous. The caput forms during labor and after the membranes have been ruptured. It is absent if the fetus is dead, the contractions are poor, or the cervix is not applied closely to the head.

The location of the caput varies with the position of the head. In OA positions, the caput forms on the vertex to the right of the sagittal suture in left (LOA), and to the left in right (ROA). As flexion becomes more pronounced during labor, the posterior part of the vertex becomes the presenting part and the caput is found in that region, a little to the right or left as before. Thus, when the position is LOA, the caput is on the posterior part of the right parietal bone, and in ROA on the posterior part of the left parietal bone.

The size of the caput succedaneum is an indication of the amount of pressure that has been exerted against the head. A large one suggests strong pressure from above and resistance from below. A small caput is present when the contractions have been weak or the resistance feeble. The largest are found in contracted pelves after long, hard labor. In the presence of prolonged labor, a large caput suggests disproportion or occipitoposterior position, and a small one indicates uterine inertia.

In performing vaginal examinations during labor, one must take care to distinguish between the station of the caput and that of the skull. The enlarging caput may make the accoucheur believe that the head is descending, when in reality it means that advancement of the head is delayed or arrested. A growing caput is an indication for reassessing the situation.

The caput is present at birth, begins to disappear immediately afterward, and is usually gone after 24 to 36 hours.

Cephalohematoma

Cephalohematoma (also spelled cephalhematoma) is a hemorrhage under the periosteum of one or more of the bones of the skull (Fig. 6-4D). It is situated on one or, rarely, both parietal bones and is similar in appearance to a caput succedaneum. A cephalohematoma is caused by trauma to the skull, including:

1. Prolonged pressure of the head against the cervix, perineum, or pubic bones
2. Damage from forceps blades or ventouse
3. Difficult manual rotation of the head
4. Rapid compression and relaxation of the forces that act on the fetal head, as in precipitous births

This injury may occur also during normal spontaneous delivery.

Because the hemorrhage is under the periosteum, the swelling is limited to the affected bone and does not cross the suture lines; this is one way of distinguishing it from a caput succedaneum. The swelling appears within a few hours of birth, and since absorption is slow, it takes 6 to

12 weeks to disappear. The blood clots early at the edges and remains fluid to the center. Rarely, ossification takes place in the clot and may cause a permanent deformity of the skull. The health of the child is not affected, and the brain is not damaged.

The prognosis is good. No local treatment is indicated, but observation of the fetus and measurement of the head circumference to ensure that the hematoma is not expanding are appropriate (to differentiate from subgaleal hematoma). Vitamin K may be given to reduce further bleeding. The area should be protected from injury, but no attempt is made to evacuate the blood. Rarely, infection ensues with formation of an abscess that must be drained. The differential diagnosis of caput succedaneum and cephalohematoma includes the following criteria:

Caput Succedaneum	Cephalohematoma
Present at birth	May not appear for several hours
Soft; pits on pressure	Soft; does not pit
Diffuse swelling	Sharply circumscribed
Lies over and crosses the sutures	Limited to individual bones; does not cross suture lines
Movable on skull; seeks dependent portions	Fixed to original site
Is largest at birth and immediately begins to grow smaller, disappearing in a few hours	Appears after a few hours, grows larger for a time, and disappears only after weeks or months

Subgaleal Hematoma

A subgaleal hemorrhage or hematoma refers to bleeding in the potential space between the periosteum of the skull and the galea aponeurosis of the scalp. These injuries are more commonly seen as a result of the traction related to vacuum-assisted vaginal delivery. This traction can rupture the connections between dural sinus and scalp veins, leading to an accumulation of blood under the aponeurosis of the scalp muscle superficial to the periosteum. The presence of the rare subgaleal hematoma should alert the clinician to seek other associated complications of head trauma such as intracranial hemorrhage or skull fracture.

Subgaleal hematoma is diagnosed based on a fluctuant boggy mass developing over the scalp and superficial skin bruising. The swelling develops gradually 12 to 72 hours after delivery, although in severe cases, it can be seen more quickly after delivery. The hematoma can slowly spread across the whole head and conceal a large quantity of blood. As such, neonates with subgaleal hemorrhage could descend into hemorrhagic shock.

As opposed to the cephalohematoma, the subgaleal hematoma can cross suture lines, and if enough blood accumulates, a visible fluid wave may be seen. The long-term prognosis is good; management consists of close observation to rule out progression and fluid resuscitation. Transfusion may be required if blood loss is significant, and the fetus should also be monitored for hyperbilirubinemia.

Meningocele

A meningocele is a hernial protrusion of the meninges. It is a serious congenital deformity and must be distinguished from caput succedaneum and cephalohematoma. The meningocele always lies over a suture or a fontanelle and becomes tense when the baby cries.

CHAPTER 7

Fetopelvic Relationships

Glenn D. Posner

Definitions

LIE Relationship of the long axis of the fetus to the long axis of the mother.

PRESENTATION The part of the fetus that lies over the inlet. The three main presentations are cephalic (head first), breech (pelvis first), and shoulder.

PRESENTING PART The most dependent part of the fetus, lying nearest the cervix. During vaginal examination, it is the area with which the finger makes contact first.

ATTITUDE Relationship of fetal parts to each other. The basic attitudes are flexion and extension. The fetal head is in flexion when the chin approaches the chest and in extension when the occiput nears the back. The typical fetal attitude in the uterus is flexion, with the head bent in front of the chest, the arms and legs folded in front of the body, and the back curved forward slightly.

DENOMINATOR An arbitrarily chosen point on the presenting part of the fetus used in describing position. Each presentation has its own denominator (i.e., occiput, sacrum, mentum, frontum).

POSITION Relationship of the denominator to the front, back, or sides of the maternal pelvis.

LIE

The two lies are: (1) longitudinal, when the long axes of the fetus and mother are parallel, and (2) transverse, or oblique, when the long axis of the fetus is perpendicular or oblique to the long axis of the mother.

All terms of direction refer to the mother in the standing position. Upper means toward the maternal head, and lower toward the feet. Anterior, posterior, right, and left refer to the mother's front, back, right, and left, respectively.

Longitudinal Lies

Longitudinal lies are grouped into: (1) cephalic, when the head comes first, and (2) breech, when the buttocks or lower limbs lead the way (Table 7-1).

TABLE 7-1: FETOPELVIC RELATIONSHIPS ACCORDING TO FETAL POSITION

Presentation	Attitude	Presenting Part	Denominator
Longitudinal lie (99.5%)			
Cephalic (96%-97%)	Flexion	Vertex (posterior part)	Occiput (O)
	Military	Vertex (median part)	Occiput (O)
	Partial extension	Brow	Forehead (frontum) (Fr)
	Complete extension	Face	Chin (mentum) (M)
Breech (3%-4%)			
Complete	Flexed hips and knees	Buttocks	Sacrum (S)
Frank	Flexed hips, extended knees	Buttocks	Sacrum (S)
Footling: single, double	Extended hips and knees	Feet	Sacrum (S)
Kneeling: single, double	Extended hips; flexed knees	Knees	Sacrum (S)
Transverse or oblique lie (0.5%)			
Shoulder	Variable	Shoulder, arm, trunk	Scapula (Sc)

Cephalic Presentations

Cephalic presentations are classified into four main groups, according to the attitude of the fetal head:

1. Flexion is present when the baby's chin is near his or her chest (Fig. 7-1A). The posterior part of the vertex is the presenting part, and the occiput is the denominator

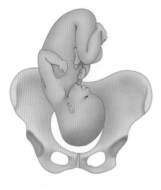

A. Flexion of head.

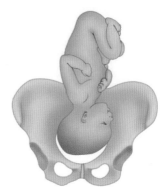

B. Military attitude.

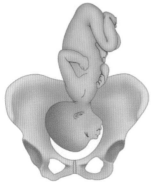

C. Brow presentation, partial
extension.

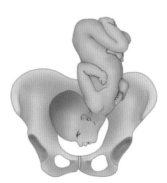

D. Face presentation,
complete extension.

FIGURE 7-1. Attitude.

2. The position with neither flexion nor extension is called the military attitude or the median vertex presentation (Fig. 7-1B). The vertex (area between the two fontanelles) presents, and the occiput is the denominator
3. In brow presentation (Fig. 7-1C), there is halfway extension. The frontum (forehead) leads the way and is also the denominator
4. When extension is complete, the presenting part is the face (Fig. 7-1D), and the denominator is the mentum (chin)

Breech Presentations

Breech or pelvic presentations are classified according to the attitudes at the hips and knees (Fig. 7-2).

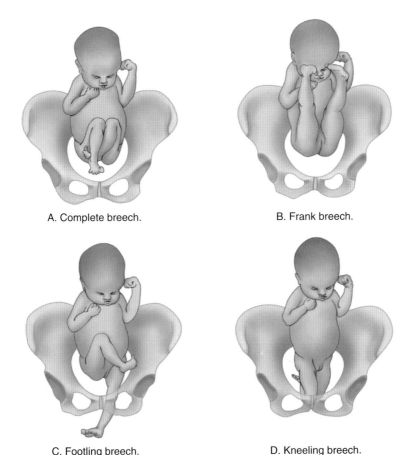

A. Complete breech.

B. Frank breech.

C. Footling breech.

D. Kneeling breech.

FIGURE 7-2. Breech.

1. The breech is complete when there is flexion at both hips and knees. The buttocks are the presenting part
2. Flexion at the hips and extension at the knees change it to a frank breech. The lower limbs lie anterior to the baby's abdomen. The buttocks lead the way
3. When there is extension both at the hips and at the knees, it is a footling breech—single if one foot is presenting and double if both feet are down
4. Extension at the hips and flexion at the knees make it a kneeling breech, single or double. Here the knees present

In all variations of breech presentation, the sacrum is the denominator.

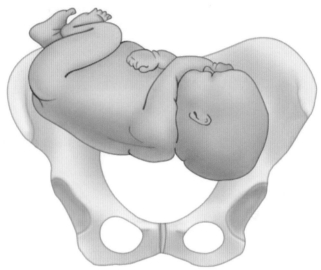

FIGURE 7-3. Transverse lie.

Transverse or Oblique Lie

Transverse or oblique lie (Fig. 7-3) exists when the long axis of the fetus is perpendicular or oblique to the long axis of the mother. Most often the shoulder is the presenting part, but it may be an arm or some part of the trunk, such as the back, abdomen, or side. The scapula is the denominator. The position is anterior or posterior depending on the situation of the scapulas and right or left according to the location of the head.

POSITION

Position is the relationship of the denominator to the front, back, or sides of the mother's pelvis. The pelvic girdle has a circumference of 360°. The denominator can occupy any part of the circumference. In practice, eight points, 45° from each other, are demarcated, and the position of the fetus is described as the relationship between the denominator and one of these landmarks.

Three sets of terms are used to describe position: (1) the *denominator;* (2) *right* or *left,* depending on which side of the maternal pelvis the denominator is in; and (3) *anterior, posterior,* or *transverse,* according to whether the denominator is in the front, in the back, or at the side of the pelvis.

With the patient lying in the lithotomy position, the pubic symphysis is anterior and the sacrum posterior. Starting at the symphysis and moving

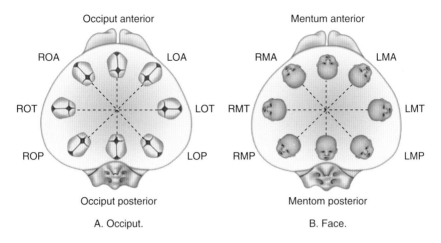

A. Occiput.

B. Face.

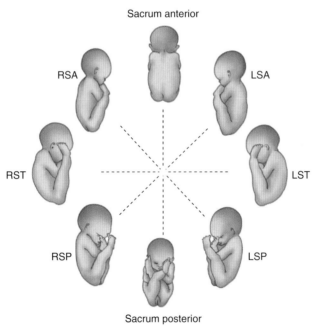

C. Breech.

FIGURE 7-4. Position.

in a clockwise direction, eight positions are described in succession, each 45° from the preceding one (Fig. 7-4A).

1. Denominator anterior (DA): The denominator is situated directly under the pubic symphysis

2. Left denominator anterior (LDA): The denominator is in the anterior part of the pelvis, 45° to the left of the midline
3. Left denominator transverse (LDT): The denominator is on the left side of the pelvis, 90° from the midline, at 3 o'clock
4. Left denominator posterior (LDP): The denominator is now in the posterior segment of the pelvis and is 45° to the left of the midline
5. Denominator posterior (DP): The denominator has rotated a total of 180° and is now in the posterior part of the pelvis, directly in the midline and directly above the sacrum
6. Right denominator posterior (RDP): The denominator is in the posterior part of the pelvis, 45° to the right of the midline
7. Right denominator transverse (RDT): The denominator is on the right side of the pelvis, 90° from the midline, at 9 o'clock
8. Right denominator anterior (RDA): The denominator is in the anterior segment of the pelvis, 45° to the right of the midline

Further rotation of 45° completes the circle of 360°, and the denominator is back under the symphysis pubis in the denominator anterior position.

This method of describing position is used for every presentation. Each presentation has its own denominator, but the basic descriptive terminology is the same.

Figure 7-4A demonstrates the various positions in which the vertex is the presenting part. The occiput (back of the head) is the denominator, and the eight positions (moving clockwise) are OA—LOA—LOT—LOP—OP—ROP—ROT—ROA—OA.

In face presentations (Fig. 7-4B), the chin (mentum) is the denominator, and the sequence of positions is MA—LMA—LMT—LMP—MP—RMP—RMT—RMA—MA.

A further example is in breech presentations in which the sacrum is the denominator (Fig. 7-4C). Here the eight positions are SA—LSA—LST—LSP—SP—RSP—RST—RSA—SA.

CEPHALIC PROMINENCE

The cephalic prominence is produced by flexion or extension (Fig. 7-5). When the head is well flexed, the occiput is lower than the sinciput, and the forehead is the cephalic prominence. When there is extension, the occiput is higher than the sinciput, and the occiput or back of the head is the cephalic prominence. The cephalic prominence can be palpated through the abdomen by placing both hands on the sides of the lower part of the

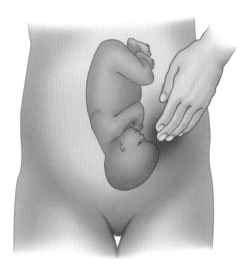

A. Flexion.

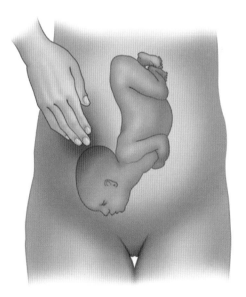

B. Extension.

FIGURE 7-5. Cephalic prominence.

uterus and moving them gently toward the pelvis. When there is a cephalic prominence, the fingers abut against it on that side and on the other side meet little or no resistance. The location of the cephalic prominence aids in diagnosing attitude. When the cephalic prominence and the back are on opposite sides, the attitude is flexion. When the cephalic prominence and the back are on the same side, there is extension. When no cephalic prominence is palpable, there is neither flexion nor extension, and the head is in the military attitude.

LIGHTENING

Lightening is the subjective sensation felt by the patient as the presenting part descends during the latter weeks of pregnancy. It is not synonymous with engagement, although both may take place at the same time. Lightening is caused by the tonus of the uterine and abdominal muscles and is part of the adaptation of the presenting part to the lower uterine segment and to the pelvis. In the latter weeks of pregnancy, the cervix is taken up and the isthmus becomes part of the lower uterine segment. As this area expands, there is more room in the lower part of the uterus, and the fetus drops into it. Symptoms include:

1. Less dyspnea
2. Decreased epigastric pressure
3. A feeling that the child is lower
4. Increased pressure in the pelvis
5. Low backache
6. Urinary frequency
7. Constipation
8. Initial appearance or aggravation of hemorrhoids and varicose veins of the lower limbs
9. Edema of the legs and feet
10. More difficulty in walking

GRAVIDITY AND PARITY

Gravidity

1. A *gravida* is a pregnant woman
2. The word *gravida* refers to a pregnancy regardless of its duration
3. A woman's *gravidity* relates to the total number of her pregnancies regardless of their duration
4. A *primigravida* is a woman pregnant for the first time

5. A *secundagravida* is a woman pregnant for the second time, although this term is rarely used in modern practice
6. A *multigravida* is a woman who has been pregnant several times, although common usage of this term is for a woman who has delivered at least once before

Parity

1. The word *para* alludes to past pregnancies that have reached viability
2. *Parity* refers to the number of past pregnancies that have gone to viability and have been delivered regardless of the number of children involved. (For example, the birth of triplets increases the parity by only one)
3. A *nullipara* is a woman who has never delivered a child who reached viability
4. A *primipara* is a woman who has delivered one pregnancy in which the child has reached viability, without regard to the child's being alive or dead at the time of birth. Alas, the common use of this term is to describe a woman who is pregnant with her first child
5. A *multipara* is a woman who has had two or more pregnancies that terminated at the stage when the children were viable, although this term is often used to describe a parturient who is delivering (at least) her second child
6. A *parturient* is a woman in labor

Nomenclature: Gravida and Para

1. A woman pregnant for the first time is a primigravida and is described as gravida 1, para 0
2. If she aborts before viability, she remains gravida 1, para 0. Specifically, she would be gravida 1, para 0, aborta 1
3. If she delivers a fetus who has reached viability, she becomes a primipara, regardless of whether the child is alive or dead. She is now gravida 1, para 1
4. During a second pregnancy, she is gravida 2, para 1
5. After she delivers the second child, she is gravida 2, para 2
6. A patient with two abortions and no viable children is gravida 2, para 0, aborta 2. When she becomes pregnant again, she is gravida 3, para 0, aborta 2. When she delivers a viable child, she is gravida 3, para 1, aborta 2
7. Multiple births do not affect the parity by more than one. A woman who has viable triplets in her first pregnancy is gravida 1, para 1

Nomenclature: The GTPAL System

A different way of describing the patient's obstetrical situation is as follows:

1. G: Gravidity
2. T: Term deliveries
3. P: Preterm deliveries
4. A: Abortions
5. L: Living children

In this nomenclature, a woman who has viable triplets born at 32 weeks in her first pregnancy is gravida 1, term 0, preterm 1, aborta 0, live 3.

CHAPTER 8

Engagement, Synclitism, Asynclitism

Glenn D. Posner

ENGAGEMENT

When the presenting part of the fetus is entirely out of the pelvis and is freely movable above the inlet, it is said to be floating (Fig. 8-1A).

When the presenting part has passed through the plane of the inlet but engagement has not occurred, it is said to be dipping (Fig. 8-1B).

By definition, engagement (Fig. 8-1C) has taken place when the widest diameter of the presenting part has passed through the inlet. In cephalic presentations, this diameter is the biparietal, between the parietal bones; in breech presentation, it is the intertrochanteric diameter.

In most women, once the head is engaged, the bony presenting part (not the caput succedaneum) is at or nearly at the level of the ischial spines. Radiologic studies have shown that this relationship is not constant and that in women with deep pelves, the presenting part may be as much as 1 cm above the spines even though engagement has occurred.

The presence or absence of engagement is determined by abdominal or vaginal examination. In primigravidas, engagement usually takes place 2 to 3 weeks before term. In multiparas, engagement may occur any time before or after the onset of labor. Engagement tells us that the pelvic inlet is adequate. It gives no information as to the midpelvis or the outlet. Although failure of engagement in a primigravida is an indication for careful examination to rule out disproportion, abnormal presentation, or some condition blocking the birth canal, it is no cause for alarm. The occurrence of engagement in normal cases is influenced by the tonus of the uterine and abdominal muscles.

STATION

Station is the relationship of the presenting part to an imaginary line drawn between the ischial spines (Fig. 8-2). The location of the buttocks in breech presentations or the bony skull (not the caput succedaneum) in cephalic presentations at the level of the spines indicates that the station is zero. Above the spines, the station is −1, −2, and so forth, depending on how many centimeters above the spines the presenting part is. At spines −5, it is at the inlet. Below the spines, it is +1, +2, and so forth. There are various relationships between station and the progress of labor.

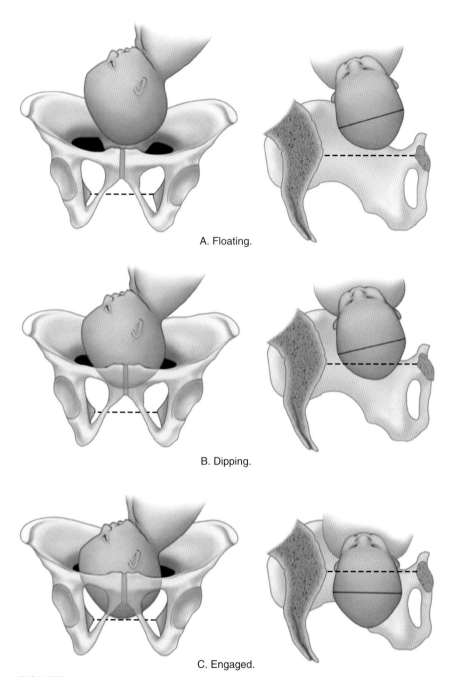

A. Floating.

B. Dipping.

C. Engaged.

FIGURE 8-1. The process of engagement.

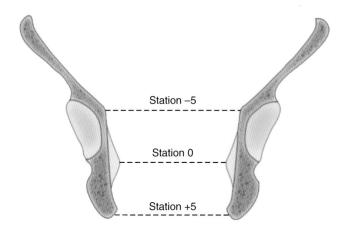

A. Anteroposterior view.

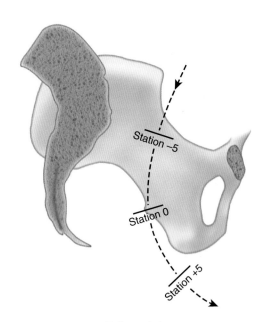

B. Lateral view.

FIGURE 8-2. Station of the presenting part.

1. In nulliparas entering labor with the fetal head well below the spines, further descent is often delayed until the cervix is fully dilated
2. In nulliparas beginning labor with the head deep in the pelvis, descent beyond the spines often takes place during the first stage of labor

3. An unengaged head in a nullipara at the onset of labor may indicate disproportion and warrants investigation. This condition is not rare, however, and in many cases, descent and vaginal delivery take place
4. The incidence of disproportion is more common when the head is high at the onset of labor
5. Patients who start labor with high fetal heads usually have lesser degrees of cervical dilatation. There is a tendency for lower stations to be associated with cervices that are more effaced and dilated, both at the onset of labor and at the beginning of the active phase
6. Other factors being equal, the higher the station, the longer the labor
7. Dysfunctional labor is more frequent when the station is high
8. A high head that descends rapidly is usually not associated with abnormal labor

SYNCLITISM AND ASYNCLITISM

Engagement in Synclitism

In cephalic presentations, engagement has occurred when the biparietal diameter has passed through the inlet of the pelvis. The fetal head engages most frequently with its sagittal suture (the anteroposterior diameter) in the transverse diameter of the pelvis. Left occiput transverse is the most common position at engagement.

When the biparietal diameter of the fetal head is parallel to the planes of the pelvis, the head is in *synclitism*. The sagittal suture is midway between the front and the back of the pelvis. When this relationship does not occur, the head is said to be in *asynclitism*.

Engagement in synclitism takes place when the uterus is perpendicular to the inlet and the pelvis is roomy (Fig. 8-3). The head enters the pelvis with the plane of the biparietal diameter parallel to the plane of the inlet, the sagittal suture lies midway between the pubic symphysis and the sacral promontory, and the parietal bosses enter the pelvis at the same time.

Posterior Asynclitism

In most women, the abdominal wall maintains the pregnant uterus in an upright position and prevents it from lying perpendicular to the plane of the pelvic inlet. As the head approaches the pelvis, the posterior parietal bone is lower than the anterior parietal bone, the sagittal suture is closer

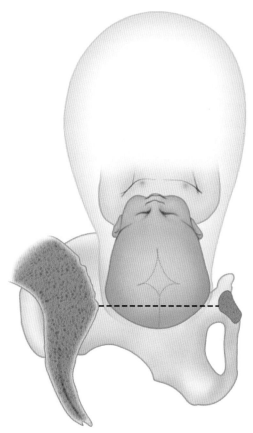

FIGURE 8-3. Synclitism at the inlet.

to the symphysis pubis than to the promontory of the sacrum, and the biparietal diameter of the head is in an oblique relationship to the plane of the inlet. This is posterior asynclitism (Fig. 8-4). It is the usual mechanism in normal women and is more common than engagement in synclitism or anterior asynclitism.

As the head enters the pelvis, the posterior parietal bone leads the way, and the posterior parietal boss (eminence) descends past the sacral promontory. At this point, the anterior parietal boss is still above the pubic symphysis and has not entered the pelvis. Uterine contractions force the head downward and into a movement of lateral flexion. The posterior parietal bone pivots against the promontory, the sagittal suture moves posteriorly toward the sacrum, and the anterior parietal boss descends past

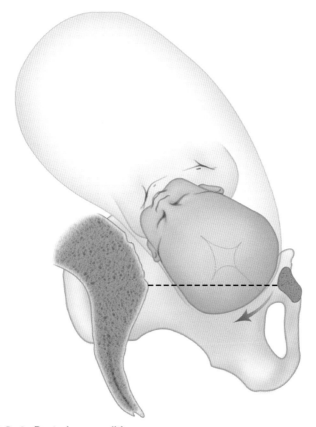

FIGURE 8-4. Posterior asynclitism.

the symphysis and into the pelvis. This brings the sagittal suture midway between the front and back of the pelvis, and the head is now in synclitism.

Anterior Asynclitism

When the woman's abdominal muscles are lax and the abdomen is pendulous so that the uterus and baby fall forward, or when the pelvis is abnormal and prevents the more common posterior asynclitism, the head enters the pelvis by anterior asynclitism (Fig. 8-5). In this mechanism, the anterior parietal bone descends first, the anterior parietal boss passes by the pubic symphysis into the pelvis, and the sagittal suture lies closer to the sacral promontory than to the pubic symphysis. When the anterior parietal bone becomes relatively fixed behind the symphysis, a movement of lateral

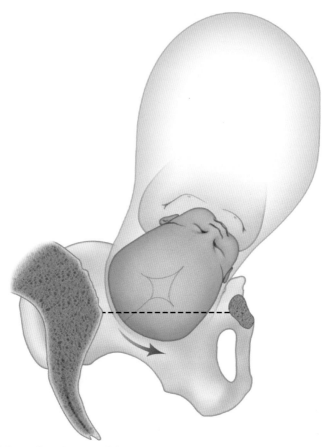

FIGURE 8-5. Anterior asynclitism.

flexion takes place so that the sagittal suture moves anteriorly toward the symphysis and the posterior parietal boss squeezes by the sacral promontory and into the pelvis. The mechanism of engagement in anterior asynclitism is the reverse of that with posterior asynclitism.

There is a mechanical advantage to the head's entering the pelvis in asynclitism. When the two parietal bosses enter the pelvic inlet at the same time (synclitism), the presenting diameter is the biparietal of about 9.5 cm. In asynclitism, the bosses come into the pelvis one at a time, and the diameter is the subsuperparietal of approximately 8.75 cm. Thus, engagement in asynclitism enables a larger head to pass through the inlet than would be possible if the head entered with its biparietal diameter parallel to the plane of the inlet (Fig. 8-6).

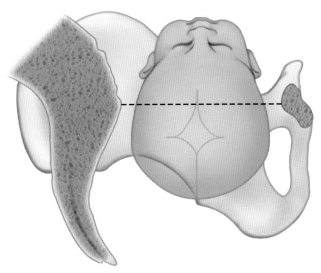

FIGURE 8-6. **Synclitism in the pelvis.**

Whenever there is a small pelvis or a large head, asynclitism plays an important part in enabling engagement to take place. Marked and persistent asynclitism, however, is abnormal. When asynclitism is maintained until the head is deep in the pelvis, it may prevent normal internal rotation.

PART II

First Stage of Labor

CHAPTER 9

Examination of the Patient

Adam Garber
Jessica Dy

Examination of the patient is important before the onset of labor to assess the fetal position with respect to the pelvis. This can be done clinically by abdominal palpation, vaginal examination, or fetal heart auscultation. Sonography can also be used to confirm fetal position in certain cases.

ABDOMINAL INSPECTION AND PALPATION (LEOPOLD'S MANEUVERS)

The position of the baby in utero is determined by inspecting and palpating the mother's abdomen, with these questions in mind:

1. Is the lie longitudinal, transverse, or oblique?
2. What presents at or in the pelvic inlet?
3. Where is the back?
4. Where are the small parts?
5. What is in the uterine fundus?
6. On which side is the cephalic prominence?
7. Has engagement taken place?
8. How high in the abdomen is the uterine fundus?
9. How big is the baby?

   The patient lies on her back with the abdomen uncovered (Fig. 9-1). To help relax the abdominal wall muscles, the shoulders are raised a little and the knees are drawn up slightly. If the patient is in labor, the examination is carried out between contractions.

First Maneuver: What Is the Presenting Part?

The examiner stands at the patient's side and grasps the lower uterine segment between the thumb and fingers of one hand to feel the presenting part (Fig. 9-2A). The other hand may be placed on the fundus to steady the

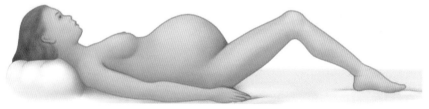

FIGURE 9-1. Position of patient for abdominal palpation.

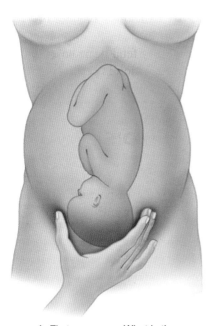

A. First maneuver: What is the
presenting part?

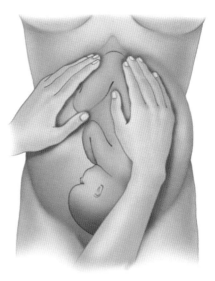

C. Third maneuver: What is in
the fundus?

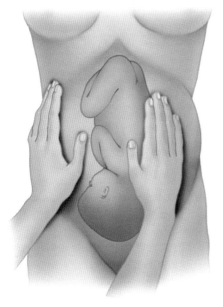

B. Second maneuver: Where is
the back?

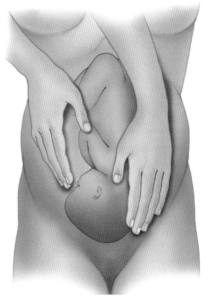

D. Fourth maneuver: What is
the cephalic prominence?

FIGURE 9-2. Abdominal palpation.

FIRST STAGE OF LABOR

uterus. This maneuver should be performed first. Since the head is the part of the fetus that can be identified with the most certainty and since it is at or in the pelvis in 90 percent of cases, the logical thing to do first is to look for the head in its most frequent location. Once it has been established that the head is at the inlet, two important facts are known: (1) that the lie is longitudinal and (2) that the presentation is cephalic. An attempt is made to move the head from side to side to see whether it is outside the pelvis and free (floating) or in the pelvis and fixed (engaged). In contrast to the breech position, the head is harder, smoother, more globular, and easier to move. A groove representing the neck may be felt between the head and the shoulders. The head can be moved laterally without an accompanying movement of the body. When the head is in the fundus and when there is sufficient amniotic fluid, the head can be ballotted.

When a floating rubber ball is forced under water, it returns to the surface as soon as it is released; so the fetal head can be pushed posteriorly in the amniotic fluid, but as soon as the pressure on it is relaxed, it rises back and abuts against the examining fingers.

Second Maneuver: Where Is the Back?

The examiner stands at the patient's side facing the patient's head. The hands are placed on the sides of the abdomen using one hand to steady the uterus while the other palpates the fetus (Fig. 9-2B). The location of the back and of the small parts is determined.

The side on which the back is located feels firmer and smoother and forms a gradual convex arch. Resistance to the palpating fingers (as pressure is exerted toward the umbilicus) is even in all regions. On the other side, the resistance to pressure is uneven, the fingers sinking deeper in some areas than they do in others. The discovery of moving limbs is diagnostic.

Third Maneuver: What Is in the Fundus?

The hands are moved up the sides of the uterus and the fundus is palpated (Fig. 9-2C). In most cases, the breech is here. It is a less definite structure than the head and is not identified as easily. The breech is softer, more irregular, less globular, and not as mobile as the head. It is continuous with the back, there being no intervening groove. When the breech is moved laterally, the body moves as well. Finding moving small parts in the vicinity of the breech strengthens the diagnosis.

Fourth Maneuver: Where Is the Cephalic Prominence?

The examiner turns and faces the patient's feet. The fingers are gently moved down the sides of the uterus toward the pubis (Fig. 9-2D). The cephalic prominence is felt on the side where there is greater resistance to the descent of the fingers into the pelvis. In attitudes of flexion, the forehead is the cephalic prominence. It is on the opposite side from the back. In extension attitudes, the occiput is the cephalic prominence and is on the same side as the back. In addition, it is noted whether the head is free and floating or fixed and engaged.

Relationship of the Head to the Pelvis

1. The floating head lies entirely above the symphysis pubis, so that the examining fingers can be placed between the head and the pubis. The head is freely movable from side to side
2. When the head is engaged, the biparietal diameter has passed the inlet, and only a small part of the head may be palpable above the symphysis. The head is fixed and cannot be moved laterally. Sometimes it is so low in the pelvis that it can barely be felt through the abdomen
3. The head may be midway between the previous two locations. Part of it is felt easily above the symphysis. It is not freely movable but is not fixed; nor is it engaged. The head is described as lying in the brim of the pelvis, or dipping

AUSCULTATION OF FETAL HEART

In most cases, there is a constant relationship between the location of the baby's heart and the fetal position in the uterus. In attitudes of flexion, the fetal heart sound is transmitted through the scapula and the back of the shoulder. It is, therefore, heard loudest in that area of the mother's abdomen to which the fetal back is closest. In attitudes of extension, the fetal heartbeat is transmitted through the anterior chest wall of the baby.

In cephalic presentations, the fetal heartbeat is loudest below the umbilicus; in anterior positions, it is clearest in one of the other lower quadrants of the mother's abdomen. The relationship of the fetal back and the fetal heart to the midline of the maternal abdomen is similar. As one comes nearer to or moves away from the midline, so does the other. In posterior positions, the fetal heart is loudest in the maternal flank on the side to

FIRST STAGE OF LABOR

which the back is related. Having the patient lie in a lateral position may bring the fetal heart closer to the midline so that the fetal heartbeat can be heard more easily in some women. In breech presentation, the point of maximum intensity of the baby's heart sound is above the umbilicus.

The position of the fetal heart changes with descent and rotation. As the baby descends, so does the fetal heart. The anterior rotation of an occiput posterior position can be followed by listening to the fetal heart as it moves gradually from the maternal flank toward the midline of the abdomen.

The location of the fetal heart (Fig. 9-3) may be used to check, but should not be relied upon to make, the diagnosis of presentation and position. Occasionally, the point of maximum intensity of the fetal heartbeat is not in the expected location for a given position. For example, it is not unusual in breech presentations for the fetal heart to be heard loudest below

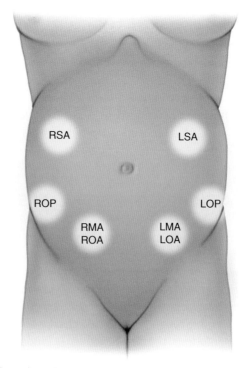

FIGURE 9-3. Location of the fetal heart beat in relation to the various positions.
LMA, left mentum anterior; LOA, left occiput anterior; LOP, left occiput posterior; LSA, left sacrum anterior; RMA, right mentum anterior; ROA, right occiput anterior; ROP, right occiput posterior; RSA, right sacrum anterior.

the umbilicus instead of above it. The diagnosis made by careful abdominal palpation is the more reliable finding. Locating the fetal heart sound in an unexpected place is an indication for reexamination by palpation of the position of the infant. If the findings on palpation are confirmed, the locale of the fetal heart tones should be disregarded.

VAGINAL EXAMINATION

Several recent studies demonstrated that there is no greater danger of infection with vaginal than with rectal examination. Points in favor of the vaginal examination in the management of labor are as follows:

1. Vaginal examination is the most accurate way to determine the condition and dilatation of the cervix. With a dilated cervix, important, accurate information on the station and position of the presenting part and relationship of the fetus to the pelvis can be obtained
2. Vaginal examination takes less time, requires less manipulation, and gives more information than the rectal approach
3. Vaginal examination causes less pain
4. Prolapse of the umbilical cord can be diagnosed early, as can compound presentations
5. Cultures taken during the puerperium from women whose vaginas were sterile on admittance to hospital showed no higher incidence of positive results in those who had vaginal examinations during labor than those who had only rectal evaluations
6. Clinical studies have shown that maternal morbidity is no higher after vaginal than after rectal examinations
7. It is important to remember that a clean or sterile glove is different from the contaminated finger of Semmelweis's time, when doctors went from infected surgical cases to the maternity ward without using aseptic precautions

The examination must be done gently, carefully, thoroughly, under aseptic conditions, and with consent. Sterile gloves should be used. We prefer the lithotomy or dorsal position, finding the examination and orientation easier. This is the best position for determining proportion between the presenting part and the pelvis.

In the past, the course of labor in normally progressing cases was followed by rectal examinations, because of fear of an increased risk of

FIRST STAGE OF LABOR

ascending infections from multiple vaginal examinations. Recent studies do not suggest increased risk of infection when a vaginal examination is properly performed. Therefore rectal examination is rarely performed today to assess labor progress unless unique circumstances, due to the advantages of vaginal examination as described above.

Palpation of Cervix

1. Is the cervix soft or hard?
2. Is it thin and effaced or thick and long?
3. Is it anterior or posterior to the fetal head?
4. Is it closed or open/dilated? If it is open, estimate the length of the diameter of the cervical ring (cervical dilatation)

Presentation

1. What is the presentation—breech, cephalic, shoulder, or compound?
2. Is there a caput succedaneum, and is it small or extensive? Is there significant molding?
3. What is the station? What is the relationship of the presenting part (not the caput succedaneum) to a line between the ischial spines? If it is above the spines, it is −1, −2, or −3 cm. If it is below the spines, it is +1, +2, or +3 cm

Position

1. If it is a breech, where is the sacrum? Are the legs flexed or extended?
2. With a cephalic presentation, identify the sagittal suture (Fig. 9-4A). What is its direction? Is it in the anteroposterior, oblique, or transverse diameter of the pelvis?
3. Is the sagittal suture midway between the pubis and the sacrum (synclitism), is it near the sacral promontory (anterior asynclitism), or is it near the pubic symphysis (posterior asynclitism)?
4. Where is the posterior fontanelle (Fig. 9-4B)? (It is Y shaped and has three sutures)
5. Is the bregma right or left, anterior or posterior? (It is diamond shaped and is the meeting point of four sutures [Fig. 9-4C])
6. Is the head in flexion (occiput lower than sinciput) or is there extension (sinciput lower than occiput)?
7. When there is difficulty in identifying the sutures, palpation of an ear (Fig. 9-4D) helps establish the direction of the sagittal suture and thus

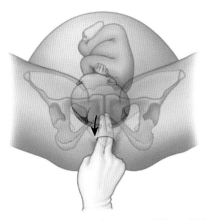

A. Determining the station and palpation of the sagittal suture.

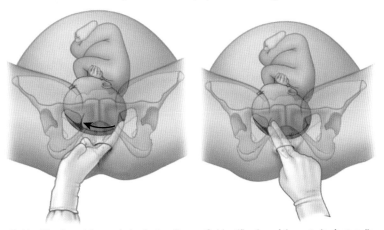

B. Identification of the posterior fontanelle.   C. Identification of the anterior fontanelle.

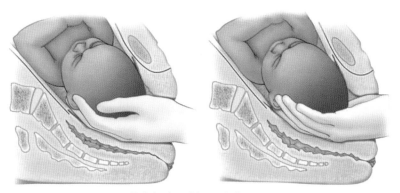

D. Palpation of the posterior ear.

FIGURE 9-4. A–D. Diagnosis of station and position. (Reproduced with permission from Douglas and Stromme, Operative Obstetrics, 4th ed, New York: McGraw Hill: Appleton-Century-Crofts, 1982.)

the anteroposterior diameter of the long axis of the head. The tragus points to the face

Membranes

Feeling the bag of waters is evidence that the membranes are intact. The drainage of fluid, passage of meconium, and palpation of fetal hair indicate that the membranes have ruptured. If membrane rupture is uncertain, a sterile speculum examination should be performed and vaginal fluid examined for the presence of ferning.

General Assessment of Pelvis

1. Can the sacral promontory be reached? The diagonal conjugate can be measured clinically. It extends from the inferior margin of the pubic symphysis to the middle of the sacral promontory, and its average length is 12.5 cm. During the vaginal examination, the promontory is palpated. When the distal end of the finger reaches the middle of the promontory, the point where the proximal part of the finger makes contact with the subpubic angle is marked (Figs. 9-5A, B, and C). The fingers are withdrawn from the vagina, and the distance between these two points is measured. By deducting 1.5 cm from the diagonal conjugate (Fig. 9-5C), the approximate length of the obstetric conjugate can be obtained. In many women, the promontory cannot be reached, and this is accepted as evidence that the anteroposterior diameter of the inlet is adequate. If the promontory can be felt, the obstetric conjugate may be short

2. Is the pelvic brim symmetrical?

3. Are the ischial spines prominent and posterior?

4. Is the sacrum long and straight or short and concave?

5. Are the side walls parallel or convergent?

6. Is the sacrosciatic notch wide or narrow?

7. Is there any bony or soft tissue encroachment into the cavity of the pelvis?

8. How wide is the subpubic angle? The distance between the ischial tuberosities (average, 10.5 cm) can be measured roughly by placing a fist between them (Fig. 9-5D). If this can be done, the transverse diameter of the outlet is considered adequate

9. Are the soft tissues and the perineum relaxed and elastic or hard and rigid?

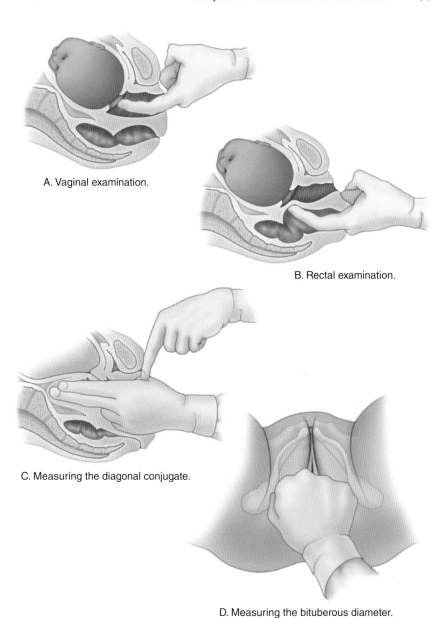

A. Vaginal examination.

B. Rectal examination.

C. Measuring the diagonal conjugate.

D. Measuring the bituberous diameter.

FIGURE 9-5. A–D. Pelvic assessment.

FIRST STAGE OF LABOR

Fetopelvic Relationship

1. How does the presenting part fit the pelvis?
2. If engagement has not taken place, can the presenting part be pushed into the pelvis by fundal and suprapubic pressure?
3. Does the presenting part ride over the pubic symphysis?

CHAPTER 10

Normal Mechanisms of Labor

Adam Garber
Jessica Dy

LEFT OCCIPUT ANTERIOR: LOA

LOA is a common longitudinal cephalic presentation (Fig. 10-1). Two-thirds of occiput anterior positions are in the LOA position. The attitude is flexion, the presenting part is the posterior part of the vertex and the posterior fontanelle, and the denominator is the occiput (O).

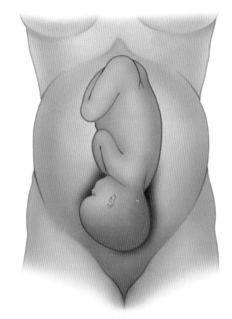

A. Abdominal view.

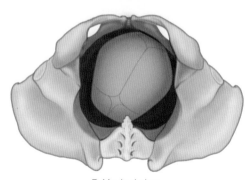

B. Vaginal view.

FIGURE 10-1. Left occiput anterior.

Diagnosis of Position: LOA

Abdominal Examination

1. The lie is longitudinal. The long axis of the fetus is parallel to the long axis of the mother
2. The head is at or in the pelvis
3. The back is on the left and anterior and is palpated easily except in obese women
4. The small parts are on the right and are not felt clearly
5. The breech is in the fundus of the uterus
6. The cephalic prominence (in this case the forehead) is on the right. When the attitude is flexion, the cephalic prominence and the back are on opposite sides. The reverse is true in attitudes of extension

Fetal Heart

The fetal heart is heard loudest in the left lower quadrant of the mother's abdomen. In attitudes of flexion, the fetal heart rate is transmitted through their back. The point of maximum intensity varies with the degree of rotation. As the fetal back approaches the midline of the maternal abdomen, so does the point where the fetal heart is heard most strongly. Therefore, in a left anterior position, it is heard below the umbilicus and somewhere to the left of the midline, depending on the exact situation of the back.

Vaginal Examination

1. The station of the head is noted—whether it is above, at, or below the ischial spines
2. If the cervix is dilated, the suture lines and the fontanelles of the fetal head can be felt. In the LOA position, the sagittal suture is in the right oblique diameter of the pelvis
3. The small posterior fontanelle is anterior and to the mother's left
4. The bregma is posterior and to the right
5. Since the head is probably flexed, the occiput is slightly lower than the brow

Normal Mechanism of Labor: LOA

The mechanism of labor as we know it today was first described by William Smellie during the 18th century. It is the way the baby adapts itself to and passes through the maternal pelvis. There are six movements, with considerable overlap:

FIRST STAGE OF LABOR

1. Descent
2. Flexion
3. Internal rotation
4. Extension
5. Restitution
6. External rotation

The following description relates to left anterior positioning of the occiput.

Descent

Descent, which includes engagement in the right oblique diameter of the pelvis, continues throughout normal labor as the baby passes through the birth canal. The other movements are superimposed on it. In primigravidas, considerable descent should have taken place before the onset of labor (Figs. 10-2A and B) in the process of engagement, provided there is no disproportion and the lower uterine segment is well formed. In multiparas, engagement may not take place until good labor has set in. Descent is brought about by the downward pressure of the uterine contractions, aided in the second stage by the bearing-down efforts of the patient and to a minimal extent by gravity.

Flexion

Partial flexion exists before the onset of labor since this is the natural attitude of the fetus in utero. Resistance to descent leads to increased flexion.

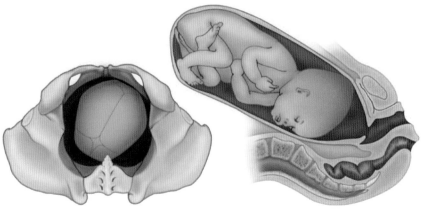

A. Vaginal view.   B. Lateral view.

FIGURE 10-2. **Mechanism of labor: left occiput anterior.**

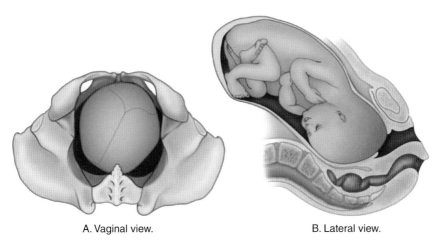

A. Vaginal view.   B. Lateral view.

FIGURE 10-3. **Descent and flexion of the head.**

The occiput descends in advance of the sinciput, the posterior fontanelle is lower than the bregma, and the baby's chin approaches his or her chest (Figs. 10-3A and B). This usually takes place at the inlet, but it may not be complete until the presenting part reaches the pelvic floor. The effect of flexion is to change the presenting diameter from the occipitofrontal of 11.0 cm to the smaller and rounder suboccipitobregmatic of 9.5 cm. Since the fit between fetal head and maternal pelvis may be snug, the reduction of 1.5 cm in the presenting diameter is important.

Internal Rotation

For the majority of pelvises, the inlet is a transverse oval. The anteroposterior diameter of the midpelvis is a little longer than the transverse diameter. The outlet is an anteroposterior oval, as is the fetal head. The long axis of the fetal head must fit into the long axis of the maternal pelvis. Hence, the head, which entered the pelvis in the transverse or oblique diameter, must rotate internally to the anteroposterior diameter in order to be born. This is the purpose of internal rotation (Fig. 10-4).

The occiput now leads the way to the midpelvis, where it makes contact with the pelvic floor (the levator ani muscles and fascia). Here the occiput rotates 45° to the right (toward the midline). The sagittal suture turns from the right oblique diameter to the anteroposterior diameter of the pelvis: LOA to occiput anterior (OA). The occiput comes to lie near the pubic symphysis and the sinciput near the sacrum.

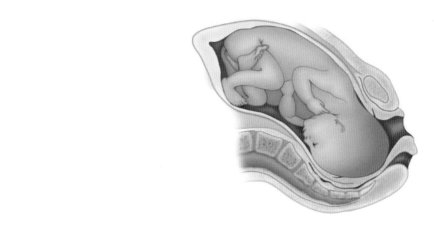

A. Lateral view.

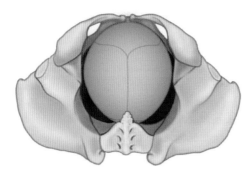

B. Vaginal view.

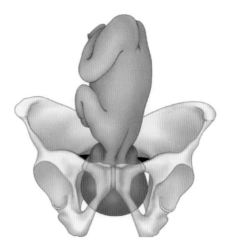

C. Anteroposterior view.

FIGURE 10-4. **Internal rotation: left occiput anterior to occiput anterior.**

The head rotates from the right oblique diameter to the anteroposterior diameter of the pelvis. The shoulders, however, remain in the left oblique diameter. Thus, the normal relationship of the long axis of the head to the long axis of the shoulders is changed, and the neck undergoes a twist of 45°. This situation is maintained as long as the head is in the pelvis.

We do not know accurately why the fetal head, which entered the pelvis in the transverse or oblique diameter, rotates so that the occiput turns anteriorly in the great majority of cases and posteriorly in so few. One explanation is based on pelvic architecture. Both the bones and the soft tissues play a part. The ischial spines extend into the pelvic cavity. The sidewalls of the pelvis anterior to the spines curve forward, downward, and medially. The pelvic floor, made up of the levator ani muscles and fascia, slopes downward, forward, and medially. The part of the head that reaches the pelvic floor and ischial spines first is rotated anteriorly by these structures. In most cases, the head is well flexed when it reaches the pelvic floor, and the occiput is lower than the sinciput. Hence the occiput strikes the pelvic floor first and is rotated anteriorly under the pubic symphysis.

This does not explain why some well-flexed heads in the left occiput transverse (LOT) and right occiput transverse (ROT) positions (proved by radiography) do not rotate posteriorly. Nor do the theories based on pelvic architecture explain the situation in which, in the same patient, the head rotates anteriorly during one labor and posteriorly in another. In truth, we do not know the exact reasons internal rotation takes place in the way it does. In most labors, internal rotation is complete when the head reaches the pelvic floor or soon after. Early internal rotation is frequent in multiparas and in patients having efficient uterine contractions. Internal rotation takes place mainly during the second stage of labor.

Extension

Extension (Fig. 10-5) is basically the result of two forces: (1) uterine contractions exerting downward pressure, and (2) the pelvic floor offering resistance. It must be pointed out that the anterior wall of the pelvis (the pubis) is only 4 to 5 cm long, but the posterior wall (the sacrum) is 10 to 15 cm. Hence, the sinciput has a greater distance to travel than the occiput. As the flexed head continues its descent, there is bulging of the perineum followed by crowning. The occiput passes through the outlet slowly, and the nape of the neck pivots in the subpubic angle. Then by a rapid process of extension, the sinciput sweeps along the sacrum, and the bregma, forehead, nose, mouth, and chin are born in succession over the perineum.

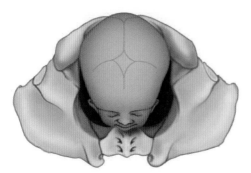

A. Vaginal view.

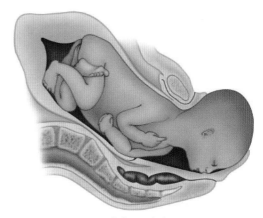

B. Lateral view.

FIGURE 10-5. Extension.

Restitution

When the head reaches the pelvic floor, the shoulders enter the pelvis (Fig. 10-6). Since the shoulders remain in the oblique diameter while the head rotates anteriorly, the neck becomes twisted. Once the head is born and is free of the pelvis, the neck untwists, and the head restitutes back 45° (OA to LOA) to resume the normal relationship with the shoulders and its original position in the pelvis.

External Rotation

External rotation of the head is really the outward manifestation of internal rotation of the shoulders. As the shoulders reach the pelvic floor, the lower anterior shoulder is rotated forward under the symphysis, and the bisacromial diameter turns from the left oblique to the anteroposterior diameter

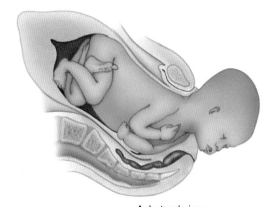

A. Lateral view.

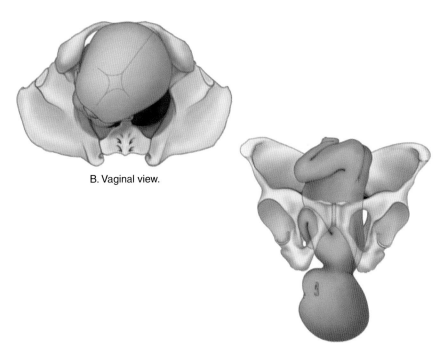

B. Vaginal view.

C. Anteroposterior view.

FIGURE 10-6. **Restitution: occiput anterior to left occiput anterior.**

of the pelvis. In this way, the long diameter of the shoulders can fit the long diameter of the outlet. The head, which had already restituted 45° to resume its normal relationship to the shoulders, now rotates another 45° to maintain it: LOA to LOT (Fig. 10-7). A summary of the mechanism of labor to this point is seen in Figure 10-8.

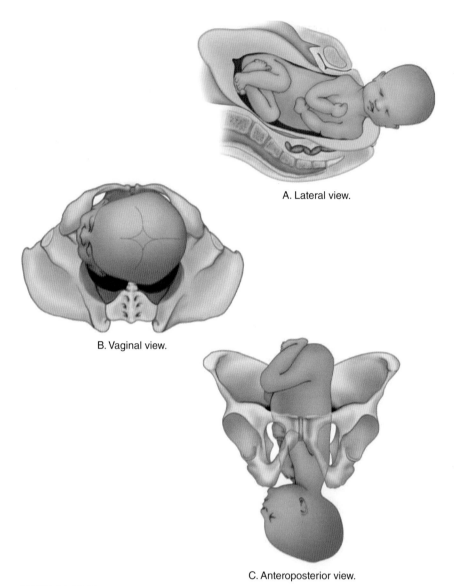

A. Lateral view.

B. Vaginal view.

C. Anteroposterior view.

FIGURE 10-7. **External rotation: left occiput anterior to left occiput transverse.**

Mechanism of the Shoulders

When the head appears at the outlet, the shoulders enter the inlet. They engage in the oblique diameter opposite that of the head. For example, in LOA, when the head engages in the right oblique diameter of the inlet, the shoulders engage in the left oblique.

The uterine contractions and the bearing-down efforts of the mother force the baby downward. The anterior shoulder reaches the pelvic floor first and rotates anteriorly under the symphysis. Anterior rotation of the shoulders takes place in a direction opposite to that of anterior rotation of the head. The anterior shoulder is born under the pubic symphysis

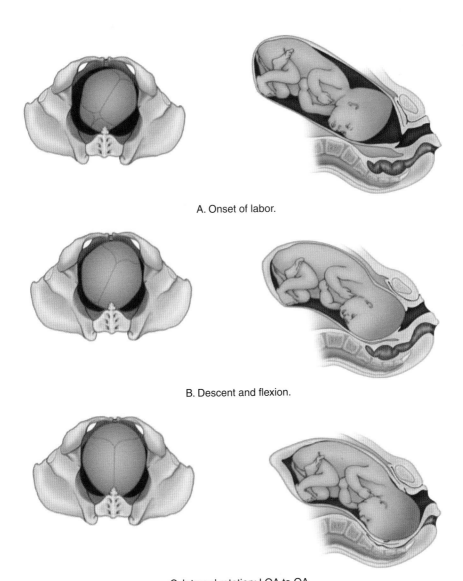

A. Onset of labor.

B. Descent and flexion.

C. Internal rotation: LOA to OA.

FIGURE 10-8. Summary of mechanism of labor: left occiput anterior.

FIRST STAGE OF LABOR

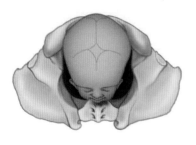
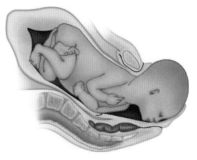

D. Extension.

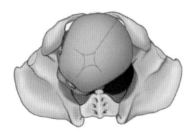
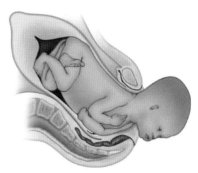

E. Restitution: OA to LOA.

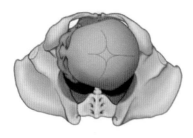
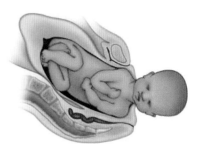

F. External rotation: LOA to LOT.

FIGURE 10-8. (*Continued*)

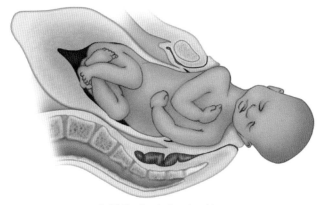

A. Birth of anterior shoulder.

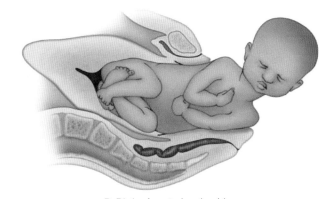

B. Birth of posterior shoulder.

FIGURE 10-9. **Delivery of the shoulders.**

FIRST STAGE OF LABOR

and pivots there (Fig. 10-9A). Then the posterior shoulder slides over the perineum by a movement of lateral flexion (Fig. 10-9B).

Birth of the Trunk and Extremities

After the shoulders have been born, the rest of the child is delivered by the mother's forcing down, with no special mechanism and with no difficulty.

Molding

In LOA, the presenting suboccipitobregmatic diameter is diminished, and the head is elongated in the verticomental diameter (Fig. 10-10).

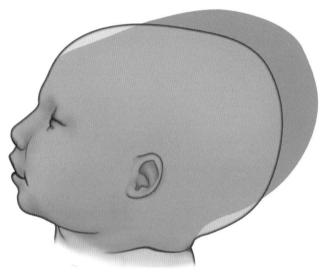

FIGURE 10-10. Molding.

BIRTH OF THE PLACENTA

Separation of the Placenta

Within a few minutes of delivery of the child, the uterine contractions begin again. Because the fetus is no longer in the uterus, the extent of the retraction of the upper segment is larger than during the first and second stages. This retraction greatly decreases the area where the placenta is attached (Fig. 10-11A). The size of the placenta itself, however, is not reducible. The resultant disparity between the size of the placenta and its area of attachment leads to a cleavage in the spongy layer of the decidua, and in this way, the placenta is separated from the wall of the uterus (Fig. 10-11B). During the process of separation, blood accumulates between the placenta and uterus. When the detachment is complete, the blood is released and gushes from the vagina; some lengthening of the umbilical cord is noted.

Expulsion of the Placenta

Soon after the placenta has separated, it is expelled into the vagina by the uterine contractions. From there, it is delivered by the bearing-down efforts of the patient. Two methods of expulsion have been described. In the Duncan method, the lower edge of the placenta comes out first, with the maternal and fetal surfaces appearing together, and the rest of the

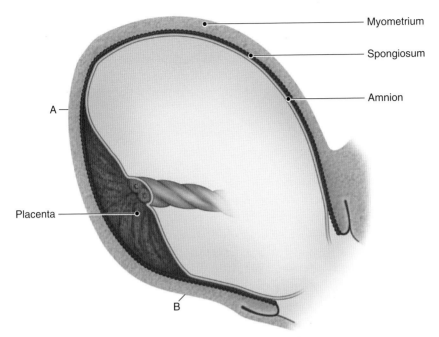

A. Placenta attached to uterine wall.

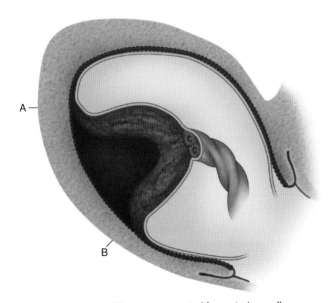

B. Placenta separated from uterine wall.

FIGURE 10-11. Birth of the placenta.

organ slides down. In the Schultze method, the placenta comes out like an inverted umbrella, the shiny fetal side appearing first and the membranes trailing after. Although the Schultze mechanism suggests fundal implantation and the Duncan method intimates that the placenta was attached to the wall of the uterus, the exact birth mechanism of the placenta is of little practical significance.

Control of Hemorrhage

The blood vessels that pass through the myometrium are tortuous and angular. The muscle fibers are arranged in an interlacing network through which the blood vessels pass. After the placenta has separated, retraction leads to a permanent shortening of the uterine muscle fibers. This compresses, kinks, twists, and closes the arterioles and venules in the manner of living ligatures. The blood supply to the placental site is effectively shut off, and bleeding is controlled. If the uterus is atonic and fails to retract properly after separation of the placenta, the vessels are not closed off, and postpartum hemorrhage may take place. It is therefore important to wait for the uterus to retract and the cleavage plane to occur before attempting to deliver the placenta.

CLINICAL COURSE OF LABOR: LOA

Almost always, an LOA turns 45° to bring the occiput under the pubic arch, from where spontaneous delivery takes place. Occasionally, because of minor degrees of disproportion, a rigid perineum, or generalized fatigue, the patient may not be able to complete the second stage. Arrests may take place in two positions:

1. It can occur after rotation to OA is complete, so that the sagittal suture is in the anteroposterior diameter
2. Rotation may fail, the fetal head remaining in the original LOA position with the sagittal suture in the right oblique diameter of the pelvis

Management of arrested occipitoanterior positions consists of the following steps:

1. If rotation to OA has occurred, forceps can be applied to the sides of the baby's head, which is then extracted. (See Chapter 25 for details of technique)

2. If rotation has failed, the forceps can be applied to the sides of the baby's head. First, the head is rotated with the forceps from LOA to OA and then it is extracted. (See Chapter 25 for details of technique)

RIGHT OCCIPUT ANTERIOR: ROA

ROA is less common than LOA. The physical findings and the mechanism of labor are similar but opposite of LOA. The difference lies in the fact that in ROA, the occiput and back of the fetus are on the mother's right side, and the small parts are on the left.

FIRST STAGE OF LABOR

CHAPTER 11

Clinical Course of Normal Labor

Susan L. Aubin

Definitions

LABOR The physiologic process by which the products of conception (fetus, amniotic fluid, placenta, and membranes) are separated and expelled from the uterus through the vagina into the outside world. It is defined by the presence of regular uterine contractions accompanied by cervical effacement and dilatation and fetal descent.

PRETERM LABOR The onset of labor in a gravid woman whose period of gestation is less than 37 completed weeks (less than 259 days) from the first day of the last menstrual period.

DYSTOCIA Delayed or arrested progress in labor.

EXPECTED DATE OF DELIVERY On an average, this is 280 days from the first day of the last menstrual period or 267 days from conception. It is calculated by going back 3 months from the first day of the last menses and adding 7 days (Naegle's rule).

ONSET OF LABOR

Causes of Onset of Labor

Hippocrates' concept that a fetus determines the time of his or her birth has been proven correct in some animals. In humans, however, it appears that the placenta and fetal membranes play the major role in the initiation of labor, while the fetus may modulate the timing of labor. Although the exact cause of and mechanism for labor are not known, evidence is mounting in support of a hormonal basis.

In sheep, it is clear that maturation of the fetal hypothalamo–hypophyseal–adrenal axis during late pregnancy is responsible for initiating labor by inducing changes in the pattern of placental steroid genesis and, ultimately, by increasing the production of intrauterine prostaglandin. Birth can be induced by infusing adrenocorticotropic hormone (ACTH) or glucocorticoids to the fetal lamb in utero before term has been reached. These preterm fetuses are viable and are able to expand their lungs, indicating that the fetal glucocorticoids play a role in pulmonary maturation as well as in parturition. In sheep as in humans, the nature of the stimulus that leads to increased pituitary–adrenal activity in late pregnancy is not known.

At the present time, there is no evidence that human fetuses play the same pivotal role in determining the time they are born as do sheep. The belief that anencephaly and adrenal hypoplasia predispose to prolongation of pregnancy has been challenged. In both humans and monkeys, the administration of glucocorticoids does not bring on labor, nor is there evidence to show that fetal cortisol sets off parturition in humans.

Estrogen

Although some evidence shows that estrogen is involved in human parturition, its mode of action has not been well defined. The placenta is the main source of estrogen biosynthesis in pregnancy. Estrogens upregulate myometrial gap junctions and receptors responsible for myometrial contractions (e.g., calcium channels and oxytocin receptors).

Progesterone

In some animals, progesterone plays a part in maintaining uterine quiescence. In primates, the role of progesterone is unclear. Recent evidence suggests that supplemental progesterone may reduce the risk of preterm birth in select women at risk of preterm labor. On the other hand, administration of progesterone receptor antagonists does not seem to induce labor at term, and progesterone withdrawal does not occur in all women before the spontaneous onset of labor. There is, to the contrary, some evidence that the levels of free progesterone may rise as parturition approaches.

Oxytocin

Maternal serum oxytocin levels do not increase before the onset of spontaneous labor; therefore, it is unlikely that oxytocin provides the trigger for the initiation of human parturition. However, the sensitivity of the uterus to oxytocin increases in late pregnancy mainly because of the 100- to 200-fold increase in the concentration of oxytocin receptors in the myometrium. And with an increase in the pulsatile release of oxytocin as labor progresses, oxytocin during labor results in stronger uterine contractions.

Prostaglandin

Three lines of evidence support the part played by prostaglandin in human parturition: (1) there is an increase in the production of prostaglandin at term; (2) myometrial contractility and preterm labor can be suppressed by the use of inhibitors of the synthesis of prostaglandin (including cyclooxygenase inhibitors such as indomethacin); and (3) exogenous prostaglandins stimulate the primate uterus to contract. Whether the primary effect of prostaglandin at term is exerted by increased biosynthesis, by increased myometrial sensitivity, or both is not yet known.

Phenomena Preliminary to the Onset of Labor

1. Lightening occurs 2 to 3 weeks before term and is the subjective sensation felt by the mother as the baby settles into the lower uterine segment
2. Engagement takes place 2 to 3 weeks before term in primigravidas
3. Vaginal secretions increase in amount
4. Loss of weight is caused by the excretion of body water
5. The mucous plug is discharged from the cervix
6. Bloody show is noted
7. The cervix becomes soft and effaced
8. Persistent backache is present
9. False labor pains occur with variable frequency

NORMAL UTERINE CONTRACTIONS

Definitions

CONTRACTION The shortening of a muscle in response to stimulus with return to its original length after the contraction has worn off.

RETRACTION The muscle shortens in response to a stimulus but does not return to its original length when the contraction has passed. The muscle becomes fixed at a relatively shorter length, but the tension remains the same. In this way, the slack is taken up, and the walls of the uterus maintain contact with the contents. Retraction is responsible for descent. Without this property, the fetus would move down with the contraction, only to return to the original level once the contraction had ceased. With retraction, on the other hand, the fetus remains at a slightly lower level each time. During contraction, it is as though three steps are taken forward and then three backward. With retraction, three steps are taken forward and then two backward. In this way, a little ground is gained each time. In the control of postpartum bleeding, retraction is essential. Without it, many patients might bleed to death.

PHYSIOLOGIC RETRACTION RING As labor and retraction proceed, the upper part of the uterus becomes progressively shorter and thicker, and the lower portion gets longer and thinner. The boundary between the two segments is the physiologic retraction ring (Fig. 11-1).

PATHOLOGIC RETRACTION RING In cases of obstructed labor, the physiologic ring becomes extreme and is known as the pathologic retraction (Bandl) ring.

CONSTRICTION RING A localized segment of myometrial spasm that grips the fetus tightly and prevents descent.

TONUS The lowest intrauterine (intra-amniotic) pressure between contractions. It is expressed in millimeters of mercury (mm Hg). The normal resting tension is 8 to 12 mm Hg.

INTENSITY Also known as amplitude, it is the rise in intrauterine pressure brought about by each contraction. It is measured from the baseline, resting pressure (tonus) rather than from zero. The normal is 30 to 50 mm Hg.

FREQUENCY Caldeyro-Barcia defined this as the number of contractions per 10 minutes. For the patient to be in good labor, the frequency must be at least two contractions per 10 minutes.

UTERINE ACTIVITY The Montevideo unit (MU) was introduced by Caldeyro-Barcia and represents the average intensity of the uterine contractions multiplied by the number of contractions observed during a 10-minute period of monitoring (intensity × frequency). To incorporate the third variation, duration of the contraction, the Alexandria unit (AU) was created. It represents the product of the average intensity of the contractions in millimeters of mercury, the frequency of contractions per 10 minutes, and the average duration of the contractions in minutes (intensity × frequency × duration).

Uterine contractions occur spontaneously in patterns that are characteristic of individuals and of various stages of gestation. The frequency, duration, and strength of the myometrial contractions can be estimated by palpation (feeling them with a hand placed on the mother's abdomen), or by electronic techniques. The latter use either a noninvasive external tocodynamometer that consists of a pressure sensor held in place on the abdomen over a prominent part of the uterus or by an internal method using an intrauterine pressure catheter placed through the cervix into the uterine cavity (IUPC). The latter is the most accurate technique of monitoring uterine contractions.

The recorded curve of a normal uterine contraction is bell shaped. The steep crescentic slope leading to the apex of the curve represents the actual power of the contraction and comprises only one-third of the total contraction. The period of relaxation makes up two-thirds of the process and is shown by a curve that is, initially, a steep decrescentic slope that becomes more horizontal in the last third, reflecting the gradualness of the final stage of relaxation.

FIRST STAGE OF LABOR

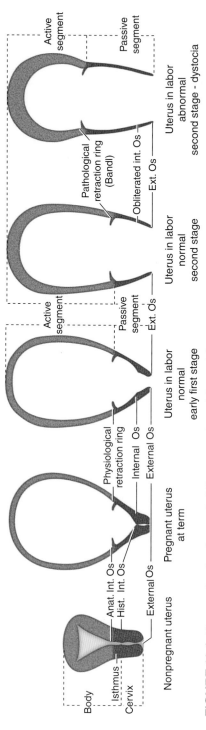

FIGURE 11-1. Progressive development of the segments and rings of the uterus at term. Note the comparison between the nonpregnant uterus, uterus at term, and uterus in labor. The passive segment is derived from the lower uterine segment (isthmus) and cervix; the physiologic retraction ring forms the anatomic internal os. The pathologic ring that forms under abnormal conditions develops from the physiologic ring. (Reproduced with permission from Pritchard, MacDonald and Gant. Williams Obstetrics, 17th ed. McGraw-Hill: Appleton-Century-Crofts; 1985.)

Caldeyro-Barcia has published a logical and understandable description of the normal uterine contraction wave.

Triple Descending Gradient of Caldeyro-Barcia

Each contraction wave has three components:

1. *The propagation* of the wave is from above downward. It starts at the pacemaker and works its way to the lower part of the uterus
2. *The duration* of the contraction diminishes progressively as the wave moves away from the pacemaker. During any contraction, the upper portion of the uterus is in action for a longer period of time than the lower
3. *The intensity* of the contraction diminishes from the top to the bottom of the uterus. The upper segment of the uterus contracts more strongly than the lower

For normal labor to take place, all parts of the triple descending gradient must perform in a coordinated fashion. The activity of the upper part dominates and is greater than that of the lower part. All parts of the uterus contract, but the upper segment does so more strongly than the lower segment; in turn, the latter's contractions are stronger than those of the cervix. Were this not so, there would be no progress.

The normal contractions are regular and intermittent. There is contraction (systole) and relaxation (diastole). The most efficient uterus is one showing moderately low tonus and strong contractions.

Pacemakers

Normally, there are two, one situated at each uterine end of the fallopian tube. Since one pacemaker is responsible for initiation of a contraction, their activities must be coordinated. In the abnormal uterus, new pacemakers may spring up anywhere in the organ, resulting in incoordinate uterine action.

Propagation

The wave begins at the pacemaker and proceeds downward to the rest of the uterus. A small wave goes up to the fundal portion of the uterus above the level of the pacemaker.

FIRST STAGE OF LABOR

Coordination

Coordination is such that, while the wave begins earlier in some areas than in others, the contraction attains its maximum in the different parts of the uterus at the same time. The places where the contraction starts later achieve their acme more rapidly. Thus, at the peak of the contraction, the entire uterus is acting as a unit. Relaxation, on the other hand, starts simultaneously in all parts of the uterus. For normal uterine action, there must be good coordination between the two halves of the uterus as well as between the upper and lower segments.

Dilatation of the Cervix

Dilatation of the cervix is caused by two mechanisms:

1. The pressure on the cervix by the presenting part: When this part of the fetus is regular and well fitting (e.g., the flexed head), it favors effective uterine action and smooth cervical dilatation. The intact amnion does not play an important role in helping promote effective contractions and rapid cervical opening
2. The longitudinal traction on the cervix by the upper part of the uterus as it contracts and retracts: After each contraction, the upper segment becomes shorter and thicker; the lower uterine segment becomes longer, thinner, and more distended; and the cervix becomes more and more dilated

Cervical dilatation is the result of a gradient of diminishing activity from the fundus through the lower uterine segment.

Round Ligament Contraction

These ligaments contain muscle, and they contract at the same time as the upper segment of the uterus. This anchors the uterus, prevents its ascending in the abdomen, and so helps force down the presenting part.

Uterine Contractions During Pregnancy

Some uterine activity goes on throughout pregnancy. During the first 30 weeks, the frequency and strength of the contractions are low, less than 20 Montevideo units.

After 30 weeks and especially after 35 weeks, the uterine activity become more frequent and may be noticed by the patient. Braxton Hicks contractions can be defined as myometrial activity that is variable in intensity, duration, and frequency that do not lead to cervical change. They may be uncomfortable but are not typically described as painful. Prelabor, as evidenced in the increasing activity of the uterus during the later weeks of pregnancy, is an integral part of the process of evacuating the human uterus. The contractions of this period are associated with steadily increasing uterine activity, cervical ripening, and general readiness for true labor. Prelabor merges into clinically recognizable labor by such small degrees that the exact point at which so-called true labor begins is difficult to determine.

PAIN OF LABOR

Pain during labor is related to contractions of the uterus. In normal labor, the pain is intermittent. It starts as the uterus contracts, becomes more severe as the contraction reaches its peak, and disappears when the uterus relaxes. The degree of pain varies in different patients, in the same patient during succeeding labors, and at different stages in the same labor. In some cases, the contractions are painless.

Causes

1. Distention of the lower pole of the uterus
2. Stretching of the ligaments adjacent to the uterus
3. Pressure on or stretching of the nerve ganglia around the uterus
4. Contractions of the muscle while it is in a relatively ischemic state (similar to angina pectoris). This occurs especially when the uterine tonus is too high or when the contractions are too frequent and last too long. Adequate amounts of blood do not get to the muscles, and they become hypoxic

Pain in the Lower Abdomen
Pain in the lower abdomen seems to be related to activity in the upper uterine segment and is present during efficient labor.

Pain in the Back
Pain in the back is related to tension in the lower uterus segment and the cervix. In normal labor, back pain is prominent only at the start of a contraction and in the early stages of cervical dilatation. When the cervix is abnormally resistant, the backache is severe. Backache is prominent also

in occiput posterior positions. In general, the less the backache, the more efficient the uterus function.

Pain in the Incoordinate Uterus

1. An excessive amount of pain is felt in the back
2. Because of persistent high tonus or spasm in some parts of the uterus, the pain seems to be present even in the intervals between contractions
3. The patient complains of pain before the uterus is felt to contract, and the pain persists even after the uterus relaxes

TRUE AND FALSE LABOR

Signs of True Labor

1. Uterine contractions occur at regular intervals. Coming every 20 or 30 minutes at the beginning, the contractions increase in frequency and occur every 3 to 5 minutes in the active phase. As labor proceeds, the contractions increase in duration and severity
2. The uterine systoles are painful
3. Hardening of the uterus is palpable
4. Pain is felt both in the back and in the front of the abdomen
5. True labor is effective in shortening and dilating the cervix
6. The presenting part descends
7. Bulging of the membranes is a frequent result

False Labor Pains

False labor pains are inefficient contractions of the uterus that usually last only a few seconds. They appear a few days to 1 month before term. Usually they start on their own. They are irregular and short and are felt more in the front than in the back. The uterus does not become stony hard and can be indented with the finger. These contractions are inefficient in pushing down the presenting part and do not bring about progressive efface-ment and dilatation of the cervix.

False labor pains can have the harmful effect of tiring the patient, so that when true labor does begin, she is in poor condition, both mentally and physically. Management is directed to the cause if there is one, or the physician can prescribe efficient analgesia that stops the false labor pains but does not interfere with true labor. It is also important to ensure that the patient has adequate hydration and rest.

TRUE LABOR	FALSE LABOR
Pains at regular intervals	Irregular
Intervals gradually shorten	No change and inconsistent
Duration and severity increase	No change and inconsistent
Pain starts in back and moves to front	Pain mainly in front
Walking increases the intensity	No change
Association between the degree of uterine hardening and intensity of pain	No relationship
Bloody show often present	No show
Cervix effaced and dilated	No change in cervix
Descent of presenting part	No descent
Head is fixed between pains	Head remains free

FIRST STAGE OF LABOR

The strength of the uterine contractions can be estimated clinically by using the criteria shown in Table 11-1.

STAGES OF LABOR

First Stage. From the onset of true labor to complete dilatation of the cervix. It is defined as regular painful uterine contractions resulting in progressive cervical change, and includes the latent and active phases.

TABLE 11-1: STRENGTH OF UTERINE CONTRACTIONS

	Frequency	Duration	Indentibility of Uterus
Good	Every 2-3 min	45-60 sec	None
Fair	Every 4-5 min	30-45 sec	Slight
Poor	Every 6+ min	<30 sec	Easy

Second Stage. From complete dilatation of the cervix to the birth of the baby. It may include passive and active stages.

Third Stage. From the birth of the baby to delivery of the placenta.

Fourth Stage. From the birth of the placenta to 1 hour postpartum.

First Stage of Labor

The first stage of labor lasts from the onset of regular painful contractions that effect cervical change, to full dilatation of the cervix. The contractions are intermittent and painful, and the uterine hardening is felt easily by a hand on the abdomen. The pains become more frequent and more severe as labor proceeds. As a rule, they begin in the back and pass to the front of the abdomen and the upper thighs.

Effacement and Dilatation of the Cervix

During most of pregnancy, the cervix uteri is about 3.0 to 4.0 cm in length and closed. Toward the end of the third trimester, progressive changes occur in the cervix, including softening, effacement (shortening), dilatation, and movement from a posterior to an anterior position in the vagina. The internal os starts to disappear as the cervical canal becomes part of the lower segment of the uterus. The extent to which these changes have taken place correlates with the proximity of the onset of labor and with the success of attempts to induce labor.

Ideally, the cervix should be ripe at the onset of labor. A ripe cervix: (1) is soft, (2) is less than 1.3 cm in length or 80% effaced, (3) admits a finger easily, and (4) is dilatable. The presence of a ripe cervix is one indication that the uterus is ready to begin labor. During labor, the cervix shortens further, and the internal os dilates. When the cervix has been completely drawn into the lower uterine segment and is no longer palpable, it is described as being fully dilated. This is on average, 10 cm in width and permits the passage of the fetal head (Fig. 11-2).

Ripening of the cervix is a gradual process that merges into labor. The rigid collagen bundles rearrange themselves in a more flexible pattern so that the fibers are able to slide over each other more freely. During pregnancy, this process takes place gradually, resulting in softening, shortening, and partial dilatation of the cervix. These changes may begin as early as the 24th to 28th week of pregnancy. The mechanisms that control cervical ripening are not well understood, but they are linked with those that control parturition. Factors that play a part include Braxton Hicks contractions

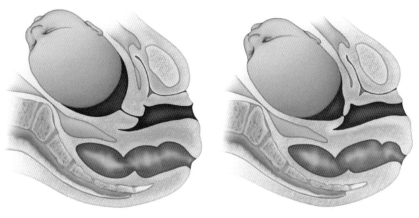

A. Cervix thick and closed.   B. Cervix effaced.

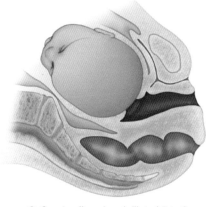

C. Cervix effaced and dilated 2 to 3 cm.

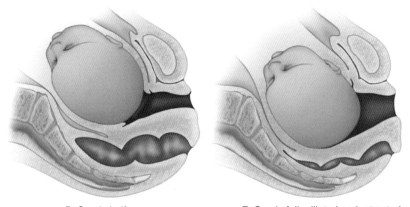

D. Cervix half open.   E. Cervix fully dilated and retracted.

FIGURE 11-2. **Dilatation of the cervix.**

FIRST STAGE OF LABOR

(usually painless) of the uterus pulling on the cervix and hormones such as estrogen, progesterone, relaxin, oxytocin, and prostaglandin.

The changes in the cervix during pregnancy can be correlated to the time of onset of labor. Women whose cervices ripen early are likely to begin labor before 40 weeks. When the cervix remains unripe until late in pregnancy, prolongation of the gestation past 40 weeks, is common.

Phases of the First Stage of Labor

The Latent Phase. The onset of the latent phase of the first stage of labor is difficult to accurately define because it begins when the patient first perceives strong, regular uterine contractions. The rate of cervical change is slow and gradual during this phase (Fig. 11-3). However, the contractions are becoming coordinated, stronger, polarized, and more efficient. At the same time, the cervix is becoming softer, pliable, and more elastic (Table 11-2). These averages can vary based on a patient's body mass index as described in updated clinical guidelines. Patients who enter labor with a ripe cervix have a shorter latent phase than those whose cervix is unripe.

The Active Phase. The diagnosis of the onset of the active phase requires an assessment of both uterine contractions and cervical changes. The dilatation of the cervix usually has reached 4 cm for nulliparas and 4 to 5 cm for multiparas and the effacement is 1 cm or less. The assessment of the cervix should also include station, consistency, and position. Although there may be no great change in the uterine contractions, the cervix has undergone important alterations that make it more responsive, and cervical dilatation proceeds more rapidly at this time.

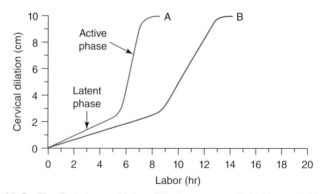

FIGURE 11-3. The first stage of labor: Friedman curve. A. Multipara. **B.** Nullipara.

TABLE 11-2: LENGTHS OF THE PHASES OF LABOR

	Nulliparas		Multiparas	
	Average	Upper Normal	Average	Upper Normal
Latent phase	8.6 hr	20 hr	5.3 hr	14 hr
Active phase	5.8 hr	12 hr	2.5 hr	6 hr
First stage of labor	13.3 hr	28.5 hr	7.5 hr	20 hr
Second stage labor	57 min	2.5 hr	18 min	50 min
Rate of cervical dilatation during active phase	1.2 cm/hr	0.5 cm/hr	1.5 cm/hr	0.8 cm/hr

The mean and upper limits of the duration of the different stages of labor were established by Friedman in the early 1950s. More recent data suggest that the upper limit of a normal active phase may be longer and rate of cervical dilatation slower than those set by Friedman. In studies by Zhang et al., nulliparous women dilated at 0.5-0.7 cm/hr, while parous women dilated at 0.5-1.3 cm/hr. Only half of nulliparous women in the active phase of the first stage of labor dilated at a rate greater than 1.2 cm/hr. These and other studies suggest that labor progress in low-risk nulliparous women who enter labor spontaneously at a rate as slow as 0.5 cm/hr should be considered normal. *With the more frequent use of regional anesthesia and an older obstetric population with higher maternal body mass index, Friedman's time parameters should only be used as a guideline.*

Descent of the Presenting Part. During the latent and early active phase of cervical dilatation, fetal descent may be minimal. When the phase of rapid cervical dilatation has begun, steady fetal descent usually begins. The greatest degree of descent takes place when the cervix nears full dilatation and in the second stage of labor. When descent begins, it should be progressive. Descent of less than 1 cm/hr in nulliparas and 2 cm/hr in multiparas is abnormal, and investigation is indicated (see Chapter 16).

Bag of Waters: Amniotic Membranes

The fetus lies in a sac with an inner layer of amnion and an outer covering of chorion. The sac is filled with the amniotic fluid. As labor proceeds and the internal os becomes effaced and opens, the membranes separate from the lower uterine segment. The lower pole of the membranes bulges a little with each contraction and may adopt various shapes:

1. The protruding part may have the shape of a watch glass (Fig. 11-4A) containing a small amount of amniotic fluid. This is called the forewaters
2. In other cases, the membranes point into the cervix like a cone (Fig. 11-4B)

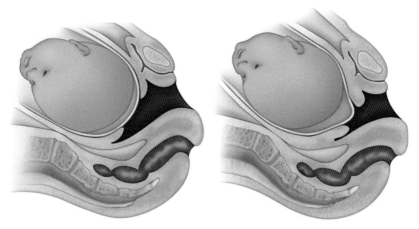

A. Forewaters: watchglass shape.   B. Forewaters: cone into the cervix.

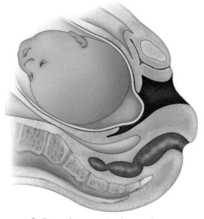
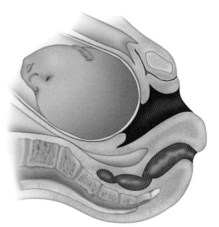

C. Bag of waters in the vagina.   D. No forewaters.

FIGURE 11-4. The membranes.

3. **The amnion may prolapse** into the vagina (Fig. 11-4C)
4. In some cases, the membranes are applied so tightly to the fetal head that no bag forms (Fig. 11-4D)

Frequently, the membranes rupture near the end of the second stage, but this event can take place at any time during or before labor. When the membranes rupture, the fluid may come away with a gush or an ongoing dribble. On occasion, it is difficult to know whether the membranes are ruptured or intact. Methods of determining whether the bag of waters has ruptured include:

1. Observation of the escape of fluid from the vagina spontaneously or as a result of manual pressure on the fundus of the uterus or simple Valsalva maneuvers
2. A sterile speculum in the vagina and directly observing amniotic fluid coming out from the cervical canal is the best method for confirming membrane rupture. The amount may be increased by pressure on the fundus of the uterus or by Valsalva maneuvers
3. The passage of meconium
4. Use of Nitrazine paper to determine the pH of the vaginal fluid. The vagina, normally acidic, becomes neutral or alkaline when contaminated with alkaline amniotic fluid. Hence, an alkaline pH in the vagina suggests that the membranes are ruptured
5. The arborization test depends on the property of dried amniotic fluid to form crystals in an arborization pattern. A few drops of vaginal fluid are obtained from the vagina and placed on a clean, dry glass slide. After waiting 5-7 minutes for drying to take place, the slide is examined under a low-power microscope for identification of the arborization (or ferning) pattern
6. The AmniSure test is a commercially available kit that detects trace amounts of placental alpha macroglobulin-1 protein in vaginal fluid with high sensitivity and specificity for membrane rupture. It is a relatively expensive test but may aid in diagnosing membrane rupture in difficult cases
7. Obstetrical ultrasound to assess for amniotic fluid volume may be used in preterm patients with inconclusive tests

After the membranes have ruptured (spontaneously or artificially), the uterine contractions are more efficient, and labor may progress faster. Routine amniotomy, however, does not accelerate spontaneous labor.

FIRST STAGE OF LABOR

A Cochrane Review compared amniotomy in the first stage to no amniotomy in over 5000 spontaneous labors and found no difference in outcomes. Also, routine amniotomy may result in more frequent variable decelerations of the fetal heart rate. Amniotomy should be avoided in women with known vasa previa, active genital herpes simplex, or an untreated HIV infection.

Indications for amniotomy include:

1. Atypical or abnormal fetal heart rate
2. To detect the presence of meconium
3. To facilitate the use of an internal scalp electrode or an internal intrauterine pressure catheter
4. To induce or augment labor

Several conditions should be present before amniotomy is performed to improve likelihood of a normal vaginal birth:

1. Labor is in progress, as indicated by presence of regular uterine contractions and observed changes in the cervix
2. The cervix is at least 3 cm dilated and effaced
3. The head is fixed in the pelvis and applied to the cervix
4. The patient does not have active genital herpes simplex virus infection or have a high HIV viral load

Passage of Meconium in Cephalic Presentations

The passage per vagina of meconium or meconium-stained amniotic fluid when the fetal presentation is cephalic may be a sign of concern. It is believed to result from relaxation of the rectal sphincter and increased peristalsis. This may be occurring as a consequence of fetal hypoxia. However, the passage of meconium may represent nothing more than fetal maturity. In most cases, no cause is found.

The incidence of meconium staining is around 5 percent. The occurrence of stillbirth when this is the only sign is very low, but the number of newborns requiring resuscitation is higher than the overall incidence.

When meconium is passed, the fetal heart must be observed closely, preferably by continuous external fetal monitoring. Should there be a significant alteration in the rate and rhythm of the fetal heart, (abnormal fetal heart tracing), immediate delivery may be needed. However, operative delivery is not indicated on the basis of meconium staining alone.

In breech presentations, the passage of meconium is caused by pressure of the uterine contractions on the fetal intestines and is not considered a sign of fetal hypoxia.

Management of the First Stage of Labor

1. As long as the patient is healthy, the presentation normal, the presenting part engaged, and the fetus in a reassuring condition, the parturient may walk about, sit in a chair, shower or bathe in a tub, or may be in bed, as she wishes. Women who are ambulatory, have frequent positional changes, and adopt a more upright position (e.g., sitting, standing, kneeling, squatting) have a shorter first stage of labor. There is also less need for analgesia and for augmentation of labor with oxytocin in women who are ambulatory during labor compared with those who remain in bed. Women should be encouraged to ambulate and to adopt whatever position they find most comfortable throughout labor

2. Continuous close supportive care should be given to the laboring patient. Appropriate support during labor may reduce the need for analgesia and decrease the rate of operative delivery. The patient should receive continual reassurance, frequent encouragement, and judicious use of analgesia

3. Breathing and relaxation techniques to help the patient cope with pain in labor should be encouraged. Such relaxation helps the patient rest, assists her in keeping control, and accelerates the progress of labor. Women reporting excessive pain or anxiety release high levels of endogenous catecholamines, which may adversely affect uterine blood flow and labor progress. Laboring in water is recommended for pain relief. When the pains are severe, inhalational, intramuscular, intravenous, or regional analgesia may be given, depending on the progress of labor and maternal and fetal well-being. Since there is a limit to the amount of opioids that can be administered without affecting the baby or interfering with labor, these must be given in logical dosage and sequence (see Chapter 36)

4. During the first stage, the patient is impressed continually with the importance of relaxing with the contractions. Bearing down must be avoided because it does not improve progress. Bearing down is needed when the cervix is fully dilated and not before. During the first stage, it may result in negative effects including:
   a. It delays cervical dilatation and can make the cervix edematous
   b. It tires the patient needlessly
   c. It forces down the uterus and stretches the supporting ligaments, predisposing to later prolapse

5. Adequate amounts of fluid and nourishment are essential. In most normal labors, isotonic drinks or clear soups can be taken by mouth. A light diet may be given in established labor. However, since solid

FIRST STAGE OF LABOR

foods remain in the stomach during labor, tend to be vomited, and increase the danger of aspiration pneumonitis, they should be avoided if the risk of a general anesthetic is high. If the patient is unable to take enough fluids orally, an intravenous infusion of crystalloid solution is given

6. Although an intravenous crystalloid infusion should not be used routinely in normal labor, a saline lock or intravenous fluids can be considered for the following reasons:

   a. Fluids and nourishment can be given without provoking emesis. A woman who cannot take adequate fluids by mouth or who is nauseated or vomiting can be maintained in a state of good hydration

   b. Analgesics in small amounts can be administered for rapid effect. Fluid preloading is also recommended if regional anesthesia is to be used to avoid hypotension

   c. When uterine action is inefficient, oxytocin added to the intravenous solution improves labor

   d. When there is excessive bleeding in the third or fourth stages, oxytocic agents can be given quickly

   e. Blood and plasma expanders may be infused without delay

   f. When hypotension has occurred, the veins often collapse, and it is difficult to insert a needle. Having an infusion already underway obviates this problem

7. The patient's condition and progress is checked periodically. The pulse, temperature, and blood pressure are measured every 4 hours or more often if necessary

8. The fetal heart should be auscultated for a minimum of 1 minute every 15-30 minutes in the active phase of the first stage of labor and every 5-10 minutes in the active second stage of labor. These should be done immediately after a contraction. If the fetal heart is abnormal by auscultation, continuous electronic fetal monitoring should be considered (see Chapter 12)

9. The progress of labor is followed by abdominal and vaginal examination to note the position of the baby, station of the presenting part, and dilatation of the cervix. A partogram should be started when a patient enters the active phase of labor. Vaginal examinations should be done at 1-4 hourly intervals and should be done only often enough to ensure safe conduct of labor

10. Artificial rupture of membranes (amniotomy). Amniotomy is an intervention and it does not accelerate spontaneous labor. It may cause harm when performed without an indication

a. Advantages of amniotomy:
   i. It enables the condition of the amniotic fluid to be observed, especially the presence or absence of meconium
   ii. When continuous fetal heart rate monitoring is indicated, the electrode can be placed directly on the fetal scalp, providing a better tracing than is obtained by an electrode on the mother's abdomen
   iii. An IUPC can be placed inside the uterus and can measure intrauterine pressure directly and accurately
   iv. It may shorten the duration of labor when performed in the setting of dysfunctional labor. It is believed that the better application of the fetal head to the cervix improves the pattern of dilatation and that direct pressure on the cervix leads to improved uterine contractions by reflex action
b. Disadvantages of amniotomy:
   i. The reduction in the amount of amniotic fluid may increase compression of the umbilical cord and result in transient reduced blood flow to the fetus and abnormal fetal heart rate patterns
   ii. There may be a slight increase in the risk of cesarean section
   iii. There may be a risk of umbilical cord prolapse if performed when the presenting part is not well applied against the cervix or in cases of unstable lie of the fetus
11. Proper hygiene measures should be implemented when caring for women in labor. Standard hand hygiene practices and single use non-sterile gloves are appropriate to reduce cross-contamination among women, babies, and health care professionals
12. Enemas should not be routinely given to the patient when she is admitted to the labor ward. Studies have shown that giving an enema made no difference in labor progress or in the incidence of fecal contamination. Many women object to having an enema
13. Over distention of the bladder is obviated by urging the patient to pass urine every few hours. Occasionally, catheterization may be necessary if epidural analgesia is in place. The distensible part of the bladder is largely abdominal during the active phase of labor, and it is rare for a full bladder to interfere with progress in a normal case. Since catheterization does not improve the progress of labor and does increase the risk of infection, it should be carried out only when absolutely necessary

FIRST STAGE OF LABOR

Second Stage of Labor

The second stage of labor lasts from the end of the first stage, when the cervix has reached full dilatation, to the birth of the baby. As the patient passes through the end of the first stage and into the second stage, the contractions become more frequent and are accompanied by some of the most intense pain of the whole labor. After the second stage has been achieved, the discomfort is less (see Chapter 16). Pushing in the second stage may start at full dilatation with an engaged presenting part, or when there is an urge to push. Delay pushing for 1-2 hours if there is a lack of urge or a high (above +2), presenting part and reassuring maternal and fetal status. The maternal position and method of pushing (spontaneous or directed with Valsalva), should follow the women's preference. The duration of the second stage (passive vs. active), and recommendations for the duration of pushing lack evidence. Hourly assessments of progress are recommended. Consider intervention after 3-4 hours depending on progress, parity, fetal status, and presence of epidural (Table 11-3).

Third Stage of Labor

Delivery of the placenta occurs in two stages: (1) separation of the placenta from the wall of the uterus and into the lower uterine segment and/or the vagina and (2) actual expulsion of the placenta out of the birth canal (see Chapter 19).

Fourth Stage of Labor

The patient is kept in the delivery suite for 1 hour postpartum under close observation. She is checked for bleeding, and her vital signs are monitored. The third stage and the hour after delivery have the greatest risk for postpartum hemorrhage.

Before the doctor leaves the patient, he or she must do the following:

1. Feel the uterus through the abdomen to be sure it is firm and not filling with blood
2. Look at the perineum and vagina to see that any lacerations have been repaired adequately and that there is no hemorrhage
3. **Assess** the mother's vital signs and ensure she is stable
4. Examine the baby to be certain that he or she is breathing well and that the color and tone are normal

TABLE 11-3: RECOMMENDATIONS IN SECOND STAGE OF LABOR BY PARITY AND USE OF EPIDURAL ANALGESIA (AFTER FULL CERVICAL DILATATION AND WITH ADEQUATE POWER)

	Nulliparous		Parous	
	No epidural	**Epidural**	**No epidural**	**Epidural**
Total duration	3 hours	4 hours	2 hours	3 hours
Passive second stage	May wait up to 2 hours prior to pushing, especially if presenting part is above +2 station, non-occiput anterior position, or no urge to push. Encourage passive descent.		Can wait up to 1 hour.	Can wait up to 2 hours before pushing, in the setting of passive descent.
Commence pushing	In presence of urge to push and not able to allow passive descent or after 2 hours of passive second stage.		In presence of urge to push or after 2 hours of passive second stage.	
Assessment	Every hour for position and descent. Reassess indication for assisted birth after 2 hours of active pushing.			

Adapted from Lee L, Dy J, Azzam H: Management of spontaneous labour at term in healthy women. J Obstet Gynaecol Can 38:9, 2016

SELECTED READING

Atwood RJ: Parturitional posture and related birth behaviour. Acta Obstet Gynecol Scand (Suppl) 57, 1976

Challis JRG, Mitchell BF: Hormonal control of preterm and term parturition. Semin Perinatal 5:192, 1981

Drover JW, Casper RF: Initiation of parturition in humans. Can Med Assoc J 128:387, 1983

Kenepp NB, Kumar S, Shelley WC, et al: Fetal and neonatal hazards of maternal hydration with 5% dextrose before cesarean section. Lancet 1:1150, 1982

Kerr-Wilson RH, Parham GP, Orr JW Jr: The effect of a full bladder on labor. Obstet Gynecol 62:319, 1983

Lee L, Dy J, Azzam H. Management of spontaneous labour at term in healthy women. J Obstet Gynaecol Can 38:843-865, 2016. https://doi.org/10.1016/j.jogc.2016.04.093

Mendiola J, Grylack LJ, Scanlon JW: Effects of intrapartum maternal glucose infusion on the normal fetus and newborn. Anesth Analg 6:32, 1982

Neal JL, Lowe NK, et al: "Active labor" duration and dilation rates among low risk, nulliparous women with spontaneous labor onset: A systematic review. J Midwifery Womens Health 55:308-318, 2010.

Shepherd JH, Knuppel RA: The role of prostaglandins in ripening the cervix and inducing labor. Clin Perinatol 8:49, 1981

FIRST STAGE OF LABOR

Smyth RM, Markham C, Dowswell T: Amniotomy for shortening spontaneous labour. Cochrane Database Syst Rev 18:6, 2013

Stewart P, Kennedy JH, Calder AA: Spontaneous labour: When should the membranes be ruptured? Br J Obstet Gynaecol 89:39, 1982

Tita AT, Rouse DJ: Progesterone for preterm birth prevention: an evolving intervention. Am J Obstet Gynecol 200:219, 2009

Smyth RM, Alldred SK, Markham C: Amniotomy for shortening spontaneous labour. Cochrane Database Syst Rev 4:CD006167, 2007

Zhang J, Landy HJ, Branch DW, et al: Contemporary patterns of spontaneous labor with normal neonatal outcomes. Obstet Gynecol 116:1281, 2010

Zhang J, Troendle JF, Yancey MK: Reassessing the labor curve in nulliparous women. Am J Obstet Gynecol 187:4, 2002

CHAPTER 12

Fetal Health Surveillance in Labor

Susan L. Aubin
Darine El-Chaâr

INDICATIONS FOR FETAL ASSESSMENT

There are numerous clinical situations in which it is important to ascertain both the maturity and the health of the fetus while it is still in utero. Among these are the following:

During Pregnancy

Patients at Risk for Uteroplacental Insufficiency

1. Diabetes mellitus
2. Hypertension and preeclampsia
3. Renal disease
4. Previous stillbirth
5. Intrauterine growth restriction, suspected
6. Postterm pregnancy (over 42 weeks)
7. Isoimmunization
8. Preterm premature rupture of membranes
9. Multiple gestation
10. History of placental abruption
11. Chronic abruption
12. Maternal obesity
13. Abnormal maternal serum screening in the absence of fetal anomaly
14. Oligohydramnios or polyhydramnios

Obstetric Reasons

1. Previous cesarean section
2. When induction of labor is necessary
   a. In the interests of the mother
   b. In the interests of the fetus

During Labor

Obstetric Reasons

1. Clinically detected abnormalities of the fetal heart rate (FHR)
2. Passage of meconium

3. Oxytocin stimulation of labor
4. Preterm labor
5. Slow progress in labor
6. Abnormal presentation

DETERMINATION OF FETAL HEALTH: ANTEPARTUM

In North America, antenatal and intrapartum deaths are rare. The reduction in the perinatal mortality rate has been achieved largely by the decrease in the rate of neonatal death. The prevention of fetal death represents a major therapeutic goal, and is the reason for antepartum fetal surveillance.

Biochemical assessment of the fetus has largely been replaced by biophysical and biometric evaluation. Fetal biophysical activities are initiated, modulated, and regulated by mechanisms of the central nervous system (CNS). A fetus compromised by hypoxia demonstrates one or both of the following changes:

1. A decrease or cessation of biophysical activity
2. A significant reduction in the volume of amniotic fluid that becomes evident as oligohydramnios on sonography

The fetal CNS is exquisitely sensitive to changes in PO_2. Hypoxia and its resultant metabolic acidosis produce pathologic CNS depression with changes in biophysical activity. Any biophysical response, however, has its own inherent periodicity and circadian (diurnal) rhythm. Hence, the absence of a given biophysical event may reflect physiologic periodicity, and a normal "sleep state" in a fetus must be differentiated from the comatose state of hypoxic CNS depression.

The important principle in antepartum testing, regardless of the method used, is that a normal test result is reliable in indicating present fetal well-being and is an accurate predictor of a good outcome. However, the diagnosis of fetal jeopardy, based on a single absent or abnormal biophysical event, is frequently inaccurate. Hence, in any scheme of antepartum testing, the goal must be to reduce and, if possible, eliminate the incidence of falsely positive results. This is achieved by increasing the period of observation for any single biophysical event and/or using multiple observations. The demonstration of several biophysical activities showing a normal pattern collectively negates a single abnormal result.

Fetal Movement

Fetal movement, first perceived by the mother at 16 to 20 weeks' gestation, may be recorded subjectively or objectively using active or passive techniques. Fetal movements are not random phenomena. Rather, they are regulated and modulated by complex CNS mechanisms and reflexes. They occur in cyclic periods or in epochs associated and integrated with respiratory, cardiac, behavioral, and "sleep" cycles. The acceleration of the FHR, which occurs after certain fetal movements, provides the basis of the nonstress test (NST). Movements lasting more than 3 seconds elicit FHR accelerations 99.8 percent of the time. Movements of lesser duration rarely do so.

It is well established that reduced fetal activity may be a good predictor of fetal compromise. Decreased placental perfusion and fetal acidosis are associated with decreased fetal movements. The significance of fetal movement counting should be discussed with all healthy pregnant women to be aware of in the third trimester. It is the only antenatal surveillance technique recommended for all pregnant women regardless of the presence or absence of risk factors. There is no evidence that fetal movement counting increases maternal stress or anxiety.

In pregnancies at increased risk for adverse perinatal outcome, daily fetal movement monitoring should be initiated from 26 to 32 weeks. In healthy pregnancies with no risk factors, fetal movement counting becomes more important in the third trimester. In these low-risk pregnancies, fetal movement count should be initiated when the woman perceives decreased movements.

Counting Methods

1. The "count to 10" method: In this simple method, the patient counts fetal movements starting at 9 AM. After 10 movements are perceived, the counting comes to an end. This routine is carried on daily, and the patient is asked to alert her physician if:
   a. Fewer than 10 movements occur after 12 hours on 2 successive days or
   b. No movements are perceived after 12 hours in a single day. In such a situation, an NST should be performed

   In most pregnancies, 10 movements are perceived within 1 hour of counting

2. Modified protocol: Counting until 6 movements are noted in 2 hours. This is more convenient for women to do daily. If the 6 movements are

not reached in a period of 2 hours, the woman should seek medical attention for further antenatal testing.

Fetal activity may be decreased in late pregnancy but only slightly in a normal fetus. The possible reasons for the reduction in fetal movement at this time include decreasing amounts of amniotic fluid and the larger fetus having less room to move in the uterus. It could also be related to sleep states, which are thought to occur for longer periods in mature fetuses. Finally, sedatives and drugs that produce autonomic blockade reduce fetal activity.

Nonstress Test

This test is performed in patients who are not in labor. It uses the observation that the occurrence of accelerations of the FHR in response to fetal movement or a uterine contraction is a reliable indicator of current healthy fetal well-being.

Advantages

1. There are no contraindications and no complications
2. The test is simple, inexpensive, and takes less time than a contraction stress test or a biophysical profile
3. It can be used in an office setting and provides immediate information
4. Performance of the test requires no special expertise

Indications

1. Patients at risk for uteroplacental insufficiency (see previous section of this chapter)
2. The absence of normal fetal movements

Instrumentation and Technique

1. An FHR tracing is obtained using a cardiotocograph for at least 20 minutes
2. The recording is obtained with the patient in the lateral recumbent position or with a lateral tilt to avoid supine hypotension. The uterus should be relaxed, and it is recommended that the woman have an empty bladder before testing

FIRST STAGE OF LABOR

Frequency of Testing

1. Weekly testing is indicated and adequate in most conditions
2. The test must be repeated immediately if any change in the clinical condition of the mother or fetus occurs
3. Certain conditions may require twice-weekly testing:
   a. Maternal diabetes
   b. Postterm pregnancy
   c. Fetal growth retardation with oligohydramnios
   d. Maternal hypertension requiring medications

Timing of Testing

In most patients, testing is instituted at 32 to 34 weeks of gestation. In selected cases, such as poor past obstetric performance or specific high-risk condition in the current pregnancy, testing may begin at 26 to 28 weeks. At this time, many fetuses may show atypical or abnormal (previously called *nonreactive*) patterns because of immaturity and the significance of the test is questionable. However, the finding of a normal (previously called *reactive*) pattern in early gestation has a reassuring value.

Classification

1. Normal NST result
   a. The presence of two or more accelerations of the FHR in a 20-minute period of observation (Fig. 12-1)
      i. Each acceleration with fetal movement must be of amplitude more than 15 beats per minute (bpm) and of duration more than 15 seconds
   b. The baseline FHR
      i. Is within the normal range of 110 to 160 bpm
   c. There is moderate FHR variability of 6 to 26 bpm
   d. There are no periodic decelerations. An occasional uncomplicated variable less than 30 seconds in duration is acceptable
2. Atypical NST result
   a. Fewer than two accelerations meeting criteria have occurred in 40 to 80 minutes
   b. The occurrence of variable decelerations lasting 30 to 60 seconds in duration

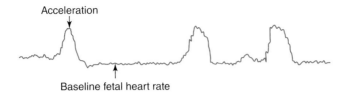

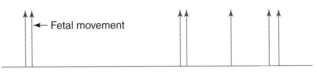

FIGURE 12-1. Normal nonstress test. Showing accelerations of fetal heart rate with fetal movement. Amplitude more than 15 bpm, duration longer than 15 seconds.

FIRST STAGE OF LABOR

   c. The baseline FHR:
      i. Is within 100 to 110 bpm
      ii. Is over 160 bpm for <30 minutes
      iii. Has a rising baseline
   d. There is absent or minimal FHR variability of 5 bpm or less for 40 to 80 minutes
3. Abnormal NST result
   a. Fewer than two accelerations meeting criteria have occurred in >80 minutes
   b. The occurrence of variable decelerations lasting >60 seconds in duration or the occurrence of late deceleration(s)
   c. The baseline FHR
      i. Bradycardia <100 bpm
      ii. Tachycardia >160 bpm for >30 minutes
      iii. Erratic baseline
   d. There is absent or minimal FHR variability ≤5 bpm for >80 minutes. There is high fetal heart variability (>25 bpm) >10 minutes or a sinusoidal FHR pattern

Significance of the Nonstress Test

1. Normal NST result: The normal (reactive) NST result is a reliable indicator of current fetal health. The risk of fetal death within 1 week of a reactive pattern is only 3.2 per 1000. Hence, the test is highly sensitive, with a false negative rate (normal test, abnormal fetus) of less than 0.5 percent

2. Atypical NST result: An atypical pattern may be caused by the following:
   a. Hypoxia
   b. Effects of drugs
      i. Sedative or tranquilizing agents
      ii. Parasympatholytic drugs (e.g., atropine)
      iii. Sympatholytic drugs (beta-blockers)
   c. Fetal immaturity
   d. Fetal sleep cycle

In contrast to the reliability of the normal NST, the false-positive (abnormal test, normal fetus) rate of an atypical NST is high. This is, almost certainly, a reflection of the normal periodicity of the function of the fetal CNS. Hence, an atypical NST result, defined as above, requires either prolonged observation or repeated testing. The primary care provider should be made aware of this to initiate further assessment as needed.

3. Abnormal NST result: This can be caused by the same reasons described above in atypical NST. This tracing requires urgent action, with an assessment of the situation, and further investigation by ultrasound or biophysical profile. This may also be an indication for immediate delivery.

Other Methods of Antenatal Fetal Assessment

In certain pregnancies with risk factors for adverse perinatal outcomes, further antenatal assessment of fetal well-being may be indicated. Where facilities and expertise exist, this may include measurement of the biophysical profile, uterine artery Doppler, and umbilical artery and fetal CNS artery Doppler through ultrasonography (see Chapter 37).

Assessment of Uterine Activity

The activity of the uterus (UA) is assessed to classify FHR patterns and identify contraction patterns that may adversely affect the fetus. Components of UA assessment include contraction frequency, duration, intensity, and resting tone. Contraction frequency is described over 10 minute intervals. The resting tone (soft or firm), and intensity (mild, moderate, or strong), are mainly assessed by palpation.

Methods

1. Maternal perception
2. Palpation
3. External: An external tocodynamometer (pressure transducer), placed on the abdominal wall
4. Internal: Intrauterine Pressure Catheter (IUPC): An IUPC, connected to a strain gauge transducer, is used to obtain and record direct pressure measurements in mm Hg

Indications for IUPC

1. Patients with a previous cesarean section undergoing a trial of labor. Sudden loss of uterine pressure may be the first sign of uterine rupture.
2. In obstructed labor, and with oxytocin augmentation, the strength of uterine contractions can be more accurately assessed.
3. Monitoring contractions in obese patients, when difficulty palpating or recording contractions externally is encountered.

Classification

1. Normal: frequency ≤5 contractions in 10 minutes, averaged over 30 minutes, duration <90 minutes, intensity palpated as mild, moderate or strong, or IUPC (25-75 mm Hg), and resting tone as soft to palpation or <25 mm Hg.
2. Tachysystole: frequency >5 contractions in 10 minutes, averaged over 30 minutes, duration >90 seconds, and <30 seconds of rest, or >25 mm Hg between contractions.

DETERMINATION OF FETAL HEALTH: INTRAPARTUM

The goal of intrapartum fetal health surveillance (FHS) is to assess fetal well-being and to intervene in a timely and effective manner to prevent perinatal morbidity/mortality. The FHR is modulated by reflex neurogenic mechanisms. A normal rate and variability of the FHR indicates an intact fetal CNS with normal cardiac responsiveness. Changes in the fetal PO_2 produce alterations in the CNS. Biochemical changes (metabolic acidosis),

FIRST STAGE OF LABOR

through their effect on the CNS, ultimately produce hemodynamic alterations including changes in the FHR.

The two modes of FHR assessment include intermittent auscultation (IA), and electronic fetal monitoring (EFM). Intrapartum FHS includes review of maternal and fetal risk factors, labor progress, uterine activity patterns, maternal heart rate (MHR), FHR characteristics and changes over time, as well as classification and interpretation of findings in light of the clinical situation. The recommended protocol for intrapartum FHS includes obtaining interpretable data, documenting the classification, interpretation, and communication of the data, as well as carrying out the appropriate response.

Intermittent Auscultation of the Fetal Heart (IA)

IA assessment includes palpating uterine activity, identifying FHR baseline, rhythm, accelerations, decelerations, and classifying as either Normal or Abnormal.

Intermittent auscultation of the fetal heart is performed with a hand-held device (fetoscope or Doppler). It is the recommended method of fetal surveillance in labor in term healthy women, without obstetric risk factors. It requires trained practitioners providing 1:1 care, be able to identify FHR sounds, and follow institutional protocols that guide the technique and interventions in a consistent manner. In the first stage of labor, the fetal heart is auscultated every 15 to 30 minutes for at least 30 to 60 seconds. In the second stage of labor, auscultation is performed every 5 minutes. Interpretation of IA requires understanding the relationship between changes in the FHR and the uterine contractions (Fig. 12-2).

Advantages of Intermittent Auscultation
This technique is inexpensive, less restrictive, more adaptable to labor positions, and has a lower intervention rate compared to EFM.

Disadvantages of Intermittent Auscultation

1. It cannot assess the type of deceleration and variable or prolonged decelerations may be missed
2. Baseline variability cannot be evaluated
3. There is no continuous record to allow for progressive analysis or retrospective evaluation
4. It may be difficult to auscultate FHR and palpate contractions in more obese patients

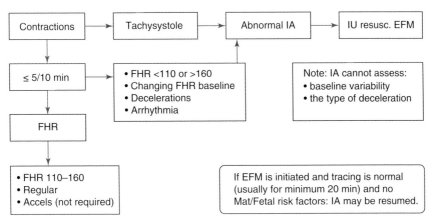

FIGURE 12-2. Intermittent auscultation classification. Accels, accelerations; EFM, electronic fetal monitoring; FHR, fetal heart rate; IA, intermittent auscultation; IU resusc., intrauterine resuscitation; Mat/Fetal, maternal–fetal.

Electronic Fetal Monitoring

All conventional FHR monitors provide a continuous record of the rate derived from serial calculations of the beat-to-beat heart rate in association with a time interval. This is then recorded on the FHR tracing in beats per minute. As the interval of each cardiac cycle changes with varying neurogenic input, the instantaneous heart rate changes constantly. This allows evaluation of intrinsic variability within the heart rate signal as well as the baseline rate.

The Role of Electronic Fetal Monitoring

Continuous FHR monitoring was developed to improve the predictive accuracy of intermittent auscultation. The clinical use of EFM is based on the assumption that there is metabolic evidence of asphyxia and hemodynamic change before permanent neurologic damage occurs. EFM during labor is a widely used and clinically accepted technique. As with most fetal assessment methods, the incidence of false-negative results is extremely low. Great care in the interpretation of abnormal tracings must be exercised, however, in order to reduce the incidence of false-positive results and subsequent increased interventions. Some institutions use fetal scalp pH assessments as an adjunct to EFM.

Indications for Electronic Fetal Monitoring

EFM is recommended for conditions associated with an increased risk of adverse fetal outcomes including:

FIRST STAGE OF LABOR

1. Clinically detected abnormalities of the FHR, tachysystole, or difficulty in reliable assessment with IA
2. Meconium in the amniotic fluid, post term pregnancy
3. Oxytocin induction or augmentation of labor
4. Slow progress in labor
5. Fetal risk factors (prematurity, IUGR, amniotic fluid alterations, cord malformations, malpresentation, abnormal biophysical profile or Doppler studies, multiple gestation)
6. Patients with risk factors for uteroplacental insufficiency (hypertensive disorders of pregnancy, diabetes, medical disease, trauma, antepartum hemorrhage)

Methods of Recording

1. Internal monitoring: a fetal scalp electrode is applied to the fetal scalp or buttocks to obtain a fetal electrocardiogram signal.
   a. Advantages:
      i. Increased accuracy in monitoring FHR with atypical external FHR patterns, maternal obesity, dystocia, high dose Oxytocin, and labor augmentation with trial of labor after Cesarean.
   b. Disadvantages:
      i. Invasive
      ii. Caution with maternal infections (HIV, genital herpes, hepatitis, intrauterine infection).
2. External monitoring: A fetal heart tracing is obtained using an ultrasound transducer. The transducer is applied to the mother's abdomen. Moving cardiac structures produce a Doppler sound wave shift in reflected frequencies that are detected by the ultrasound crystals in the monitor and converted to an electronic signal.
   a. Advantages:
      i. Noninvasive
      ii. Suitable in patient with intact membranes or a closed cervix
      iii. Allows for antepartum monitoring
   b. Disadvantages:
      i. High level of artifact, including MHR, doubling or halving of input signal, variable quality of signal, and challenges with tracing interpretation (intra and inter observer variability)
      ii. May artificially increase FHR variability

    iii. Need for readjustment with maternal or fetal movement
    iv. Difficult to obtain clear tracing in obese women and in polyhydramnios

Components of the FHR Tracing

1. Baseline fetal heart rate
2. Baseline variability
3. Periodic changes:
    a. Accelerations
    b. Decelerations
4. Uterine Activity

Interpretation of External EFM

In interpreting the FHR patterns (Fig. 12-3), the following features are significant:

1. The baseline and variability of the FHR
2. Changes (accelerations, decelerations) in the FHR in response to a uterine contraction
3. Patterns over time—i.e., repetitive decelerations.

Baseline FHR

The baseline FHR is the average FHR over 2 minutes observed between uterine contractions and excluding periodic changes. The mean FHR is obtained by rounding to increments of 5 beats per minute within a 10 minute window. It must be differentiated from MHR. A change in baseline is defined as alterations in FHR lasting more than 10 minutes.

Definitions

1. Normal range: 110 to 160 bpm
2. Baseline Tachycardia
    a. Atypical: >160 bpm for >30 minutes to <80 minutes
    b. Abnormal: >160 bpm for >80 minutes

FIRST STAGE OF LABOR

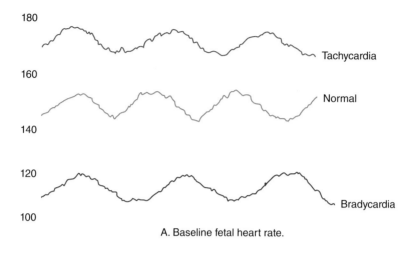

A. Baseline fetal heart rate.

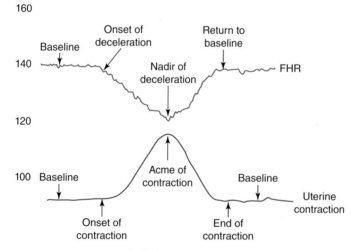

B. Early deceleration.

FIGURE 12-3. Fetal heart rate patterns. A. Baseline fetal heart rate. **B.** Early deceleration. **C.** Late deceleration. **D.** Variable deceleration.

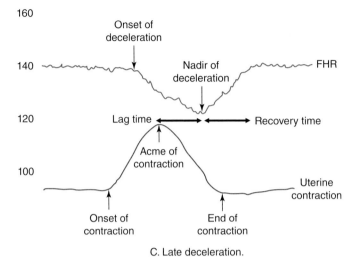

C. Late deceleration.

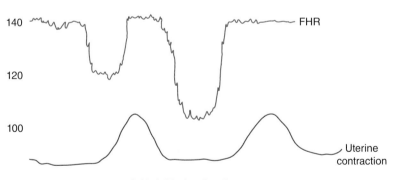

D. Variable deceleration.

FIGURE 12-3. (*Continued*)

3. Baseline Bradycardia
   a. Atypical: 100 to 110 bpm
   b. Abnormal: <100 bpm

The baseline FHR decreases with advancing gestational age, reflecting increased parasympathetic control of the sinoatrial node. The baseline FHR is the least sensitive indicator of the degree of fetal oxygenation, but concern for asphyxia should be considered.

Tachycardia. A FHR over 160 bpm is defined as tachycardia. It reflects increased adrenergic tone with decreased vagal input. Tachycardia is usually accompanied by some decrease in heart rate variability.

1. Causes of tachycardia
   a. Fetal hypoxia
   b. Fetal anemia
   c. Fetal cardiac failure
   d. Fetal tachyarrhythmia
   e. Prematurity
   f. Maternal fever (and therefore elevated fetal temperature)
   g. Maternal anxiety
   h. Maternal or fetal hyperthyroidism
   i. Chorioamnionitis
   j. Parasympatholytic drugs (atropine, phenothiazines)
   k. Betamimetic drugs (salbutamol)
2. Outcome
   a. The outcome is good if decelerations are absent and FHR variability is normal
   b. The outcome is poor if decelerations, with or without a decrease in FHR variability, are present

Tachycardia alone is not a good indicator of fetal infection or asphyxia. It may, however, be an early sign of hypoxia when accompanied by periodic changes and absent or minimal variability.

Bradycardia. A FHR less than 110 bpm is defined as bradycardia. Any bradycardia in the presence of moderate FHR variability is usually benign. Bradycardias are distinguished from prolonged decelerations by duration (>10 minutes).

1. Causes of bradycardia:
   a. Asphyxia (usually a late sign)
   b. Physiologic
   c. Arrhythmia
   d. Drug effect
   e. Maternal hypotension
   f. Maternal position
   g. Congenital heart block (maternal systemic lupus erythematous)
   h. Umbilical cord compression
2. Outcome: Fetal bradycardia is a late sign of fetal compromise when:
   a. Variability and accelerations are absent
   b. Presence of late decelerations. In a severely compromised fetus, late decelerations may be absent because the fetus is so acidotic that it cannot change its heart rate

Baseline Variability of the FHR

Variability is the beat to beat fluctuation of FHR from baseline excluding accelerations and decelerations. It is assessed over at least 1 minute. In the normal FHR, there is a variation of 6 to 25 bpm. It indicates an intact fetal CNS capable of controlling the FHR (Fig. 12-3A).

In predicting the immediate status of the fetus, variability of the baseline FHR is a most significant parameter. Moderate variability suggests normal fetal acid–base balance and correlates well with intrapartum fetal scalp pH and cord blood gases. Transient decreases in variability may be physiologic (i.e., fetal sleep), but persistent loss of variability may indicate metabolic acidosis and fetal compromise. FHR variability may be difficult to interpret if external EFM quality is poor. A fetal scalp electrode (IFM) can be applied to improve the assessment. Absence of variability on external EFM is significant because the true variability is never more than that displayed on the monitor.

Classification of FHR Variability:

Absent: undetectable change in amplitude
Minimal: ≤5 bpm in range
Moderate: range of 6 to 25 bpm
Marked: >25 bpm in range

Sinusoidal—smooth repetitive pattern (sine wave like), 5 to 15 bpm amplitude occurring 3 to 5 cycles per minute

FIRST STAGE OF LABOR

1. Changes in Variability
   a. Marked variability: If high variability (>25 bpm) persists over 10 minutes the FHR tracing is abnormal. There are several possible explanations:
      i. Mild fetal hypoxia. Marked variability may be an early FHR sign of a decrease in fetal oxygenation
      ii. Fetal hemorrhage. In this case, there is usually an accompanying tachycardia. A Kleihauer test may reveal fetal red blood cells in the maternal circulation. Assessment of the hematocrit from a fetal scalp sample will show anemia
      iii. Sinusoidal. Persistence of this smooth wave like pattern for >20 minutes is associated with fetal anemia or hypoxia and is considered abnormal.
   b. Absent or minimal variability: A tracing is atypical if variability is ≤5 bpm for 40 to 80 minutes and abnormal if the variability is decreased longer than 80 minutes. Decreased variability is associated with several factors:
      i. Fetal sleep. In labor, this lasts 20 to 40 minutes.
      ii. Fetal hypoxia or acidemia. This is the most serious situation
      iii. Medications (beta-blockers, steroids), CNS depressant drugs (narcotics, sedatives, magnesium sulphate)
      iv. Parasympatholytic drugs cause decreased variability and tachycardia
      v. Sympatholytic drugs lead to decreased variability and bradycardia
2. Interpretation: When absent or minimal variability is the result of hypoxia, there are often periodic changes (decelerations) in the FHR with or without a change in the baseline rate. Decreased variability occurs during fetal sleep, and if the tracing is normal in other respects, only continued observation is indicated. A difficult pattern to evaluate is one in which the variability is minimal but the FHR is within the normal range and there are no abnormal periodic changes. Possible causes include:
   a. Congenital anomalies of the heart or CNS
   b. Prematurity
   c. Previous hypoxia
   d. Some cases are idiopathic, and no etiologic factor is identifiable. Consider internal fetal monitoring or fetal scalp pH sampling if available

Periodic Changes in the FHR

Accelerations.   An acceleration is defined as an abrupt change (<30 seconds), of the FHR of 15 bpm or greater above the baseline lasting over 15 seconds but less than 2 minutes (10 bpm for >10 seconds at <32 weeks). Atypical FHR tracing have an absence of accelerations despite fetal scalp stimulation. Abnormal FHR tracings usually lack accelerations.

There are two possible physiologic mechanisms for accelerations:

1. They represent an intact CNS in a state of arousal, indicating a healthy fetus
2. Partial cord occlusion results in compression of the umbilical vein while the umbilical artery remains patent. This decreases fetal cardiac output and causes transient fetal hypotension. Hypotension elicits a baroreceptor response, resulting in an acceleration. These accelerations are often seen at the start of a uterine contraction and often precede a variable deceleration

Decelerations.   A deceleration is a decrease in FHR (abrupt or gradual), from the baseline lasting <30 seconds to <10 minutes. Three types (early, late, or variable), are described according to their shape and temporal relationship to uterine contractions and may be periodic, episodic, repetitive, and prolonged.

CLASSIFICATION OF DECELERATIONS

1. Uniform: gradual deflection of the FHR from baseline associated with uterine contractions
   a. Early deceleration (Fig. 12-3B)
   b. Late deceleration (Fig. 12-3C)
2. Variable: abrupt deflections of the FHR from baseline not necessarily associated with uterine activity (Fig. 12-3D). They can be divided into two groups, defined later in this section
   a. Uncomplicated
   b. Complicated

EARLY DECELERATION OF FHR

1. Characteristics: All the following must apply (Fig. 12-3B):
   a. The shape of the deceleration is gradual (>30 seconds from baseline to nadir)

FIRST STAGE OF LABOR

    b. The pattern of the FHR mirrors that of the contraction, with onset occurring early in the contraction cycle, nadir with the peak of contraction and return to baseline prior to end of contraction

    c. The amplitude is usually <30 bpm and the nadir rarely falls below 100 bpm

    d. The pattern is repetitive in most cases

    e. Baseline variability is maintained

2. Proposed mechanism: Early decelerations are believed to be the result of fetal head compression, resulting in altered cerebral blood flow initiating a vagal reflex and cardiac slowing

3. Interpretation: This is a benign FHR pattern associated with active labor, fetal descent or full dilation. It is not usually associated with baseline changes or loss of FHR variability. It is not associated with fetal hypoxia, acidosis, or low APGAR scores

4. Management: Continue observation

LATE DECELERATION OF FHR

1. Characteristics: All the following must apply (Fig. 12-3C):

    a. The shape of the deceleration is gradual (>30 seconds from baseline to nadir)

    b. The onset of the deceleration occurs late in the uterine contraction cycle, 20 to 30 seconds after the start of the contraction

    c. The FHR does not return to baseline until after the end of the uterine contraction. The deceleration may persist for 30 to 60 seconds after the contraction

    d. The lag time (interval between the acme of the uterine contraction and nadir of the FHR) is >20 seconds

    e. The duration of the deceleration of the FHR is proportional to the uterine contraction

    f. The amplitude of the deceleration is usually 20 to 30 bpm. Rarely does it exceed 40 bpm

    g. The pattern is usually repetitive (occurring after >50% of the contractions)

2. Proposed mechanism:

    a. Decreased uterine blood flow (uteroplacental insufficiency or tachysystole)

    b. Reduction of Po_2 below a critical level during the peak of contraction

    c. Initially mediated by hypoxic depression of CNS (chemoreceptor response with secondary baroreceptor response)

    d. Severe hypoxia also leads to direct depression of fetal myocardium

3. Interpretation: Late decelerations are potentially ominous, and a repetitive pattern may lead to fetal acidosis. Management depends on the stage of labor, associated risk factors and whether the cause of the uteroplacental insufficiency is potentially reversible

    a. Potentially reversible causes:

        i. Tachysystole with oxytocic agents

        ii. Maternal hypotension

            i. Supine position

            ii. Associated with epidural anesthesia

            iii. Maternal hypovolemia

    b. Usually irreversible causes:

        i. Fetal growth restriction

        ii. Diabetes

        iii. Hypertension

        iv. Postmaturity

        v. Placental abruption

4. Management:

    a. Corrective measures:

        i. Intrauterine resuscitation—check maternal vital signs, relief of maternal hypotension by turning the patient on her side, consider a vaginal examination

        ii. Reduction of uterine tachysystole by discontinuing oxytocin

        iii. Consider IV fluid bolus if hypotension or hypovolemia

        iv. Consider supplemental oxygen if maternal hypoxia or hypovolemia confirmed

    b. If the pattern persists for >15 minutes after resuscitative measures, prepare for delivery

    c. The presence of moderate FHR variability would indicate the absence of fetal acidosis. Consider digital fetal scalp stimulation or fetal scalp pH and close monitoring. Fetal scalp stimulation involves lightly stroking the fetal scalp for 15 seconds and observing the FHR. An acceleration suggests an absence of acidosis. A lack of acceleration does not predict fetal compromise, but repeat assessment should be considered

    d. Persistent late decelerations accompanied by baseline changes (bradycardia or tachycardia) and decreased FHR variability, indicate significant fetal distress and acidosis and delivery is indicated (cesarean section or assisted vaginal birth)

e. If late decelerations persist with normal heart rate variability or scalp pH, delivery by cesarean section may still be performed in situations of suspected uteroplacental insufficiency

VARIABLE DECELERATION OF FHR

1. Characteristics:
   a. Abrupt deceleration (<30 seconds) from baseline to nadir. The shape of the deceleration is variable, i.e., may be U, V, or W shaped (Fig. 12-3D)
   b. Variable in onset, amplitude and duration
   c. May be periodic or episodic and may or may not be repetitive
   d. May be preceded or followed by accelerations ("shoulders")
2. Proposed mechanism:
   a. Cord compression obstructing the umbilical vein causes a transient fall in fetal cardiac output, leading to hypotension, and a baroreceptor response. This response initiates a period of FHR acceleration
   b. As umbilical cord compression continues, the flow through the umbilical artery is also occluded. This isolates the fetal cardiovascular system from the low-pressure placental unit and increases peripheral vascular resistance in the fetus. The subsequent increase in fetal blood pressure provokes a vagal reflex response which slows the FHR. If cord compression is sustained and persistent, it may eventually lead to hypoxia and metabolic acidosis. Variable decelerations have two components:
      i. A neurogenic or reflex vagal deceleration, usually accompanied by a reversible respiratory acidosis caused by the accumulation of carbon dioxide and increased Pco_2 in the fetus
      ii. A late component caused by hypoxic depression of the CNS if sustained or persistent cord compression. When this occurs, metabolic acidosis will supervene
3. Interpretation: Variable decelerations are the most common periodic change observed in labor. There is a higher incidence in association with a nuchal, short, or prolapsed cord and when oligohydramnios is present. The potential for cord compression exists each time there is fetal movement or a uterine contraction

Variable Deceleration Categories. Variable decelerations can be divided into two types: uncomplicated and complicated

a. Uncomplicated: Abrupt decelerations 15 bpm below baseline lasting >15 seconds. They often occur with "shoulders," brief accelerations, before and after the deceleration. This type of variable deceleration is not associated with low APGAR scores or fetal acidosis

b. Complicated: Abrupt decelerations with any of the following features and may be a predictor of fetal hypoxia particularly if repetitive
   i. Prolonged deceleration to <60 bpm for >60 seconds
   ii. Minimal variability in the baseline FHR and in the trough of the deceleration
   iii. Overshoot acceleration after deceleration lasting >20 bpm for >20 seconds
   iv. Slower or lack of return to baseline FHR
   v. Associated with baseline fetal bradycardia or tachycardia

4. Management: Uncomplicated variable decelerations can be managed by continuing surveillance and do not require intervention. Complicated variable decelerations require assessment of the patient, intrauterine resuscitation and consideration of delivery depending on the severity, persistence, and response of the FHR to the interventions.

   Tracing Classification: Intrapartum EFM tracings are classified as normal, atypical, or abnormal. Most normal FHR tracing will have occasional uncomplicated variables or early decelerations. A tracing becomes atypical when there are three or more uncomplicated variable decelerations in a 20-minute tracing. Atypical tracing may also have occasional late decelerations or a single prolonged deceleration over 2 minutes but less than 3 minutes.
   An abnormal tracing is defined as having three or more complicated variable decelerations, recurrent late decelerations or if there is a single prolonged deceleration over 3 minutes but less than 10 minutes. Abnormal tracings require timely assessment and intervention.

a. A patient in the first stage of labor with an abnormal tracing or persistently atypical tracing not responding to resuscitative measures and/or additional risk factors is best managed by cesarean section

b. In the second stage of labor, atypical tracings with uncomplicated variable decelerations may be managed expectantly. Repetitive variable decelerations (>60 seconds), during pushing in the second stage, are frequently seen. If FHR baseline and variability are normal, it is unlikely that fetal acidosis is present. Determine the significance,

FIRST STAGE OF LABOR

duration of effect, reserve of the fetus, and the labor progress. Expedite delivery if FHR deteriorates or progress is lacking

Summary

1. A normal FHR tracing with moderate variability indicates a healthy fetus and is usually associated with normal APGAR scores
2. FHR changes represent a hemodynamic response to a fetal *stress* and should not be interpreted to mean the presence of fetal *distress*. According to the 2020 SOGC Clinical Practice Guideline No. 396 on Intrapartum Fetal Health Surveillance, external EFM tracings are categorized as normal, atypical, or abnormal (Table 12-1):
   a. **Normal FHR** patterns: Associated with fetal well-being. No interventions are required
      i. Baseline rate: 110 to 160 bpm
      ii. Baseline FHR variability: moderate (6-25 bpm)
      iii. Late or complicated variable decelerations: absent
      iv. Early decelerations or nonrepetitive uncomplicated variables: present or absent
      v. Accelerations: present or absent
   b. **Atypical FHR** patterns: May be associated with fetal acidemia. Requires evaluation, vigilance and continued surveillance, depending on clinical scenario
      i. Baseline rate <110 bpm or baseline >160 bpm
      ii. Minimal <5 bpm for 40 to 80 min, or marked variability
      iii. Rising baseline or fetal arrhythmia
      iv. Absence of accelerations after fetal stimulation
      v. Prolonged decelerations (>2 minutes but <10 minutes)
      vi. Intermittent late decelerations
      vii. Repetitive uncomplicated variables, nonrepetitive complicated variable decelerations
   c. **Abnormal FHR** patterns: Consistently associated with fetal acidemia. This requires prompt evaluation and management, including intrauterine resuscitation, discontinue labor stimulus, or emergency delivery
      i. Baseline <100 bpm or >160 for >80 minutes
      ii. Minimal or absent variability
      iii. Repetitive complicated variable decelerations
      iv. Recurrent late decelerations or single prolonged deceleration >3 minutes
      v. Sinusoidal pattern

TABLE 12-1: CLASSIFICATION OF INTRAPARTUM EFM TRACINGS

	Normal	Atypical	Abnormal
Uterine acitivity	• Normal contraction pattern	• Tachysystole may be present with normal, atypical, or abnormal tracings; monitor closely for concerning FHR characteristics	
Baseline	• 110–160 bpm	• 100–110 bpm • >160 bpm for 30–80 minutes • Rising baseline • Arrhythmia (Irregular rhythm)	• <100 bpm • >160 bpm for >80 minutes • Erratic baseline
Variability	• 6–25 bpm • ≤5 bpm for <40 minutes	• ≤5 bpm for 40–80 minutes	• ≤5 bpm for >80 minutes • ≥25 bpm for >10 minutes • Sinusoidal
Accaleration	• Spontaneous accelerations but not required • Acceleration with scalp stimulation	• Absence of acceleration with scalps stimulation	• Usually absent (accelerations, if present, do not change classification of tracing)
Deceleration	• None • Non-repetitive uncomplicated variable decelerations • Early decelerations	• Repetitive uncomplicated variables • Non-repetitive complicated variables • Intermittent late decelerations • Single prolonged deceleration ≥2 minutes but <3 minutes	• Repetitive complicated variables • Recurrent late decelerations • Single prolonged decelerations ≥3 minutes but <10 minutes
Interpret clinically (in light of total situation)	• No evidence of fetal compromise	• Physiologic response	• Possible fetal compromise

(Continued)

FIRST STAGE OF LABOR

TABLE 12-1: CLASSIFICATION OF INTRAPARTUM EFM TRACINGS (*Continued*)

	Normal	Atypical	Abnormal
Terminology	**Recurrent:** Decelerations occur with ≥50% of uterine contractions in any 20-mintue window. **Intermittent:** Decelerations occur with <50% of uterine contractions in any 20-minutes segment. **Repetitive:** ≥3 in a row **Non-repetitive:** 1 or maximally 2 in a row		

EFM: electronic fetal monitoring; FHR: fetal heart rate.

Reproduced with permission from Dore S, Ehman W. No. 396-Fetal Health Surveillance: Intrapartum Consensus Guideline. J Obstet Gynaecol Can 2020;42(3):316-348.e9.

PSYCHOLOGICAL RESPONSE TO FETAL MONITORING

Proper use of both IA and continuous EFM, in both high- and low-risk patients, should include an explanation to the patient of the purpose of these examinations and a discussion with her about her concerns and wishes. Ideally, this should take place during the prenatal visits and again upon her admittance to the labor suite. As valuable as the fetal monitor is, it transforms the labor room into an intensive care environment, and some patients manifest strong reactions.

Positive Response

Many women find that their state of anxiety is relieved, the machine providing valuable information that is otherwise unavailable. The clicking of the monitor confirms that the baby is alive. Both the patient and her partner can tell when the next contraction is coming and are able to prepare for it. Women who have had a fetal loss in a previous pregnancy are strongly in favor of fetal monitoring.

Negative Response

Patients complain about the discomfort from the abdominal transducers or from the wires of an intravaginal electrode. They are concerned with decreased mobility, the loss of privacy, and loss of control. Some are concerned that the electrode may injure the baby or become anxious by variations in the FHR. Some may resent care givers paying attention to the equipment.

The solution lies in education. Fetal monitoring is an important topic for prenatal classes and can be reviewed at antenatal visits. During labor, the use of fetal monitors including wireless models should be explained, and the patient's mobility, comfort, and privacy be of paramount importance.

BIOCHEMICAL ANALYSIS OF FETAL CAPILLARY BLOOD

When significant fetal hypoxia occurs, metabolic acidosis develops. As anaerobic metabolism proceeds, increasing amounts of lactic acid progressively lower the pH of fetal blood. A fetal scalp blood sample can be obtained to assess the fetal pH or lactate. Fetal scalp lactate testing has become a preferred approach to fetal scalp pH testing to assess fetal hypoxia because it is easier to do as point-of-care testing, requires less blood volume, has faster results, and samples are less likely to clot.

Indications

1. Atypical or abnormal FHR pattern unresolved with intrauterine resuscitation or fetal scalp stimulation
2. Uncertainty with the EFM interpretation
3. Delivery not imminent and gestational age more than 34 weeks

Contraindications include noncephalic/breech presentations, history of bleeding disorders, and maternal infections.

Technique

Fetal capillary blood sampling requires an organized routine, availability of equipment for immediate analysis, and operators with expertise. The membranes must be ruptured, the presenting part fixed in the pelvis, the position known, the cervix dilated more than 3 cm, and good lighting available. Under aseptic conditions and with the patient lying preferably in the left lateral position, an amnioscope is introduced into the posterior fornix of the vagina and into the cervix. The amnioscope must press lightly against the fetal scalp (or rarely, the buttocks). The site for sampling is wiped clean of maternal blood and amniotic fluid, and a thin layer of silicone gel is applied to induce beading of blood to aid in its collection. The commercially available scalpels are preset so that the depth of incision is

FIRST STAGE OF LABOR

3 mm. A cruciate incision is made, and a brief, moderate flow of blood follows. The volume collected is depending on the commercial kit used. The samples must be analyzed immediately. Excessive or prolonged bleeding is rare; it is easily controlled by pressure. In fewer than 1 percent of cases, a mild localized infection occurs.

Correlation Between FHR Patterns, Fetal pH, and Outcome

A normal fetus has a pH of 7.25 to 7.35 before the start of labor. During labor, there is a gradual shift in pH toward 7.25. If fetal hypoxia produces metabolic acidosis, fetal pH falls through preacidosis (7.20-7.24) to frank acidosis (<7.20).

Certain correlations between fetal pH and neonatal condition have been observed:

1. pH over 7.25: Most neonates will be healthy, with high APGAR scores and would have shown normal FHR patterns during labor
2. pH between 7.20 and 7.24: This level indicates mild preacidosis. It is often associated with a prolonged second stage of labor and mild hypoxemia. FHR patterns often demonstrate late or variable decelerations, but FHR variability is normal. Most of these neonates have high APGAR scores. Operative intervention is not indicated, but the sampling should be repeated in 30 minutes
3. pH less than 7.20: This is usually indicative of significant fetal acidosis. In 80 percent of neonates, the APGAR score is under 6. FHR patterns often show persistent late or persistent severe variable decelerations with loss of FHR variability
4. pH less than 7.10: This indicates profound asphyxia. Significant neonatal depression is present in most cases

A low fetal pH should not be interpreted in isolation. A full review of the entire blood gas picture must be carried out. An assessment of the P_{CO_2}, bicarbonate, and base deficit values are required to substantiate a diagnosis of metabolic acidosis. Interpreted in isolation of other acid–base parameters and the clinical context can lead to unnecessary intervention.

Factors Affecting Fetal Scalp pH Results

1. Normal scalp pH >7.20, but low APGAR score can occur in association with sedative drugs, anesthesia, obstruction of the airway, congenital

anomalies, prematurity, hypoxia subsequent to the sampling, trauma of delivery, or a previous episode of asphyxia
2. Low scalp pH <7.20, but normal APGAR score may occur in the presence of maternal acidosis

Management During Labor

1. An abnormal FHR is an indication for prompt assessment that may include fetal scalp pH
2. If the pH is over 7.25, labor continues, and the analysis is repeated if the FHR remains abnormal
3. When the pH is 7.20 to 7.24, repeat sampling in 30 minutes or consider delivery
4. With the pH under 7.20, delivery is indicated

Fetal Scalp Lactate Parameters

1. Lactate <4.2: Normal value, repeat fetal scalp blood sampling in 30 minutes if FHR abnormality persists
2. Lactate 4.2 to 4.8: Borderline, repeat fetal scalp blood sampling within 30 minutes or consider delivery if significant fall in pH or rise in lactate
3. Lactate >4.8: Abnormal, delivery is indicated

SELECTED READING

Cordero L, Anderson CW, Zuspan FP: Scalp abscess: A benign and infrequent complication of fetal monitoring. Am J Obstet Gynecol 146:126, 1983

Dore S, Ehman W: No. 396-Fetal Health Surveillance: Intrapartum consensus guideline. J Obstet Gynaecol Can 42:316-348.e9, 2020

Elias S: Fetoscopy in prenatal diagnosis. Clin Perinatol 10:357, 1983

Electronic fetal heart rate monitoring: research guidelines for interpretation. National Institute of Child Health and Human Development Research Planning Workshop. Am J Obstet Gynecol 177:1385, 1997

Freeman RK, Garite TJ: Fetal Heart Rate Monitoring. Baltimore/London: Williams and Wilkins, 1981, pp 84-112

Leveno KJ, William ML, DePalma RT, Whalley PJ: Perinatal outcome in the absence of antepartum fetal heart acceleration. Obstet Gynecol 61:347, 1983

Liston R, Sawchuck D, Young D: Fetal health surveillance: antepartum and intrapartum consensus guideline. J Obstet Gynaecol Can 29 (9 Suppl 4) S3, 2007

Macones GA, Hankins GD, Spong CY, et al: The 2008 National Institute of Child Health and Human Development Workshop Report on Electronic Fetal Monitoring: Update on definitions, interpretation, and research guidelines. Obstet Gynecol 112:661, 2008

Madanes AE, David D, Cetrulo C: Major complications associated with intrauterine pressure monitoring. Obstet Gynecol 59:389, 1982

Manning FA, Lange IR, Morrison I, Harman CR: Determination of fetal health: Methods for antepartum and intrapartum fetal assessment. Curr Prob Obstet Gynecol 7, 1983

Miller RC: Meconium staining of the amniotic fluid. Clin Obstet Gynecol 6:359, 1979

Molfese V, Sunshine P, Bennett A: Reactions of women to intrapartum fetal monitoring. Obstet Gynecol 59:705, 1982

Pearson JF, Weaver JB: Fetal activity and fetal wellbeing: an evaluation. Br Med J, 1:1305, 1976

Young DC, Gray JH, Luther ER, et al: Fetal scalp blood pH sampling: Its value in an active obstetric unit. Am J Obstet Gynecol 136:276, 1980

Induction of Labor

Amanda Black
Innie Chen

Induction of labor (IOL) is the process of artificially stimulating the uterus to start labor. IOL should be considered only in cases where there is a clear medical indication and the expected benefits of an earlier delivery outweigh the potential harms. A careful and well-documented discussion should occur between the health care provider and the patient and should include the reason for induction, method of induction, and risks associated with IOL. Depending on the indication for induction, IOL has been associated with higher rates of complications such as bleeding, operative vaginal deliveries, cesarean deliveries, uterine hyperstimulation, and adverse perinatal outcomes.

Some common indications and contraindications for IOL are discussed below.

MATERNAL INDICATIONS

PRELABOR SPONTANEOUS RUPTURE OF MEMBRANES (PROM) If membrane rupture occurs beyond 37 weeks and labor does not begin within 24 hours of PROM, IOL is appropriate and recommended to reduce the risk of infection to both the mother and the baby. In the case of maternal GBS colonization, IOL should be considered immediately rather than choosing expectant management.

PRETERM PRELABOR RUPTURE OF MEMBRANES (PPROM) If membrane rupture occurs prior to 37 weeks gestational age, IOL should be considered after 34 weeks in the context of the patient's complete clinical picture.

PREECLAMPSIA IOL should be considered in women with severe preeclampsia at any gestational age. IOL should also be considered for patients with gestational hypertension ≥38 weeks in the context of other clinical findings.

ANTEPARTUM BLEEDING IOL may be indicated in cases of significant but stable antepartum bleeding.

MATERNAL DIABETES Insulin-dependent diabetes is associated with an increased risk of in utero fetal death during the later weeks of pregnancy. In cases of preexisting diabetes, insulin-dependent diabetes, or in the presence of complications associated with diabetes, labor induction is indicated. Maternal glucose control may dictate the urgency of IOL. The timing of induction should be individualized. Unless otherwise indicated, IOL for gestational diabetes (GDM) that is controlled with diet and exercise only should not occur before 39 weeks.

INTRAUTERINE FETAL DEATH (IUFD) In cases of IUFD where there is evidence of ruptured membranes, infection, bleeding, or coagulopathy, immediate IOL is recommended. If the woman is otherwise well, labor induction may be delayed. IOL may also be considered in women with a history of IUFD near term in past pregnancies. The timing of induction should be individualized but is usually carried out 1 week prior to the gestation of a previous stillbirth.

ADVANCED MATERNAL AGE (AMA) AMA is associated with an increase in antenatal and intrapartum stillbirth. The risk at 39 weeks in a 40-year-old is equivalent to the risk at 41 weeks in a 24- to 29-year-old, although the *absolute risk* is still low. IOL should be offered at 39 weeks for mothers above the age of 40.

CHOLESTASIS OF PREGNANCY Due to the increased risk of stillbirth associated with obstetrical cholestasis, IOL should be offered at 37 weeks gestational age.

MATERNAL OBESITY IOL may be considered ≥39 weeks gestation in an attempt to reduce the risk of cesarean section. However, there is a correlation between increasing BMIs and longer labors, need for repeated cervical ripening agents, more oxytocin use, and increased cesarean section rates.

FIRST STAGE OF LABOR

FETAL INDICATIONS

POSTTERM PREGNANCY There is strong evidence to support a recommendation of IOL between 41^{+0} and 42^{+0} weeks of gestation. Delivery after 42^{+0} weeks is associated with an increase risk of NICU admission, perinatal death, macrosomia, shoulder dystocia, postmaturity syndrome, and meconium aspiration. After 42^{+0} weeks, the risk of maternal complications also increases, including perineal lacerations, infections, postpartum hemorrhage, and cesarean deliveries. The risk of cesarean section is reduced when IOL is carried out between 41^{+0} and 42^{+0} weeks gestation.

INTRAUTERINE GROWTH RESTRICTION (IUGR) Depending on other clinical parameters and ultrasound findings, IOL should be considered in cases of suspected IUGR at or near term to reduce the risk of stillbirth. Ultrasound findings of decreasing growth velocity, MCA redistribution, and absent/reverse end diastolic flow may dictate the urgency of induction.

MACROSOMIA There is a higher risk of shoulder dystocia and brachial plexus injury when the birthweight is above 4500 g. This risk is increased if the mother has diabetes or if a previous delivery had shoulder dystocia. However, due to the potential in error for ultrasound estimation of fetal weight, IOL solely for suspected macrosomia should not be carried out routinely before 39 weeks. Cesarean section may be recommended when the estimated fetal weight is >4500 g in the presence of diabetes or > 5000 g in the absence of diabetes.

CHORIOAMNIONITIS IOL is indicated in cases of suspected chorioamnionitis.

ISOIMMUNIZATION When the fetus is being sensitized or when there has been isoimmunization or fetal death in utero during previous pregnancies, IOL is indicated. The timing of induction should be individualized.

OLIGOHYDRAMNIOS There is no evidence to support routine IOL in otherwise uncomplicated pregnancies with isolated oligohydramnios. However, some experts advocate IOL to reduce perinatal mortality and morbidity. In cases of oligohydramnios associated with IUGR, postterm pregnancy, or other abnormal maternal/fetal findings, IOL should be offered.

POLYHYDRAMNIOS There is no evidence to support routine IOL in otherwise uncomplicated pregnancies with polyhydramnios. IOL is sometimes carried out if an unstable lie places the woman at high risk for an umbilical cord prolapse if the membranes rupture spontaneously.

TWIN PREGNANCIES IOL should be considered in uncomplicated dichorionic twin pregnancies past 38 weeks gestation, and for monochorionic twin pregnancies after 37 weeks gestation.

When IOL is being carried out for the convenience of the patient and/or the health care provider in the absence of medical indications, it is called an *elective induction*. Elective inductions should be avoided as much as possible. In exceptional circumstances (e.g., a history of rapid labors or the patient lives far from a hospital), induction may be considered at or after 40 weeks.

CONTRAINDICATIONS FOR LABOR INDUCTION

PLACENTA PREVIA OR VASA PREVIA When the placenta and associated blood vessels are in close proximity to the cervix.

NONCEPHALIC PRESENTATION IOL is contraindicated if the baby is in a transverse lie or is a footling breech. It is generally not recommended if the baby is in a breech presentation.

UMBILICAL CORD PROLAPSE

PRIOR CLASSICAL CESAREAN SECTION OR INVERTED T UTERINE INCISION

PRIOR SIGNIFICANT UTERINE SURGERY (e.g., full-thickness myomectomy)

PRIOR UTERINE RUPTURE

PELVIC STRUCTURAL DEFORMITIES

ACTIVE GENITAL HERPES

INVASIVE CERVICAL CARCINOMA

RISKS ASSOCIATED WITH LABOR INDUCTION

FAILURE TO ESTABLISH LABOR

IATROGENIC PRETERM OR LATE PRETERM BIRTH It is important to confirm the estimated gestational age prior to IOL, preferably with the results of an early ultrasound performed prior to 24-week gestational age.

INCREASED OPERATIVE VAGINAL DELIVERY

PROLONGED LABOR

INCREASED CESAREAN DELIVERY

UMBILICAL CORD PROLAPSE

FIRST STAGE OF LABOR

TACHYSYSTOLE (excessive uterine activity) with or without fetal heart rate changes

ABNORMAL FETAL HEART RATE PATTERNS

UTERINE RUPTURE in a scarred or unscarred uterus

CHORIOAMNIONITIS

POSTPARTUM HEMORRHAGE

PREREQUISITES AND CONDITIONS FOR SUCCESSFUL LABOR INDUCTION

PRESENTATION The presentation should be cephalic. Labor should not be induced with a transverse lie or compound presentations. IOL is not usually performed in breech presentations.

STATION Amniotomy should only be performed when the head is engaged to avoid umbilical cord prolapse. The lower the head, the easier and safer the procedure.

CERVICAL RIPENESS Prelabor status of the cervix (including cervical effacement, dilation, position, and firmness) is an important predictor of induction success. Preferably the cervix is effaced, soft, dilated, open to admit at least one or two fingers, and the firm ring of the internal os is not present. The Bishop's score may be used to document cervical ripeness.

PARITY The success rate for vaginal delivery within 24 hours is better for multiparous women than nulliparous women.

MATERNAL HEIGHT AND WEIGHT Successful induction is associated with women who are taller and have a lower body mass index.

GESTATIONAL AGE Usually, the closer the gestation is to term, the more favorable the cervix, and the greater likelihood of successful IOL. When preterm IOL is necessary, tests for fetal lung maturity can be performed.

PREINDUCTION CERVICAL RIPENING

The changes in the uterine cervix that take place before the onset of labor include physically detectable softening, shortening, and dilatation of the cervical os. This process is known as *ripening*. The collagen fibrils become disaggregated and no longer tightly bound by the glycosaminoglycans so that they will slide apart more readily and allow the cervix to dilate.

In most pregnancies, the cervix is ripe at the onset of labor. A ripe cervix is soft, less than 1.3 cm in length, admits a finger easily, and is dilated. The length of labor and the success of induction in both nulliparous and multiparous women depend on the degree of cervical ripeness. There are many situations, however, in which labor and vaginal delivery are indicated when the cervix is not ripe. In such cases, the cervix is unlikely to respond favorably to uterine activity.

Evaluation of the Cervix

Before inducing labor or using a modality to prime or ripen a cervix, the physical characteristics of the cervix should be assessed to determine the best modality for IOL. The Bishop scoring system (Fig. 13-1). has been utilized to apply a numerical score to the physical examination characteristics of the cervix, including dilation, effacement, consistency, and position of the cervix in the vagina. Of all these parameters, dilation is the most significant. The maximum Bishop score is 13. When the score is 9 or more, there is a high likelihood that IOL will be successful. When the score is 4 or less, failure of induction is common, and preinduction cervical priming should be performed.

		Points		
	0	1	2	3
Dilation of cervix (cm)	0	1–2	3–4	5–6
Effacement of cervix (%)	0–30	40–50	60–70	80
Consistency of cervix	Firm	Medium	Soft	
Position of cervix in the vagina	Posterior	Mid	Anterior	
Station	−3	−2	−1, 0	+1, +2

(Factor)

FIGURE 13-1. Bishop score.

Station	−3	−2	−1, 0	+1, +2
Points	0	1	2	3
Dilation of cervix (cm)	0	1–2	3–4	>4
Points	0	2	4	6
Length of cervix (cm)	3	2	1	0
Points	0	1	2	3

FIGURE 13-2. Lange score.

Lange and associates suggested that the factor of crucial significance to inducibility of labor is the condition of the cervix and that cervical dilatation should be weighted by at least twice the value given it by Bishop (Fig. 13-2). The results of their modified score are the same as those achieved by other methods, but theirs is simpler in that only three parameters are used: station of the presenting part, dilatation of the cervix, and length of the cervix. When the score is 5 to 7, the rate of successful induction is over 75 percent. When it is under 4, the rate of success is much lower.

METHODS OF CERVICAL PRIMING

Mechanical Methods of Cervical Priming

Mechanical methods for cervical ripening have the advantage of lower cost, stability at room temperature, low risk of tachysystole, and few systemic side effects. However, there is generally a small increased risk of infection (depending on the type of mechanical method used) to both the mother and the baby.

Hygroscopic Dilators

Hygroscopic dilators are safe and effective for dilating the cervix but are inadequate for IOL. Hygroscopic dilators may be synthetic or made from dried natural seaweed (laminaria tents). They are primarily used for pregnancy termination rather than for preinduction cervical ripening of term pregnancies.

Hygroscopic dilators expand when they come in contact with moisture. They gradually swell within the cervical canal to three to five times its original diameter, which causes gradual softening and dilatation of the cervix. The most rapid swelling occurs in the first 4-6 hours, and the maximal effect is achieved in 24 hours. The effect is entirely local and uterine hyperactivity is rare.

In the evening before the day of induction, two to five laminaria are placed in the cervix taking care not to rupture the membranes. The number depends on the capacity of the cervix. Insertion of multiple small-diameter hygroscopic dilators (2 or 3 mm) is better than using a few large ones. One or two 4 × 4 sterile gauze are placed against the cervix to hold the laminaria in place. The number of dilators and gauze inserted should be documented. The dilators are removed the next morning and amniotomy is performed when the presenting part is well applied against the cervix. An oxytocin infusion may be started immediately, although some obstetrical providers prefer to use oxytocin only if labor does not begin after a few hours.

Possible side effects/complications of hygroscopic dilators include pelvic cramping, cervical bleeding, and infection. The risk of infection increases if the interval between the insertion of the tents and the emptying of the uterus is prolonged.

Intracervical Balloon Catheters

Commercially available balloons for cervical ripening or a regular Foley catheter (#16 with a 30-80 cc balloon) can be used. Use of a balloon catheter results in a mean change of 3.3 to 5.3 in the Bishop score. They are generally as effective as prostaglandins (PGs) for cervical ripening. Compared with women receiving PGs, women who had balloon catheters for cervical ripening required more use of oxytocin for labor induction and augmentation. Balloon catheters are associated with less uterine hyperstimulation or tachysystole compared with PGs. Balloon catheters for cervical ripening are generally reserved for use in women with intact membranes. There is a small increased risk in maternal infection.

Method of Balloon Catheter Insertion. With a speculum in the vagina and the cervical os well visualized, a deflated balloon catheter is passed through the internal cervical os and into the extra-amniotic space. Ring forceps can be used to aid in passing the catheter through the cervical os.

FIRST STAGE OF LABOR

When in the extra-amniotic space, the balloon is filled with 30 to 60 cc of saline or water. Tension is placed on the catheter by pulling on it until the balloon rests against the internal os. The catheter is left in place until it spontaneously falls out (usually when the cervix is more favorable and about 2-3 cm dilated). This usually occurs within 12-24 hours of catheter placement. If the catheter does not fall out spontaneously after 24 hours, the method of IOL should be reassessed. An amniotomy is performed or oxytocin induction is usually started after the balloon catheter has been removed.

Pharmacologic Methods of Cervical Priming

Prostaglandins

Prostaglandin (PG) preparations are widely used for cervical ripening. PGs bring about biochemical changes in the collagenous matrix of the cervix that result in softening, effacement, and partial dilatation of the cervix and may also stimulate uterine activity. The E class of prostaglandins are bronchodilators and thus are not contraindicated in patients with asthma.

PGE2 preparations are available as a controlled-release vaginal mesh as well as an intravaginal or intracervical gel. Locally administered PG preparations (intravaginal or endocervical) appear to have good clinical response while minimizing systemic side effects and are therefore the preferred routes. Potential maternal side effects include fever, vomiting, and diarrhea. They are associated with a risk of uterine tachsystole and associated fetal heart changes. Fetal heart rate (FHR) monitoring should be performed continuously for at least 30 minutes after administration of PG. The mesh is easier to remove than the gel in cases of uterine tachsystole with FHR changes. Higher dose PGE2 vaginal preparations should not be inserted into the cervical canal. PGE2 should not be used in a TOLAC due to low certainty about its effect on potential uterine rupture. If an abnormal FHR occurs with tachsystole, the PG should be removed from the vagina if possible. Nitroglycerin 50 mcg IV may be considered; however, it may cause profound hypotension.

PGE1 (misoprostol) is approved for the treatment and prevention of peptic ulcers; however, it is an effective pharmacologic agent for cervical ripening and labor induction (off label use). It has been studied in thousands of women worldwide for over 15 years. Benefits of PGE1 include stability at room temperature, low cost, multiple options for route of administration, and cervical ripening/labor induction actions. The dose required for cervical ripening and labor induction in the third trimester is much lower than in the first or second trimester because the myometrium has increased sensitivity to PGs with advancing gestational age. When given orally, serum levels fall and uterine activity ends within 1-2 hours of the dose. The increased resting tone after vaginal or sublingual dosing is usually replaced by rhythmic contractions after 1-2 hours and lasts for 3 hours (after sublingual dose) or 4 hours (after vaginal dose). The recommended dose is 25-50 mcg vaginally every 4 hours or 25-50 mcg orally every 2 hours. If necessary, oxytocin may be initiated no earlier than 4 hours after the last misoprostol dose if given vaginally or no less than 2 hours after the last oral misoprostol dose.

In all PGE2 and PGE1 preparations, contractions of low amplitude can begin within a couple of hours. These are similar to the contractions of early spontaneous labor. Not infrequently, active labor begins during the period of cervical ripening, so that use of oxytocin is less when PGs are used. PGs should be administered in settings where uterine activity and FHR patterns can be monitored. Both PGE1 and PGE2 can be used in case of term PROM.

If labor has not started within 24 hours but the cervix has become favorable, amniotomy is performed and, if necessary, an oxytocin infusion can be initiated. When the cervix does not respond, the case must be reevaluated. An additional dose of PG may be required.

Oxytocin

Oxytocin induces contractions of the pregnant myometrium but it has not been proven to be an efficient cervical priming agent. An intravenous oxytocin infusion does improve the Bishop score but to a much smaller extent than that achieved by PGs or mechanical balloon catheters.

METHODS OF INDUCING LABOR

Complementary Approaches

Although there have been no randomized studies, castor oil (30-60 cc mixed with juice) may decrease the need for IOL in multiparous women. Sexual intercourse at term is not harmful for most pregnancies but a meta-analysis concluded that it does not significantly increase the rate of spontaneous labor. Nipple stimulation or breast compression may help to stimulate labor within 72 hours.

FIRST STAGE OF LABOR

Membrane Stripping

Membrane stripping or sweeping after 38 weeks can increase the release of local prostaglandins and is a common practice. Membrane sweeping involves examining the cervix, reaching beyond the internal cervical os with the examining finger, and rotating the finger circumferentially to detach the fetal membranes from the lower uterine segment. When performed at 40 weeks of gestation, membrane stripping may reduce the need for labor induction for postterm pregnancy because a majority of women enter spontaneous labor within 72 hours. A meta-analysis found low certainty evidence that membrane sweeping reduced the need for induction compared to expectant management without adverse maternal or fetal outcomes aside from minor bleeding and discomfort. Membrane sweeping alone or prior to insertion of PGE2 vaginally or amniotomy has been associated with shorter induction to birth time, less oxytocin use, and decreased cesarean section rates, even when accounting for parity.

Artificial Rupture of Membranes

Artificial rupture of membranes, or amniotomy, may be performed during the induction process but there is limited evidence to support amniotomy alone as a method of induction. It may be considered when the cervix is favorable and the presenting part is well applied against the cervix. Amniotomy alone may not be enough to initiate labor, and oxytocin infusion is usually required to establish labor. In women with a high BMI, early amniotomy increases the risk of cesarean section proportional to the BMI. In women desiring TOLAC, amniotomy at less than 4 cm increases the rate of cesarean section. Amniotomy is a commitment to delivery so it should only be performed when the indication for induction is compelling.

Technique for Performing Amniotomy

The fetal heart is checked first. A vaginal examination is performed to **determine the Bishop's score.** With a finger placed between the cervix and the bag of waters, the cervix is rimmed, stripping the membranes away from the lower uterine segment. If necessary, pressure is maintained on the uterine fundus through the abdomen to keep the head well down. Using a uterine dressing forceps, an Allis forceps, a Kelly clamp, or a membrane hook, the amniotic sac is punctured. A gush of fluid from the vagina is evidence of success. The fetal heart is checked carefully after successful amniotomy to ensure that there is no evidence of umbilical cord prolapse.

Contraindications to Artificial Rupture of the Membranes

1. High presenting part
2. Presentation other than vertex
3. Unripe cervix
4. Active genital herpes and HIV infection with high viral load

Oxytocin

Oxytocin, an octapeptide, is produced in the supraoptic and paraventricular nuclei of the hypothalamus. The hormone migrates down the supraoptic–neurohypophyseal nerve pathways and is stored in the posterior pituitary gland. Secretion seems to occur in a pulsatile fashion. It binds to uterine receptors to produce uterine contractions. Oxytocin has a half-life of 1 to 6 minutes (decreased in late pregnancy) and reaches steady state plasma concentration in 40 minutes. Maternal levels of oxytocin increase throughout gestation. The uterus becomes more responsive to oxytocin as pregnancy progresses due to increasing oxytocin receptors on the myometrium. With prolonged labor, the uterus becomes decreasingly receptive due to saturation of the receptors. Oxytocin has no direct effect on the cervix. Oxytocin-releasing stimuli include: (1) cervical dilatation; (2) coitus; (3) emotional reactions; (4) suckling; and (5) drugs such as acetylcholine, nicotine, and certain anesthetics.

The exact role of oxytocin in human labor is not known. It may be that oxytocin has only a facilitating role in the physiology of uterine activity during pregnancy and not a primary role in the initiation and maintenance of labor. Synthetic oxytocin does not cross the maternal blood brain barrier.

Cardiovascular and Renal Effects of Oxytocin

HEART RATE A small to moderate increase.

SYSTEMIC ARTERIAL BLOOD PRESSURE A decrease results mainly from a lowering of peripheral resistance.

CARDIAC OUTPUT Given as a single dose, oxytocin causes a rise in cardiac output followed by a fall; continuous infusion results in an increased cardiac output.

RENAL BLOOD FLOW No significant change.

SKIN The blood vessels are sensitive to the vasodilatory action of oxytocin, and flushing of the face, neck, and hands may occur.

UTERINE FLOW The decrease is caused mainly by the extravascular resistance around the uterine blood vessels as the result of the increased uterine contractions.

ANTIDIURESIS Resorption of water from the renal distal convoluted tubules and the collecting ducts. Renal blood flow is not reduced.

Administration

For IOL or labor augmentation, a dilute solution of oxytocin is administered as a controlled IV infusion with a constant rate infusion pump. Although various modes of administration have been used in the past, controlled rate IV administration is the gold standard so precise titration can be performed to minimize the risk of serious adverse effects. Potential adverse effects are primarily dose related and include: uterine tachysystole, abnormal FHR, maternal hypotension, water intoxication, and uterine rupture (rare). Both high- and low-dose oxytocin regimens are appropriate and may be considered for labor induction (see Table 13-1). Once oxytocin infusion is initiated, ongoing monitoring of the oxytocin infusion rate, uterine response, and FHR should be performed.

Technique of Intravenous Administration

A test dose at a rate of 1.0 mU/min is suggested to test for untoward reactions. If none occurs, the oxytocin infusion should be gradually increased by 1 to 2 mU/min or 4 to 6 mU/min at 20- to 30-minute intervals until adequate uterine contractions are achieved. In most cases, doses of less than 10 mU/min are adequate. The aim is to bring about strong uterine contractions lasting 40 to 50 seconds and recurring every 2 to 3 minutes. Once a dose of 20 mU/min has been reached, the situation should be reassessed. Tachysystole should be avoided due to the associated risk of uterine rupture, placental separation, and fetal asphyxia. If excessive uterine contractions occur, or if there is fetal bradycardia (<100 bpm), tachycardia (>160 bpm), or irregularity of the heart, the oxytocin should be stopped.

A solution of 20 units of oxytocin in 1 L of crystalloid solution (e.g., normal saline or Ringer's lactate) administered through a constant rate infusion pump is recommended to avoid fluid overload. Because solution

TABLE 13-1: LOW-DOSE VERSUS HIGH-DOSE OXYTOCIN PROTOCOLS

	Low-Dose Protocol	High-Dose Protocol
Initial dose of oxytocin	1-2 mU/min	4-6 mU/min
Interval between dose increments	15-40 minutes	15-40 minutes
Dose increments	1-2 mU	4-6 mU
Maximum dose before reassessment	30 mU/min	30 mU/min
Benefits	Less tachysystole Lower total dose	Shorter time to delivery
Risks	Longer time to delivery	More tachysystole +/– FHR changes

concentrations vary, the rate of infusion should always be documented in mU/min rather than mL/hour. An infusion pump should be used because accurate control of the rate of infusion flow is essential. When used for induction or augmentation of labor, it is advisable to maintain the infusion for 1-hour postpartum to obviate uterine atony.

Prerequisites for the Use of Oxytocin

1. The presenting part should be well engaged
2. The cervix must be ripe, effaced, soft, and partially dilated
3. There must be no fetopelvic disproportion
4. There should be a normal fetal heart rate
5. Adequate personnel available to monitor the patient and respond to emergency situations
6. Examination before the oxytocin is started

Contraindications to the Use of Oxytocin

1. Absence of proper indication
2. Absence of the prerequisites
3. Disproportion, generally contracted pelvis, or obstruction by tumors
4. Instances where vaginal delivery or trial of labor is contraindicated, e.g., previous classical cesarean section or extensive myomectomy, placenta previa

5. Hypertonic or incoordinate uterus: The hypertonic or incoordinate uterus is made worse by oxytocin and may lead to a constriction ring
6. Abnormal FHR pattern
7. Abnormal presentation and position of all types
8. Unengaged head
9. Congenital anomalies of the uterus

Adverse Effects of Oxytocin

Maternal Dangers

1. Tachysystole is defined as having more than five contractions in 10 minutes over a 30-minute period. This can be associated with a normal or abnormal FHR pattern. Prolonged or excessive uterine contractions can occur with the use of PGs and oxytocin
2. Uterine rupture. Tetanic contractions may be significant enough to lead to uterine rupture. The risk of uterine rupture is doubled when the patient has had a previous cesarean section
3. Uterine atony and postpartum hemorrhage may develop when the oxytocin is discontinued, most commonly in cases of prolonged labor
4. Abruptio placentae
5. Water intoxication

Water Intoxication

Oxytocin has an antidiuretic effect that begins when the rate of infusion is 15 mU/min and is maximal at 45 mU/min. Single doses have no effect; the antidiuretic activity seems to depend on the maintenance of a constant and critical level. The action is on the distal convoluted tubules and collecting ducts of the kidneys, causing increased resorption of water from the glomerular filtrate. The combination of oxytocin and large amounts of electrolyte-free glucose in water leads to retention of fluid, low serum levels of sodium chloride, and often progressive oliguria.

The symptoms range from headache, nausea, vomiting, mental confusion, and seizures to coma and death. These have been attributed to edema and swelling of the brain.

Prevention and Management of Water Intoxication. To prevent water intoxication, a more concentrated solution of oxytocin (20 units in 500 cc of crystalloid solution) is recommended. Patients receiving an oxytocin infusion should not receive more than 1 L of electrolyte-free fluid in 24 hours.

For mild cases of water intoxication, discontinue the oxytocin and withhold all fluids. Severe cases will also require intravenous infusion of hypertonic (3.0%) sodium chloride (3.0% NaCl). This will withdraw fluid from the tissues and bring about a diuresis. The rate of infusion must be slow and should be discontinued when the diuretic phase ends to avoid overcorrection, lest the cerebral effects of hypernatremia be imposed upon those of water intoxication

UNSUCCESSFUL INDUCTION OF LABOR

A proposed definition of failed IOL is one of the following two scenarios:

1. **With ruptured membranes:** If regular contractions and cervical change do not occur after at least 12 to 18 hours of oxytocin administration following membrane rupture
2. **With intact membranes:** If regular contractions are not occurring approximately every 3 minutes and cervical change does not occur after at least 24 hours of oxytocin administration

These times do not include the time devoted to cervical ripening. A failed IOL does not necessarily mean that a cesarean section is required. Subsequent management options include a further attempt to induce labor (the timing should depend on the clinical situation and the patient's wishes) or cesarean delivery. If labor does not progress after attempting induction and the patient and fetus are doing well, the situation should be reevaluated and a decision made whether to continue IOL or not. If the patient and fetus are doing well after attempting induction and membrane are intact, it may be reasonable to send the patient home and schedule another time to attempt IOL again. If there are fetal or maternal concerns or the membranes have been ruptured, then a cesarean section may be indicated.

SELECTED READING

ACOG Practice Bulletin No. 107: Induction of labor. Obstet Gynecol 114:386-397, 2009

ACOG Practice Bulletin No. 146: Management of late-term and postterm pregnancies. Obstet Gynecol 124:390-396, 2014

Bakker R, Pierce S, Myers D: The role of prostaglandins E1 and E2, dinoprostone, and misoprostol in cervical ripening and the induction of labor: a mechanistic approach. Arch Gynecol Obstet 296:167-179, 2017

FIRST STAGE OF LABOR

Binkin NJ, Schulz KF, Grimes DA, Cates W: Urea-prostaglandin versus hypertonic saline for instillation abortion. Am J Obstet Gynecol 146:947, 1983

Crane JM: Factors predicting labour induction success: A critical analysis. Clin Obst Gynecol 49:3, 2006

Gower RH, Toraya J, Miller JM: Laminaria for preinduction cervical ripening. Obstet Gynecol 60:617, 1982

Hogg BB, Owen J: Laminaria versus extra-amniotic saline solution infusion for cervical ripening in second-trimester labor inductions. Am J Obstet Gynecol 184:1145-1148, 2001

Lange AP, Secher NJ, Westergaard JG, et al: Prelabour evaluation of inducibility. Obstet Gynecol 60:137, 1982

Mozurkewich E, Chilimigras J, Koepke E, King V: Indications for induction of labour: A best-evidence review. BJOG 116:626-636, 2009

National Institute for Health and Care Excellence: Inducing Labour. Clinical Guideline. https://nice.org.uk/guidance/cg70, 2008

Pandis GK, Papageorghiou AT, Otigbah CM, Howard RJ, Nicolaides KH: Randomized study of vaginal misoprostol (PGE(1)) and dinoprostone gel (PGE(2)) for induction of labor at term. Ultrasound Obstet Gynecol 18:629-635, 2001

SOGC Clinical Practice Guidelines. Induction of Labour. J Obstet Gynecol Can 2022.

Taylor DR, Doughty AS, Kaufman H, Yang L, Iannucci TA: Uterine rupture with the use of PGE2 vaginal inserts for labor induction in women with previous cesarean sections. J Reprod Med 47:549-554, 2002

Tenore JL: Methods for cervical ripening and induction of labor. Am Fam Physician 67:2123-2128, 2003

Thomas J, Fairclough A, Kavanagh J, Kelly AJ: Vaginal prostaglandin (PGE2 and PGF2a) for induction of labour at term. Cochrane Database Syst Rev 6:CD003101, 2014

Tsakiridis I, Mamopoulos A, Athanasiadis A, Dagklis T: Induction of Labor: An Overview of Guidelines. Obstet Gynecol Surv 75:61-72, 2020

Vaknin Z, Kurzweil Y, Sherman D: Foley catheter balloon vs. locally applied prostaglandins for cervical ripening and labour induction: A systematic review and metaanalysis. Am J Obstet Gynecol 203:418, 2010

World Health Organization: WHO Recommendations: Induction of Labour at or Beyond Term. https://apps.who.int/iris/bitstream/handle/10665/277233/9789241550413-eng.pdf, 2018

CHAPTER 14

Labor Dystocia

Roxanna Mohammed
Darine El-Chaâr

Labor dystocia refers to a slow and abnormal progression of labor. It is the most common problem associated with labor and primarily affects nulliparous women. A Danish study reported a 37-percent incidence of dystocia among uncomplicated pregnancies in nulliparous women. Labor dystocia is the leading indication for primary cesarean sections.

DEFINITION

The definition of *dystocia* is based on the deviations from the normal labor curve established by Friedman. Because it is difficult in many cases to be certain exactly when labor began, dystocia is rarely diagnosed with absolute certainty. A commonly accepted definition of dystocia is a rate of cervical dilatation less than 0.5 cm/hr over 4 hours in the active phase of the first stage of labor or fetal descent of less than 1 cm/hr in the second stage. These definitions are based on the 95th percentile for duration of labor in low-risk women with spontaneous labor. The term *failure to progress* has also been commonly used and refers to either a lack of progressive cervical dilatation or a lack of fetal descent or both.

ETIOLOGY AND RISK FACTORS

The principal causes of dystocia are related to the 4 Ps: power, passenger, passage, and psyche.

Power

Uterine contractions may be infrequent, hypotonic, or incoordinate such that they are unable to dilate the cervix. This is commonly seen in primary dysfunctional labor. Normal uterine contractions in the active phase have been defined as uterine contraction pressures greater than 200 Montevideo units. Maternal exhaustion or dense motor blockage from regional anesthesia can result in ineffective maternal expulsive efforts in the second stage.

Passenger

Fetal malposition and malpresentation (e.g., asynclitism, persistent occiput posterior, brow presentation) are associated with dystocia. If the fetus is disproportionately large relative to the maternal pelvis or if there is a congenital anomaly (hydrocephalus), prolonged labor can also ensue.

Passage

Examination of the pelvis may reveal an inadequate pelvis. Any prominent ischial spines, a narrow pubic arch, or other soft tissue mass (e.g., tumors, septums) may impede progressive descent of the fetus. True *cephalopelvic disproportion* refers to a disparity between the pelvic architecture or size and the fetal head that precludes vaginal delivery.

Inlet Contraction

Inlet contraction is present when the anteroposterior diameter (obstetric conjugate) is less than 10 cm or the transverse diameter is less than 12 cm. Inlet contraction may result from rickets or from generally poor development.

Effects on the fetus are:

1. Failure of engagement
2. Increase in malpositions
3. Deflexion attitudes
4. Exaggerated asynclitism
5. Extreme molding
6. Formation of a large caput succedaneum
7. Prolapse of the umbilical cord. This becomes a complication because the presenting part does not fit the inlet well

Effects on labor include:

1. Dilatation of the cervix is slow and often incomplete
2. Premature rupture of the membranes is common
3. Inefficient uterine action is a frequent accompaniment

Midpelvic Contraction

Midpelvic contraction is basically a reduction in the plane of least dimensions, the one that passes from the apex of the pubic arch through the ischial spines to meet the sacrum usually at the junction of the fourth and fifth segments.

When the distance between the ischial spines is less than 9.0 cm or when the sum of the interspinous (normal, 10.5 cm) and the posterior sagittal (normal, 4.5-5.0 cm) distances is less than 13.5 cm (normal is 15.0-15.5 cm), contraction of the midpelvis is probably present. To obtain accurate measurement of these diameters, x-ray pelvimetry is essential. Clinical suspicion of a small midpelvis is aroused by the finding on manual examination of a small pelvis, the palpation of large spines that jut into the cavity, and the observation that the distance between the ischial tuberosities is less than 8.0 cm.

Midpelvic contraction is a common cause of dystocia and operative delivery. It is more difficult to manage than inlet contraction because if the fetal head cannot even enter the inlet, there is no doubt that abdominal delivery is necessary. However, when the head has descended into the pelvis, one is loath to perform cesarean section, hoping that the head will come down to a point where it can be extracted with forceps. A danger here is that with molding and caput formation, the head may appear lower than it actually is. Instead of the projected midforceps delivery, one is engaged in a high forceps operation, often with disastrous results for both the mother and infant.

Midpelvic contractions may prevent anterior rotation of the occiput and may direct it into the hollow of the sacrum. Failure of rotation and deflexion attitudes are associated frequently with a small pelvic cavity.

Outlet Contraction

Outlet contraction is present when the distance between the ischial tuberosities is less than 8.0 cm. Dystocia may be expected when the sum of the intertuberous diameter and the posterior sagittal diameter is much less than 15.0 cm. Diminution of the intertuberous diameter and the subpubic angle forces the head backward, so the prognosis depends on the capacity of the posterior segment, the mobility at the sacrococcygeal joint, and the ability of the soft tissues to accommodate the passenger. The sides of the posterior triangle are not bony. Although outlet contraction causes an increase in perineal lacerations and a greater need for forceps deliveries, only rarely is it an indication for cesarean section. Because the bituberous diameter can be measured manually, however, and since it may warn us that there is contraction higher in the pelvis, it should always be assessed as part of the routine examination.

Psyche

Pain, anxiety, and stress can inhibit progressive cervical dilatation, especially in the latent phase.

Other Risk Factors for Labor Dystocia

Other risk factors associated with labor dystocia include:

1. Advanced maternal age
2. Obesity
3. Nulliparity
4. Short maternal stature (<150 cm)
5. Medical complications in pregnancy
6. Induction of labor
7. Prelabor rupture of membranes
8. Prolonged latent phase
9. Epidural anesthesia
10. Chorioamnionitis
11. Postterm pregnancy (>41 weeks)
12. Estimated fetal weight large for gestational age
13. Malpositioning or malpresentation (occiput posterior position, face presentation)

These factors may act alone or in concert. A marked abnormality of one or a minor deviation in several can prevent successful spontaneous vaginal birth. Whereas normal delivery is impossible in the presence of absolute cephalopelvic disproportion, a mild disparity between the size of the pelvis and that of the fetus can be overcome by strong and effective uterine contractions. The pelvis may be sufficiently large to accommodate an occipitoanterior presentation but too small for an occipitoposterior one. It is a matter of balance.

COMPLICATIONS OF LABOR DYSTOCIA

Although prolonged labor is worrisome, maternal and neonatal outcomes are generally good. However, if labor dystocia is not recognized and proper interventions are not carried out, it can be associated with serious maternal and neonatal morbidity.

Maternal Complications

1. Postpartum hemorrhage
2. Chorioamnionitis

FIRST STAGE OF LABOR

3. Injuries to the pelvic floor (especially from a prolonged second stage)
4. Increased risk of operative deliveries

Neonatal Complications

Prolonged labor has been associated with a higher risk of meconium-stained fluid at the time of delivery and an increased risk of neonatal infection and bacteremia. There may also be an increased incidence of transient depression at birth requiring immediate resuscitation of the newborn. However, most studies looking at neonatal outcomes in labors with dystocia report overall good neonatal outcomes with no increased risk for fetal asphyxia, lower APGAR scores, or admission to neonatal intensive care unit.

GRAPHIC ANALYSIS OF LABOR

Friedman described a graphic analysis of labor, also called a *partogram* (Fig. 14-1), correlating the duration of labor with the rate of cervical dilatation. On graph paper, the cervical dilatation in centimeters is placed on the ordinate, and the time in hours is plotted on the abscissa. Joining the points of contact makes a sigmoid curve. The rate of cervical dilatation, as shown by the slope of the curve, is described in centimeters per hour.

    Once the active phase of labor begins, changes in cervical dilatation usually proceed at a much faster rate, and labor is closely monitored to ensure adequate progress. The partogram is the documentation of serial assessments of the cervical dilatation and fetal descent as soon as the active phase of labor begins. It is an easy and simple way of visually summarizing

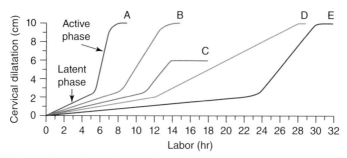

FIGURE 14-1. Normal and abnormal labor during the first stage. A. Average multipara. **B**. Average primigravida. **C**. Secondary arrest of dilatation. **D**. Primary dysfunctional labor. **E**. Prolonged latent phase.

the progress of labor, or the lack of progress, and allows early and objective identification of labor that has deviated from the normal labor curve.

The mean and longest acceptable duration of labor and rates of cervical dilatation were historically established by Friedman in the early 1950s based on a mixed population of women, including women who were in spontaneous and induced labor and fetuses in breech presentations. Friedman's data showed a nonlinear (sigmoid) curve of labor progress in the active phase that encompassed dilatation of the cervix from 2.5 to 10 cm. The average duration of the active phase of labor for nulliparous women was 4.6 hours, and the longest normal duration (mean +2 standard deviation) was 11.7 hours. The average rate of cervical dilatation was 3 cm/hr, and the slowest acceptable rate was 1.2 cm/hr.

Data from the Consortium on Safe Labor have been used to revise the definition of contemporary normal labor progress. This study was conducted at 19 U.S. hospitals, and the duration of labor was analyzed in 62,415 parturient women, each of whom delivered a singleton vertex fetus vaginally and had a normal perinatal outcome. The 95th percentile rate of active phase dilation was substantially slower than the standard rate derived from Friedman's work, carrying from 0.5 cm/hr to 0.7 cm/hr for nulliparous women and from 0.5 cm/hr to 1.3 cm/hr for multiparous women. The data from this study highlights two important features of contemporary labor progress:

1. From 4 to 6 cm, nulliparous and multiparous women dilated at essentially the same rate, and more slowly than historically described. Beyond 6 cm, multiparous women dilated more rapidly
2. The maximal slope in rate of change in cervical dilation over time (i.e., the active phase) often did not start until at least 6 cm

The data from this study suggest that neither active phase protraction or labor arrest should be diagnosed before 6 cm.

CLASSIFICATION OF PROLONGED LABOR

Prolonged Latent Phase

False labor and the latent phase of labor initially share similar characteristics, so determining the actual duration of the latent phase accurately is problematic. The latent phase begins with the onset of true labor and lasts

TABLE 14-1: AVERAGE DURATION OF THE PHASES OF LABOR

	Primigravidas		Multiparas	
	Average	Upper Normal	Average	Upper Normal
Latent phase (hr)	8.6	20	5.3	14
Active phase (hr)	5.8	12	2.5	6
First stage of labor (hr)	13.3	28.5	7.5	20
Rate of cervical dilatation during active phase (cm/hr)	1.2	0.5	1.5	0.8

until the beginning of the active phase of cervical dilatation, when the cervix has usually reached 3 to 4 cm (and even up to 6 cm in newer studies) dilatation in nulliparous women. In nulliparous women, the average length of the latent phase is 8.6 hours, with the upper limit of normal at 20 hours (Table 14-1). For multiparas, the figures are 5.3 and 14 hours. In general, a latent phase that exceeds 20 hours in a nullipara or 14 hours in a multipara is considered prolonged and abnormal.

Wide variations occur, and a prolonged latent period does not necessarily mean that the active phase will be abnormal. The unripe cervix prolongs only the latent phase, and most cervices open normally once effacement is achieved. Even when the latent phase lasts more than 20 hours, many patients advance to normal cervical dilatation when the active phase begins. A diagnosis of labor dystocia should not be made before the onset of the active phase when the cervix is less than 4 cm.

Risk factors for prolonged latent phase include: (1) an unripe cervix at the onset of labor, (2) abnormal position of the fetus (occiput transverse or posterior positions), (3) cephalopelvic disproportion, (4) dysfunctional labor, (5) induction of labor, (6) prelabor rupture of amniotic membranes, and (7) early administration of regional anesthetic with heavy motor block. Maternal age, infant birth weight, pelvic capacity, and gestational age do not affect the duration of the latent phase.

Prolonged Active Phase

The active period lasts from the end of the latent phase to full dilatation of the cervix. The curve changes from the almost horizontal slope of the latent phase to a nearly vertical incline representing a period of steady and rapid cervical dilatation. Recent studies on contemporary labor patterns suggest that this phase is actually more gradual than that suggested by Friedman's curve and in some cases may not actually start until cervical dilatation has reached 5 to 6 cm in a nulliparous woman.

There is considerable variation in the duration of labor and rate of cervical dilatation in the active phase of labor. An active phase longer than 12 hours in a nullipara and longer than 6 hours in a multipara was considered abnormal based on Friedman's data on normal labor. More important than the length of this phase is the speed of cervical dilatation. According to Friedman's data, a rate less than 1.2 cm/hr in nulliparas and 1.5 cm/hr in multiparas is evidence of some abnormality and should alert the attendant.

A recent systematic review of labor duration in nulliparous women in spontaneous labor shows that the upper limit of a normal active phase appears to be longer and rate of cervical dilatation appears to be slower that those set by Friedman. Only half of nulliparous women in the active phase dilated at a rate greater than 1.2 cm/hr. For all of these labor curves, it is evident that the duration of labor varies from woman to woman, and the rate of cervical change is faster in the active first stage and in parous women. These studies suggest that in low-risk nulliparous women with a spontaneous onset of labor, labors progressing at a rate greater than 0.5 cm/hr should be considered normal.

According to newer data, arrest of labor in the first stage is defined as more than or equal to 6-cm dilation with membrane rupture and one of the following:

1. 4 hours of more of adequate contractions (i.e., >200 Montevideo units)
2. 6 hours of more of inadequate contractions and no cervical changes

Accurate assessment of the situation and diagnosis of etiology is vital. Keeping in mind that inefficient uterine action is often associated with disproportion and abnormal position of the fetus, one must not blame the lack of progress on poor contractions until mechanical factors have been ruled out. When ineffective labor (often myometrial fatigue) is the sole cause, half the patients resume progress after no more than treatment with rest and adequate hydration. In this group, amniotomy and oxytocin stimulation work well. When there are complications such as disproportion or abnormal position, the treatment must be aimed in their direction.

FIRST STAGE OF LABOR

Descent of the Presenting Part

Once active descent begins late in the first stage of labor, it should advance progressively throughout the course of the second stage. Interruption of descent usually suggests malpositioning, cephalopelvic disproportion, or abnormalities of uterine action. Diagnosis is based on the demonstration of there being no change in the station of the fetal presenting part over the period of at least 2 hours. Cesarean section and assisted vaginal deliveries are frequently associated with this problem. With difficult or failed operative vaginal deliveries, maternal and fetal trauma are common.

Prolonged Second Stage

Prolonged labor in the second stage was formerly defined as labor exceeding 2 hours in a nullipara and 1 hour in a multipara. Because of the concept of passive and active second stage, these time limits are no longer appropriate definitions of dystocia in the second stage (see Chapter 16). In general, birth should be expected to occur within 3 hours of the start of the active second stage in a nullipara and within 2 hours in a multipara. Delay in the active second stage should therefore be recognized and diagnosed when it has lasted 2 hours in the nullipara and 1 hour in the multipara. Labor dystocia in the second stage has also been defined as a lack of descent or descent less than 1 cm/hr of the fetal presenting part in the active phase of the second stage of labor.

Etiology of Prolonged Second Stage

1. Cephalopelvic disproportion
    a. Small pelvis
    b. Large baby
2. Malpresentation and malposition
3. Ineffective labor
    a. Primary inefficient uterine contractions
    b. Myometrial fatigue: secondary inertia
    c. Constriction (Bandl's ring)
    d. Inability or refusal of the patient to bear down (maternal exhaustion)
    e. Excessive motor block from regional anesthesia
4. Soft tissue dystocia
    a. Narrow vaginal canal
    b. Rigid perineum

Under conditions of good fetal well-being, the second stage can be extended if there appears to be good progress being made and vaginal delivery is likely. Factors that affect the duration of second stage include:

1. Parity
2. Regional anesthesia
3. Duration of first stage of labor
4. Maternal height and weight
5. Fetal weight
6. Fetal position

A prolonged second stage is associated with increased maternal risks, including chorioamnionitis, postpartum hemorrhage, operative vaginal delivery, and third- and fourth-degree perineal lacerations.

MANAGEMENT OF LABOR DYSTOCIA

Management of labor includes several components, including a strict and disciplined approach to the diagnosis of labor, regular assessment of maternal and fetal well-being, and careful monitoring of labor progress. Once labor dystocia is recognized and confirmed, management depends on the etiology and stage or phase of labor. Appropriate and timely intervention with oxytocin augmentation may reduce maternal and neonatal morbidity.

Prevention Strategies

1. Good prenatal care and preparation for childbirth reduce the incidence of prolonged labor. Continuous close support during labor has also been shown to prevent the incidence of labor dystocia
2. Labor should not be induced in the absence of a medical indication for induction and/or when the cervix is not favorable
3. The patient's general physical and mental condition is assessed with respect to fatigue, morale, hydration, and nourishment
4. False labor is treated by adequate rest, hydration, and support. Judicious use of appropriate analgesia in the early phase of labor should also be given
5. Admission to the birthing unit should be delayed until the woman has entered the active phase of labor as long as maternal and fetal well-being are confirmed
6. Avoid routine amniotomy, especially in the latent phase of labor

7. Avoid a diagnosis of labor dystocia in the latent phase of labor. Newer studies suggest cervical dilation of 6 cm to be considered the threshold for active phase of most women in labor
8. Assess adequacy of labor progress. By charting the progress of labor on a partogram (see Fig. 14-1), we can ascertain whether cervical dilatation is occurring at a normal rate, too slowly, or has ceased altogether. The type of abnormality can be diagnosed, and the point at which intervention is necessary is indicated

Vaginal Examination

Once labor dystocia is diagnosed and confirmed (Table 14-2), vaginal examination should be performed at 2-hour intervals in the first stage and 1-hour intervals in the second stage of labor to ensure adequate progress in labor. A careful assessment of the cervix and fetal station and position is performed.

TABLE 14-2: LABOR DYSTOCIA CHECKLIST

1. Diagnosis of Dystocia/Arrest Disorder (all three should be present)
- Cervix 6 cm or greater
- Membranes ruptured, then
- No cervical change after at least 4 hours of adequate uterine activity (e.g., strong to palpation or Montevideo units >200), or at least 6 hours of oxytocin administration with inadequate uterine activity

2. Diagnosis of Second Stage Arrest (only one needed)
No descent or rotation for:
- at least 4 hours of pushing in nulliparous woman with epidural
- at least 3 hours of pushing in nulliparous woman without epidural
- at least 3 hours of pushing in multiparous woman with epidural
- at least 2 hour of pushing in multiparous woman without epidural

3. Diagnosis of Failed Induction (both needed)
- Bishop score ≥6 for multiparous women and ≥8 for nulliparous women, before the start of induction (for nonmedically indicated/elective induction of labor only)
- Oxytocin administered for at least 12-18 hours after membrane rupture, without achieving cervical change and regular contractions. *note: at least 24 hours of oxytocin administration after membrane rupture is preferable if maternal and fetal statuses permit

Adapted from ACOG/SMFM criteria

Reproduced with permission from Smith H, Peterson N, Lagrew D, Main E. 2016. Toolkit to Support Vaginal Birth and Reduce Primary Cesareans: A Quality Improvement Toolkit. Stanford, CA: California Maternal Quality Care Collaborative.

Cervix

Has there been any progress or further dilatation since the last examination? Is the cervix swollen suggestive of obstructed labor? Is an anterior cervical lip caught between the head and the symphysis?

Station of Presenting Part

The station of the bony presenting part is determined. Is it at, above, or below the spines? Has engagement taken place? Is there a caput? Is molding excessive?

Position

The position must be diagnosed accurately. In all cases of prolonged labor, malpositions such as brow presentation and occiput posterior should be kept in mind.

Failure of Descent

What seems to be holding up the presenting part? Is the cause of arrest in the bony pelvis or the cervix? Is the head too big for the pelvis? Or is the problem not the pelvis, the cervix, or the fetus, but in the uterine contractions, and will a few hours of really good labor achieve progress to successful delivery?

Uterine Contractions

The uterine contractions are assessed in terms of strength and frequency. Is the basic problem in the type of labor, or is the main problem elsewhere and the poor uterine action a secondary complication? If the contractions are judged to be efficient, then the reason for the failure of progress must be in another field. Because inefficient uterine action is almost entirely a disorder of primigravidas, multiparas with prolonged labors must be investigated for other factors carefully before a diagnosis of poor labor is made. A woman who has delivered a 7-pound baby with no trouble may not be able to do the same with a 9-pound baby.

The strength of the contractions may be assessed manually or with the use of an electronic external or internal uterine pressure monitoring system.

Dystocia in the First Stage

Mechanical factors must be ruled out. In some cases, there is cephalopelvic disproportion, and cesarean section is indicated. For the rest, hypotonic uterine contractions account for the majority of slowly progressive labor, and medical management is carried out as long as the fetus and mother are in good condition. Nothing is done to complicate the situation further. Slow progress is accepted. Support, reassurance, rest, fluids, and analgesia are provided. Premature and traumatic vaginal operations are not recommended.

Therapeutic Rest

Therapeutic rest involves providing pain relief by effective support and analgesia. Some women who experience excessive pain or anxiety during labor produce high endogenous catecholamines, which has a direct inhibitory effect on uterine contractions. This leads to a vicious cycle of inefficient uterine contractions, poor labor progress, increased anxiety, and higher catecholamines. Nonpharmacologic and pharmacologic options for pain management should be provided.

Parenteral narcotics with a short half-life are effective in providing short-term pain relief. Epidural anesthesia has an advantage of providing effective pain relief for the duration of labor and allows women to rest (see Chapter 36). In particular, it allows the administration of oxytocin augmentation for women with labor dystocia without increasing the amount of labor pain significantly.

Epidural anesthesia is associated with prolonged labor in the first and second stages of labor, an increased incidence of fetal malposition, an increased use of oxytocin augmentation, and an increased risk of assisted vaginal deliveries. It has not been shown to increase the risk of cesarean section, although studies are conflicting.

Amniotomy

Amniotomy alone when used in the latent phase of labor is usually insufficient to result in significant augmentation of labor. Routine and early amniotomy has also not been shown to accelerate spontaneous labor or increase the chance of a successful vaginal delivery. However, in the setting of prolonged or delayed labor in the active phase, amniotomy is recommended in all women with intact membranes. Performing an amniotomy increases local prostaglandin levels and may increase the strength and frequency of uterine contractions. Amniotomy in this setting has also been shown to shorten the duration of the first stage of labor.

Oxytocin

When all other more conservative measures have been attempted to stimulate more effective contractions and in the setting of stable maternal and fetal conditions, it is recommended that labor augmentation be started with oxytocin before a caesarean delivery being performed for "failure to progress." Oxytocin should be initiated in cases of labor dystocia caused by inadequate of inefficient uterine contractions. Oxytocin, when administered intravenously as a constant infusion, increases the frequency, force, and duration of uterine contractions. Several studies have shown that oxytocin augmentation decreases the duration of labor and increases the rate of successful spontaneous vaginal delivery.

It should be used with caution when cephalopelvic disproportion is suspected, in cases of hypersensitivity to oxytocin, uteroplacental insufficiency, abnormal fetal heart rate (FHR), and previous cesarean section.

When oxytocin is used, an initial dose of 1-2 mU/min of oxytocin is started. It should be titrated slowly to achieve a contraction pattern of four or five contractions in 10 minutes. This should be done gradually with a 30-minute interval between dose increases. While most patients achieve a response to stimulation at oxytocin concentrations between 4 and 10 mU/min, a proportion of nullipara require higher doses of oxytocin. When 20 mU/min of oxytocin is reached, a careful reevaluation of the labor progress and maternal and fetal well-being should be carried out before further increases in oxytocin titration. Continuous electronic fetal heart rate monitoring (EFM) should be implemented whenever oxytocin is used.

Tachysystole

Oxytocin use is associated with an increased incidence of tachysystole. *Tachysystole* is defined as a contraction frequency of more than five contractions in 10 minutes with less than 60 seconds of resting tone or uterine contractions lasting for more than 2 minutes. It can occur with or without FHR abnormalities. Persistent uterine tachysystole with FHR abnormalities can lead to fetal hypoxia if not corrected. Appropriate use and titration of the oxytocin dose to achieve minimally effective strength and frequency of uterine contractions, without causing too much, is usually sufficient to correct tachysystole.

Uterine tachysystole is associated with (1) high-dose oxytocin titration regimens (4-6 mU/min oxytocin increments) and (2) when incremental increases in oxytocin dose are increased at intervals of less than 30 minutes.

Fetal Heart Rate Monitoring

Continuous FHR monitoring should be offered when labor dystocia is diagnosed. Whenever oxytocin is used, continuous external or internal FHR monitoring should be used (see Chapter 12).

FIRST STAGE OF LABOR

Cervical Dystocia

The cervix may be holding up progress. A thick anterior lip or a thin, soft rim of cervix may be caught between the head and the symphysis pubis. This can be pushed over the head during a contraction, especially in multiparous women.

Arrest of Labor in the Second Stage

Clinical reassessment of labor progress should be done at hourly intervals in the second stage. It is vital that mechanical factors be ruled out carefully. These include malpositions and malpresentations as well as cephalopelvic disproportion. Cesarean section is performed in most cases of cephalopelvic disproportion.

Maternal and fetal well-being should be monitored carefully. Continuous EFM is recommended when there is a delay in the second stage to ensure that the fetus is tolerating labor. In the setting of good fetal well-being, support, rest, and adequate pain relief for the exhausted mother may be beneficial in the second stage. A passive second stage (or delayed pushing) allows for fetal descent to occur mainly from the action of the uterine contractions without exhausting the mother. Where membranes are still intact in the second stage, they should be artificially ruptured.

Oxytocin should be started as soon as labor dystocia is recognized in the second stage. The same principles for oxytocin use in the first stage of labor are applied in the second stage. It should be used with caution when cephalopelvic disproportion is suspected and in cases of hypersensitivity to oxytocin, uteroplacental insufficiency, abnormal FHR, and previous cesarean section.

If progress is being made and vaginal delivery is expected, the duration of the second stage alone should not mandate intervention with operative delivery.

Operative Delivery

Delivery by cesarean section or assisted vaginal delivery is indicated when there is no further progress despite oxytocin augmentation. In the first stage of labor, an adequate trial of oxytocin augmentation with a minimum of 4 hours of minimally effective uterine contractions should be given before operative delivery is considered. Minimally effective uterine contractions is defined either as uterine contractions achieving 200 or more Montevideo units or three or four strong contractions every 10 minutes.

In spontaneously laboring women with slow progress of labor at term, oxytocin augmentation for 4 hours can result in vaginal deliveries in approximately 80 percent of nulliparous women and 95 percent of multiparous women with no adverse effect on the mother or baby. After an adequate trial of oxytocin augmentation and complete arrest of dilatation of the cervix occurs in the first stage of labor (dilatation arrests at less than 10 cm), vaginal delivery is impossible at this time, and cesarean section must be performed.

When arrest of labor in the second stage is established, operative delivery is indicated when there is no further descent of the presenting part after 1 hour of active pushing with adequate contractions. If the presenting part is low in the pelvis, there is no disproportion, and the baby may be delivered by forceps or vacuum if the presentation is cephalic and by cesarean section if he or she is a breech. The decision to proceed with an assisted vaginal delivery versus a cesarean section should be made on the basis of the clinical assessment of the mother and fetus and the skill of the obstetrician.

At any sign fetal or maternal distress, early intervention and operative delivery are indicated. Preparations should be at hand for the treatment of postpartum hemorrhage and fetal distress.

SELECTED READING

American College of Obstetricians and Gynecologists: Dystocia and Augmentation of Labor. ACOG Practice Bulletin No. 49. Obstet Gynecol 102:1445-1454, 2003

American College of Obstetrics and Gynecology, Society for Maternal-Fetal Medicine: Obstetric care consensus no. 1: Safe prevention of the primary cesarean delivery. Obstet Gynecol 123:693-711, 2014

Drouin P, Nasah BT, Nkounawa F: The value of the Partogramme in the management of labor. Obstet Gynecol 53:741, 1979

Friedman EA: Disordered labor. Objective evaluation and management. J Family Pract 2:167, 1975

Friedman EA, Sachtleben MR: Station of the fetal presenting part. Arrest in nulliparas. Obstet Gynecol 47:129, 1976

Kjaergaard H, Olsen J, Ottesen B, Dykes AK: Incidence and outcomes of dystocia in the active phase of labor in term nulliparous women with spontaneous labor onset. Acta Obstet Gynecol Scand 88:402, 2009

Maltau JM, Anderson HT: Epidural anesthesia as an alternative to cesarean section in the treatment of prolonged, exhaustive labour. Acta Anesthesiol Scand 19:349, 1975

National Institute for Health and Clinical Excellence: Intrapartum Care, care of healthy women and their babies during childbirth. http://guidance.nice.org.uk/CG55/Guidance, 2007

FIRST STAGE OF LABOR

Neal JL, Lowe NK, Ahijevych KL et al: Active labor duration and dilation rates among low-risk, nulliparous women with spontaneous labor onset: A systematic review. J Midwifery Womens Health 55:308-318, 2010

Rouse DJ, Owen J, Savage KG, Hauth, JC: Active phase labor arrest: oxytocin augmentation for at least 4 hours. Obstet Gynecol 93:323, 1999

Spong CY, Berghella V, Wenstrom KD, Mercer BM, Saade GR: Preventing the first cesarean delivery: summary of a joint Eunice Kennedy Shriver National Institute of Child Health and Human Development, Society for Maternal-Fetal Medicine, and American College of Obstetricians and Gynecologists Workshop. Obstet Gynecol 120:1181-1193, 2012

Zhang J, Landy HJ, Branch DW, et al: Contemporary patterns of spontaneous labor with normal neonatal outcomes. Obstet Gynecol 116:1281, 2010

CHAPTER 15

Abnormal Cephalic Presentations

Roxanna Mohammed
Darine El-Chaâr

MALPRESENTATIONS

The fetus enters the pelvis in a cephalic presentation approximately 95 to 96 percent of the time. In these cephalic presentations, the occiput may be in the persistent transverse or posterior positions. In about 3 to 4 percent of pregnancies, there is a breech-presenting fetus (see Chapter 25). In the remaining 1 percent, the fetus may be either in a transverse or oblique lie (see Chapter 26), or the head may be extended with the face or brow presenting.

Predisposing Factors

Maternal and Uterine Factors

1. Contracted pelvis: This is the most common and important factor
2. Pendulous maternal abdomen: If the uterus and fetus are allowed to fall forward, there may be difficulty in engagement
3. Neoplasms: Uterine fibromyomas or ovarian cysts can block the entry to the pelvis
4. Uterine anomalies: In a bicornuate uterus, the nonpregnant horn may obstruct labor in the pregnant one
5. Abnormalities of placental size or location: Conditions such as placenta previa are associated with unfavorable positions of the fetus
6. High parity

Fetal Factors

1. Large baby
2. Errors in fetal polarity, such as breech presentation and transverse lie
3. Abnormal internal rotation: The occiput rotates posteriorly or fails to rotate at all
4. Fetal attitude: Extension in place of normal flexion
5. Multiple pregnancy
6. Fetal anomalies, including hydrocephaly and anencephaly
7. Polyhydramnios: An excessive amount of amniotic fluid allows the fetus freedom of activity, and he or she may assume abnormal positions
8. Prematurity

Placenta and Membranes

1. Placenta previa
2. Cornual implantation
3. Premature rupture of membranes

Effects of Malpresentations

Effects on Labor

The less symmetrical adaptation of the presenting part to the cervix and to the pelvis plays a part in reducing the efficiency of labor.

1. The incidence of fetopelvic disproportion is higher
2. Inefficient uterine action is common. The contractions tend to be weak and irregular
3. Prolonged labor is seen frequently
4. Pathologic retraction rings can develop, and rupture of the lower uterine segment may be the end result
5. The cervix often dilates slowly and incompletely
6. The presenting part stays high
7. Premature rupture of the membranes occurs often
8. The need for operative delivery is increased

Effects on the Mother

1. Because greater uterine and intra-abdominal muscular effort is required and because labor is often prolonged, maternal exhaustion is common
2. There is more stretching of the perineum and soft parts, and there are more lacerations
3. Bleeding is more profuse, originating from:
   a. Tears of the uterus, cervix, and vagina
   b. Uterine atony from prolonged labor
4. There is a greater incidence of infection. This is caused by:
   a. Early rupture of the membranes
   b. Excessive blood loss
   c. Tissue damage
   d. Frequent rectal and vaginal examinations
   e. Prolonged labor

FIRST STAGE OF LABOR

5. The patient's discomfort seems out of proportion to the strength of the uterine contractions. She complains bitterly of pain before the uterus is felt to harden and continues to feel the pain after the uterus has relaxed
6. Paresis of the bowel and bladder add to the patient's suffering

Effects on the Fetus

1. The fetus fits the pelvis less perfectly, making passage through the pelvis more difficult and leading to excessive molding
2. The long labor is harder on the baby, with a greater incidence of a low arterial cord pH at the time of delivery. Without appropriate and timely intervention, this can lead to anoxia, brain damage, asphyxia, and intra-uterine death
3. There is a higher incidence of operative delivery, increasing the danger of trauma to the baby
4. Prolapse of the umbilical cord is more common than in normal positions

TRANSVERSE POSITIONS OF THE OCCIPUT

Left Occiput Transverse: LOT

Engagement is more frequent in the transverse diameter of the inlet than in the oblique. LOT is the most common position at the onset of labor (Fig. 15-1).

Diagnosis of Position: LOT

Abdominal Examination

1. The lie is longitudinal
2. The head is at or in the pelvis
3. The back is on the left and toward the mother's flank
4. The small parts are on the right and sometimes can be felt clearly
5. The breech is in the fundus of the uterus
6. The cephalic prominence (forehead) is on the right

Fetal Heart. The fetal heart is heard loudest in the left lower quadrant of the mother's abdomen.

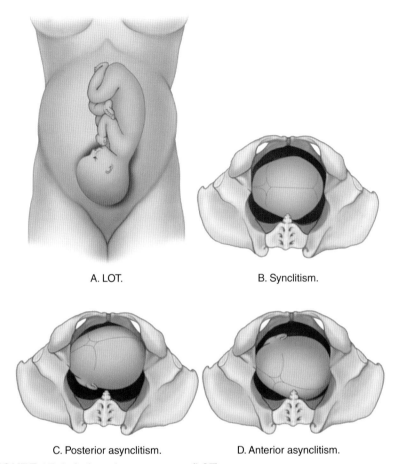

A. LOT.   B. Synclitism.

C. Posterior asynclitism.   D. Anterior asynclitism.

FIGURE 15-1. Left occiput transverse (LOT).

FIRST STAGE OF LABOR

Vaginal Examination

1. The sagittal suture is in the transverse diameter of the pelvis. If the head is in synclitism (Fig. 15-1B), the sagittal suture is midway between the symphysis pubis and the promontory of the sacrum. If there is posterior asynclitism (Fig. 15-1C), the sagittal suture is closer to the pubic symphysis. With anterior asynclitism (Fig. 15-1D), the sagittal suture is closer to the sacral promontory
2. The small posterior fontanel is toward the mother's left at 3 o'clock
3. The bregma is on the right at 9 o'clock
4. If there is flexion, the occiput is lower than the brow. If flexion is poor, the occiput and brow are almost at the same level in the pelvis

Mechanism of Labor: LOT

Descent. Descent includes engagement, which may have taken place before labor (Figs. 15-2A and B). Descent continues throughout labor.

Flexion. Resistance to descent causes the head to flex (Fig. 15-2B) so that the chin approaches the chest. This reduces the presenting diameter by 1.5 cm. The occipitofrontal diameter of 11.0 cm is replaced by the sub-occipitobregmatic diameter of 9.5 cm.

Internal Rotation. The head enters the pelvis with the sagittal suture in the transverse diameter of the inlet and the occiput at 3 o'clock. The occiput then rotates 90° to arrive under the pubic symphysis. The sinciput comes to lie anterior to the sacrum. The sequence is LOT to left occiput anterior (LOA) to occiput anterior (OA) (Figs. 15-2A to 2D). The shoulders lag behind 45° so that when the sagittal suture of the head is in the anteroposterior diameter of the pelvis, the shoulders are in the left oblique. Thus, the neck is twisted.

Extension. Birth is by extension (Figs. 15-2E and F). The nape of the neck pivots under the pubis, while the vertex, bregma, forehead, face, and chin are born over the perineum.

Restitution. When the head has made its exit, the neck untwists, and the head turns back 45° to the left, resuming the normal relationship with the shoulders—OA to LOA (Fig. 15-2G).

External Rotation. The shoulders now rotate 45° to the left to bring their bisacromial diameter into the anteroposterior diameter of the pelvis. The head follows the shoulder and rotates externally another 45° to the left—LOA to LOT (Fig. 15-2H).

Birth of Shoulders, Trunk, and Placenta. Birth of the shoulders, trunk, and placenta is the same as described in Chapter 10, "Normal Mechanism of Labor." A summary of the mechanism of labor (LOT) is presented in Figure 15-3.

Clinical Course of Labor: LOT

Most fetuses who begin labor in the LOT position rotate the head 90° (LOT to LOA to OA) to bring the occiput under the pubic symphysis, from which position spontaneous delivery takes place.

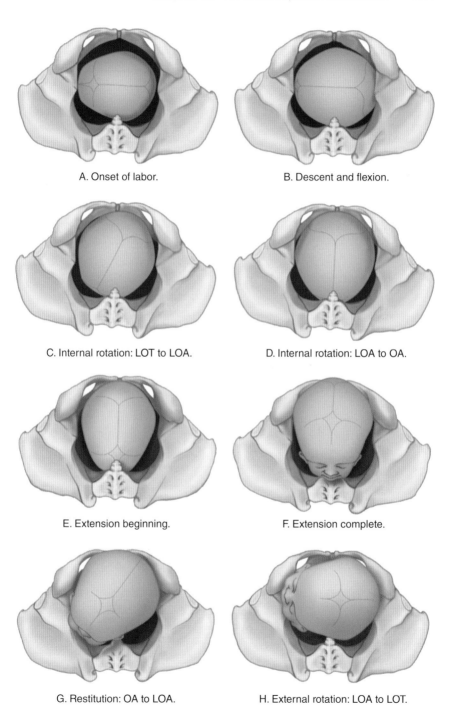

A. Onset of labor.

B. Descent and flexion.

C. Internal rotation: LOT to LOA.

D. Internal rotation: LOA to OA.

E. Extension beginning.

F. Extension complete.

G. Restitution: OA to LOA.

H. External rotation: LOA to LOT.

FIRST STAGE OF LABOR

FIGURE 15-2. Mechanism of labor: left occiput transverse (LOT). LOA, left occiput anterior; OA, occiput anterior.

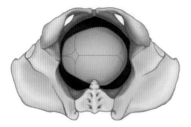

A. At onset of labor.

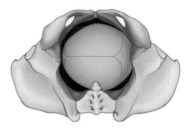

B. Descent and flexion.

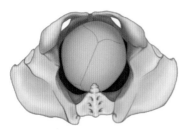

C. Internal rotation: LOT to LOA.

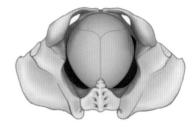

D. Internal rotation: LOA to OA.

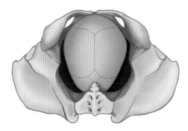

E. Extension beginning.

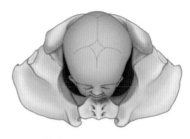

F. Extension complete.

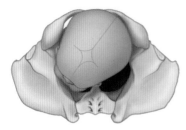

G. Restitution: OA to LOA.

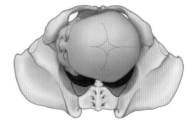

H. External rotation: LOA to LOT.

FIGURE 15-3. Summary of the mechanism of labor: left occiput transverse (LOT).
LOA, left occiput anterior; OA, occiput anterior.

Arrest of Progress. Arrest of progress can occur in any of these situations:

1. Anterior rotation of 90° to the OA position but spontaneous delivery does not take place
2. Anterior rotation of 45° with cessation of progress in the LOA position
3. No rotation. The head is arrested with the sagittal suture in the transverse diameter of the pelvis. This is known as transverse arrest
4. In the rare case posterior rotation takes place, LOT to left occiput posterior (LOP). The mechanism of labor then becomes that of occipitoposterior positions

Management of Arrested Cases. Providing the prerequisites for operative vaginal delivery are present (see Chapter 17), the following treatment is carried out:

1. Arrest in OA position: Forceps or vacuum are applied to the sides of the fetal head, which is then extracted
2. Arrest as LOA: Forceps or vacuum are applied to the fetal head, which is then rotated 45° to the OA position and extracted
3. Transverse arrest: LOT: Two operative techniques are available
   a. Manual rotation, 90°, LOT to LOA to OA, followed by forceps or vacuum extraction
   b. Application of the forceps to the sides of the baby's head, rotation by the forceps of 90°, LOT to LOA to OA, and then extraction by the forceps or vacuum
4. Arrest as an occiput posterior is treated like other occiput posterior deliveries

Right Occiput Transverse: ROT

ROT is similar to LOT. The difference is that the back and occiput are on the mother's right, and the limbs are on her left.

POSTERIOR POSITIONS OF THE OCCIPUT

General Considerations

Definition
The occiput and the small posterior fontanel are in the rear segment of the maternal pelvis, and the brow and bregma are in the anterior segment.

FIRST STAGE OF LABOR

Incidence

The incidence of this position is 15 to 30 percent of all cephalic presentations and is more common in nulliparous women. The exact incidence of posterior positions is difficult to ascertain since most of them rotate anteriorly and are considered erroneously as being originally occipitoanterior. The posterior positions that rotate anteriorly with no difficulty are often not diagnosed, and only the persistent posteriors are recognized regularly. Right occiput posterior (ROP) is five times as common as LOP.

Etiology

The etiology of posterior positions of the occiput is the same as the etiology of other abnormal positions. Cephalopelvic disproportion is a frequent and serious complicating factor that must be considered at all times. The shape of the pelvic inlet influences the position of the occiput. Where the forepelvis is narrow, there is a tendency for the back of the head with its long biparietal diameter to be pushed to the rear, so that the front of the head with its short bitemporal diameter can be accommodated by the small forepelvis. Hence, posterior positions of the occiput are found often in android and anthropoid pelvises.

Right Occiput Posterior: ROP

Diagnosis of Position: ROP

Abdominal Examination

1. The lie is vertical. The long axis of the fetus is parallel to the long axis of the mother (Fig. 15-4)
2. The head is at or in the pelvis
3. The fetal back is in the right maternal flank. In most cases, it cannot be outlined clearly
4. The small parts are easily felt anteriorly on the left side. The maternal abdomen has been described as being alive with little hands and feet
5. The breech is in the fundus of the uterus
6. The cephalic prominence is on the left. It is not felt as easily as in anterior positions because flexion is less marked

Fetal Heart. Fetal heart tones are transmitted through the scapula and hence are heard in the right maternal flank on the same side as the baby's back. Frequently, the fetal heart sounds are indistinct. They can be

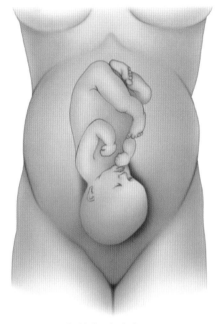

A. Abdominal view.

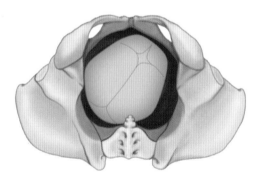

B. Vaginal view.

FIGURE 15-4. **Right occiput posterior.**

transmitted through the baby's chest and in some cases are loudest in the left anterior lower quadrant of the abdomen. The location of the fetal heart sounds is not a reliable sign in determining how the baby is placed; hence, a carefully made diagnosis of posterior position should not be changed because of the situation of the fetal heart. As the back rotates anteriorly, the fetal heart tones approach the midline of the abdomen.

Vaginal Examination

1. The sagittal suture is in the right oblique diameter of the pelvis
2. The small posterior fontanel is in the right posterior segment of the pelvis
3. The bregma is anterior and to the left of the symphysis pubis
4. Since flexion is imperfect, the fontanels may be close to the same level in the pelvis
5. Where there is difficulty in diagnosis, the pinna (auricle) of the ear is found pointing to the occiput

Mechanism of Labor: ROP

Rotation of varying degree and direction can take place:

1. Anterior rotation:
   a. Long arc rotation of 135°, ROP to ROT to right occiput anterior (ROA) to OA. This occurs in 90 percent of occipitoposterior positions. The baby is born as an occipitoanterior
   b. Rotation of 90°, ROP to ROT to ROA
   c. Rotation of 45°, ROP to ROT. The result is deep transverse arrest
2. No rotation. The position remains ROP
3. Posterior rotation of 45°, ROP to OP with the occiput turning into the hollow of the sacrum

Spontaneous delivery can take place after:

1. Anterior rotation to OA with normal birth
2. Posterior rotation to OP with face to pubis delivery

Arrest of labor can occur:

1. High in the pelvis, with failure to engage. These are often problems of disproportion
2. In the midpelvis, with complete or partial failure of rotation
   a. Deep transverse arrest, ROT
   b. Arrest with the sagittal suture in the right oblique diameter of the pelvis, ROP
   c. Arrest with the occiput in the hollow of the sacrum, OP
3. Arrest at the outlet

Long Arc Rotation: 135° to the Anterior

DESCENT. The head enters the inlet with the sagittal suture in the right oblique diameter (Fig. 15-5A), and unless obstruction is encountered descent continues throughout labor. Engagement may be delayed, and the entire labor may take longer than in normal anterior positions.

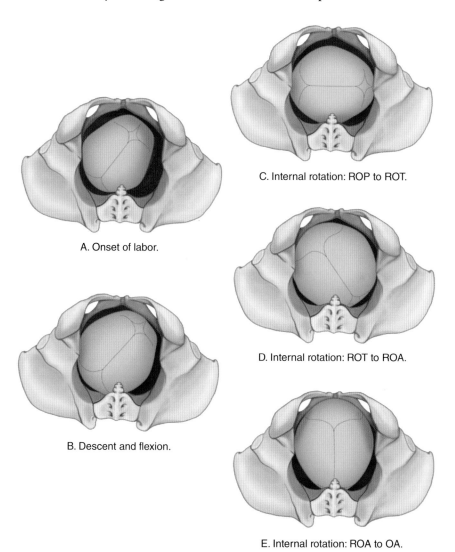

A. Onset of labor.

B. Descent and flexion.

C. Internal rotation: ROP to ROT.

D. Internal rotation: ROT to ROA.

E. Internal rotation: ROA to OA.

FIRST STAGE OF LABOR

FIGURE 15-5. Right occiput posterior (ROP): long arc rotation. OA, occiput anterior; ROA, right occiput anterior.

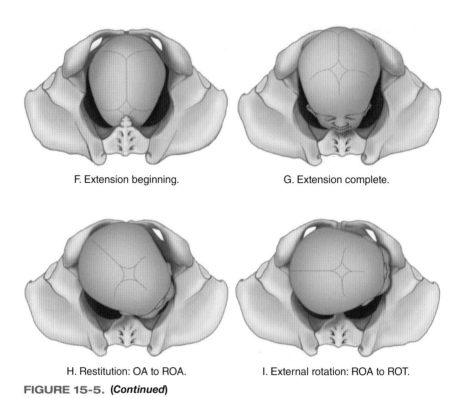

F. Extension beginning.

G. Extension complete.

H. Restitution: OA to ROA.

I. External rotation: ROA to ROT.

FIGURE 15-5. *(Continued)*

FLEXION. Flexion (Fig. 15-5B) is imperfect and often is not complete until the head reaches the pelvic floor. The partial flexion and the resulting larger diameter of the presenting part contribute to the labor being longer and harder for both the mother and child.

INTERNAL ROTATION. The occiput rotates 135° anteriorly under the symphysis pubis—ROP to ROT to ROA to OA (Figs. 15-5C to E).

EXTENSION. The nape of the neck pivots in the subpubic angle, and the head is born by extension (Figs. 15-5F and G). The bregma, forehead, nose, mouth, and chin pass over the perineum in order.

RESTITUTION. Restitution (OA to ROA) takes place to the right (Fig. 15-5H). The extent of restitution depends on how far the shoulders have followed the head during internal rotation. In most cases, the shoulders turn with the head, lagging behind only 45°, and restitution is the usual 45°.

Occasionally, the shoulders may lag behind more or may swing back. The head then restitutes 90° or even 135°.

EXTERNAL ROTATION. The anterior shoulder strikes the pelvic floor and rotates 45° toward the pubic symphysis so that the bisacromial diameter of the shoulders is in the anteroposterior diameter of the outlet. The head follows the shoulders, and the occiput rotates 45° to the right transverse position—ROA to ROT (Fig. 15-5I).

Short Arc Rotation: 45° to the Posterior

DESCENT. The head enters the inlet with the sagittal suture in the right oblique (Fig. 15-6A). Descent continues throughout labor.

FLEXION. Flexion (Fig. 15-6B) is imperfect, resulting in a longer presenting diameter.

INTERNAL ROTATION. The occiput turns posteriorly 45° (ROP to OP) into the hollow of the sacrum (Fig. 15-6C). The sagittal suture is in the antero-posterior diameter of the pelvis. The bregma is behind the pubis.

BIRTH OF HEAD. Birth of the head is by a combination of flexion and extension (Fig. 15-6D-G).

There are two mechanisms of flexion:

1. Where there is good flexion, the area anterior to the bregma pivots under the symphysis pubis. The presenting diameter is the suboccipi-tofrontal of 10.5 cm. The bregma, vertex, small fontanel, and occiput are born by further flexion
2. Where flexion is incomplete, the root of the nose pivots under the sym-physis. The presenting diameter is the larger occipitofrontal of 11.5 cm. This bigger diameter is more traumatic than the smaller one. By flexion, the forehead, bregma, vertex, and occiput are born over the perineum

After the top and back of the head have been born by flexion, the occiput falls back toward the anus, and the nose, mouth, and chin are born under the symphysis pubis by extension (Figs. 15-6H and I).

Restitution of the occiput is 45° to the right oblique (OP to ROP) to resume the normal relationship of the head to the shoulders (Fig. 15-6J).

FIRST STAGE OF LABOR

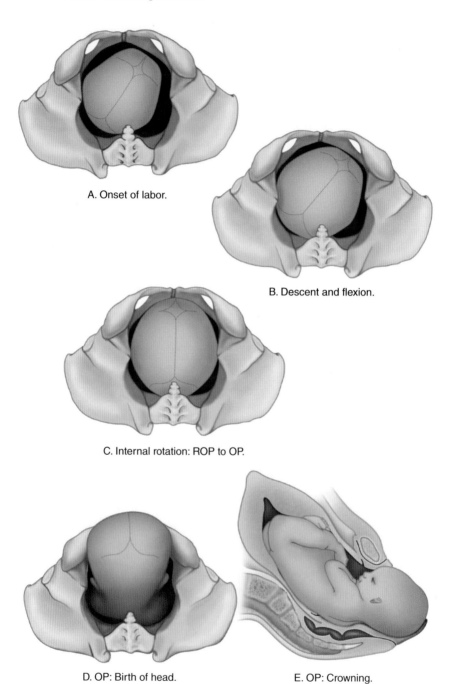

A. Onset of labor.

B. Descent and flexion.

C. Internal rotation: ROP to OP.

D. OP: Birth of head.

E. OP: Crowning.

FIGURE 15-6. Right occiput posterior (ROP): short arc rotation. OP, occiput posterior; ROT, right occiput transverse.

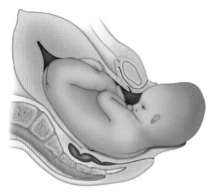

F. OP: Flexion beginning.

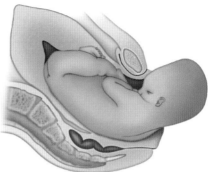

G. OP: Flexion complete.

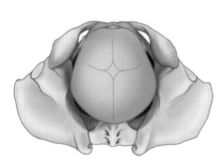

H. Extension: Vaginal view.

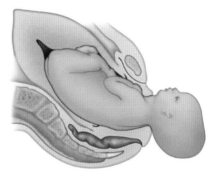

I. Extension: Lateral view.

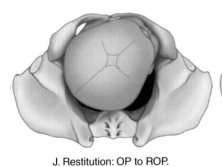

J. Restitution: OP to ROP.

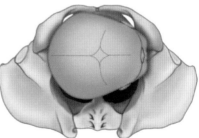

K. External rotation: ROP to ROT.

FIGURE 15-6. (Continued)

FIRST STAGE OF LABOR

The anterior shoulder strikes the pelvic floor and rotates 45° toward the symphysis pubis to bring the bisacromial diameter of the shoulders into the anteroposterior diameter of the pelvis (external rotation). The head follows, and the occiput rotates 45° to the right transverse position— ROP to ROT (Fig. 15-6K).

Molding. In persistent occipitoposterior positions, the head is shortened in the occipitofrontal and lengthened in the suboccipitobregmatic and mentobregmatic diameters. The head rises steeply in front and in back. The caput succedaneum is located over the bregma. Molding (Fig. 15-7) and extensive edema of the scalp make accurate identification of the sutures and fontanels difficult, thereby obscuring the diagnosis.

Summaries. Summaries of both long arc and short arc rotations may be reviewed in Figures 15-8 and 15-9, respectively.

Management of the Persistent Occiput Posterior Position

1. Expectant observation is the best policy. Given sufficient time, most posterior positions of the occiput rotate anteriorly, and the baby is delivered spontaneously or by low forceps or vacuum. Thus, as long as the fetus and mother are in good condition and labor is progressing, there is no justification for interference. The safe and wise rule is to

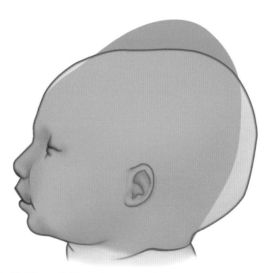

FIGURE 15-7. Molding: right occiput posterior.

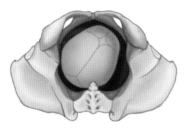

A. ROP: Onset of labor.

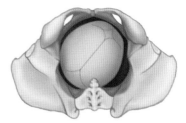

B. Descent and flexion.

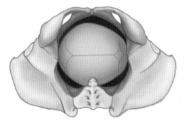

C. Internal rotation: ROP to ROT.

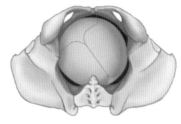

D. Internal rotation: ROT to ROA.

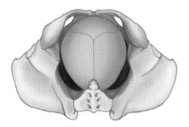

E. Internal rotation: ROA to OA.

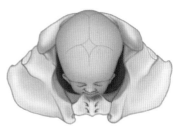

F. Extension.

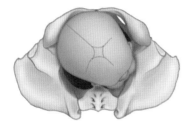

G. Restitution: OA to ROA.

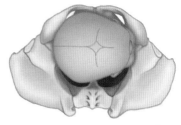

H. External rotation: ROA to ROT.

FIGURE 15-8. Summary of long arc rotation: right occiput posterior (ROP) toocciput posterior (OP). OA, occiput anterior; ROA, right occiput anterior; ROT, right occiput transverse.

FIRST STAGE OF LABOR

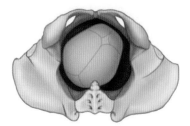

A. ROP: Onset of labor.

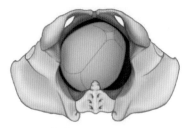

B. Descent and flexion.

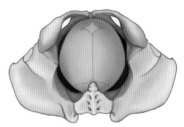

C. Internal rotation: ROP to OP.

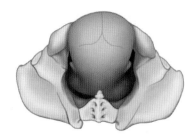

D. Birth by flexion.

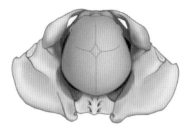

E. Head falls back in extension.

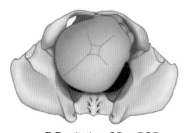

F. Restitution: OP to ROP.

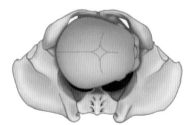

G. External rotation: ROP to ROT.

FIGURE 15-9. Summary of short arc rotation: right occiput posterior (ROP) to occiput posterior (OP). ROT, right occiput transverse.

leave occipitoposterior positions to nature, supplying only supportive measures until there is a definite indication for intervention

2. Placing the mother in forward-leaning or side-lying positions may help the rotation of the occiput. Forward-leaning positions such as kneeling, straddling, and hands and knees positions may enhance the rotation and reduce back pain. It is believed that anterior rotation is helped by the mother's lying on the same side toward which the occiput is already directed. So if the fetus is in the ROP position, the mother lies on her right side

3. Because the labor may be long and difficult for mother and child, care must be exercised to ensure adequate intake of fluids and nourishment. More judicious use of analgesia and sedation is required than in normal occipitoanterior positions

4. If effective labor does not begin, the uterus may be stimulated using an intravenous oxytocin infusion as per protocol developed in each institution. The drip is started slowly at a rate of about 1 to 2 milliunits/hr and then increased every half an hour by either 1 to 2 milliunits/hr. During this time, the effect on the contractions and the fetal heart is observed. The aim is to achieve good uterine contractions every 2 to 3 minutes, lasting 45 to 60 seconds (see Chapter 14)

5. Intact membranes do not always help labor and often even seem to delay it. Therefore, before the progress of labor can be considered halted, the membranes should be ruptured artificially and the patient given a further trial of labor. With these measures, the patient frequently makes good progress in rotation and descent, and spontaneous delivery takes place

6. When the head is delivered in the posterior position (face to pubis), the large back part of the head (biparietal diameter, 9.5 cm) causes greater stretching and more lacerations of the perineum than does the narrow anterior part of the head (bitemporal diameter, 8.0 cm). For this reason, an episiotomy may sometimes be helpful. Frequently, there is arrest at the perineum, and low forceps or vacuum is the management of choice

7. With forceps or vacuum, the fetal head can be delivered in the posterior position or can be rotated to the anterior position before being extracted. The various maneuvers are described in Chapter 17. If an attempt at operative vaginal delivery fails, cesarean section is performed

8. If there has been no progress in the face of efficient uterine contractions and a diagnosis of fetopelvic disproportion has been made, cesarean section should be performed

Indications for Intervention

Although the basic strategy of nonintervention is, up to a point, a wise one, it is not safe to wait too long; fine judgment is needed to decide the point at which further delay is undesirable or even harmful. When the standard signs of fetal concern or maternal distress are present, the decision to interfere is based on clear-cut grounds.

Maternal Distress. Maternal distress is fatigue or exhaustion and is accompanied by the following signs:

1. Pulse >100 bpm
2. Temperature >100°F
3. Dehydration, dry tongue, dry skin, concentrated urine
4. Loss of emotional stability

Fetal Distress. Fetal distress is shown by:

1. Irregular fetal heart rate
2. Fetal heart rate <100 or >160 bpm between uterine contractions
3. Passage of meconium in a vertex presentation

Lack of Progress. The cessation of descent and/or rotation indicates that labor is arrested and that interference is mandatory. Reasons for failure of descent and rotation include:

1. Cephalopelvic disproportion
2. Android midpelvis
3. Ineffective uterine contractions
4. Deflexion of the head
5. Uterine contraction ring preventing the shoulders from rotating anteriorly
6. Multiparity, pendulous abdomen, poor abdominal and uterine tone
7. A weak pelvic floor, failing to guide the occiput anteriorly

BROW PRESENTATIONS

General Considerations

Definition

Brow presentation is an attitude of partial (halfway) extension in contrast to face presentation in which extension is complete. The presenting part is the area between the orbital ridges and the bregma. The denominator is the forehead (frontum: Fr). The presenting diameter is the verticomental, which, at 13.5 cm, is the longest anteroposterior diameter of the fetal head.

Incidence

The incidence is under 1 percent, ranging from one in 500 to one in 1400. Primary brow presentations—those that occur before labor has started—are rare. The majorities are secondary—that is, they occur after the onset of labor. Often the position is transitory, and the head either flexes to an occiput presentation or extends completely and becomes a face presentation.

Etiology

The causes are similar to those of face presentation and include anything that interferes with engagement in flexion.

1. Cephalopelvic disproportion is of great significance
2. Some fetal conditions prevent flexion
   a. Tumors of the neck (e.g., thyroid)
   b. Coils of umbilical cord around the neck
   c. Fetal anomalies
3. Increased fetal mobility
   a. Polyhydramnios
   b. Small or premature baby
4. Premature rupture of membranes when the head is not engaged. It is trapped in an attitude of extension
5. Uterine abnormalities
   a. Neoplasm of lower segment
   b. Bicornuate uterus
6. Abnormal placental implantation: placenta previa
7. Iatrogenic: external version

Left Frontum Anterior: LFrA

Diagnosis of Position: LFrA

Abdominal Examination

1. The lie is longitudinal (Fig. 15-10A)
2. The head is at the pelvis but is not engaged

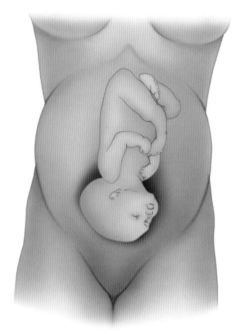

A. Abdominal view.

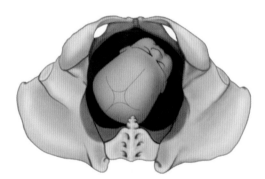

B. Vaginal view.

FIGURE 15-10. **Left frontum anterior.**

3. The back is on the mother's right and posterior; it may be difficult to palpate. The small parts are on the left and anterior
4. The breech is in the fundus of the uterus
5. The cephalic prominence (occiput) and the back are on the same side (the right)

Fetal Heart. Fetal heart sounds are heard best in the left lower quadrant of the maternal abdomen.

Vaginal Examination

1. The anteroposterior diameter of the head is in the right oblique diameter of the pelvis (Fig. 15-10B)
2. The brow, the area between the nasion and the bregma, presents and is felt in the left anterior quadrant of the pelvis
3. The vertex is in the right posterior quadrant
4. The bregma (anterior fontanel) is palpated easily
5. The frontal suture is felt, but the sagittal suture is usually out of reach
6. Identification of the supraorbital ridges is a key to diagnosis

Late and Failed Diagnosis. The difference, on vaginal examination, between the hard, smooth dome of the skull and the soft, irregular face is great enough to diagnose the abnormal position or at least to suspect it. On the other hand, the feel of the vertex and that of the forehead may be similar, and molding and edema add to the difficulty of differentiation. Hence, anything short of a most careful abdominal and vaginal examination with a high index of suspicion fails to identify the malposition. A good rule is that whenever there is failure of progress, one should examine the patient thoroughly, keeping brow presentation in mind.

Mechanism of Labor: LFrA

The presenting diameter is the verticomental, measuring 13.5 cm. It is the longest anteroposterior diameter of the head. When engagement takes place, it is accompanied by extensive molding, and when progress occurs, it is slow.

Spontaneous delivery is rare and can take place only when there is the combination of a large pelvis, strong uterine contractions, and a small baby. In these cases, the following mechanism of labor occurs (Fig. 15-11):

Extension. The head extends and the verticomental diameter presents, with the forehead leading the way.

Descent. Descent is slow and late. Usually the head does not settle into the pelvis until the membranes have ruptured and the cervix has reached full dilatation.

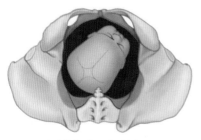

A. LFrA: Onset of labor.

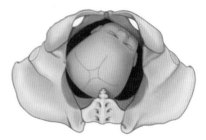

B. Descent.

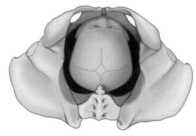

C. Internal rotation: LFrA to FrA.

FIGURE 15-11. Labor: left frontum anterior (LFrA). Descent, internal rotation. FrA, frontum anterior.

Internal Rotation. The forehead rotates anteriorly 45° so that the face comes to lie behind the pubic symphysis (LFrA to frontum anterior [FrA]). A considerable amount of internal rotation may take place between the ischial spines and the tuberosities.

Flexion. The face impinges under the pubis, and as the head pivots round this point, the bregma, vertex, and occiput are born over the perineum (Figs. 15-12A to C).

Extension. The head then falls back in extension (Figs. 15-13A and B), and the nose, mouth, and chin slip under the symphysis.

Restitution. The neck untwists, and the head turns 45° back to the original side (Fig. 15-14A).

External Rotation. As the shoulder rotates anteriorly from the oblique to the anteroposterior diameter of the pelvis, the head turns back another 45° (Fig. 15-14B).

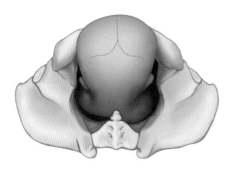

A. Birth by flexion.

B. Flexion beginning.

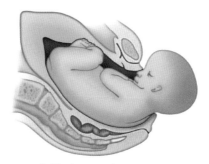

C. Flexion complete.

FIGURE 15-12. **Birth of brow and head by flexion.**

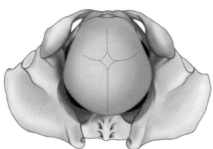

A. Vaginal view.

B. Lateral view.

FIGURE 15-13. **Head falls back in extension.**

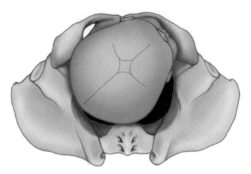

A. Restitution: FrA to LFrA.

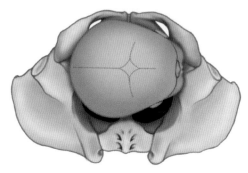

B. External rotation: LFrA to LFrT.

FIGURE 15-14. Restitution, external rotation. FrA, frontum anterior; LFra, left frontum anterior; LFrT, left frontum transverse.

Molding. Molding is extreme (Fig. 15-15). The verticomental diameter is compressed. The occipitofrontal diameter is elongated markedly so that the forehead bulges greatly. The face is flattened, and the distance from the chin to the top of the head is long. This is exaggerated by the large caput succedaneum that forms on the forehead.

Prognosis: Brow Presentations

Labor

In most cases, brow presentations do not deliver spontaneously. If the malposition is detected early in labor and if appropriate therapeutic measures are undertaken, the fetal and maternal results are good. Failure to recognize the problem leads to prolonged and traumatic labor.

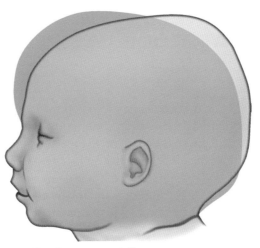

FIGURE 15-15. Molding: brow presentation.

Mother

Passage of a brow through the pelvis is slower, harder, and more traumatic to the mother than any other presentation. Perineal laceration is inevitable and may extend high into the vaginal fornices or into the rectum because of the large diameter offered to the outlet.

Fetus

The fetal mortality rate is high. The excessive molding may cause irreparable damage to the brain. Mistakes in diagnosis and treatment are the main causes of the poor fetal prognosis.

Management of Brow Presentations

1. *Trial of labor:* Since brow presentation may be transitory, a trial of labor is permissible in the hope that flexion to an occiput presentation or complete extension to a face presentation will take place
2. *Persistent brow presentation:* Since brow presentations cannot deliver spontaneously, operative interference is necessary
   a. Cesarean section is the treatment of choice, giving the best results for both the mother and child
   b. Flexion of the head may be attempted, especially in multiparas. This procedure is carried out when the cervix is dilated and soon after the membranes have ruptured. If success is not immediate, the procedure must be abandoned in favor of cesarean section without delay

MEDIAN VERTEX PRESENTATIONS: MILITARY ATTITUDE

Definition

There is neither flexion nor extension; the occiput and the brow are at the same level in the pelvis. The presenting part is the vertex. The denominator is the occiput. The presenting diameter is the occipitofrontal, which at 11.0 cm is longer than the more favorable suboccipitobregmatic of 9.5 cm. Hence the progress is slower, and arrest is a little more frequent. In many cases, the military attitude is transitory, and the head flexes as it descends. Occasionally, extension to a brow or face presentation takes place.

Diagnosis of Position: Median Vertex Presentation

Abdominal Examination

1. The long axes of the fetus and mother are parallel (Fig. 15-16A)
2. The head is at or in the pelvic inlet
3. The back is in one flank, the small parts on the opposite side
4. The breech is in the fundus
5. Since there is neither flexion nor extension, there is no marked cephalic prominence on one side or the other

Fetal Heart

The fetal heart tones are heard loudest in the lower quadrant of the mother's abdomen on the same side as the fetal back.

Vaginal Examination

1. The sagittal suture is felt in the transverse diameter of the pelvis, as LOT or ROT (Fig. 15-16B)
2. The two fontanels are equally easy to palpate and identify. They are at the same level in the pelvis

Mechanism of Labor: Median Vertex Presentation

Engagement takes place most often in the transverse diameter of the inlet. The head descends slowly, with the occiput and the brow at the same level (there is neither flexion nor extension) and with the sagittal suture in the

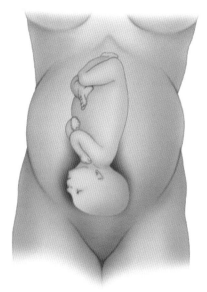

A. Abdominal view.

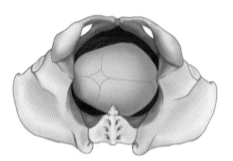

B. Vaginal view.

FIGURE 15-16. Median vertex presentation: left occiput transverse.

transverse diameter of the pelvis until the median vertex reaches the pelvic floor. Then several terminations are possible:

1. Most often the head flexes, the occiput rotates to the anterior, and delivery takes place as an occipitoanterior position
2. The head may become arrested in the transverse diameter of the pelvis. Operative assistance is necessary for deep transverse arrest
3. The head may rotate posteriorly with or without flexion. The occiput turns into the hollow of the sacrum and the forehead to the pubis. The

mechanism is that of persistent occipitoposterior positions. Delivery may be spontaneous or by operative methods
4. In rare instances, delivery can occur with the sagittal suture in the transverse diameter
5. Occasionally, the head extends, and the mechanism becomes a face or brow presentation

Prognosis: Median Vertex Presentation

Although labor is a little longer and harder than normal on the mother and child, the prognosis is reasonably good. Many cases flex and proceed to normal delivery.

Management of Median Vertex Presentation

1. Since flexion occurs so frequently, there should be no interference as long as progress is being made
2. When flexion takes place, the management is that of occipitoanterior or occipitoposterior positions
3. Cases in which the head extends are treated as face or brow presentations
4. When arrest occurs in the military attitude and the head is low in the pelvis, vaginal delivery may be attempted by flexing the head manually, rotating the occiput to the anterior, and extracting the head by forceps or vacuum (see Chapter 17)
5. When there is disproportion, when the head is high in the pelvis, or when an attempt at vaginal delivery fails, cesarean section should be performed

FACE PRESENTATION

General Considerations

Definition
The lie is longitudinal, the presentation is cephalic, the presenting part is the face, the attitude is one of complete extension, the chin (mentum, M) is the denominator and leading pole, and the presenting diameter is the subment-obregmatic of 9.5 cm. In face presentations, the part between the glabella and chin presents; in brow presentations, it is the part between the glabella and bregma. However, positions intermediate to these are seen.

Incidence

The incidence is less than 1 percent (one in 600-800) and is higher in multiparas than primigravidas. Primary face presentations are present before the onset of labor and are rare. Most face presentations are secondary, extension taking place during labor generally at the pelvic inlet. About 70 percent of face presentations are anterior or transverse, while 30 percent are posterior.

Etiology

Anything that delays engagement in flexion can contribute to the etiology of attitudes of extension. There is an association between attitudes of extension and cephalopelvic disproportion, and since this is a serious combination, the presence of a small pelvis or a large head must be ruled out with certainty. Prematurity is another etiology; as with smaller head dimensions, preterm infants can engage before conversion to vertex position. Rare causes of extension include thyroid neoplasms, which act by pushing the head back; multiple coils of cord around the neck, which prevent flexion; and spasm or shortening of the extensor muscles of the neck. Anencephalic fetuses frequently present by the face. In many cases, no cause can be found.

Anterior Face Presentations

The following descriptions apply to the left mentum anterior (LMA) presentation. The mechanism for the right mentum anterior (RMA) presentation is similar to that for LMA except that the chin, small parts, and fetal heart are on the right side, and the back and cephalic prominence are on the left.

Diagnosis of Position: LMA

Abdominal Examination

1. The long axes of the fetus and mother are parallel (Fig. 15-17)
2. The head is at the pelvis. Early in labor, the head is not engaged
3. The back is on the right side of the mother's abdomen, but since it is posterior, it is often felt indistinctly. The small parts are on the left and anterior. Extension of the spine causes the chest to be thrown out and the back to be hollowed
4. The breech is in the fundus

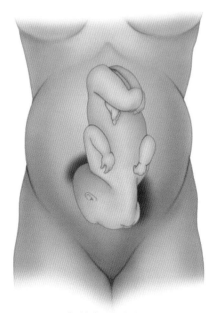

A. Abdominal view.

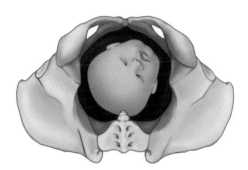

B. Vaginal view.

FIGURE 15-17. Left mentum anterior.

5. The cephalic prominence (the occiput) is on the right. An important diagnostic sign of extension attitudes is that the back and the cephalic prominence are on the same side. When flexion is present, the cephalic prominence and the back are on opposite sides

6. It must be kept in mind that in anterior face presentations, the baby's back and occiput are posterior. When the chin is posterior, on the other hand, the back and occiput are anterior

Fetal Heart. The fetal heart tones are transmitted through the anterior chest wall of the fetus and are heard loudest in the left lower quadrant of the maternal abdomen on the same side as the small parts.

Vaginal Examination

1. The clue to diagnosis is a negative finding—that is, absence of the round, even, hard vertex. In place of the dome of the skull with its identifying suture lines and fontanels, there is a softer and irregular presenting part. One suspects a face or breech presentation. Identification of the various parts of the face clinches the diagnosis. After prolonged labor, marked edema may confuse the picture
2. The long axis of the face is in the right oblique diameter of the pelvis (Fig. 15-17B)
3. The chin is in the left anterior quadrant of the maternal pelvis
4. The forehead is in the right posterior quadrant of the pelvis
5. Vaginal examination must be performed gently to avoid injury to the eyes
6. Ultrasonography can be useful for radiographic demonstration of the hyperextended head with the facial bones at or below the pelvic inlet

Late Diagnosis. Because most face presentations make good progress, the diagnosis may not be made until the face has reached the floor of the pelvis or until advance has ceased.

Mechanism of Labor: LMA

Extension. For some reason, the head does not flex. Instead, it extends (Fig. 15-18), so that in place of an LOP or ROP, there is an RMA or an LMA. The baby enters the pelvis chin first. The presenting diameter in face presentations (submentobregmatic) and in well-flexed head presentations (suboccipitobregmatic) is 9.5 cm in each case. This is one of the reasons why most anterior face presentations come to spontaneous delivery.

Descent. With the chin as the leading part, engagement takes place in the right oblique diameter of the pelvis. Descent is slower than in flexed attitudes. The face is low in the pelvis before the biparietal diameter has passed the brim. When the forward leading edge of the presenting face is felt at the level of the ischial spines, the tracheobregmatic diameter is still above the inlet.

FIRST STAGE OF LABOR

Internal Rotation. With descent and molding, the chin reaches the pelvic floor, where it is directed downward, forward, and medially. As it rotates 45° anteriorly toward the symphysis (LMA to mentum anterior [MA]), the long axis of the face comes into the anteroposterior diameter of the pelvis (Figs. 15-18C and D). With further descent, the chin escapes under the symphysis. The shoulders have remained in the oblique diameter, so the neck is twisted 45°. An essential feature of internal rotation is that the chin must rotate anteriorly and under the symphysis, or spontaneous delivery is impossible. Anterior rotation does not take place until the face is well applied to the pelvic floor and may be delayed until late in labor. The attendant must not give up hope too soon.

Flexion. The head is born by flexion (Figs. 15-18E to G). The submental region at the neck impinges under the symphysis pubis. With the head pivoting around this point, the mouth, nose, orbits, forehead, vertex, and occiput are born over the perineum by flexion. The head then falls back (Figs. 15-18H and I).

Restitution. As the head is released from the vagina, the neck untwists, and the chin turns 45° back toward the original side (Fig. 15-18J).

External Rotation. The anterior shoulder reaches the pelvic floor and rotates toward the symphysis to bring the bisacromial diameter from the oblique to the anteroposterior diameter of the outlet. The chin rotates back another 45° to maintain the head in its correct relationship to the shoulders (Fig. 15-18K).

Molding. Molding (Fig. 15-19) leads to an elongation of the head in its anteroposterior diameter and flattening from above downward. The forehead and occiput protrude. The extension of the head on the trunk disappears after a few days.

Prognosis: Anterior Face Presentations

Labor. Because the face is a poor dilator and because attitudes of extension are less favorable, labor takes longer than in normal occipitoanterior positions. The labor is conducted with this in mind. Delay takes place at the inlet, but when the face presentation and the labor are well established, steady progress is the rule. More than 90 percent of anterior face presentations deliver per vagina without complications. Figure 15-20 summarizes the mechanism of labor with the LMA presentation.

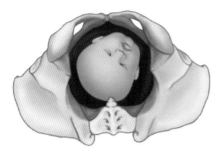

A. LMA: Onset of labor.

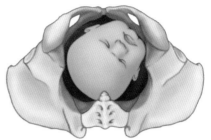

B. Extension and descent.

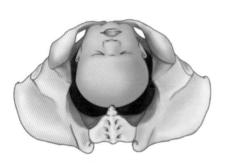

C. Vaginal view.

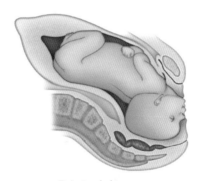

D. Lateral view.

C and D. Internal rotation: LMA to MA.

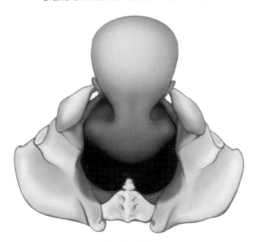

E. Flexion.

FIGURE 15-18. A to **D.** Mechanism of labor. **E** to **G**. Birth of the face and head by flexion. **H** and **I.** Head falls back in extension. **J** and **K.** Restitution and external rotation. LMA, left mentum anterior; LMT, left mentum transverse; MA, mentum anterior.

FIRST STAGE OF LABOR

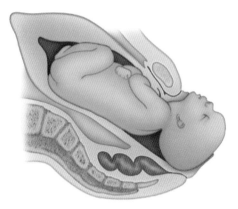

F. Flexion beginning.

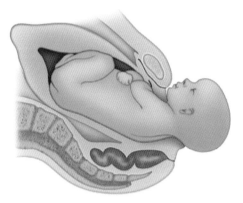

G. Flexion complete.

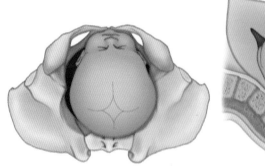

H. Vaginal view.

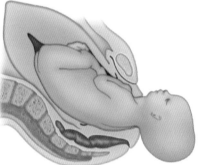

I. Lateral view.

FIGURE 15-18. (*Continued*)

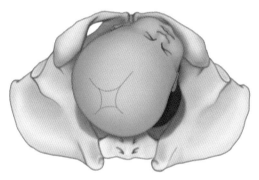

J. Restitution: MA to LMA.

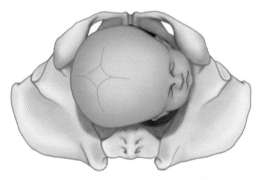

K. External rotation: LMA to LMT.

FIGURE 15-18. (*Continued*)

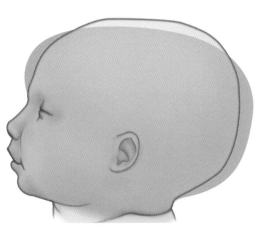

FIGURE 15-19. Molding: face presentation.

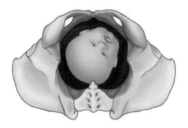

A. LMA: Onset of labor.

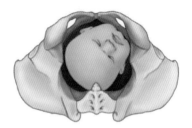

B. Extension and descent.

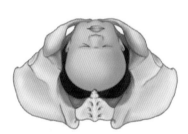

C. Internal rotation: LMA to MA.

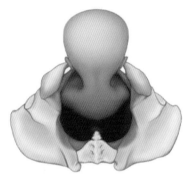

D. Flexion.

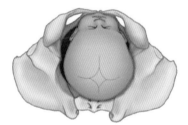

E. Extension.

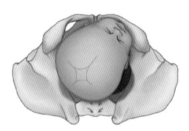

F. Restitution: MA to LMA.

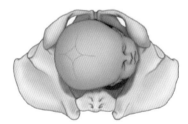

G. External rotation: LMA to LMT.

FIGURE 15-20. **Summary of mechanism of labor: left mentum anterior (LMA).** LMT, left mentum transverse; MA, mentum anterior.

Mother. The mother has more work to do, has more pain, and receives greater lacerations than in normal positions.

Fetus. The baby does well in most cases, but the prognosis is less favorable than in normal presentations. The outlook for the child can be improved by early diagnosis, carefully conducted first and second stages of labor, and the restriction of operative vaginal deliveries to easily performed procedures. Cesarean section is preferable to complicated, difficult, and traumatic assisted vaginal deliveries. The membranes rupture early in labor, and the face takes the brunt of the punishment so that it becomes badly swollen and misshapen. Its appearance is a great worry to the parents. The edema disappears gradually, and the infant takes on a more normal appearance. Edema of the larynx may result from prolonged pressure of the hyoid region of the neck against the pubic bone. For the first 24 hours, the baby must be watched carefully to detect any difficulty in breathing.

Management of Anterior Face Presentations

1. *Disproportion*: Disproportion is managed by cesarean section
2. *Normal pelvis*: In a normal pelvis, anterior face presentations are left alone for these reasons:
   a. Most deliver spontaneously or with the aid of low forceps
   b. If conversion (flexion) is successful, the anterior face presentation is replaced by an occipitoposterior one (LMA to ROP or RMA to LOP). This does not improve the situation and may make it worse
   c. If conversion is partially successful, the face is changed to a brow presentation. In this case, a face presentation, which usually delivers spontaneously, is replaced by a brow presentation, which cannot
3. *Arrest*:
   a. Low in the pelvis, well below the ischial spines: Extraction with low forceps
   b. High in the pelvis: Cesarean section

Transverse Face Presentations

The long axis of the face is in the transverse diameter of the pelvis, with the chin on one side and the forehead on the other (Fig. 15-21).

The following descriptions apply to the left mentum transverse (LMT) presentation. The mechanism of labor for the right mentum transverse

FIRST STAGE OF LABOR

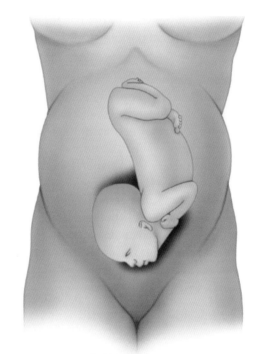

A. Abdominal view.

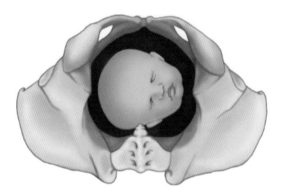

B. Vaginal view.

FIGURE 15-21. Left mentum transverse.

(RMT) presentation is the same as that for LMT except that the chin, small parts, and fetal heart are on the right, and the back and cephalic prominence are on the left.

Diagnosis of Position: LMT

Abdominal Examination

1. The long axis of the fetus is parallel to that of the mother
2. The head is at the pelvis
3. The back is on the right, toward the maternal flank. The small parts are on the left side
4. The breech is in the fundus
5. The cephalic prominence (the occiput) is on the right, the same side as the back

Fetal Heart. The fetal heart is heard loudest in the left lower quadrant of the mother's abdomen.

Vaginal Examination

1. The long axis of the face is in the transverse diameter of the pelvis
2. The chin is to the left at 3 o'clock
3. The forehead is to the right at 9 o'clock

Mechanism of Labor: LMT

A summary of the mechanism of labor for the LMT presentation is given in Figure 15-22.

Extension. Extension to LMT occurs instead of flexion to ROT.

Descent. Engagement takes place in the transverse diameter of the pelvis. Descent is slow.

Internal Rotation. The chin rotates 90° anteriorly to the midline (LMT to LMA to MA). The chin comes under the symphysis.

Flexion. The submental region of the neck impinges in the subpubic angle. Birth is by flexion, after which the head falls backward.

Restitution. As the neck untwists, the head turns back 45°.

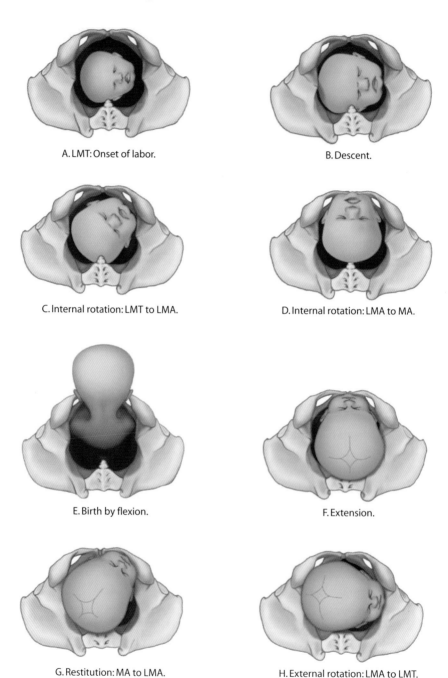

A. LMT: Onset of labor.

B. Descent.

C. Internal rotation: LMT to LMA.

D. Internal rotation: LMA to MA.

E. Birth by flexion.

F. Extension.

G. Restitution: MA to LMA.

H. External rotation: LMA to LMT.

FIGURE 15-22. Mechanism of labor: left mentum transverse (LMT). LMA, left mentum anterior; MA, mentum anterior.

External Rotation. The shoulders turn from the oblique into the antero-posterior diameter of the pelvis, and the head rotates back another 45°.

Clinical Course of Labor and Management: LMT

1. Anterior rotation takes place in the majority of cases, LMT to LMA to MA. The treatment is the same as LMA. Delivery is spontaneous or assisted by low forceps
2. Arrest as LMT low in the pelvis
   a. Rotation to LMA manually or by forceps followed by extraction of the head by forceps
   b. If rotation is difficult or fails, cesarean section is performed
3. Arrest as LMT high in the pelvis is treated by cesarean section

Posterior Face Presentations

Some 30 percent of face presentations are posterior. Most of these rotate anteriorly. The flexed counterpart of the posterior face is the anterior occiput; thus, LMP flexes to ROA and RMP to LOA. Persistent posterior face presentations become arrested because they cannot deliver sponta-neously. The descriptions here are for the left mentum posterior (LMP) presentation.

Diagnosis of Position: LMP

Abdominal Examination

1. The long axis of the fetus is parallel to the long axis of the mother (Fig. 15-23)
2. The head is at the pelvis
3. The back is anterior and to the right. The small parts are on the left and posterior
4. The breech is in the fundus of the uterus
5. The cephalic prominence (occiput) is to the right and anterior. It is on the same side as the back

Fetal Heart. The fetal heart tones, transmitted through the anterior shoulder, are heard loudest in the left lower quadrant of the mother's abdomen.

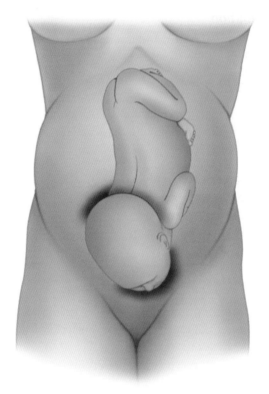

A. Abdominal view.

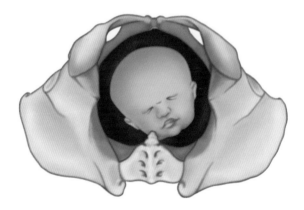

B. Vaginal view.

FIGURE 15-23. **Left mentum posterior.**

Vaginal Examination

1. The long diameter of the face is in the left oblique diameter of the pelvis
2. The chin is in the left posterior quadrant of the pelvis (Fig. 15-23B)
3. The forehead is in the right anterior quadrant

Mechanism of Labor: LMP

There are two basic mechanisms:

1. Long arc rotation, with the chin rotating 135° to the anterior. About two-thirds of posterior face presentations do this and deliver spontaneously or with the aid of low forceps
2. Short arc rotation of 45° to the posterior, with the chin ending up in the hollow of the sacrum. These cases become arrested as persistent posterior face presentations

Long Arc Rotation: 135° to the Anterior

Extension. Extension to LMP (Fig. 15-24) occurs instead of flexion to ROA.

Descent. Descent is slow. The presenting part remains high while the essential molding takes place. Without extreme molding, the vertex cannot pass under the anterior part of the pelvic inlet.

Internal Rotation. The slow descent continues; the marked molding enables the chin to reach the pelvic floor, where it rotates 135° to the anterior and comes to lie under the symphysis. Since the original position was LMP, the sequence is LMP to LMT to LMA to MA in rotations of 45° between each step (Figure 15-24B to D).

Flexion. The submental area pivots under the symphysis, and the head is born by flexion. The head then falls backward.

Restitution. The chin rotates back 45° as the neck untwists.

External Rotation. With the rotation of the shoulders from the oblique into the anteroposterior diameter of the pelvis, the chin turns back another 45°.

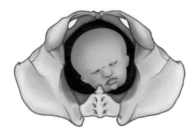

A. LMP: Descent.

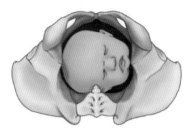

B. Internal rotation: LMP to LMT.

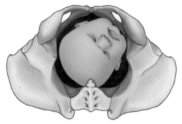

C. Internal rotation: LMT to LMA.

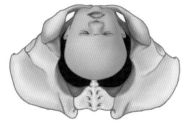

D. Internal rotation: LMA to MA.

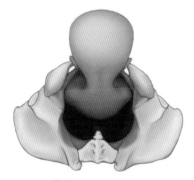

E. Birth by flexion.

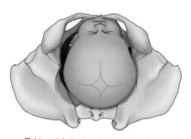

F. Head falls back in extension.

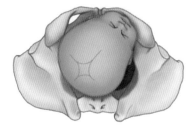

G. Restitution: MA to LMA.

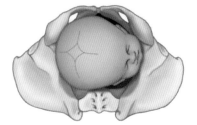

H. External rotation: LMA to LMT.

FIGURE 15-24. Left mentum posterior (LMP): long arc rotation. LMA, left mentum anterior; LMT, left mentum transverse; MA, mentum anterior.

Short Arc Rotation: 45° to the Posterior

Extension. Extension to LMP takes place (Fig. 15-25).

Descent. Descent occurs with the help of extreme molding.

Internal Rotation. The chin rotates 45° posteriorly into the hollow of the sacrum (LMP to MP). Impaction follows, and the progress of labor comes to a halt. Flexion cannot take place and further advancement is not possible, except in the rare situation in which the baby is so small that the shoulders and head can enter the pelvis together.

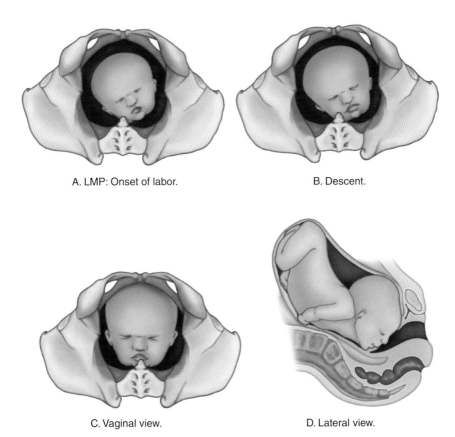

A. LMP: Onset of labor.

B. Descent.

C. Vaginal view.

D. Lateral view.

C. and D. Internal rotation: LMP to MP.

FIGURE 15-25. Left mentum posterior (LMP): short arc rotation. MP, mentum posterior.

Prognosis: Posterior Face Presentations

The prolonged labor and difficult rotation are traumatic to both the baby and mother. When the chin rotates posteriorly, the prognosis is poor unless the situation is corrected. Maternal morbidity is directly proportional to the degree of difficulty of the birth. High forceps or version and extraction carry with them the most morbid postpartum courses.

Management of Posterior Face Presentations

1. *Disproportion:* Disproportion is managed by cesarean section
2. *Trial of labor:* Since two-thirds of posterior faces rotate anteriorly and deliver spontaneously, and since internal rotation may not be completed until later in labor when the face is distending the pelvic floor, plenty of time should be allowed for the rotation to be accomplished. Interference must not be premature
3. *Persistent posterior face:* Since face presentations that have remained posterior cannot be delivered spontaneously, operative delivery is necessary
   a. Cesarean section is the modern treatment of choice, giving the best results for both the mother and child
   b. Flexion (conversion) from mentoposterior to occipitoanterior may be considered if cesarean section cannot be performed. One method of accomplishing this is by the *Thorn maneuver* (Fig. 15-26). The cervix must be fully dilated. With the vaginal hand, the operator flexes the fetal head. With the other hand, the operator pushes on the breech to flex the body. At the same time, an assistant presses against the baby's thorax or abdomen to try and jack-knife the infant's body. This procedure is performed under anesthesia and must be done soon after the membranes rupture. If the amniotic fluid has drained away, the dry uterine cavity and snug fit of the uterus around the baby make it difficult or impossible to carry out this treatment. Once flexion has been accomplished, the head is pushed into the pelvis and held in place
   c. Rotation to mentum anterior can sometimes be achieved by the use of forceps, but the operation is difficult and may be traumatic

Management Summary

In the setting of a normal pelvis and effective contractions, successful vaginal delivery with face presentation is usually possible. It is important to monitor fetal heart rate with external devices because internal

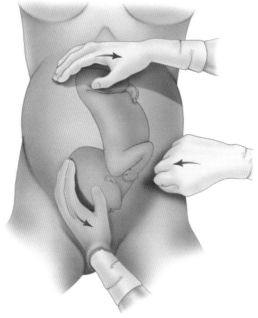

FIGURE 15-26. **Thorn maneuver.**

monitoring may cause injury to the face and eyes. In the presence of pelvic inlet contraction and posterior face presentation, cesarean delivery is usually indicated.

SELECTED READING

Benedetti TJ, Lowensohn RI, Truscott AM: Face presentation at term. Obstet Gynecol 55:199, 1980

Cruikshank DP, White CA: Obstetric malpresentations: twenty years' experience. Am J Obstet Gynecol 116:1097, 1973.

Cunningham FG, Gant NF, Leveno KJ, et al: Abnormal labour. In: *Williams Obstetrics*, 23rd ed. New York: McGraw-Hill, 2010, pp 452-454

Duff P: Diagnosis and management of face presentation. Obstet Gynecol 57:105, 1981

Shaffer BL, Cheng YW, Vargas JE et al: Face presentation: Predictors and delivery route. Am J Obstet Gynecol 194:e10, 2006

PART III

Second Stage
of Labor

CHAPTER 16

The Second Stage of Labor

Lawrence Oppenheimer
Amanda Black

DEFINITION OF THE SECOND STAGE OF LABOR

The second stage of labor lasts from the end of the first stage, when the cervix has reached full dilatation, to the birth of the baby. There are two phases: (1) the passive stage during which the fetus descends through the maternal pelvis, and (2) the active phase of maternal pushing. The duration of the normal second stage of labor is mainly influenced by parity and the presence of an epidural. The median durations of the second stage are given in Table 16-1, but there is a large range in duration.

Second Stage in the Absence of Epidural Analgesia

In the absence of an epidural, a woman will often experience more intense and frequent contractions as she approaches full dilatation. This is sometimes referred to as *transition*. The patient should be discouraged from pushing (bearing down) before full dilatation. Breathing deeply and slowly during each contraction may help in coping with the pain. Once the head reaches the perineum, the maternal desire to bear down may become difficult to resist. The following are possible indicators of the onset of the second stage, although they are not exclusive to the second stage:

1. There is an increase in bloody show
2. The woman wants to bear down with each contraction

TABLE 16-1: DURATION OF SECOND STAGE IN MINUTES

| Parity | Epidural | | No Epidural | |
	Median	IQ Range	Median	IQ Range
0	82	45-134	45	27-76
1	36	20-77	15	10-25
2	25	14-60	11	7-20
3	23	12-53	10	5-16
≥4	22	9-30	10	5-15

IQ, interquartile range (25%-75% of the population).

3. She feels pressure on the rectum accompanied by the desire to defecate
4. Nausea and vomiting may occur as the cervix reaches full dilatation

The cervical dilation, station of the presenting part, and fetal position must be confirmed by vaginal examination.

Second Stage with Epidural Analgesia

In the presence of epidural analgesia, the duration of the second stage is approximately twice the duration of a nonepidural second stage. This is because the neurohumoral reflex of oxytocin release due to the perineal pressure of the head, which assists the urge to bear down, may be interrupted. The incidence of instrumental vaginal delivery, but not cesarean section, is also increased twofold. For this reason, it is important for the obstetrical care provider to have an understanding of how to best manage the second stage under epidural.

Passive Phase of the Second Stage

During the passive phase of the second stage, the cervix is fully dilated, but there are no voluntary or involuntary expulsive efforts. The head usually has not yet reached the pelvic floor (thus the station is +1 or higher). The rotation of the occiput to the optimal position of occipitoanterior may not yet be completed, and the head may be in an oblique or transverse position. There is usually no urge to bear down even in the absence of epidural analgesia.

Active Phase of the Second Stage

During the active (pushing) phase of the second stage, the cervix is fully dilated, and the woman begins to push either voluntarily or involuntarily. The woman may begin pushing because she experiences a strong urge to push or bear down. The active phase may also commence when a woman is instructed to start pushing regardless of the head station. Women with an epidural may not have a strong urge to push.

Fetal Monitoring in the Second Stage of Labor

Fetal health surveillance is discussed in depth in Chapter 12. In the active portion of the second stage, fetal heart rate (FHR) auscultation should be carried out immediately after a contraction for 1 minute at 5-minute intervals. In some instances, continuous electronic fetal monitoring (EFM) may be indicated. These would include higher risk situations, for example, fetal growth restriction, preeclampsia, and oxytocin use for augmentation of labor. FHR abnormalities are common in the second stage of labor but are generally well tolerated by the fetus if the FHR was normal throughout the first stage of labor. A prolonged second stage must be avoided if there are persistent FHR abnormalities, particularly when there are other risk factors that may impact the degree of fetal reserve.

The maternal pulse should be carefully palpated throughout the second stage to ensure there is no confusion between the fetal and maternal heart rates. The effort of pushing will raise the maternal heart rate into the fetal range in around 50 percent of women. The FHR transducer monitor may display maternal pulse instead of fetal heart rate, particularly where there are significant decelerations or a fetal bradycardia, and true FHR abnormalities may be masked by an apparently normal looking tracing. The use of a handheld doppler for intermittent auscultation can also be subject to the same artifact. Clues regarding maternal heart rate artifact include the maternal pulse shows a uniform acceleration with every contraction caused by the Valsalva maneuver associated with pushing; sudden changes in baseline or switching between maternal and fetal rates; and improvement of a previously persistently abnormal FHR pattern. Current fetal monitors have the capability to continuously display the maternal pulse (MHR) as well as the FHR, and provide coincidence alerts when these rates overlap. If EFM is being utilized, the use of such MHR displays in the second stage is suggested. If maternal artifact is suspected, application of a fetal scalp electrode or direct visualization of the FHR with ultrasound, if available, will help to clarify the situation.

Situations of particular concern include repetitive severe variable decelerations with pushing that may be associated with cord compression or a nuchal cord. This can be followed by a prolonged bradycardia as the cord tightens in the late second stage. Late-stage bradycardia may also be caused by head compression. A fetus with a previously normal tracing can withstand a bradycardia for a few minutes and if the head is crowning, it does not require immediate instrumental delivery. Uterine contraction frequency must be recorded. Hypersystole/too frequent contractions, especially when oxytocin is being used, on top of the maternal Valsalva maneuver from pushing, further diminishes uterine blood flow and can exhaust even a healthy fetus over a period of time. Suggested guidelines for delaying pushing in the second stage of labor apply only in instances with ongoing evidence of fetal well-being.

MANAGEMENT OF THE SECOND STAGE OF LABOR

There are very few comprehensive evidence-based clinical practice guidelines for management of the second stage of labor; however, the ideal management of the second stage of labor should maximize the probability of vaginal delivery while minimizing the risk of maternal and neonatal morbidity and mortality. The fundamental principles of care in the second stage include: (1) establishing fetal and maternal well-being and fetal head position at the onset; (2) performing hourly vaginal assessments in the second stage by a consistent examiner to assess fetal position and station; (3) informing the primary health care provider when the cervix is fully dilated, if there is a lack of progress in any 1-hour block, and at the end of 2 hours; and (4) regularly assessing the bladder to ensure that a full bladder is not obstructing progress.

Whether to start pushing immediately once full dilation is achieved or to delay pushing to allow for further head descent and rotation is controversial. The practice of delayed pushing is based on the theory that a woman receiving an epidural anesthetic is able to have a period of rest once she reaches 10 cm, thereby allowing the fetus to passively rotate and descend while conserving the patient's energy for when she starts to push. Previous studies found that delaying maternal pushing for a maximum of up to 2 hours, particularly in primigravidas, reduced the incidence of operative vaginal deliveries and cesarean sections at the expense of an increased duration of second stage. More recent studies in nulliparous women under epidural found that delayed pushing did not significantly improve the likelihood of spontaneous vaginal birth and there was no reduction in the rate of operative vaginal delivery or cesarean section. The risks of delayed pushing include an increased incidence of chorioamnionitis (in one study) when compared to immediate pushing (9.1% vs. 6.6%), postpartum hemorrhage, and umbilical cord pH less than 7.10 (2.7% vs. 1.3%); however, there was no difference in Apgar scores less than 7 at 5 minutes or in NICU admissions. This suggests that a delay in the onset of pushing of more than 1 hour may not be beneficial, and the options/risks of delayed pushing versus immediate pushing should be discussed with nulliparous women with an epidural. A shorter delay while waiting for a dense epidural block to wane may be acceptable for some women who find it hard to push. Few multiparous women were included in the above studies. Their progress in the second stage is generally much quicker.

The Ottawa Hospital utilizes a second stage protocol that allows up to 4 hours total duration of the second stage in primigravidas under epidural

TABLE 16-2: THE OTTAWA HOSPITAL SECOND STAGE PROTOCOL

	Hour Begins			
	1	2	3	4
Primigravida, epidural	Wait	Wait	Wait/push*	Push
Primigravida, no epidural	Wait	Wait	Push	
Multigravida, epidural	Wait	Wait	Push	
Multigravida, no epidural	Wait	Push		

*Waiting for a third hour may be appropriate if the active phase is not yet reached but there is continuous progress.

and 3 hours for multiparas (Table 16-2). The protocol recommends to wait 2 hours before pushing in all women with epidural anesthesia who have no urge to push, or in whom the station of the presenting part is above +2, or in whom the fetus is in the occipitoposterior (OP) or occipitotransverse (OT) position. If the fetus is in the OP or OT positions, manual rotation to the occipitoanterior (OA) position is attempted and the patient is repositioned to optimize fetal rotation and/or maintain the OA position. After 2 hours, the woman should be instructed to push regardless of head station. The duration of pushing within the total time frame should preferably not exceed 2 hours because the pH of the fetus will gradually fall during active pushing, although absolute time limits cannot be stipulated because of a lack of conclusive evidence.

Studies show that around 10 to 20 percent of nulliparous women under epidural will have a second stage greater than 3 hours but only 2 percent will exceed 4 hours. There is a lack of consensus to support an absolute time limit to end the second stage with an intervention, and care providers must be aware of the benefits and risks of intervention versus continued expectant management in the second stage.

Recommendations from the National Institute for Health and Care Excellence (NICE) regarding the total duration of the second stage are summarized in Table 16-3. We suggest consideration of operative vaginal delivery at the end of these time limits unless spontaneous delivery is thought to be imminent (i.e., the head is visible and there is continued progress with contractions). In those cases, it is not necessary to impose an absolute limit on the duration of the second stage. There are, however, some important caveats:

TABLE 16-3: RECOMMENDATIONS FOR DURATION OF THE SECOND STAGE OF LABOR

Parity	Recommendation
Nulliparous women	• Birth would be expected to take place within 3 hours of the start of the active second stage in most women. • A diagnosis of delay in the active second stage should be made when it has lasted 2 hours and a health care professional trained to undertake an operative vaginal birth should be consulted if birth is not imminent.
Parous women	• Birth would be expected to take place within 2 hours of the start of the active second stage in most women. • A diagnosis of delay in the active second stage should be made when it has lasted 1 hour and a health care professional trained to undertake an operative vaginal birth should be consulted if birth is not imminent.

Recommendations from National Institute for Health and Care Excellence: Intrapartum care for healthy women and babies. Clinical Guideline. 2017.

1. The fetus is healthy, term, and in an uncomplicated cephalic presentation
2. There is no uterine scar (e.g., no previous cesarean section)
3. The fetal heart, assessed by intermittent auscultation or electronic monitoring, and other tests of fetal well-being are normal and reassuring
4. There is continued progress as evidenced by gradual descent of the head on hourly assessments

If these conditions are not met or if there are concerns about fetal or maternal health, management should be individualized. This usually means shortening the above time parameters or earlier consideration of operative delivery.

Dystocia in the Second Stage

There is no clear consensus on what constitutes delay in the second stage of labor. In general, no change in the head station during any 1-hour interval warrants careful evaluation for dystocia. An active (pushing) phase longer than 2 hours in a primigravida or 1 hour in a multigravida warrants assessment by a health care professional trained in operative vaginal delivery unless birth is imminent. Oxytocin may be started at any time during the second stage, particularly when contractions are inadequate, or there is a lack of progress. Women who are already on oxytocin at the onset of the second stage should continue to receive it provided that there are no concerns regarding the FHR or uterine tachysystole. *Assessing fetal position at the start of the second stage of labor, prior to the development of caput and molding, is of paramount importance.* Malposition of the fetal head is a frequent cause of delay in the second stage and may be associated with infrequent or insufficient uterine contractions. Failure to determine fetal head position at the start of the second stage can lead to a prolonged second stage, difficulty assessing fetal head position accurately as the second stage progresses, and the inability to perform an operative vaginal delivery if the fetal head position is not known. Maternal positioning and manual fetal head rotations may be important interventions when fetal malposition is identified. In some cases, the fetal head position may be difficult to determine. In these instances, transvaginal ultrasonography, if available, can be helpful in determining head position with great accuracy. If malposition is identified at the start of the second stage, *manual rotation* to the OA position should be considered in order to avoid a prolonged second stage with lack of fetal descent, progressive worsening of fetal head impaction, and increasing molding and caput formation.

Second stage management should be individualized depending on the clinical situation. In some situations, it may be appropriate to wait longer for spontaneous head rotation, but in other situations, it may be preferable to shorten the timeline for waiting and pushing to avoid the additional complications of a prolonged second stage when operative delivery may be required. Caution should be exercised in the infrequent situation of failure of head descent in a multipara with an occipitoanterior presentation and strong, frequent contractions. This clinical picture may represent true cephalopelvic disproportion, in which the fetus may be significantly larger than in the patient's previous deliveries. In this case, excessive uterine activity for too long a period could lead to complications. Around 80 percent of multiparas under epidural analgesia will deliver within 3 hours and almost all within 90 minutes without an epidural.

Well-grown fetuses that are not compromised during the first stage of labor and are carefully monitored in the second stage seldom develop asphyxia, even when the second stage is prolonged. One should avoid a traumatic forceps or vacuum delivery just because an arbitrary time point has passed. However, the decision to allow labor to continue should be based on evidence of continued progress of descent or rotation.

Pushing in the Second Stage

During the second stage of labor, the expulsive powers include: (1) involuntary uterine contractions, (2) voluntary efforts of the abdominal, thoracic and diaphragmatic muscles, and (3) action of the levator ani muscles. In general, the more effectively the mother bears down, the shorter the second stage. This action may be more efficient if the woman braces herself against a solid object, such as a hand bar or birthing bars. When the contraction begins, the woman takes one or two deep breaths and then holds her breath to fix the diaphragm. She then pulls on the hand bars (or on her own legs with her hands behind her knees) and at the same time bears down as hard and for as long a period as she can. In general, she should be encouraged not to push beyond the time of completion of each uterine contraction.

Although many obstetrical care providers encourage pushing that incorporates a Valsalva maneuver, the use of "physiologic bearing down" instead of sustained breath holding during expulsive efforts may be equally effective. Physiologic bearing down (making several short pushes without breath-holding, the "open glottis technique"), although resulting in a slightly longer second stage, may result in improved maternal–fetal gas exchange and maternal satisfaction with the birth experience. In general, women should be guided by their own urge to push provided that their pushing efforts are productive. Guided pushing, whereby the birth attendant performs a vaginal exam and depresses the posterior vaginal wall while the patient is pushing to provide guidance and feedback on pushing efforts, may be helpful, particularly when a patient first starts pushing, to establish whether the maternal expulsive efforts are productive and to assess for progress.

Positioning in the Second Stage of Labor

There is no single correct position for delivery. Patients should choose a position that is comfortable for them and enhances their pushing efforts. It has been traditional practice for women to be positioned and to push in the horizontal (dorsal), semi-Fowler's (head and back elevated at 30 degrees), or lithotomy position during the second stage of labor (Fig. 16-1A to D). Use of these positions is often dictated by interventions such as epidural analgesia, EFM, or intravenous lines and pumps that limit mobility. Upright or vertical positions such as squatting, semi-recumbency, standing, and upright kneeling generate up to 30 percent more intraabdominal pressure and increased anteroposterior and transverse diameters of the pelvic outlet. Positioning may be important when lack of progress is identified in the second stage. Frequent changes in position may help when fetal malposition is identified or to relieve back pain. It is recommended that women should not lie supine or semi-supine during the second stage (in which case a firm wedge should be inserted under the woman's right side to prevent supine hypotension) and should adopt any other position that is comfortable for her and enhances pushing efforts.

In women with epidural analgesia and especially in women with any degree of motor neuron blockade, appropriate positioning is important to prevent injury associated with lack of sensation, poor alignment, or unnatural positioning of joints (e.g., hyperflexion of hips). Women with epidural anaesthesia do not need to remain horizontal. More upright positions can be used when local anesthetic is combined with narcotics to minimize motor blockade.

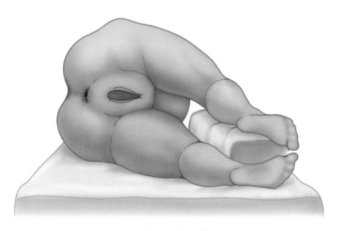

A. Left lateral position.

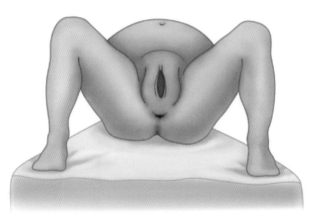

B. Dorsal position.

FIGURE 16-1. Positions for delivery.

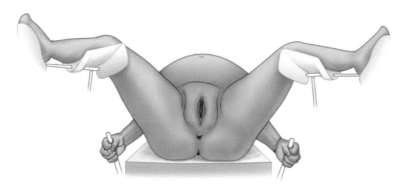

C. Lithotomy position.

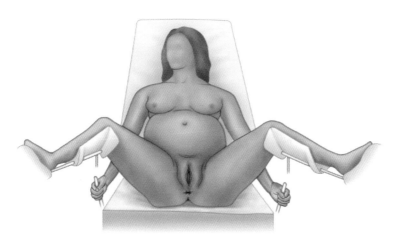

D. Back elevated: semisitting position.

FIGURE 16-1. **(Continued)**

Postural Supine Hypotension

Laboring women should avoid supine positioning. When a pregnant, term or near-term woman lies on her back, the uterus bulges over the vertebral column and compresses the inferior vena cava. This leads to an increased blood volume in the lower limbs but decreased return to the heart, lowered pressure in the right atrium, diminished cardiac output, and hypotension. Reduced perfusion of the uterus and placenta leads to fetal hypoxia and changes in the FHR.

Supine hypotension may be exacerbated by an epidural caused by the sympathetic blockade and venous pooling in the lower body. The pregnant woman may not display any signs or symptoms, but significant impairment of uterine blood flow can result. It is important to use a wedge, preferably under the right flank or buttock, for any woman in late pregnancy if she is required to lie supine for delivery or surgery.

DELIVERY OF THE FETUS

Descent, Crowning, and Spontaneous Birth of the Head

With each contraction, the head advances and then recedes as the uterus relaxes. Each time a little ground is gained. The introitus becomes an antero-posterior slit, then an oval, and finally a circular opening (Fig. 16-2A to C).

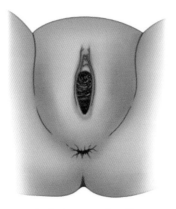

A. Anteroposterior slit.

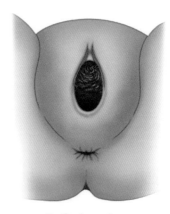

B. Oval opening.

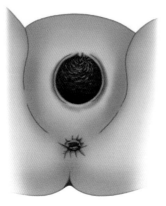

C. Circular shape.

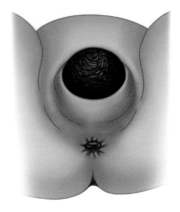

D. Crowning.

FIGURE 16-2. Dilatation of the introitus and birth of the head.

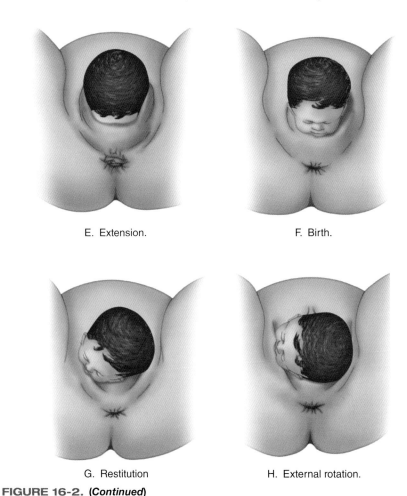

E. Extension.

F. Birth.

G. Restitution

H. External rotation.

FIGURE 16-2. *(Continued)*

With each contraction, the perineum bulges increasingly, and the pressure of the head thins out the perineum. Feces may be forced out of the rectum. With descent, the occiput comes to lie under the pubic symphysis. The head continues to advance and recede with each contraction until a strong contraction forces the largest diameter of the head through the vulva (*crowning*), as seen in Figure 16-2D. Manual perineal protection is recommended at this point. The perineum becomes very thin, and spontaneous laceration may occur. Routine episiotomy is not recommended. The fetal head is then delivered by a process of extension (Fig. 16-2E) as the bregma, forehead, nose, mouth, and chin sequentially appear over the perineum (Fig. 16-2F). The head then falls posteriorly back toward the anus.

SECOND STAGE OF LABOR

After the fetal head is out of the vagina, it restitutes (Fig. 16-2G), and assumes a transverse position. External rotation takes place (Fig. 16-2H) as the shoulders move from the oblique to the anteroposterior diameter of the pelvis.

Controlled Birth of the Head

The presence of a birth attendant allows for immediate action to be undertaken if complications arise during the birth process and also reduces the incidence of large and uncontrolled maternal lacerations. Procedures designed to encourage a slowly progressive delivery of the fetal head should be performed. A sudden, rapid, and uncontrolled emergence of the fetal head should be avoided because it may lead to large lacerations, including third- and fourth-degree lacerations into the anal sphincter and rectum.

1. *Management of bearing-down efforts*: The two forces responsible for delivery are uterine contractions and bearing-down forces. Uterine contractions are involuntary but maternal bearing-down forces can be controlled. Strong and effective bearing-down efforts are important. Initially, the patient must bear down during the uterine contractions to expedite progress. However, during the actual delivery, having the patient pant rapidly during the contractions may help to avoid a too rapid emergence of the fetal head. When the patient breathes in and out rapidly, the diaphragm moves, making it impossible for effective intraabdominal pressure to be built up, and so the power to bear down is lost

2. *Manual pressure*: In most cases, the speed of delivery can be reduced by gentle manual pressure against the baby's head. Manual perineal protection (MPP) helps to prevent abrupt head deflexion and subsequent perineal injury. Occasionally, the propulsive force is so great that it is impossible to try slowing the birth. The head should never be held back forcibly

3. *Ritgen maneuver*: The objective of this maneuver is to slow down the head and control deflexion with one hand while gently lifting the fetal chin over the posterior perineum with the other hand. This procedure is performed ideally between uterine contractions. During this interval, the head can be delivered slowly, gradually, and under the attendant's control. The maneuver can be done when the fetal head is extending the introitus about 5 cm and not moving back between contractions, that is, when the suboccipitofrontal diameter is ready to be born. It cannot be carried out before the occiput has come under the symphysis. The head is slowly delivered by its smallest diameter, carefully avoiding abrupt emergence, while the forehead is delivered during the pause

between two contractions. The same procedure is performed while delivering the posterior shoulder with perineal support because inappropriate perineal support while delivering the posterior shoulder can also result in extensive perineal tears.

The birth attendant's hand, covered with a towel or a pad, is placed so that the fingers are over the posterior perineum between the maternal anus and the coccyx (Fig. 16-3). The attendant's other hand is placed on the fetal occiput to exert pressure superiorly against the occiput and to help control the speed of its delivery. Pressing against the baby's face, preferably the chin, through the rectum, furthers extension of the fetal head. The bregma, forehead, and face are born in that order. The other hand is placed against the baby's occiput to control the speed of its delivery.

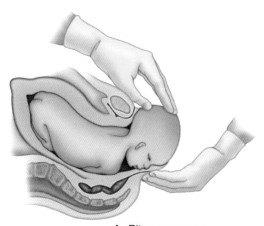

A. Ritgen maneuver.

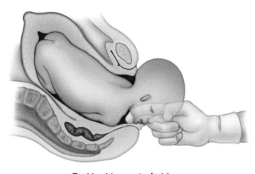

B. Hooking out of chin.

FIGURE 16-3. Birth of the head.

SECOND STAGE OF LABOR

4. *Episiotomy*: The routine use of episiotomy is discouraged. Allowing the perineum to tear spontaneously usually results in less postpartum pain and discomfort. When an episiotomy is required because of instrumental birth or suspected fetal compromise, the recommended technique is a mediolateral episiotomy originating at the vaginal fourchette and usually directed to the right side (a right lateral episiotomy) rather than a midline episiotomy to avoid an extension into the anal sphincter. The angle to the vertical axis should be between 45° and 60° at the time of the episiotomy.

After Delivery of the Head

1. The head should be supported as it restitutes and rotates externally
2. Routine aspiration of mucus and/or meconium from the baby's upper airways (mouth, nose, and throat) is no longer recommended because a normal, vigorous baby will clear its airway spontaneously. To prevent meconium aspiration syndrome if meconium is present, a skilled attendant should be present who can perform neonatal laryngoscopy, endotracheal intubation, and suction meconium from beneath the glottis (at or below the level of the vocal cords) under direct visualization if required. Meconium should be suctioned out before any resuscitative measures, such as positive-pressure ventilation, are performed.
3. The neck should be examined to determine if a nuchal cord (a coil of umbilical cord looped around the fetal neck) is present. Nuchal cords occur in approximately 25 percent of births. If the cord is around the neck loosely, the fetus may be able to deliver through the loop of cord or the cord may be slipped over the fetal head. In the event of a tight nuchal cord that doesn't easily reduce, it must be clamped doubly, cut between the clamps, and then unwound.

Birth of the Body and Shoulders

By the time the shoulders are ready for delivery, restitution has occurred, and external rotation is taking place. During a uterine contraction, the patient is asked to bear down. The sides of the head are grasped with two hands, and gentle downward traction is applied with the head depressed toward the rectum until the anterior shoulder appears under the pubic arch (Fig. 16-4A). The head of the baby is usually grasped with both hands on the parietal bones. If the anterior shoulder does not deliver easily with gentle downward traction, the birth attendant should consider the possibility of shoulder dystocia and use the appropriate maneuvers for managing

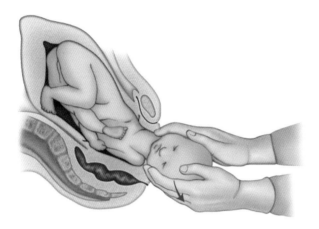

A. Downward traction of the fetal head.

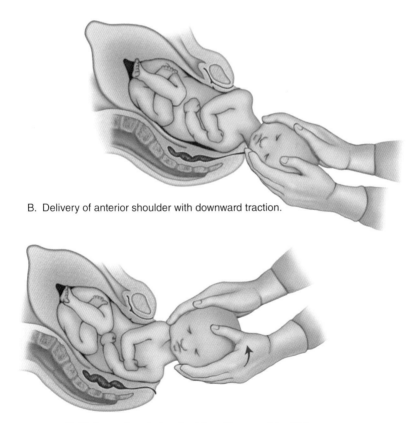

B. Delivery of anterior shoulder with downward traction.

C. Delivery of posterior shoulder with upward traction.

FIGURE 16-4. Delivery of the posterior shoulder with gentle upward traction.

SECOND STAGE OF LABOR

shoulder dystocia. Once the anterior shoulder has emerged from under the symphysis pubis (Fig. 16-4B), the head is raised upward so that the posterior shoulder can be born over the perineum (Fig. 16-4C). The birth attendant merely lowers and lifts the baby's head to facilitate birth of the shoulders. They *must not* exert excessive traction because of the risk of damaging the nerve plexus in the neck. The force that actually pushes out the shoulder is provided by the bearing-down efforts of the mother if she is awake or by pressure on the fundus by an assistant if the mother is unable to push.

Trunk and Lower Limbs
Once the head and shoulders have been delivered, the rest of the body usually slips out easily, often with a gush of amniotic fluid.

Clamping the Umbilical Cord
Unless there are significant fetal and/or neonatal concerns requiring urgent intervention, immediate skin-to-skin with the mother is recommended due to its many benefits for both mother and baby. The infant should be placed directly on the mother's skin and covered with a warm blanket, being careful not to apply excessive tension on the umbilical cord. Delayed cord clamping of 1 to 2 minutes is recommended for most term infants during which time the newborn can be dried and stimulated. If cord clamping is delayed for at least 30 to 60 seconds, an average of 80 cc of blood may be shifted from the placenta to the infant. In term infants, delayed umbilical cord clamping increases hemoglobin levels at birth and improves initial iron stores, which may have a favorable effect on developmental outcomes; however, there may be an increased risk of neonatal hyperbilirubinemia and mechanisms should be in place to monitor and treat neonatal jaundice. Prolonged delay in cord clamping is not routinely recommended. The umbilical cord should be cut between a cord clamp placed 2 to 3 cm from the fetal abdomen and another clamp just distal to the first clamp.

SELECTED READING

American College of Obstetrics and Gynecology: Approaches to limit intervention during labor and birth. ACOG Committee Opinion Number 766. February 2019

American College of Obstetrics and Gynecology: Delayed umbilical cord clamping after birth: ACOG Committee Opinion Number 814. December 2020

American College of Obstetrics and Gynecology: Delivery of a newborn with meconium-stained amniotic fluid. ACOG Committee Opinion Number 689. March 2017 (reaffirmed 2021)

Di Mascio D, Saccone G, Bellussi F, Al-Kouatly HB, Brunelli R, Benedetti Panici P, et al: Delayed versus immediate pushing in the second stage of labor in women with neuraxial analgesia: A systematic review and meta-analysis of randomized controlled trials. Am J Obstet Gynecol 223:189-203, 2020

National Collaborating Centre for Women's and Children's Health: Intrapartum care: Care of healthy women and their babies during childbirth. London, UK: RCOG Press; 2017. https://www.nice.org.uk/guidance/cg190

National Institute for Health and Care Excellence: Intrapartum care for healthy women and babies. Clinical Guideline. 2017

Patterson C, Saunders N St G, Wadsworth J: The characteristics of the second stage of labour in 25,069 singleton deliveries in the North West Thames Health Region, 1988. Br J Obstet Gynecol 99:377, 1992

Society of Obstetricians and Gynecologists of Canada: Fetal health surveillance: Intrapartum consensus guideline. Clinical Practice Guideline No. 396. March 2020

Society of Obstetricians and Gynecologists of Canada: Obstetrical Anal Sphincter Injuries (OASIS): Prevention, recognition, and repair. Clinical Practice Guideline No. 330. December 2015

Sprague AE, Oppenheimer L, McCabe L, Brownlee J, et al: The Ottawa Hospital's clinical practice guideline for the second stage of labour. J Obstet Gynaecol Can 28:769, 2006

CHAPTER 17

Operative Vaginal Birth

Gihad Shabib
Amanda Black

Assisted or operative vaginal birth refers to the use of a vacuum or forceps to achieve a vaginal birth in the second stage of labor for fetal or maternal indications. When deciding whether to perform an assisted vaginal birth (AVB), considerations must include indications and contraindications to the procedure, timing and choice of instrument, the maternal or fetal risks of using either instrument, the urgency of the need to expedite delivery, the experience and skills of the birth attendant, and the risks associated with the alternative choice of cesarean section in the second stage of labor. Regardless of the instrument used, the indications for AVB are the same. The operator should assess the safety and likelihood of success by considering the estimated fetal weight, adequacy of the maternal pelvis, fetal station, fetal position, and adequacy of anesthesia prior to use of either forceps or the vacuum. AVB should only be attempted if there is a reasonable chance of success, and a backup plan should be in place in case the attempt is not successful. Forceps or vacuum extraction is contraindicated if the fetal head is not engaged in the pelvis or if the fetal position cannot be determined.

RATES OF ASSISTED VAGINAL BIRTH

The rate of AVB in North America has decreased over time, while the rates of primary cesarean birth have been increasing. The rates of vacuum-assisted vaginal birth are higher than the rates of forceps-assisted vaginal birth. Reasons for declining rates of forceps use may include increased litigation, unfavorable publicity regarding forceps, decreasing family size, and improved safety of cesarean section. The decrease in forceps use and the increase in cesarean section rates may also be secondary to a decrease in operator skills required to perform a forceps delivery because obstetric trainees now receive less exposure to forceps training.

Many international colleges and societies have advocated for increased use of AVB in order to reduce the increasing rate of cesarean births. The current challenge for promoting AVB is ensuring adequate health care provider training and skills. It is widely accepted that obstetrical trainees should receive appropriate comprehensive training in AVB and deemed competent prior to independent practice. This maintains a high standard of care and the highly skilled *Art of Obstetrics* in the next generation of care providers.

CHOICE OF INSTRUMENT

Whether to use forceps or a vacuum extractor (and the specific instrument) will depend on the clinical circumstances, provider preference based on experience and training, and the patient's choice. Informed consent is an essential part of an AVB. The indications for vacuum and forceps are the same, although it is believed that vacuum extraction is easier to learn. Vacuum may be preferred when asynclitism prevents proper forceps placement, while forceps provide a more secure application and are used to rotate the fetal head to the occipitoanterior (OA) or occipitoposterior (OP) position. Forceps are associated with a higher likelihood of achieving a vaginal birth but are also associated with a higher likelihood of third- and fourth-degree tears. Although the safe lower limit for gestational age has not been established, vacuum extraction is generally discouraged at gestational ages less than 34 weeks and should be used with caution between 34 and 36 weeks. Overall, both vacuum and forceps are associated with relatively low rates of serious maternal and/or neonatal morbidity and mortality when performed by skilled operators in appropriately selected circumstances. As the second stage of labor progresses, the balance of risks between AVB and cesarean delivery changes continuously. A second-stage cesarean delivery may have higher risks compared to an AVB or a cesarean section done in the first stage of labor.

Current evidence suggests that sequential use of forceps and vacuums (i.e., the use of an alternative instrument after the first instrument has failed) should generally be avoided due to increased risk of neonatal complications. However, the vacuum is also associated with an increased risk of noncompletion of vaginal deliveries (30% failure rate in cohort studies) thus requiring forceps to complete the delivery (40% for rotational delivery). Knowing this, an experienced operator may preferentially choose forceps for an AVB. Due to the increasing use of the vacuum, sequential use of instruments may become more common.

The use of manual rotation from OP or occipitotranverse (OT) to a more optimal OA position may be up to 90 percent effective in rotating to OA. When successful, it is associated with a significant reduction in the need for cesarean section, decreased use of instruments to achieve a vaginal birth, and an increased rate of vaginal birth. It may also improve the likelihood of a successful AVB. The operator uses their hand to rotate the presenting fetal head. Although it is generally performed at full dilation (10 cm), it may be considered prior to full dilation in some clinical scenarios to facilitate labor progress.

OBSTETRIC FORCEPS

The obstetric forceps are instruments designed to extract the fetal head. Forceps cradle the parietal and malar bones of the fetal skull and apply traction to these areas as they displace maternal tissue laterally. There are many varieties of forceps, but the basic design and purpose are the same. They may be used to provide traction, rotation, flexion, and extension.

All forceps consist of two crossing branches. Each branch consists of four parts: the blade, shank, lock, and handle. Each blade has two curves: the cephalic curve that conforms to the shape of the fetal head and the pelvic curve that conforms to the shape of the birth canal. Some blades are fenestrated and some are solid (Fig. 17-1A).

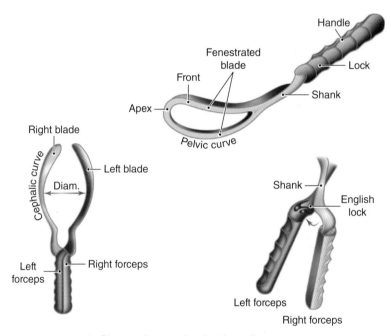

A. Simpson forceps showing the various parts.

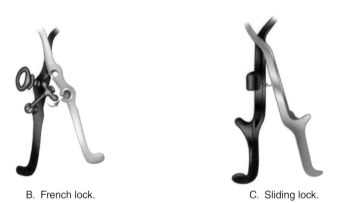

B. French lock.   C. Sliding lock.

FIGURE 17-1. Obstetric forceps.

Parts of the Forceps

1. *Handles:* These are used to grip the forceps
2. *Lock:* This holds the forceps together. It is constructed so that the right one fits on over the left. For this reason, the left blade should usually be applied first. The main types of lock are:
   a. The *English lock* (e.g., Simpson forceps) has a shoulder and flange in each shank that fits into each other. Articulation is fixed at a given point
   b. The *French lock* (e.g., Tarnier and De Wees) has a pinion and screw. The left shank bears a pivot fitting into a notch on the right shank. After articulation, the pivot is tightened by screwing it in (Fig. 17-1B)
   c. The *sliding lock* (e.g., Kielland). The articulation is not fixed. This allows the shanks to move forward and backward independently so can be useful to correct an asynclitic head (common in deep transverse arrest) (Fig. 17-1C)
3. *Shank:* This connects the handle to the blade. The shanks are either parallel as in the Simpson forceps or overlapping as they are in the Tucker-McLane forceps. A short-shanked instrument such as the Wrigley's forceps can be used only when the fetal head (not the caput) is on the perineum (≥+3 station). When the head has not reached the perineum, longer shanks are needed. The shank of the Piper forceps is noticeably longer to allow for ventral application to the after-coming head.
4. *Blades:* These enclose the fetal head and may be solid (e.g., Tucker-McLane forceps) or fenestrated (e.g., Simpson forceps). They are designed to grasp the head firmly but without excessive compression. The solid blades may cause less maternal tissue trauma. The fenestrated blades are lighter, grip the fetal head better, and are less likely to slip. The edges are smooth to reduce damage to the soft tissues. A single blade can also be used to scoop out the head during cesarean delivery.
   a. *Right and left forceps:* The forceps are designated right or left depending on the side of the maternal pelvis to which it is applied. Since most forceps cross at the lock, the handle of the right forceps is held in the operator's right hand, and the right blade fits the right side of the pelvis. The left blade fits the left side of the maternal pelvis, and its handle is held in the left hand of the operator. This does not apply in Kielland forceps where there is a minimal pelvic curve

    b. *Curves:* The forceps has two curves. The cephalic curve fits the shape of the baby's head and reduces the danger of compression. The diameter is the widest distance between the cephalic curves of the blades (~7.5 cm). The pelvic curve follows the direction of the birth canal. It makes application and extraction easier and decreases damage to the maternal tissues. The pelvic curve is minimal in Kielland forceps.

Types of Forceps

There are many forceps and some have specialized functions (Figs. 17-2A to E). Rotational forceps or forceps for the after-coming head at breech delivery require specific forceps. Birth attendants should learn to use one instrument and become thoroughly skilled and comfortable with that instrument before learning the use of another instrument.

1. *Simpson forceps* (Figs. 17-1A, 17-2A): This is the most commonly used forceps. It has a cephalic curve, an ample pelvic curve, a fenestrated blade, and a wide straight shank in front of an English lock. This is a good general-duty forceps and is used widely for direct obstetric forceps operations (when the sagittal suture is in the midline anteroposterior [AP] diameter)

2. *DeLee forceps:* This is the Simpson forceps with some minor modifications. The shank is a little longer to keep the handle away from the anus. The handle is changed to secure lightness, a better grip, and ease of cleaning

3. *Luikart forceps* (Fig. 17-2B): This is a modified Simpson forceps with a semi-fenestrated blade

4. *Wrigley's forceps:* This is similar to Simpson forceps but has very short (or no) shanks. It can be used only when the fetal head (not the caput) is on the perineum (>+3 station) (i.e., no downward traction is required). A single blade can be used to scoop out the head during cesarean delivery

5. *Kielland forceps* (Fig. 17-2C): The pelvic curve is minimal, which makes these forceps ideal for rotating the fetal head. Rotation can be accomplished simply by twisting the closed handles instead of sweeping them through a wide arc, as is necessary when using forceps with a deep pelvic curve. The sliding lock allows for simultaneous correction of asynclitism before rotation. On each handle there is a small knob (on the side of the minimal pelvic curve) that indicates the direction of the occiput. Delivery can be accomplished with the same instrument; no reapplication is needed. There is also a unique perineal curve that rests

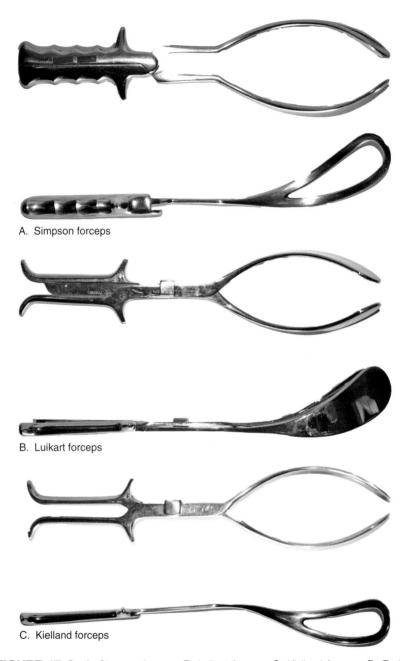

A. Simpson forceps

B. Luikart forceps

C. Kielland forceps

FIGURE 17-2. A. Simpson forceps. **B.** Luikart forceps. **C.** Kielland forceps. **D.** Tucker-McLane forceps. **E.** Piper forceps.

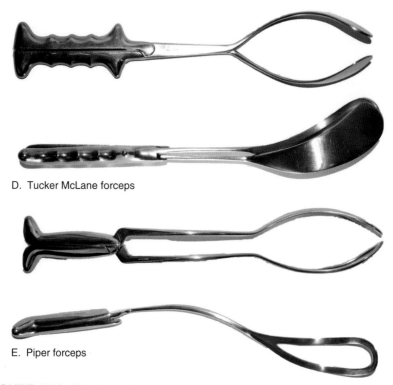

D. Tucker McLane forceps

E. Piper forceps

FIGURE 17-2. (*Continued*)

on the perineal body and can aid in the downward traction in midforceps application in substitution for the axis-traction piece. The shanks are usually long to allow for the anterior wandering method of application. In the absence of Piper forceps, Kielland forceps can be used to deliver an after-coming head in breech presentation

6. *Tucker-McLane forceps* (Fig. 17-2D): The blades are solid and have a more rounded cephalic curve. Some operators use this forceps for rotation because its pelvic curve is smaller than that of Simpson forceps

7. *Piper forceps* (Fig. 17-2E): These are used for the delivery of the after-coming head at breech delivery. The blade of these forceps is similar to the Simpson forceps. The shank is longer and curved downward so that the handles are lower than the blades. This forceps has a prominent perineal curve, which facilitates application to the after-coming head from underneath the fetal body in breech presentations

8. *Axis-traction piece:* These forceps are designed to direct traction efforts into the pelvic curve. A traction apparatus can be attached either to:

- The blades at the base of the fenestrae (Tarnier and Milne-Murray) or
- The handles (DeWees or Barnes-Neville)
  In the past, they were used for difficult high and midforceps deliveries but they are rarely used in modern obstetrics

USE OF FORCEPS

Indications for Use of Forceps

Forceps may be used for fetal or maternal indications. An AVB may be indicated if there is a threat to the mother or fetus that may be relieved by delivery. When signs of fetal compromise are present and delivery can be expedited by an easy forceps delivery, this should be done as quickly as possible. On the other hand, one should avoid panicky attempts to deliver a fetus with possible anoxia because these attempts may in fact be damaging to the fetus if a difficult, traumatic, and sometimes needless or inappropriate forceps traction is attempted.

Fetal Indications

1. Suspicion of fetal compromise in the second stage of labor
2. Fetal head malposition, such as direct occipitoposterior (DOP), occipitotransverse (ROT or LOT), or persistent occipitoposterior (POP)
3. After-coming head in breech vaginal delivery

Maternal Indications

1. Shortening of the second stage because of maternal conditions that preclude repetitive Valsalva maneuvers such as:
   a. Cardiac or pulmonary disease as heart failure, severe hypertension, risk of aortic dissection, or history of spontaneous pneumothorax
   b. Certain neurological conditions, such as elevated intracranial tension, cerebral aneurysms, spinal cord injuries with risk of autonomic dysreflexia, spinal tap, and Myasthenia gravis.
   c. Certain ophthalmological conditions such as proliferative retinopathy
2. Maternal exhaustion resulting in a lack of effective maternal effort

SECOND STAGE OF LABOR

Prolonged Active Second Stage

Lack of progress in the second stage includes failure of descent and failure of internal rotation. The chance of fetal compromise increases with prolonged pushing in the second stage or when the presenting part is low on the perineum for an extended period of time. Pelvic floor injury becomes more common as the duration of the second stage increases. After more than 3 hours in primigravida and 2 hours in multigravida of synchronized pushing aided by adequate uterine contractions, AVB should be considered if there is no other evidence of cephalopelvic disproportion (CPD). Situations that may predispose to a prolonged second stage include:

1. Poor uterine contractions
2. Minor degrees of relative disproportion
3. Fetal macrosomia
4. Abnormal fetal position, such as occiput posterior position, or attitudes (deflexion). Manual rotation may be attempted to turn the fetal head to a more optimal OA position and when successful, has been shown to increase the rate of vaginal birth
5. Rigid perineum that the advancing head cannot thin out
6. A lax pelvic floor that inhibits proper rotation of the head, as with deep epidural block

Contraindications to the Use of Forceps

1. Nonvertex or brow presentation. Forceps can be used for face presentation and after-coming head of the breech presentation. Vacuum cannot be used for a face presentation
2. Unengaged or high fetal head
3. Incompletely dilated cervix
4. Inability to determine the presentation and fetal head position or pelvic adequacy
5. Fetal bleeding disorder (e.g., alloimmune thrombocytopenia), or predisposition to fracture (e.g., osteogenesis imperfecta)
6. Gestation less than 34 weeks. Vacuum extraction should not be performed under 34 weeks and used only with caution between 34 and 36 weeks because its safety in this gestational age range is uncertain
7. Cephalopelvic disproportion (CPD)
8. Absence of a proper indication
9. Any contraindication to vaginal delivery
10. Absence of adequate anesthesia. A pudendal block may be sufficient for vacuum or outlet forceps

11. Inadequate facilities and support staff to do an urgent cesarean section in case of failure
12. Inexperienced operator

Morbidity Associated with Forceps Delivery

Risks of AVB should be compared to risks of second stage cesarean birth because cesarean birth is the clinical alternative.

Maternal Risks
Maternal risks tend to increase significantly with rotational and midcavity births.

1. Lacerations of the vulva, vagina, and cervix, and extension of episiotomy
2. Third- and fourth-degree lacerations (Obstetric Anal Sphincter Injuries [OASIS]) with possible long-term anal sphincter dysfunction
3. Postpartum hemorrhage secondary to lacerations and uterine atony
4. Vaginal and vulvar hematomas
5. Postpartum urinary retention and bladder dysfunction. Bladder atony usually starts as sensory atony secondary to pain from the perineal injuries or prolonged postpartum epidural effect such as with a top-up prior to forceps application. Inability to feel the bladder fullness causes overdistension of the bladder. This leads to motor atony with high postvoid residuals and subsequent urinary infections. After a difficult AVB, bladder rest via a Foley catheter insertion followed by bladder training usually leads to a return to normal function after a few days
6. Genital tract infection and perineal wound dehiscence

The role of routine episiotomy for AVBs is controversial. Evidence shows that performing a mediolateral or lateral episiotomy in women having their first vaginal birth reduces the risk of OASIS in both vacuum- and forceps-assisted births (24% fewer OASIS with forceps AVB and 16% fewer OASIS with vacuum AVB). Thus, episiotomy should be considered in the context of the clinical scenario.

Fetal Risks
The type and frequency of neonatal injuries vary to some degree with the instrument used.

1. Fetal facial marks, facial lacerations (1%).
2. Facial nerve palsies (<1%)

3. Minor external ocular trauma (2.3%)
4. Retinal hemorrhage and corneal abrasion (abrasion more common with forceps; retinal hemorrhage more common with vacuum)
5. Cephalohematoma (5% of vacuum assisted births): A deeper collection of blood between the skull bone and periosteum that is typically benign and resolves over time. Neonatal hyperbilirubinemia may occur secondary to resorption of hemoglobin in approximately 5 percent of vacuum deliveries
6. Subaponeurotic/subgaleal hemorrhage due to tearing of the large emissary veins below the scalp aponeurosis. (0.1-0.3% of vacuum deliveries, potentially life threatening due to rapid loss of volume and neonatal hypovolemia and shock)
7. Intracranial hemorrhage (0.1-0.2%)
8. Neurological injuries (0.2-0.5%)
9. Fetal scalp laceration
10. Shoulder dystocia (if lack of progress and anticipated macrosomia or prolonged second stage in a multigravida)
11. Fetal skull fractures (very rare)
12. Brachial plexus injury (0.05%)
13. Cervical spine injury (rare, 0.07% of rotational forceps births)
14. Cord compression

Complications do not appear to be substantially greater than with cesarean section performed in labor. Evidence suggests that some injuries (such as intracranial hemorrhage) attributed to AVB are actually associated with the indication for delivery rather than the procedure itself, and that the alternative of cesarean birth does not lessen the risk. In the clinical scenario of signs of fetal compromise in the second stage of labor, timely and skilled use of AVB potentially decreases the exposure to ongoing intrauterine insults and intrapartum factors that could lead to neonatal encephalopathy and hypoxic-ischemic encephalopathy.

Serious fetal injuries with forceps AVB consist mainly of damage to the falx cerebri, the tentorium cerebelli, and the associated venous sinuses and other vessels. These injuries are associated mainly with deliveries from the midpelvis or higher and are caused by excessive force and excessive compression. This trauma is extremely rare in modern obstetrics. The dangers are especially great when: (1) the forceps are poorly applied (applied in other than the biparietal diameter [BPD]), (2) the fetal head is forced downward through the least favorable diameters of the pelvis, (3) forceful rotation is made at the wrong level of the pelvis or against the fetal back, and (4) excessive force is used in other than the correct line of the axis of the pelvis.

Classification of Forceps Operations

Forceps delivery may be classified into one of four categories: outlet, low, mid, or high forceps (Fig. 17-3). Most cases fit into these categories. However, when there is extreme molding, marked asynclitism, a large caput succedaneum, or an abnormal pelvis, the operator may make the error of thinking that the station is lower than it really is. In general, high forceps deliveries are contraindicated in modern obstetrics.

Outlet forceps	• Fetal scalp is visible on the vulva without separating the labia • Fetal skull (not caput) has reached the pelvic floor (+3 station) • Fetal head is at or on the perineum • Sagittal suture is in the AP diameter (OA or OP) or rotation does not exceed 45° (LOA, ROA, LOP, ROP)
Low forceps	The leading point of the skull (not caput) is at +2 station The leading point is not on the pelvic floor Rotation of <45° (LOA, ROA, LOP, ROP)
Midforceps	Fetal head is engaged (<1/5 palpable abdominally) The leading point of the fetal skull is <+2 station but not above the ischial spines A. Rotation of 45 degrees or less from OA position B. Rotation of >45° from OA position (OT to OA or DOP to DOA)
High forceps	• Fetal head is not engaged. The station is above the ischial spines and the head palpable 2/5 or more abdominally • Contraindicated in modern obstetrics

Prerequisites for an Assisted Vaginal Birth

- Consent
- No fetal contraindications
- Examination: Abdominal and vaginal
- Cervix fully dilated and membranes ruptured
- Engaged fetal head
- Exact fetal head position known
- Estimation of fetal weight
- Adequate maternal pelvis
- Adequate anesthesia
- Empty bladder. Remove indwelling catheter or deflate balloon
- Adequate staff: skilled operator, staff skilled in neonatal resuscitation, anesthesia aware and available
- Appropriate location for delivery
- Willingness to abandon attempt at AVB. Backup plan in place if AVB attempt is unsuccessful

SECOND STAGE OF LABOR

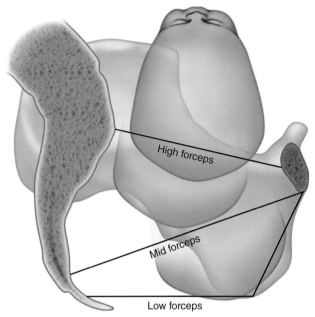

FIGURE 17-3. Classification of forceps operations according to station.

1. The head must be deeply engaged in the pelvis (i.e., the vault bone must be >1 cm below the ischial spines). Assessing engagement of the bony skull in relation to the ischial spines should not be confused with caput succedaneum. Abdominal assessment using the fourth Leopold maneuver can be used to ensure that the BPD has passed the pelvic brim. Less than 1/5 of the head should be palpable abdominally

   "If you feel the fetal head abdominally, deliver it abdominally."

2. The fetus must present as a vertex or as mentum anterior in a face presentation
3. The exact position of the fetal head must be known
   a. Suspect malposition of the head if labor progress was slow, when there is a prolonged decelerative phase of labor (the cervix is 9 cm for more than 1 hour), or when there are repeated early decelerations on the fetal heart tracing. This is usually the result of vagal stimulation secondary to compression of the anterior fontanelle of the deflexed head against the pelvic floor
   b. Abdominal examination (Leopold's maneuvers) can be used to diagnose OP malposition in early labor:

- Flattening of the abdomen below the umbilicus
- Fetal limbs may be felt over the front of the uterus
- The fetal back is not palpated in the flank but rather laterally
- The fetal heart is best heard on the outer third of a line between the umbilicus and anterior superior iliac spine

c. Pelvic examination during labor: Use the fontanelles and sutures to determine the position (Figs. 17-4A to C). This is not always easy at the end of the second stage because of skull molding and scalp caput
  - If you can feel a fontanelle easily, then it is more likely to be the anterior fontanelle. The anterior fontanelle is merely a bony defect with four surrounding sutures meeting as an X
  - The posterior fontanelle is a potential space, not a palpable soft spot. Feel for three sutures meeting as a Y
  - Locate the sagittal suture. If the suture is not in the AP diameter, then check for the fetal ear under the symphysis pubis. This is usually palpable in OT malposition
  - Check for asynclitism. In anterior asynclitism, the sagittal suture is easily palpable (common in primigravida). The sagittal suture is difficult to palpate in posterior asynclitism (common in multigravidas)
  - Ultrasound evaluation is a useful tool if the exact position of the head is uncertain by clinical evaluation

"Correct determination of the position is the most important step before forceps application."

4. The cervix must be fully dilated and retracted
5. The membranes must be ruptured. If they are not, there is an increased chance of the blades slipping and there is danger of pulling the placenta away from the uterine wall
6. There should be no suspicion of CPD
7. Informed consent must be obtained
8. The mother must have adequate anesthesia. Topping up the epidural anesthesia with a perineal block dose is often used. A pudendal block may be useful for a vacuum or outlet forceps but is not sufficient for mid or rotational forceps
9. The maternal bladder is empty. It is also advisable to drain the bladder for a few hours after a rotational or difficult forceps delivery, especially if the patient received an epidural top-up immediately before delivery
10. Adequate facilities and backup personnel should be available

SECOND STAGE OF LABOR

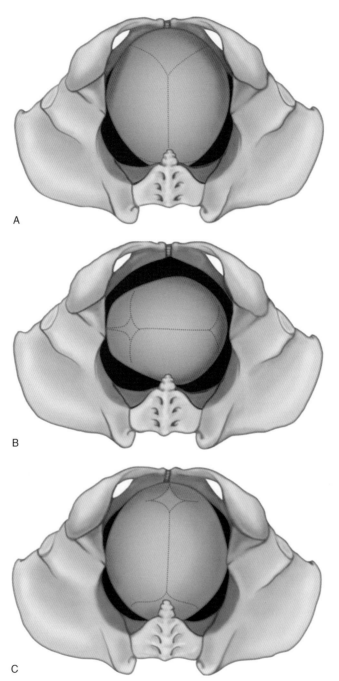

A

B

C

FIGURE 17-4. A. Direct occipitoanterior (OA) position. **B.** Left occipitotransverse (LOT) position. **C.** Direct occipitoposterior (OP) position.

11. The operator should be fully competent and have the knowledge, experience, and skill necessary to use the instruments, recognize when to stop, and manage complications that may arise

APPLICATION OF FORCEPS

Cephalic Application

A cephalic application is made to fit the baby's head (Fig. 17-5A). An ideal cephalic application in OA positions is along the occipitomental diameter, with the fenestrae including the parietal bosses and the zygomo-temporal arch with its tips lying over the cheeks. The convex edges are toward the face.

With this application, pressure on the head causes the least damage. Forceps marks lateral to the eyes and over the ear or the mastoid bone indicate good application. If the forceps are applied so that one blade lies over the face and the other over the occiput (bad application), any degree of compression may cause fetal tentorial tears, intracranial hemorrhage, and facial soft tissue damage. This type of poor application is almost always the result of an inability to determine with certainty the exact position of the fetal head in the pelvis.

Pelvic Application

A pelvic application is made to fit the maternal pelvis (Fig. 17-5B), regardless of how the forceps grip the fetal head. The pelvic application alone is associated with a high risk of fetal injuries. The term pelvic application is used when:

1. The left blade is next to the left side of the pelvis
2. The right blade is on the right side of the pelvis
3. The concave margin is near the symphysis pubis
4. The convex margin is in the hollow of the sacrum
5. The diameter of the forceps is in the transverse diameter of the pelvis.

Perfect Application

A perfect (cephalopelvic) application (Fig. 17-5C) is achieved when both the cephalic and pelvic requirements have been fulfilled. A perfect

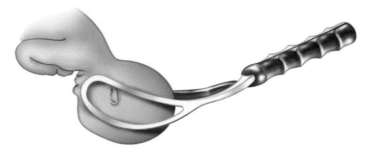

A. Cephalic application.

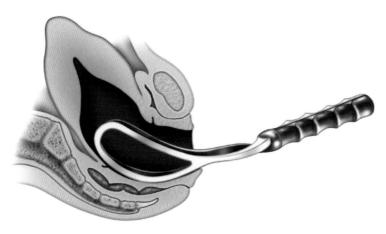

B. Pelvic application.

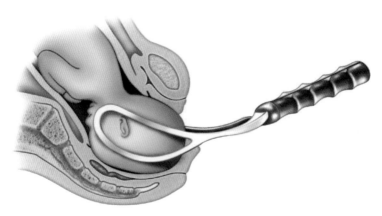

C. Perfect application.

FIGURE 17-5. **A**. Cephalic application of obstetric forceps. **B.** Pelvic application of obstetric forceps. **C.** Perfect application of obstetric forceps.

application is possible in direct OA (DOA) positions when the occiput has already rotated to be directly under the symphysis pubis and the sagittal suture is in the AP diameter.

THE USES OF OBSTETRIC FORCEPS

Direct Occipitoanterior Forceps Delivery

In other than expert hands, the use of forceps should be restricted to that of direct application and traction. Simpson or Tucker-McLane forceps are useful for simple direct application and traction.

Application

1. Recheck that the prerequisite conditions and indications have been met (a checklist is helpful)
2. Perform a vaginal examination to accurately diagnose the position and station of the head, whether there is flexion or extension, and the presence of synclitism or asynclitism
3. Perform a phantom application. The locked forceps are held outside the vagina in front of the perineum in the way they are to be applied to the fetal head in the pelvis
4. The left blade is inserted first. The left blade is held in the left hand (pencil grip). At first the blade is in an almost vertical position. Gently introduce the blade into the left lower side of the pelvis (5 o'clock position) using the back of the right index and middle fingers to retract the vaginal wall laterally while the right thumb is directing the blade on the hollow of the sacrum then upward opposite to the ala of the sacrum (Fig. 17-6A)
5. The handle is lowered slowly to the horizontal and toward the midline by pushing downward on the handle. This should help to complete the last part of the head rotation from left occipitoanterior (LOA) to DOA (Fig. 17-6B)
6. The right blade is then held in the right hand, and the fingers of the left hand are inserted in the right side of the vagina between the fetal head and the vaginal wall. The right blade is gently introduced over the left forceps between the operator's fingers and the fetal head at about 7 o'clock (Fig. 17-6C). The right handle is lowered to the horizontal and toward the midline. At the same time, the vaginal fingers move the blade up over the right side of the head to the occipitomental

position. The fingers of the left hand are then removed from the vagina (Fig. 17-6D)

7. Lock the blades. They should fall into place without any excessive force. The handles must never be forced together. If the blades do not lock easily, suspect a *bad application*. Remove the forceps and reevaluate the fetal head position (Fig. 17-7)

   In ROA (<45 degrees): Introduce the right blade first and push the handle downward to help the rotation to DOA then apply the left blade as usual. They will not spontaneously articulate. The operator must rotate the left handle around the right to bring the lock into proper position.

8. Final evaluation to confirm a *good application*

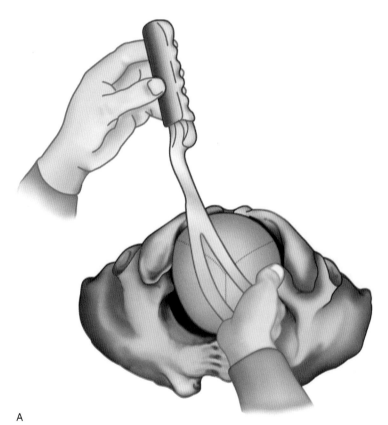

A

FIGURE 17-6. **A.** Insertion of left blade between fetal head and left side of pelvis. **B.** Handle of left forceps is lowered and the blade moved up over the left parietal bone. **C.** Insertion of right blade between fetal head and right side of pelvis. **D.** Handle of right forceps is lowered and the blade moved up over the right parietal bone.

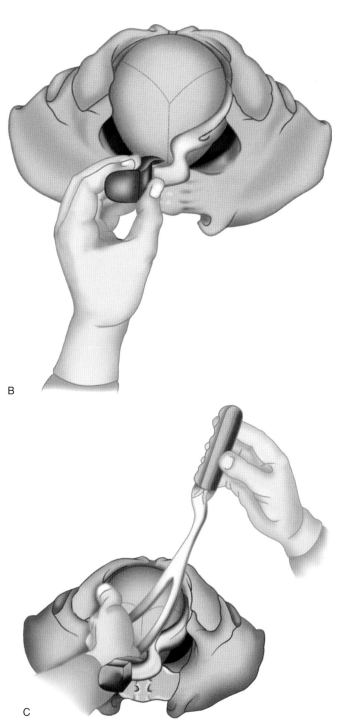

B

C

FIGURE 17-6. (*Continued*)

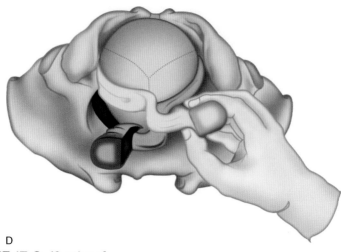

D

FIGURE 17-6. (*Continued*)

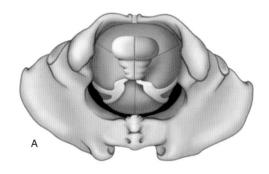

A

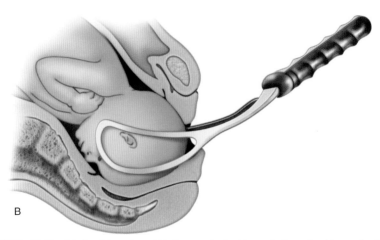

B

FIGURE 17-7. OA: Locking. A and B. Forceps locked in cephalic and pelvic application.

    a. The posterior fontanelle should be midway between the blades, and the lambdoid sutures should be one finger above the shanks. If this is too far, suspect head deflexion that would increase the risk of maternal injuries

    b. The sagittal suture should be perpendicular to the plane of the shanks, and the blades should be equidistant from the sagittal suture. An asymmetrical relationship indicates that one of the blades was applied in a higher or a lower position in relation to the fetal face and subsequently increases the risks of fetal injury

    c. The fenestration of the blades is barely felt and is equal. If you can easily introduce your finger, suspect a short application and a subsequent higher risk of fetal injury

Traction and Delivery

It is preferable to provide traction with each contraction. The head should be allowed to recede in intervals between contractions.

1. The direction of traction is along the pelvic curvature (backward-tilted L-shape with the lower end pointed up 45°). As the station changes during descent, so will the line of traction (Fig. 17-8A)

2. Gentle, slow, downward traction is applied during uterine contractions until the vault of the fetal skull is at +3 station or the head is on perineum and visibly distending the vulva

3. At that point, the direction should change to upward (Fig. 17-8B) and then toward the mother's abdomen as the head reaches the perineum and becomes visible within the vulva and the parietal bones emerge. This will allow for delivery of the head by extension. This step should be undertaken very slowly in order to minimize maternal soft tissue trauma

4. Episiotomy should not be performed routinely for operative vaginal deliveries. If it is deemed necessary, a mediolateral episiotomy may have a lower risk of anal sphincter injury than midline episiotomy but it is associated with an increased likelihood of long-term perianal pain and dyspareunia

5. The forceps are removed when the head is crowning just prior to the full delivery of the head in a process, that is, the reverse of their application. The handle of the right blade is raised toward the mother's left groin and the blade slides around the head and out of the pelvis (Fig. 17-9). Then, the same is done with the left forceps by raising the handle toward the maternal right groin. This allows for spontaneous

SECOND STAGE OF LABOR

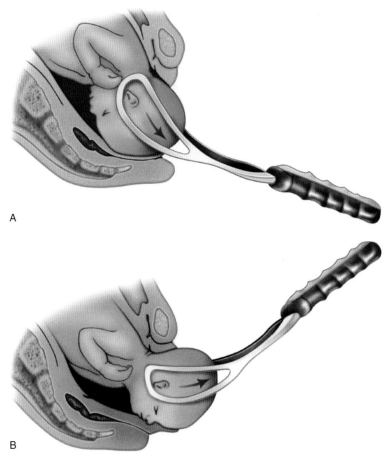

A

B

FIGURE 17-8. **A.** Traction is made outward and posteriorly until the nape of the neck is under the pubic symphysis. **B.** The direction of traction is changed to promote extension of the fetal head.

delivery and helps to minimize perineal lacerations. Delivery can also be aided by the unlocked forceps blades (modified Ritgen maneuver)

Left Occipitoanterior Forceps Delivery

The principles of forceps application with an LOA presentation are similar to those with a DOA position with the exception that the head is rotated with the use of the forceps from an LOA to OA position. In many cases, the head may rotate spontaneously from LOA to OA as traction is applied, but

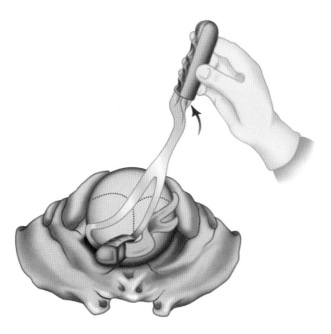

A. Removal of right forceps.

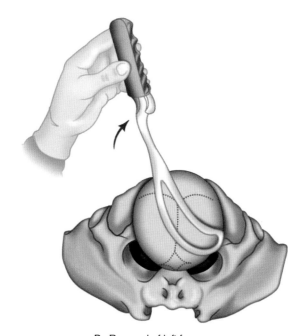

B. Removal of left forceps.

FIGURE 17-9. Removal of forceps.

if not, the operator must rotate the occiput 45° to the anterior at the same time that they are exerting traction (Fig. 17-10).

Direct Occipitoposterior Forceps Delivery

In DOP positions, delivering the head by direct application and traction using Simpson or Tucker-McLane forceps is possible. However, the risk of perineal trauma, including fourth-degree tears, is high as the wider part of the head, the occiput, lies against the perineum. The head is delivered in flexion. It is advisable to change the direction of traction to upward earlier than in OA presentations before the occiput fills the posterior half of the vulva.

Orientation and Desired Application: The Perfect Cephalopelvic Application

The cephalic application:

1. The blades of the forceps are over the parietal bones in an occipitomental application. The left blade is on the right parietal bone, and the right blade is on the left parietal bone
2. The front of the forceps (concave edges) point to the face. In an ideal cephalic application, they point to the occiput
3. The convex edges point to the occiput. In the ideal application, they point to the face

The pelvic application:

1. The diameter of the forceps is in the transverse diameter of the pelvis
2. The sides of the blades are next to the sidewalls of the pelvis, the left blade near the left side and right blade near the right side
3. The concave edges point to the pubis
4. The convex edges point to the sacrum (Fig. 17-11)

Extraction of the Head

1. Traction is made outward and posteriorly until the area between the bregma and the nasion lies under the pubic arch (Fig. 17-12A)
2. The direction is changed to outward and anterior (Fig. 17-12B). As the handles of the forceps are raised, the occiput is born over the perineum

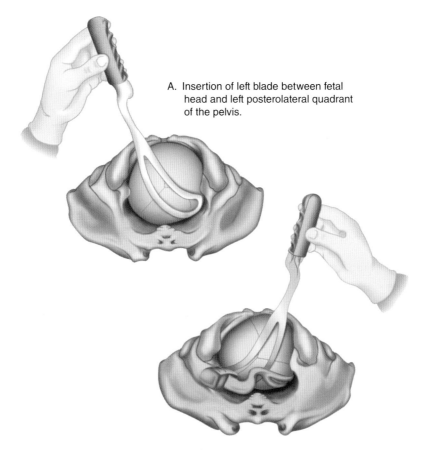

A. Insertion of left blade between fetal head and left posterolateral quadrant of the pelvis.

B. Insertion of right blade between fetal head and right posterolateral quadrant of the pelvis, followed by upward movement of the blade to right anterolateral quadrant of the pelvis.

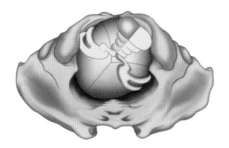

C. Locking of forceps in cephalic application.

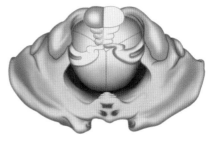

D. Head is rotated from LOA to OA. It is now ready for extraction.

FIGURE 17-10. Application of forceps in left occipitoanterior position.

by flexion. The forceps are then slipped off the head and out of the vagina. Using a modified Ritgen maneuver and carefully supporting the perineum, flexion is increased until the occiput has cleared the perineum completely

3. The head then falls back in extension. The nose, face, and chin are delivered under the pubis

4. If the head cannot be delivered as a posterior presentation without using an excessive amount of force, this method of delivery should be abandoned and an anterior rotation of the occiput carried out

Long Anterior Rotation in the Event of a Failed DOP Assisted Delivery

If the head is arrested in the midpelvis or if direct application and traction fails, a *long forceps rotation by Kielland* forceps can be performed by an

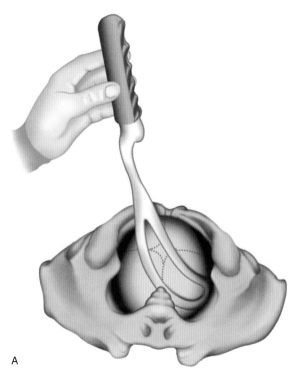

A

FIGURE 17-11. Application of forceps in the occipitoposterior position.

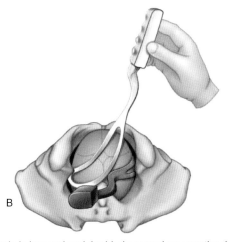

Handle of left blade is lowered and the blade moved up over the right parietal bone. Insertion of right blade between fetal head and right side of pelvis.

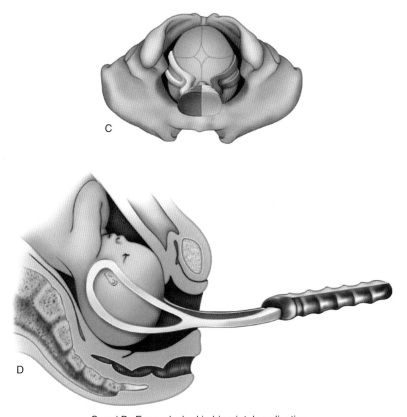

C and D. Forces locked in biparietal application.

FIGURE 17-11. (Continued)

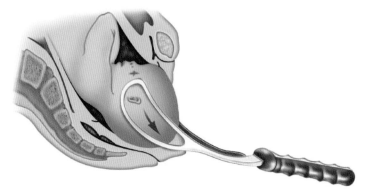

A. Traction is made outward and posteriorly until the area between
the bregma and nasion lies under the pubic arch.

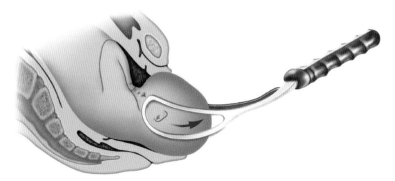

B. Traction is made outward and anteriorly to promote flexion.

FIGURE 17-12. **Extraction of the fetal head in the occipitoposterior position.**

experienced operator. On each handle of the Kielland forceps is a small
knob that indicates the direction of the occiput.

1. The operator should determine the position of the fetal back (right or left)
2. Perform a phantom application where the Kielland forceps are assem-
   bled with the knobs on the handles directed downward toward the
   occiput. The blades are then introduced directly on each side of the
   head with the pelvic curve in an inversed position
3. The head is then rotated gently toward the fetal back. Forceful rotation in the opposite direction of the fetal back may violently twist the
   baby's neck and may result in fatal axis fracture. *Rotation must only be*

performed between contractions when the uterus is relaxed. The rotation is counterclockwise if the back is on the left and clockwise if the back is on the right. It is advisable that the operator rotates the forceps from lower than the patient's bed level as the rotation takes place in the mid-pelvic plane (the upper limb of the 45° backward tilted L-shape pelvic curvature). Gentle and easy rotation should be performed in two stages:

a. From DOP to OT, bringing the knobs toward the position of the fetal back

b. The forceps application should be checked, and the fetal heart rate should be evaluated. Then, rotate OT to OA, bringing the knobs upward

ROTATIONAL FORCEPS FROM TRANSVERSE POSITIONS

Rotation from Transverse Positions (ROT or LOT to DOA)

Single Application for Rotation and Traction: Kielland Forceps

Deciding Which Is the Anterior Blade. Kielland forceps do not have a right or left blade, so the operator has to use the *phantom application* to determine the anterior and posterior blades. This is performed by holding the forceps outside the patient while directing the knobs on the shanks toward the fetal occipital bone.

Applying the Anterior Blade (Wandering Method). Between uterine contractions, the anterior blade is applied first by guiding it into the pelvis posteriorly (as in the direct forceps application). The operator then kneels down while pushing the blade deep in the pelvis. The blade is then rotated upward and laterally around the occiput or the face (clockwise or counterclockwise) according to the position of the occiput (left occipitotransverse [LOT] or right occipitotransverse [ROT]). Then, gently ease the blade concavity over the head in the occipitomental diameter, where it lays immediately under the symphysis pubis. This maneuver is called the *wandering method.*

There are other (obsolete) methods of applying the anterior blade, but these are rarely used in modern obstetrics. These include:

1. *Direct method:* The anterior blade is pushed directly below the symphysis pubis with the concavity over the side of the head. This can cause significant damage to the urethro-vesical sphincter and subsequent stress incontinence or urinary fistulae
2. *Classical method:* The anterior blade is introduced with its concavity under the symphysis pubis and pushed upward inside the uterus, above the head, and then twisted to bring the cephalic curve inward and downward over the fetal head. This maneuver has become obsolete because of the high risk of uterine rupture

Applying the Posterior Blade.   This is applied and guided directly into the hollow of the sacrum. Now it lays directly under the fetal zygomo-temporal arch with its tips lying over the cheek.

Correction of Asynclitism, Rotation, and Delivery

1. In between uterine contractions, the forceps blades are locked. The handles appear unequal outside the vulva with the posterior blade seeming longer in cases of anterior asynclitism (the reverse in posterior asynclitism.) Using the *sliding lock*, the longer handle is pushed inward in order to bring the blades opposite to each other. This motion will correct the asynclitism and would disengage the head slightly to allow for the rotation. The head is then rotated gently between contractions from OT to OA, to bring the knobs upward. Rotate clockwise to rotate the head from ROT to DOA or rotate anticlockwise to rotate the head from LOT to DOA
2. If the head is low in the pelvis, rotation may bring it to the "crowning" stage. The forceps can be removed because further traction is not required. More often traction is needed and should be carried out during uterine contraction after first checking the application is correct as in the direct forceps delivery
3. *The Modified Ritgen Maneuver* is highly recommended in rotational forceps to minimized perineal lacerations and anal sphincter injuries

Double Application of Forceps: "Scanzoni Maneuver"

Tucker-McLane or Simpson forceps can be applied to rotate the occiput anteriorly (Fig. 17-13). The handles should be maneuvered through a wide arc to reduce the arc of the blades and to lower the incidence and extent

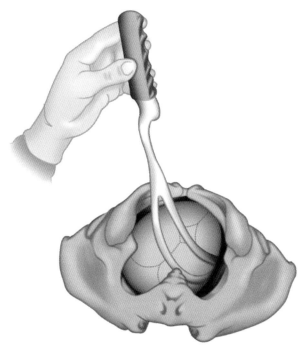

A. Insertion of left blade between fetal head and left posterolateral quadrant of pelvis.

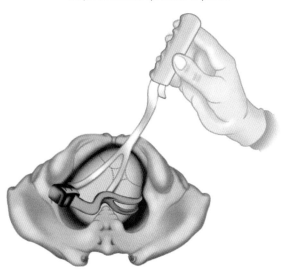

B. Handle of left blade is lowered. Insertion of right blade between fetal head and right posterolateral quadrant of pelvis, followed by upward movement of blade to right anterolateral quadrant of pelvis.

FIGURE 17-13. Application of forceps in the right occipitoposterior position for the Scanzoni maneuver.

SECOND STAGE OF LABOR

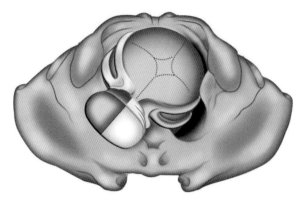

C. Locking of forceps in biparietal application.

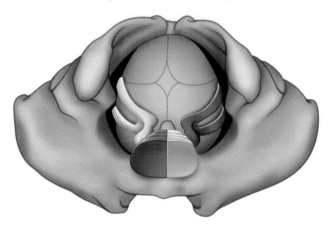

D. Posterior rotation ROP to OP (45°)

FIGURE 17-13. (*Continued*)

of vaginal lacerations (Fig. 17-14). The handles of the forceps are raised toward the opposite groin (in right occipitoposterior [ROP] toward the left groin), which favors flexion of the fetal head. Without traction, the handles are carried around in a large circle so that they point first to the left groin (ROP), next toward the left thigh (ROT), then toward the left ischial tuberosity, and finally toward the anus and pelvic floor. With the wide sweep of the handles, the blades turn in a small arc and do not deviate from the same axis during the process of rotation.

At this point, the forceps are not in a suitable position to extract the head (Fig. 17-15), and adjustments are necessary. The forceps are then unlocked and removed. The right blade is removed first by depressing the handle further so that the blade slides around the head and out of the vagina (Fig. 17-16). The left blade is then removed in the same way.

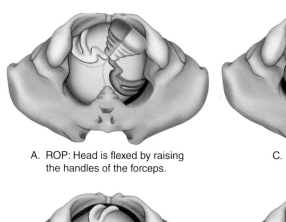
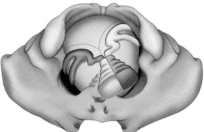
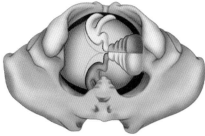
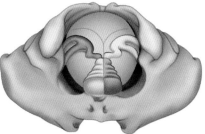

A. ROP: Head is flexed by raising the handles of the forceps.

C. ROT to ROA (45°).

B. Anterior rotation by forceps: ROP to ROT (45°).

D. ROA to OA (45°).

FIGURE 17-14. Scanzoni maneuver from right occipitoposterior (ROP) to occipito-anterior (OA). ROA, right occipitoanterior; ROT, right occipitotransverse.

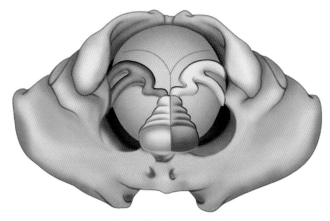

New position: OA. Forceps upside down.

FIGURE 17-15. New position: occipitoanterior (OA). Forceps upside down.

SECOND STAGE OF LABOR

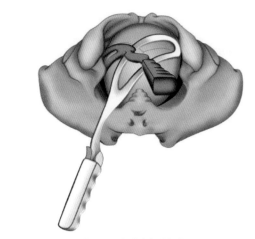

A. Removal of right blade.

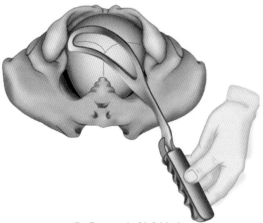

B. Removal of left blade.

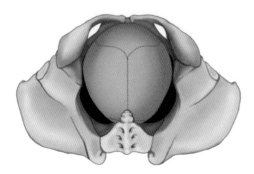

C. New position: OA

FIGURE 17-16. **Scanzoni maneuver: removal of forceps.** OA, occipitoanterior.

A vaginal examination is performed to confirm the position. The forceps are then reapplied so that the pelvic curve of the forceps is directed anteriorly (as in a DOA application) (Figs. 17-17A to C) and the head is extracted in the usual way. Some operators use Kielland forceps (or Tucker-McLane or Simpson) for rotation and then remove the blade on the left side of the pelvis to apply the left blade of a Tucker-McLane or Simpson forceps; then the same is repeated on the right side (Fig. 17-18). This modification, called a two-forceps maneuver, is useful to avoid rotation of the fetal head back to the transverse or posterior position.

Long Anterior Rotation of DOP to DOA

Single Application for Rotation and Traction: Kielland Forceps

This should be a trial of forceps in the operating room with all necessary preparations made to undertake immediate cesarean section if the procedure fails.

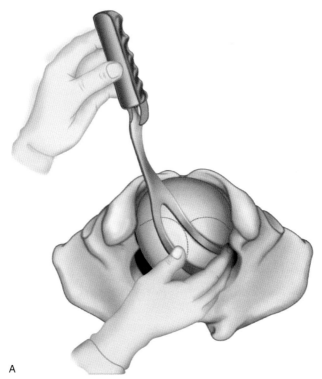

A

FIGURE 17-17. A. Reapplication of left blade between fetal head and left side of pelvis. **B.** Reapplication of right blade between fetal head and right side of pelvis. **C.** Locking of forceps in biparietal cephalic and pelvic application.

SECOND STAGE OF LABOR

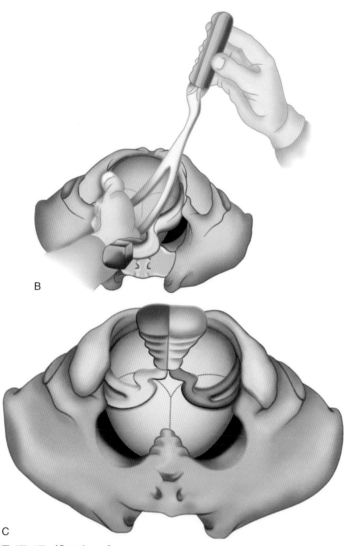

B

C

FIGURE 17-17. *(Continued)*

Determine the Position of the Fetal Back (Right or Left). This the most important step as forceful rotation in the opposite direction of the fetal back may violently twist the baby's neck and potentially result in fatal axis (C2) fracture.

Clinical evaluation is used however, the use ultrasound can be used just before application to identify the direction of the fetal spines and confirm the DOP by identifying both orbits (eye sockets) underneath the symphysis pubis.

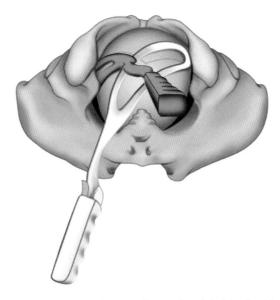

A. Removal of right Simpson forceps from left side of pelvis.

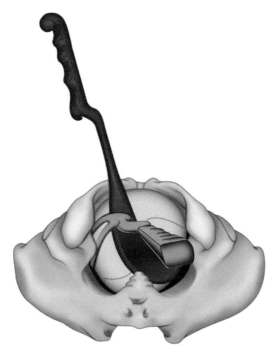

B. Insertion of left Tucker-McLane forceps between fetal head
    and left side of pelvis. The left Simpson is still in place.

FIGURE 17-18. Two-forceps maneuver.

SECOND STAGE OF LABOR

Phantom Application: The knobs on the Kielland's forceps knobs are directed downward outside the patient (*phantom application).* Between contractions, the blades are then inserted directly on each side of the head with the pelvic curves directed downward in an *inverted position.*

Long Anterior Rotation (180 degrees)

1. Rotate from lower level

   It is advisable that the operator rotates the forceps while kneeling to be in a lower plane than the patient's bed level. The head rotation naturally takes place in the midpelvic plane (the upper limb of the 45° backward-tilted L-shape pelvic curvature)
2. Gentle and easy rotation should be performed in two stages as outlined below. In between the uterine contractions, the head is gently rotated toward the fetal back. If the back is on the right, rotate *clockwise.* If the back is on the left, rotate *anticlockwise*

STAGE 1: ROTATE FROM DOP TO ROT OR LOT (90 DEGREES). The knobs (and the fetal back) are now directed to the either right or left side of the mother. Now, *pause* and recheck the forceps application and the fetal heart pattern.

STAGE 2: RESUME ROTATION BETWEEN CONTRACTIONS FROM ROT OR LOT TO DOA (ANOTHER 90 DEGREES). Now the knobs are directed upward. All these maneuvers take place while the operator is in a lower level from the pelvis.

Traction and Delivery. If traction is needed it should be carried out during a uterine contraction after first checking the application as in the DOA forceps delivery. The *Modified Ritgen maneuver* is highly recommended in rotational forceps to minimized perineal lacerations and anal sphincter injuries.

Manual Rotation of the Head

Manual rotation is associated with a significant reduction in the need for an operative birth, including cesarean section. It is best to perform it early in the second stage before the head is lodged in the pelvis. Prophylactic rotation in the first stage of labor may help but can be difficult. At the operator's discretion, manual rotation may be attempted first and if it is not successful, consider proceeding to the use of Kielland forceps. There are two techniques for manual rotation:

TECHNIQUE NUMBER 1

1. The operator places their entire hand in the woman's vagina behind the occiput with their palm facing up. The fetal head is flexed and dislodged
2. The operator rotates the fetal occiput anteriorly between contractions by pronating or supinating their forearm. If OP, the operator pronates their dominant hand on exam. If ROP, the operator pronates their left hand clockwise. If LOP, the examiner pronates their right hand counterclockwise
3. The fetal head should be held in place for a few contractions or until the forceps or vacuum are applied

TECHNIQUE NUMBER 2

1. The examiner's fingers are placed along the lambdoid sutures
2. The fetal head can be rotated to an OA position with mild pressure and a dialing motion
3. The fetal head should be held in place for a few contractions or until the vacuum or forceps is applied

Manual rotation can be used as an alternative to forceps rotation. However, it may not be successful and/or need to be repeated, may strain the examiner's hand, joints, and tendons, and is less effective if there is a deep transverse arrest.

Forceps for After-Coming Head

Piper forceps are ideal for delivery of the after-coming head in a breech presentation. Kielland forceps can be used as a substitute.

1. After delivering the body and with the appearance of the nape of the baby's neck outside the vulva, an assistant gently lifts the fetus upward. The body should not be lifted too much because excessive stretching can damage the fetal neck structures
2. The right hand is introduced into the vagina between the head and the left posterolateral wall of the vagina. The left blade is held in the left hand and guided into the vulva from underneath the body and around the right side of the fetal face. This is a mento-occipital application. The right blade is then introduced in the same manner around the left side of the fetal face

3. The handles are then locked underneath the fetal chest, and the fetal body is allowed to rest on the operator's forearms. Vaginal examination is performed to be certain that the application is correct (Fig. 17-19)

4. Traction is applied outward and posterior until the nape of the neck is in the subpubic angle. Downward traction is rarely needed to ensure complete delivery of the neck

5. After delivery of the nape, the direction of traction is changed upward toward the mother's abdomen to deliver the head in flexion. This step should be performed very slowly to avoid sudden decompression. As the face appears, it is advisable to wipe the nose and mouth clean before delivering the occiput

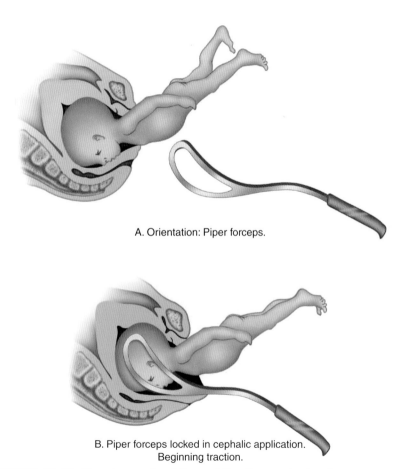

A. Orientation: Piper forceps.

B. Piper forceps locked in cephalic application.
Beginning traction.

FIGURE 17-19. Piper forceps for delivery of the after-coming head.

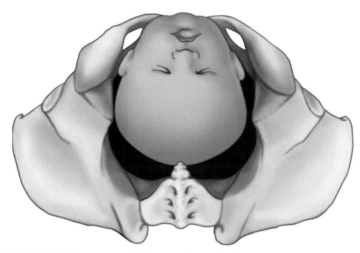

FIGURE 17-20. Face presentation, mentum anterior.

Some advocate an elective forceps delivery for the after-coming head at all breech deliveries. This is because the forceps are applied on the parietal bone, so there is reduced chance of soft tissue trauma that may result from difficult after-coming head delivery using the jaw-flexion shoulder-traction technique.

Forceps for Face Presentation

Direct mentum anterior face presentations (Fig. 17-20) can be delivered using Simpson or Tucker-McLane forceps (Fig. 17-21). The forceps blades are applied to the sides of the head along the occipitomental diameter with the pelvic curve directed toward the neck. Forceps should *not* be applied

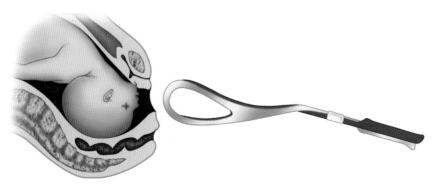

FIGURE 17-21. Face presentation phantom application.

to mentum posterior presentations because the head is at maximum extension. Mentum transverse face presentations usually spontaneously rotate to mentum anterior positions. In rare occasions, an expert operator may attempt to rotate a mentum transverse to a mentum anterior with Kielland forceps.

In the direct mentum anterior position, the forceps are applied, and their position is verified. Then the handles of the forceps are depressed toward the floor to deflex the head completely. Traction is made in an outward, horizontal, and slightly posterior direction until the chin appears under the symphysis pubis and the submental region of the neck impinges on the subpubic angle (Fig. 17-22). With further descent, the face and forehead appear, and the direction of traction is changed to outward and anterior (upward). This brings about both descent and flexion, and the vertex and occiput are born over the perineum.

TRIAL OF FORCEPS AND UNSUCCESSFUL FORCEPS

All midpelvic forceps and rotational forceps should be considered a trial of forceps. The rate of failed AVB ranges between 2.9 and 6.5 percent. Higher rates of unsuccessful AVB attempts are associated with maternal body mass index greater than 30 kg/m^2, estimated fetal weight greater than 4000 grams, OP positions, and midpelvic procedures. However, after controlling for operator experience, the most common reasons for failed AVB are fetal macrosomia and prolonged second stage of labor. AVB attempts that have a lower likelihood of success should be considered a trial of instrumental delivery and performed in and/or close to an operating room with anesthesia present so that the team can proceed immediately to cesarean section if necessary ("double setup").

The principle of trial of forceps is that after successful application of the forceps, fetal head descent should be achieved with gentle traction performed during contractions. If descent does not occur with traction, the attempt at AVB should be abandoned and the operator should proceed to immediate cesarean delivery.

There is limited data to determine the number of pulls (or vacuum cup popups) that should be allowed before abandoning the attempted AVB. In general, if there is failure in application or there is no descent with moderate traction after the first 2-3 traction attempts, then the situation should be reappraised and there should be a low threshold for abandoning the procedure.

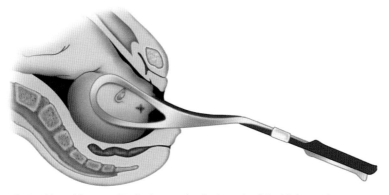

A. Locking of forceps. Beginning traction in the axis of the birth canal.

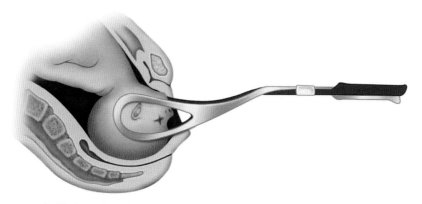

B. Horizontal traction.

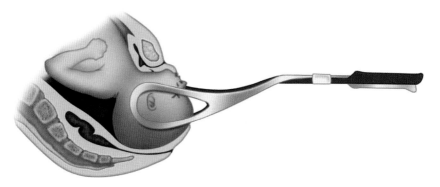

C. Delivery by flexion of the head.

FIGURE 17-22. Forceps delivery of mentum anterior.

SECOND STAGE OF LABOR

Cesarean section after failed AVB is associated with higher fetal and maternal complications. Maternal complications include extensions of the lower uterine segment incision, severe intraoperative bleeding, and maternal tissue damage, particularly if the head was deeply impacted in the pelvis. The rate of fetal subdural and cerebral hemorrhage, admission to Neonatal Intensive Care Unit (NICU), seizures, and mechanical ventilation are higher after failed AVB attempts compared to successful AVB or cesarean birth in the second stage without a trial of forceps. However, secondary analysis of National Institute of Child Health and Human Development data found that fetal morbidities associated with cesarean birth after failed forceps were confined to the subgroup of patients with nonreassuring fetal heart rate patterns as an indication for the AVB. Thus, trial of AVB is a reasonable option if the operator believes it has a good chance of success.

CAUSES OF CATASTROPHIC FORCEPS

An attempt to deliver the baby by forceps may not be successful, may produce a damaged baby, and may cause significant maternal lacerations. Pitfalls that contribute to making an inappropriate decision to attempt an AVB include the following:

1. Misunderstanding the significance and the relationship of station and the level of the BPD. Station zero means that the presenting part has reached the level of the ischial spines. In most women, when the station is zero, the BPD is at or just through the pelvic inlet. Thus, when forceps are applied at station zero, the procedure does not simply involve extracting the presenting part from the midpelvis; rather, the BPD must be pulled all the way from the inlet, through the midpelvis, and the outlet. This is a difficult and potentially dangerous procedure. On the other hand, when the station is +2 and the BPD is at or below the spines, a midforceps operation is often easy and safe. One must always consider both the *station of the presenting part and the level of the BPD.*
2. Unrecognized disproportion caused by:
   a. A small or abnormal pelvis
   b. A large baby. This is particularly concerning in a multipara who had a normal delivery previously. An AVB in this instance may be complicated by a difficult forceps extraction, shoulder dystocia, vaginal and cervical lacerations, postpartum hemorrhage, and potentially a

damaged infant. Whenever progress has ceased, the size of the baby must be reassessed before any action is taken

3. Misdiagnosis of station because of:
   a. Caput succedaneum (scalp edema) In prolonged labor, the caput may be 1-2 cm thick, and hence the bony skull is at a correspondingly higher level in the pelvis. It is important to ascertain the station of the skull and not the edematous scalp. A large caput indicates strong contractions, great resistance, or both. A small or absent caput suggests that the contractions or the resistance of the pelvic tissues are weak
   b. Molding. Excessive molding makes the head pointed by lengthening its long axis; therefore, the BPD is at a greater distance from the leading part of the skull. In these situations, engagement may not have taken place when the station is zero. Not only is the forceps operation difficult, but also the pressure of the instrument on a brain already under stress increases the risk of damage. Extreme molding and lack of progress are very concerning
4. Misdiagnosis of position. In descending order of importance, the steps in the use of forceps are: diagnosis of position, application, and traction. It is obvious that if the exact position of the fetal head is not known, the forceps cannot be applied correctly. Difficulty in applying forceps demands a complete reevaluation of the situation, not forceful delivery. Whenever labor ceases to advance, the possibility of an abnormal position or a malpresentation (e.g., brow) must be kept in mind
5. Misdiagnosis of inefficient uterine action. The erroneous assumption that the lack of progress is the result of poor contractions leads to trouble in two ways: (1) forceps are applied too soon, and (2) an oxytocin infusion may dilate the cervix and jam the fetal head into the pelvis just far enough to encourage the performance of a misguided forceps extraction
6. Premature interference. This involves the use of forceps either before the patient is ready and the prerequisites are fulfilled or when there are no valid indications. Modern management of the second stage is a good way to prevent this problem

VACUUM EXTRACTOR

A vacuum extractor applies suction and traction to an area of the fetal scalp covered by a suction cup in order to assist maternal expulsive efforts. It is not a device for applying rotational forces, although rotation may

SECOND STAGE OF LABOR

occur with descent of the vertex. Vacuum cups can be metal, plastic, or silicone and can be rigid or soft. They are usually 50 or 60 mm in diameter. The vacuum extractor should not be considered as an easier alternative to forceps or for use by less skilled operators. It is not likely to succeed in the absence of maternal expulsive efforts and the vacuum has been found to be more likely to fail as the instrument of delivery than forceps.

The vacuum has some advantages over forceps. It does not encroach on the space in the pelvis, reducing the incidence of damage to maternal tissues. The fetal head is not fixed by the application, so it can go through the rotations that the configurations of the birth canal require. The fetal head is allowed to find the path of least resistance.

Indications for Use of a Vacuum

The indications for vacuum-assisted vaginal birth are much the same as those for forceps delivery. These include fetal indications, such as an atypical or abnormal fetal heart tracing, maternal indications (e.g., indications to avoid Valsalva maneuver), inadequate progress of labor, and lack of effective maternal expulsive efforts.

Contraindications to Use of a Vacuum

1. Noncephalic presentation such as face or brow presentation
2. Fetal conditions such as bleeding disorder or demineralization disorder
3. Any contraindication to a vaginal birth
4. Less than 34 weeks of gestation
5. Fetal congenital anomalies such as hydrocephalus
6. Evidence of CPD
7. Dead fetus: suction and traction are not efficient in this case
8. Need for operator-applied rotation
9. An incompletely dilated cervix with an unengaged head. Note: Although it is preferable for the cervix to be fully dilated and the head to be engaged, in some circumstances with a multiparous patient, a vacuum delivery may still be performed, but only when the benefits significantly outweigh the risks and when there is no viable alternative

Previous fetal scalp sampling is not a contraindication to a vacuum-assisted vaginal birth.

Morbidity and Mortality with Vacuum-Assisted Vaginal Births

Many studies have reported that maternal injury is less frequent and less extensive with the use of vacuum cups compared with forceps. Potential maternal complications include cervical lacerations, severe vaginal lacerations, vaginal hematomas, and third- and fourth-degree tears.

Potential fetal complications are similar to those seen with forceps. These include fetal scalp trauma, subgaleal hemorrhage, intracranial hemorrhage, hyperbilirubinemia, and retinal hemorrhage.

1. The formation of a pronounced caput succedaneum is a part of the procedure and is seen in almost all cases. The caput usually disappears within a few hours
2. Abrasions, necrosis, and ulceration of the scalp at the site of application of the cup. The longer the cup is on, the greater the chance of scalp trauma. These should be treated by gentle cleansing and antibiotic ointments. The skin at the site of the suction must be handled carefully to avoid rubbing off the friable superficial layer
3. Cephalohematoma. This occurs in 10 to 15 percent of cases and is higher than that reported for spontaneous births and forcep deliveries. Cephalohematoma is more common as the duration of vacuum application increases, with a rate of 28 percent when the time from application to delivery exceeds 5 minutes. Reducing the vacuum pressure between contractions does not appear to reduce the incidence of fetal scalp injury. Serious complications are rare and the prognosis is good; however, neonatal care providers should be aware of the vacuum delivery so the neonate can be monitored for instrument-related injuries
4. Subaponeurotic or subgaleal hemorrhage may occur from beneath the galea aponeurotica layer of the scalp. Sometimes, it is not evident until a couple of days after birth. The bleeding may be massive and life threatening because the subaponeurotic space is continuous across the cranium without periosteal attachments. A hematoma in this space can dissect across the cranial vault, elevating part of or the entire scalp. If there is a suspicion of or increased risk for a subgaleal hemorrhage, head circumferences should be closely monitored. To minimize the risk of a subgaleal hemorrhage, avoid "rocking" the vacuum, which can increase shearing forces on the scalp
5. Retinal hemorrhage occurs more frequently than with spontaneous births or forceps deliveries. There seems to be no residual damage

SECOND STAGE OF LABOR

Prerequisites for a Vacuum-Assisted Vaginal Birth

The same criteria as for a forceps delivery must be met before an attempt at a vacuum-assisted vaginal birth. These include:

1. Informed consent
2. No fetal contraindications
3. Appropriate analgesia and anesthesia
4. Cervix fully dilated and membranes ruptured
5. Vertex presentation
6. Vertex engaged
7. Adequate uterine contractions
8. No evidence of CPD
9. Empty maternal bladder
10. Experienced operator; adequate facilities and resources available
11. Properly functioning equipment
12. Ongoing maternal and fetal assessment
13. Backup plan in place in case the procedure is unsuccessful

Application of the Vacuum and Delivery

The patient is positioned and prepared just as for a forceps delivery. The largest cup that fits is used. When soft cups are used, they are inserted by compressing the cup in an AP direction and then introducing it into the posterior fourchette while making space and protecting the maternal tissue with the opposite hand. When a hard cup is used, it is slid sideways into the vagina and then flipped onto the fetal skull. Once in the vagina, the cup is moved anteriorly to a position centred over the sagittal suture and anterior to the posterior fontanelle (~2 cm) to ensure that the smallest diameter of the head will travel through the pelvis. This is called the *flexion point*. Verification of a good placement is then required, including ensuring that no maternal tissue is trapped between the cup and the fetal head.

Slowly, the negative pressure is pumped up until it reaches 500-600 mm Hg (0.6-0.8 kg/cm^2). An artificial caput succedaneum, a "chignon," is formed. The vacuum pressure may be released between contractions to resting pressures of between 100 and 200 mm Hg (0.1-0.3 kg/cm^2). However, there is no evidence that there is a difference in neonatal outcome if the vacuum is maintained, with or without traction, between contractions.

Traction is then applied with the right hand pulling downward on the tube or handle of the vacuum while the left hand presses on the cup and the fetal head to ensure a continuous good seal (Fig. 17-23). This produces

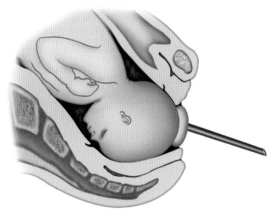

A. Traction outward and posteriorly.

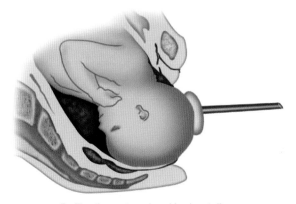

B. Traction outward and horizontally.

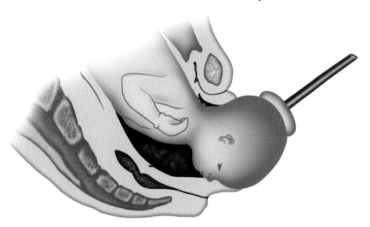

C. Traction outward and anteriorly.

FIGURE 17-23. **Vacuum-assisted vaginal delivery.**

SECOND STAGE OF LABOR

a force along the direction of the birth canal. Traction should be synchronized with an adequate uterine contraction and maximum maternal pushing effort. Traction is applied in the direction of the pelvic curve, initially downward and then upward. No rotational force should be applied, but the fetal head may rotate on its own with descent. The operator's free hand should verify adequate descent with each pull. When the head is crowning, the direction of the pulling is changed to upward and toward the mother's abdomen. The left hand then moves to support the perineum. A common mistake is to extend the head prematurely, thereby increasing the diameter that must pass over the perineum and increasing the likelihood of fetal–maternal trauma and a vacuum pop-off. Rocking motions may also increase the possibility of scalp damage and subgaleal hemorrhage.

Pop-offs (i.e., when the suction cup loses it seal on the fetal head and is inadvertently pulled away by the operator) should not be considered a normal event in a vacuum-assisted vaginal birth. Causes of pop-offs include:

1. Poor seal causing a vacuum leak
2. Excessive traction force
3. Unrecognized CPD
4. Midpelvic application
5. OP presentation
6. Deflexed attitude
7. Paramedian application
8. Improper angle of traction causing shearing
9. Impingement of maternal soft tissue

When to Abandon an Attempted Vacuum-Assisted Vaginal Birth

It is important that the operator knows when to abandon an attempted AVB. The operator should abandon the procedure if any of these three circumstances occur:

1. After three pulls over three contractions with no progress or descent
2. After three pop-offs without obvious cause
3. After 20 minutes if delivery is not imminent

In these instances, the vacuum should be removed, and a different method of delivery should be considered. In most instances, this would be achieved by cesarean section, although a forceps-assisted delivery may also be considered. The risk of complications increases with the sequential use of different instruments. The following table provides a brief "ABC" mnemonic to help guide operators at a vacuum-assisted vaginal birth.

A	Address Anesthesia Assistance	• The patient • Adequate relief • Neonatal support
B	Bladder	• Empty
C	Cervix	• Fully dilated • Membranes ruptured
D	Determine	• Position, station, pelvic adequacy • Anticipate shoulder dystocia
E	Equipment	• Inspect cup, pump, tubing, pressure
F	Fontanel (posterior)	• Under or posterior to cup
G	Gentle traction	• With contractions
H	Halt	• If no progress after: Three contractions Three pop-offs 20 minutes
I	Incision	• Consider episiotomy

Adapted from Bachman J: A forceps needs to be documented in the same manner as any other operative procedure. Forceps Delivery Correspondence. J Am Acad Fam Pract 29:4, 1989

DOCUMENTATION OF AN ASSISTED VAGINAL BIRTH

Clear documentation is important throughout labor and birth, particularly in the case of an AVB. Cognitive checklists, such as those proposed by the Society of Maternal Fetal Medicine for (1) preparation and performance of the procedure and (2) documentation after the procedure, are useful tools to ensure that the team is familiar with the elements of the procedure and that documentation is complete. The following points should be clearly documented after an AVB:

1. Indication for intervention
2. Discussion with the woman of the risks, benefits, and options

3. Position and station of the fetal head as well as how it was assessed (i.e., vaginally, abdominally, or both)
4. Amount of molding and caput present
5. Assessment of maternal pelvis
6. Assessment of fetal heart and contractions
7. Type of vacuum or forceps used
8. Number of attempts and ease of application of vacuum or forceps
9. Duration of traction (forceps) or duration of application (vacuum) and force used
10. Condition of newborn at delivery. Description of maternal and neonatal injuries

MATERNAL CARE AFTER AN ASSISTED VAGINAL BIRTH

Prophylactic Antibiotics after an Assisted Vaginal Birth

Based on the ANODE trial results, prophylactic antibiotics should be considered for women who undergo an AVB to reduce the risk of postpartum infection, particularly if an episiotomy was performed. The recommended regimen is amoxicillin-clavulanate intravenously 1000 mg + 200 mg. Oral antibiotics may be given if there is no intravenous access (amoxicillin-clavulanate 875/125 orally). In the case of a penicillin allergy, cephazolin 2 g IV or clindamycin 600 mg IV can be used as an alternative. A single dose of IV antibiotics should be given in cases of third- or fourth-degree lacerations.

Postnatal Care Following an Assisted Vaginal Birth

Postnatal care following AVB should include a discussion about reasons for the AVB, management of complications, and prognosis for future pregnancies. Success rates for spontaneous vaginal births in subsequent pregnancies range from 78 to 91 percent. Other topics to address include the potential need for thromboembolic prophylaxis, analgesia, voiding function, and pelvic floor rehabilitation.

Thromboprophylaxis should be initiated based on a venous thromboembolism risk profile. Regular acetaminophen and nonsteroidal anti-inflammatory drugs (NSAIDs) should be offered. If pain is not adequately controlled, complications such as hematoma formation and infection should be ruled out by clinical examination. An indwelling catheter for 12 hours after delivery may be considered due to the increased risk of urinary retention following AVB, particularly if a spinal or epidural top up has been used. Postpartum bladder function should be carefully observed to avoid bladder overdistension and long-term bladder dysfunction. If urinary retention is suspected, postvoid residual volumes should be measured. Pelvic floor exercises such as Kegel's exercises should be encouraged in the postnatal period. Physiotherapy may also be helpful.

SELECTED READING

American College of Obstetricians and Gynecologists: ACOG Practice Bulletin No. 219: Operative vaginal birth. Obstet Gynecol 135:e149-e159, 2020

Bachman J. A forceps needs to be documented in the same manner as any other operative procedure. Forceps Delivery Correspondence. J Am Acad Fam Pract 29:4, 1989

Gei AF, Pacheco, LD: Operative vaginal deliveries: practical aspects. Obstet Gynecol Clin North Am 38: 323, 2011

Goplani S, Bennet K, Critchlow C: Factors predictive of failed operative vaginal delivery. Am J Obstet Gynecol 191:892, 2004

Healy DL, Quinn MA, Pepperell RJ: Rotational delivery of the fetus: Kielland's forceps and two other methods compared. Br J Obstet Gynaecol 89:501, 1982

Ingardia CJ, Cetrulo CL: Forceps—use and abuse. Clin Perinatol 8:63, 1981

Knight M, Chiocchia V, Partlett C, Rivero-Arias O, Hua X, Hinshaw K, et al: Prophylactic antibiotics in the prevention of infection after operative vaginal delivery (ANODE): A multicentre randomised controlled trial. ANODE collaborative group. Lancet 393:2395-403, 2019

Majoko F, Gardner G: Trial of instrumental delivery in theatre versus immediate caesarean section for anticipated difficult vaginal births. Cochrane DataBase Syst Rev 4: CD005545, 2012

O'Mahony F, Homier GJ, Menon V: Choice of instruments for assisted vaginal delivery. Cochrane Database Syst Rev 11:CD005455, 2010

Patient Safety and Quality Committee, Society for Maternal-Fetal Medicine. Staat B, Combs CA: SMFM Special Statement: Operative vaginal delivery: Checklists for performance and documentation. Am J Obstet Gynecol 222:B15, 2020

Royal Australian and New Zealand College of Obstetricians and Gynaecologists: Instrumental vaginal birth. https://ranzcog.edu.au/RANZCOG_SITE/media/RANZCOG-MEDIA/Women%27s%20Health/Statement%20and%20guidelines/Clinical-Obstetrics/Instrumental-vaginal-birth-(C-Obs-16)-Review-March-2020.pdf, March 2020

Simpson AN, Gurau D, Secter M, Hodges R, Windrim R, Higgins M: Learning from experience: Development of a cognitive task list to perform a safe and successful non-rotational forceps delivery. J Obstet Gynecol Can 37:589-597, 2015

Society of Obstetricians and Gynaecologists of Canada: Clinical Practice Guideline No. 381. Assisted vaginal birth. J Obstet Gynecol Can 41:870-882, 2019

CHAPTER 18

Shoulder Dystocia

Yaa A. Amankwah

GENERAL CONSIDERATIONS

Definition of Shoulder Dystocia

Shoulder dystocia occurs when the fetal head is delivered but the shoulders cannot be spontaneously delivered by the usual method of gentle downward traction. The fetus must be in the cephalic presentation. Shoulder dystocia occurs when the anterior fetal shoulder is obstructed by the maternal pubic symphysis or, less commonly, from impaction of the posterior fetal shoulder on the maternal sacral promontory. Additional obstetric maneuvers are required to help deliver the fetal shoulders. Retraction of the delivered head against the maternal perineum, the "turtle sign," is suggestive of shoulder dystocia but not diagnostic. Shoulder dystocia is an unpredictable and unpreventable obstetrical emergency, thus obstetrical care providers should have the knowledge and ability to perform additional obstetrical maneuvers promptly.

Incidence of Shoulder Dystocia

The general incidence of shoulder dystocia is between 0.2 and 3.0 percent of vaginal births. The variation in reported incidence is due to differences in the definition of shoulder dystocia, characteristics of the study populations, varied clinical scenarios, reliance on the health care provider's clinical judgment, and the consistency and accuracy of reporting. Approximately 50 percent of shoulder dystocias occur in women without risk factors.

Mechanism of Shoulder Dystocia

In most cases of normal labor and delivery, the fetal shoulders enter the pelvis in an oblique diameter. As labor progresses, the shoulders descend and rotate the bisacromial diameter toward the anteroposterior (AP) diameter of the pelvis. By this mechanism, the anterior shoulder comes under the pubic symphysis a little to the side of the midline and is then delivered.

Impaction of the shoulders occurs when the fetus attempts to enter the pelvis with the bisacromial diameter in the AP diameter of the inlet (Fig. 18-1) instead of one of the oblique diameters. Rarely do both shoulders impact above the pelvic brim. Usually, the posterior shoulder can negotiate its way past the sacral promontory, but the anterior shoulder becomes wedged against the pubic symphysis.

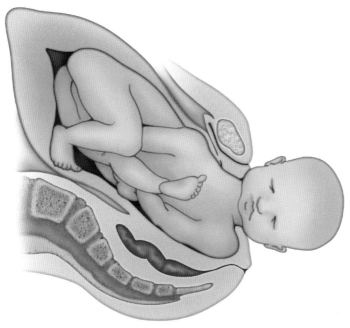

FIGURE 18-1. Shoulder dystocia: bisacromial diameter in the anteroposterior diameter of the pelvis.

CLINICAL PRESENTATION

When the anterior shoulder, or less commonly the posterior shoulder, is impacted against the symphysis pubis/sacral promontory in the AP diameter, the remainder of the body is unable to be delivered by the usual methods. The head remains tight against the perineum (the "turtle sign"), spontaneous restitution does not occur, and the baby does not deliver with the usual maternal effort and gentle downward traction. In 1955, Morris described the classic picture of shoulder dystocia as follows:

> The delivery of the head with or without forceps may have been quite easy, but more commonly there has been a little difficulty in completing the extension of the head. The hairy scalp slides out with reluctance. When the forehead has appeared it is necessary to press back the perineum to deliver the face. Fat cheeks eventually emerge. A double chin has to be hooked over the posterior vulvar commissure, to which it remains tightly opposed. Restitution seldom occurs spontaneously, for the head seems incapable of movement as a result of friction with the girdle of contact of the vulva. On the other hand, gentle manipulation of the head sometimes results in

sudden 90-degree restitution as the head adjusts itself without descent to the AP position of the shoulders.

Time passes. The child's head becomes suffused. It endeavours unsuccessfully to breathe. Abdominal efforts by the mother or by her attendants produce no advance; gentle head traction is equally unavailing.

Usually equanimity forsakes the attendants. They push, they pull. Alarm increases. Eventually by greater strength of muscle or by some infernal juggle the difficulty appears to be overcome, and the shoulders and trunk of a goodly child are delivered. The pallor of its body contrasts with the plum-colored cyanosis of the face, and the small quantity of freshly expelled meconium about the buttocks. It dawns upon the attendants that their anxiety was not ill-founded, the baby lies limp and voiceless, and too often remains so despite all efforts at resuscitation.

Differential Diagnosis

There are exceptional situations that prevent spontaneous delivery of the fetal shoulder and body after the delivery of the head. These are not considered "true" shoulder dystocia and include:

1. Short umbilical cord
2. Tight nuchal cord
3. Abdominal or thoracic enlargement of the infant (anasarca, abdominal or back neoplasms)
4. Locked or conjoined twins
5. Uterine constriction ring

RISK FACTORS FOR SHOULDER DYSTOCIA

Shoulder dystocia cannot be accurately predicted or prevented; however, health care providers should be aware of possible risk factors for shoulder dystocia in order to better prepare for deliveries at higher risk. Most risk factors for shoulder dystocia have extremely poor positive predictive values; shoulder dystocia is unpredictable in 50 to 70 percent of occurrences.

Risk factors include fetal macrosomia, maternal diabetes, maternal obesity (BMI $\geq$30 kg/m^2), prior history of shoulder dystocia, induction of labor, and operative vaginal delivery. Prolonged second stage is not a risk factor itself but may be associated with other individual risk factors and interventions that are associated with an increased risk of shoulder dystocia.

The main risk factors appear to be previous shoulder dystocia and fetal macrosomia. The ultrasound-derived fetal abdominal diameter–biparietal diameter difference has not been found to be clinically useful as a predictor for shoulder dystocia. Although maternal diabetes and increasing birthweight are associated with an increased incidence of shoulder dystocia, most cases will occur in women without diabetes and with normal weight infants. Only 16 percent of newborns that experienced a shoulder dystocia–related morbidity had a known risk factor.

Fetal Macrosomia

Although there is a relationship between fetal size and shoulder dystocia, this is not an accurate predictor. In 48 percent of shoulder dystocia cases, infants weigh less than 4000 g at birth. Interestingly, a large proportion of infants with birth weights of 4500 g or more do not develop shoulder dystocia. In babies weighing over 4500 g, shoulder dystocia is encountered 22.6 percent of the time. Macrosomic infants tend to deposit their excess weight in the chest and abdominal regions, causing these areas to be significantly out of proportion to the head. In postterm babies, as well as babies of diabetic mothers, the size of the baby's chest and trunk can potentially increase and result in shoulder dystocia. This disproportion between the shoulder and head dimensions is much more pronounced in babies of mothers with diabetes.

Maternal Diabetes Mellitus

Fetal macrosomia in the setting of maternal diabetes increases the risk of shoulder dystocia; however, these factors combined predict only about 55 percent of shoulder dystocia cases. In addition to the disproportionately larger shoulder-to-head circumference generally noted in macrosomic infants, babies born to mothers with diabetes have more body fat, which tends to be deposited in the arms and folds of the triceps, contributing to shoulder dystocia.

Maternal Obesity

Obesity in pregnancy (prepregnancy maternal BMI >30 kg/m^2) is associated with fetal macrosomia and in some situations, macrosomic infants may be at risk for shoulder dystocia. Patients should be encouraged to adhere to guidance on recommended weight gain during pregnancy:

11.5 to 16 kg for normal BMI patients, 7 to 11 kg for overweight patients, and 5 to 9 kg in obese patients.

Previous Shoulder Dystocia

A prior history of shoulder dystocia is one of the more accurate predictors for recurrent shoulder dystocia. The recurrence rate is quoted as up to 16.7 percent, although most say at least 10 percent. This translates to a 10- to 20-fold increased risk compared with baseline. When shoulder dystocia results in fetal injury, the likelihood of recurrent shoulder dystocia and fetal injury in subsequent pregnancies is greater. It is therefore important for the delivering provider to accurately document the details of delivery and clearly explain the events surrounding the delivery to the patient, including the risk of recurrence. Universal elective cesarean delivery is not recommended for patients who have a history of shoulder dystocia because most subsequent deliveries will not be complicated by shoulder dystocia. However, clinical information, future pregnancy plans, and patient preference should be considered and careful birth planning is recommended.

Other Risk Factors

Multiparity, postterm pregnancy, labor dystocia, and assisted vaginal delivery are have been linked to shoulder dystocia. It is unclear what the direct causes are in the cases; however, fetal macrosomia is often present in these scenarios and may explain their association with shoulder dystocia.

PREVENTION OF SHOULDER DYSTOCIA

Because shoulder dystocia cannot be predicted, studies have been done to determine if it can be prevented with induction of labor or with a planned cesarean delivery. Induction of labor and planned cesarean section are not recommended in most instances because it does not decrease the rate of shoulder dystocia and does not improve maternal or fetal outcomes.

To date, no study has proven that correcting the stated risk factors, with the exception of gestational diabetes, will reduce the risk of shoulder dystocia. In the general population, physical exercise is recommended before and during pregnancy to reduce the risk of gestational diabetes, excessive maternal weight gain during pregnancy, and fetal macrosomia.

In overweight or obese patients, physical activity coupled with dietary management is recommended to reduce maternal weight gain and fetal macrosomia. In situations of gestational diabetes, a diabetic diet, glucose monitoring, and insulin therapy if required are used to reduce the risk of fetal macrosomia and shoulder dystocia.

Most macrosomic fetuses that deliver vaginally do not have a shoulder dystocia. Different approaches to birth planning for macrosomic fetuses have been suggested to decrease the risk of shoulder dystocia:

1. Elective cesarean delivery if the estimated fetal weight is ≥4500 g for diabetic women and 5000 g for nondiabetic women
2. Expectant management; however, children with birth weight ≥4500 g had significantly increased risk of perinatal mortality, neonatal asphyxia, trauma, and cesarean delivery
3. Induction of labor, reducing the possibility of further fetal growth, risk of cesarean delivery for cephalopelvic disproportion, and shoulder dystocia
4. Cesarean section during labor, in case of fetal macrosomia and failure to progress in the second stage, when the fetal head station is above +2

Due to the very high number of cesarean sections that would be required to prevent one permanent fetal injury, elective cesarean delivery should only be considered for nondiabetic women with suspected macrosomia and an estimated fetal weight of ≥5000 g, and for diabetic women whose fetuses have an estimated fetal weight of ≥4500 g.

Induction of labor between 38 and 40 weeks' gestation for suspected fetal macrosomia is controversial. Two small trials did not show maternal or neonatal benefit with induction of labor for fetal macrosomia. However, a meta-analysis found that compared with expectant management, labor induction for suspected fetal macrosomia significantly reduced the risk of shoulder dystocia and any type of fracture and that there was no change in the risk of cesarean delivery, assisted vaginal delivery, or brachial plexus injury. It is not certain if that reduction in shoulder dystocia would persist if labor induction occurred after 39 weeks' gestation, hence induction solely for fetal macrosomia is discouraged. At this time, there is not enough evidence to make recommendations regarding labor induction in patients with gestational diabetes and suspected macrosomia on the incidence of shoulder dystocia. If induction of labor is considered, it should not be performed before 39 completed weeks of pregnancy unless otherwise medically indicated.

SECOND STAGE OF LABOR

SEQUELAE OF SHOULDER DYSTOCIA

Complications of shoulder dystocia include fetal, neonatal, and maternal injuries. The rate of transient or permanent neonatal injury is up to 20 percent. Fetal injuries include brachial plexus injuries, neonatal encephalopathy, asphyxia and possible death, fracture (clavicle and/or humerus), contusions, and lacerations. Maternal morbidities include genital tract lacerations, uterine rupture, obstetric anal sphincter injuries (OASIS), and postpartum hemorrhage secondary to uterine atony or lacerations.

Birth Asphyxia

Birth asphyxia is the most dreaded complication of shoulder dystocia because it may result in permanent neurologic damage and even death. Shoulder dystocia alone is not an accurate predictor of neonatal asphyxia or death. Fortunately, neonatal encephalopathy and death in cases of shoulder dystocia are infrequent (0.08-1 percent).

With each uterine contraction, large amounts of blood are transferred from the baby's trunk to their head. The angulation of the neck and the compression of the chest interfere with cardiac function and impair the venous return. The intracranial vascular system of the fetus cannot compensate for the excessive intravascular pressure. Compression of the umbilical cord between the baby's body and the maternal birth canal results in a further reduction of blood flow and oxygenation to the fetus. This results in increasing fetal acidosis and asphyxia. Under these conditions, anoxia develops and may be accompanied by hemorrhagic effusions. If this condition persists too long, the baby may sustain irreversible brain damage. The infant may die during the attempts at delivery or in the neonatal period. Studies suggest that after abrupt cessation of umbilical blood flow, babies not delivered within 5 to 10 minutes will have permanent neurologic damage or death. This is a result of the increasing acidosis with the umbilical artery pH declining at a rate of 0.04 units/min in the presence of total cord occlusion. In shoulder dystocia, there may be some preservation of maternal–fetal circulation and a less rapid drop in pH unless the cord has previously been clamped and cut. This underscores the reason for not routinely cutting a nuchal cord in the presence of suspected shoulder dystocia.

Brachial Plexus Injury

Transient or permanent brachial plexus injury (BPI) occurs in between 10 and 20 percent of all shoulder dystocia deliveries, although rates of 4 to

40 percent have been reported. It may be associated with extreme lateral traction being applied to the fetal head by the birth attendant. However, it can occur regardless of which procedure is used to disimpact the shoulders because all of the maneuvers can increase the stretch on the brachial plexus. Brachial plexus injuries can also occur in the absence of shoulder dystocia, after breech deliveries, and in uncomplicated cesarean sections. BPI is *not* evidence that a shoulder dystocia has occurred. A brachial plexus injury most commonly involves the C5 and C6 nerve roots, resulting in the classical Erb-Duchenne palsy (waiter's tip sign). When the damage involves C8 and T1, it is called Klumpke's brachial plexus palsy ("claw hand" sign). BPI is occasionally accompanied by diaphragmatic paralysis, Horner syndrome, and facial nerve injuries.

The majority of brachial plexus birth injuries are transient and most resolve by 3 months. If there is residual impairment by the end of the first month of life, the infant should be referred for a specialist assessment. Approximately 5 to 22 percent result in some degree of permanent injury.

Fetal Fractures and Bruising

Fetal clavicle fractures occur in 10 percent of deliveries complicated by shoulder dystocia. After the delivery of the fetal head, excessive pressure may be applied to the shoulders in an attempt to complete the delivery with a resultant fracture to the clavicle. In some cases, the attendant deliberately fractures the clavicle to reduce the diameter of the fetal chest and intershoulder distance to facilitate delivery. Humeral fractures occur in approximately 4 percent of infants with shoulder dystocia deliveries. They tend to heal quickly with no long-term complications.

Bruises on the fetal body may result from pressure of the attendant's hands on the fetus while performing various maneuvers to effect delivery. Such bruises may also occur during routine deliveries that are not complicated by shoulder dystocia.

Maternal Morbidity

Shoulder dystocia is associated with an increased risk of maternal morbidity. Complications include vulvar, vaginal, and cervical lacerations, as well as episiotomy extensions. The rate of fourth degree lacerations is 3.8 percent. The rate of postpartum hemorrhage with shoulder dystocia is approximately 11 percent and may be the result of genital tract lacerations, uterine atony, and, rarely, uterine rupture. Prolonged and intense pressure on the bladder from the fetal anterior shoulder may cause bladder atony and temporary urinary retention. Extreme hyperflexion of the maternal legs required for maneuvers to help resolve shoulder dystocia can cause a lateral femoral cutaneous neuropathy as well as separation of the maternal pubic symphysis. Heroic measures, such as the Zavanelli maneuver and symphisiotomy, are associated with a high incidence of significant maternal morbidity.

DIAGNOSIS

Diagnosis can be made only after the head has been delivered. The following signs may then appear:

1. The fetal head delivers but restitution does not take place spontaneously. Because of friction with the vulva, the head seems incapable of movement
2. The head recoils back against the perineum after it comes out from the vagina ("turtle sign")
3. The shoulders fail to deliver with maternal expulsive efforts and gentle downward traction from below

MANAGEMENT OF SHOULDER DYSTOCIA

Shoulder dystocia cannot be reliably predicted; therefore, all deliveries should be considered to have the potential for a shoulder dystocia. If a woman is considered at risk for shoulder dystocia, the woman, her support person, and the birth attendant's team should prepare for a shoulder dystocia in advance of delivery of the fetal head. Preparing the team for the possibility of flattening the bed, the McRoberts maneuver, suprapubic pressure, and rolling over can increase cooperation in the event of a shoulder dystocia. In addition, a stool placed at the side of the bed corresponding to the fetal back helps to indicate to the team the location to apply oblique suprapubic pressure. Low-fidelity simulation exercises may be used to improve the aspects of teamwork that may be helpful for the management of shoulder dystocia.

As soon as shoulder dystocia is recognized, several measures have to be taken. The attendant must seek help from other health care personnel.

If an obstetrician is not present, he or she should be notified to proceed to the delivery room. An anesthesia and neonatal team should also be called. The most responsible birth attendant should be constantly informed of the time that has elapsed since delivery of the head. An effective way of ensuring this is to designate a timekeeper to document the timing of events. In all instances, one should avoid pulling on the head, pushing on the fundus, panicking, and pivoting (severely angulating the fetal head using the coccyx as a fulcrum). It is important to ask the woman to *stop pushing* until maneuvers to relieve the shoulder dystocia are carried out.

Several obstetric maneuvers can be used to resolve shoulder dystocia, including the McRoberts maneuver, suprapubic pressure, delivery of the anterior shoulder, delivery of the posterior shoulder and arm, the Wood's screw maneuver, deliberate fracture of the fetal clavicle or humerus, the Zavanelli maneuver, and maternal symphysiotomy.

The McRoberts maneuver should be attempted first. Delivery of the posterior shoulder appears to be associated with the highest rate of delivery compared with the other maneuvers; thus, it should be considered after the McRoberts maneuver and suprapubic pressure. The need for additional maneuvers is associated with higher rates of neonatal injury. Despite historical recommendations to perform an episiotomy at the time of a diagnosed shoulder dystocia to prevent a brachial plexus injury, the literature does not support a benefit to this practice.

McRoberts Maneuver and Suprapubic Pressure

These two maneuvers are often used simultaneously as the first steps to help resolve shoulder dystocia. About 50 to 60 percent of shoulder dystocias resolve using a combination of McRoberts maneuver and suprapubic pressure, thereby eliminating the need for further maneuvers.

The McRoberts maneuver involves flexing the legs sharply upon the maternal abdomen. This causes the symphysis pubis to rotate cephalad and the sacrum to be straightened with flattening of the lumbar lordosis, thus allowing the fetal shoulder to slide out beneath the maternal pubic bone anteriorly.

An assistant can perform suprapubic pressure (*not* fundal pressure) by applying oblique pressure (downward toward the pubic bone and laterally toward the fetus's face or sternum) just above the maternal pubic bone with the heel of their clasped hands against the posterior aspect of the shoulder to dislodge it (Mazzanti maneuver). A stool may be useful to facilitate this maneuver, particularly in the case of a shorter assistant. It is necessary to know the position of the occiput so that pressure is applied from the correct side and is most effective. Shoulder dystocia is caused by an infant's shoulders entering the pelvis in a direct AP axis instead of the physiologic oblique axis; therefore, pushing the baby's anterior shoulder to one side or the other from above can often change his or her position to the oblique, thus allowing its delivery.

The birth attendant may also attempt to manually dislodge the anterior shoulder from behind the symphysis pubis. One may place a hand deep in the vagina behind the anterior shoulder and attempt to rotate the axis of the shoulders into the oblique diameter of the pelvis (Fig. 18-2). Firm traction is then applied to the fetal head, deflecting it toward the floor.

Posterior Arm and Shoulder Delivery

If McRoberts maneuver and suprapubic pressure are not successful, the obstetrical care provider should then attempt to deliver the posterior arm. This requires the least amount of force to deliver the baby and results in the lowest amount of stretch on the brachial plexus. The fetal arm is usually flexed at the elbow, and if it is not, pressure in the antecubital fossa can assist with flexion. The hand can then be grasped and swept across the chest and delivered.

1. The hand of the operator is placed deeply into the vagina along the curvature of the sacrum and behind the posterior shoulder of the fetus. If the back of the fetus is toward the operator's right side, the left hand is used. If the back is toward the operator's left, the right hand is preferred (Fig. 18-3A)
2. The antecubital fossa of the posterior arm is located and using the pressure of a finger, an attempt is made to flex the arm in a fashion similar to the Pinard maneuver in a breech extraction
3. The forearm is swept across the chest and face, the hand is then grasped, and the arm is extended along the fetal face and delivered (Fig. 18-3B)
4. Once this has been accomplished, the anterior shoulder delivers in most cases. If it does not, the body is rotated 180° so that the anterior shoulder is now posterior. It is then extracted by the same maneuver. This maneuver tends to increase the risk of fracturing the humerus; however, most humeral fractures heal quickly with no permanent damage. In view of this, it is worth trying this maneuver to resolve the shoulder dystocia of an infant in a life-threatening situation when the other maneuvers have not worked

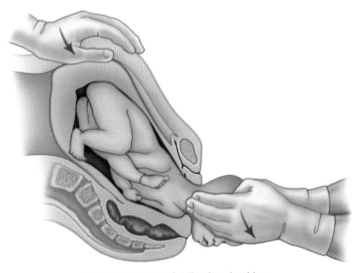

A. Basic method of delivering shoulders.

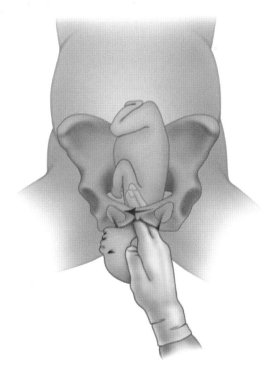

B. Shoulder dystocia: Rotation of bisacromial diameter from
anteroposterior diameter pelvis into the oblique.

FIGURE 18-2. **A** and **B.** Delivery of anterior shoulder.

SECOND STAGE OF LABOR

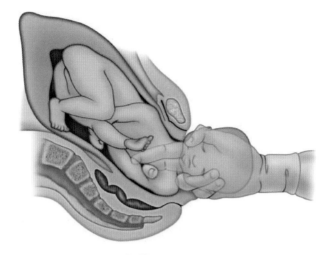

A. First step.

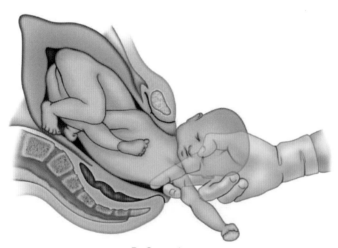

B. Second step.

FIGURE 18-3. A and **B.** Extraction of the posterior shoulder and arm.

Wood's Screw and Rubin Maneuvers

The Wood's screw and Rubin maneuvers are rotational maneuvers that can be attempted after a failure of delivery of the posterior arm. In the Rubin maneuver, the birth attendant places their hand vaginally on the back surface of the most easily accessible fetal shoulder (anterior or posterior) and rotates it toward the fetal face. This flexes the shoulders across the chest and decreases the distance between the shoulders, thus decreasing the dimension of the fetal chest that must fit out through the pelvis.

In the Wood's screw maneuver, the birth attendant pushes the posterior shoulder through a 180° arc by applying pressure on the anterior surface of the posterior shoulder to turn the fetus until the anterior shoulder emerges from under the maternal symphysis. The idea is to progressively rotate the posterior shoulder in a corkscrew fashion to release the opposite impacted anterior shoulder. To perform this maneuver, the posterior shoulder must have passed the spines for this maneuver to be successful. In a situation in which the fetal head position is left occiput transverse (LOT), two fingers of the left hand are placed on the anterior aspect of the posterior shoulder. Pressure is made against the shoulder so that it moves counterclockwise, the posterior aspect leading the way (Fig. 18-4). It is turned 180°, past 12 o'clock. In this way, the posterior shoulder is delivered under the pubic arch. The head has turned from LOT to right occiput transverse (ROT). This should result in delivery of the posterior shoulder, and the anterior shoulder should now be posterior.

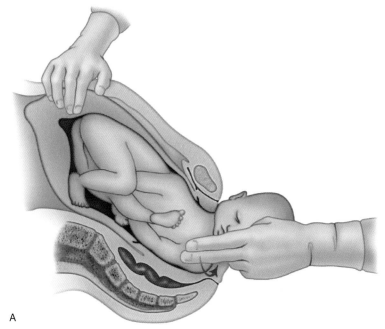

A

FIGURE 18-4. Wood's screw maneuver.

SECOND STAGE OF LABOR

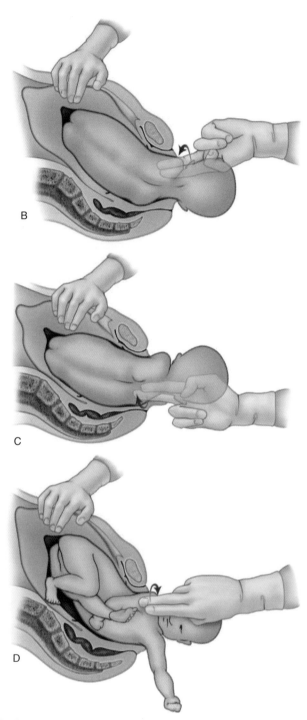

FIGURE 18-4. *(Continued)*

Fetal Clavicle Fracture

Although this maneuver is often described in shoulder dystocia literature, it is rarely performed. The fetal clavicle is a strong bone and not that easy to deliberately fracture. The clavicle may be deliberately fractured by pressing the anterior clavicle against the pubic ramus. The fractured clavicle decreases the bisacromial diameter, facilitating resolution of the dystocia. Serious fetal consequences that may occur include damage to the lungs and major blood vessels.

Rolling Over to "All Fours" Position

Moving the mother onto all fours on her hands and knees (the Gaskin maneuver) may increase the effective pelvic dimensions and allow the fetal position to shift, thereby freeing the impacted shoulder. With gentle downward traction on the posterior shoulder (the shoulder against the maternal sacrum), the anterior shoulder may become more impacted (with gravity) but will facilitate the freeing up of the posterior shoulder.

Zavanelli Maneuver

This maneuver is reserved for catastrophic cases and is associated with a significantly increased risk of fetal morbidity and mortality and maternal morbidity. This is a cephalic replacement maneuver whereby cardinal movements of labor are reversed; the head must first be rotated back to its pre-restitution position, flexed, pushed up, rotated to the transverse, and disengaged, and then a cesarean section is performed. Constant firm pressure is applied from below while the head is pushed back into the vagina. A general anesthetic is often administered in addition to tocolytics to produce uterine relaxation required for this maneuver. Cesarean delivery must be performed immediately after replacement of the head.

Symphysiotomy

This procedure is rarely performed and is usually reserved for areas with no quick access to performing cesarean sections. It involves dividing the ligaments between the right and left pubic symphyseal bones. This results in an increase in the transverse diameter of the pubis by adding about 3 cm to the circumference of the pelvis. The major risk involves potential injury to maternal soft tissues especially the bladder and urethra.

SECOND STAGE OF LABOR

DOCUMENTATION OF SHOULDER DYSTOCIA

Contemporaneous documentation of cases of shoulder dystocia is recommended, starting with the time that shoulder diagnosis is first diagnosed. Checklists or standardized documentation forms are encouraged to record facts, findings, and observations about the dystocia and its sequelae. This informs patients and health care providers about the event as well as assists with counselling for future births.

RISK MANAGEMENT

Obstetrical simulation and practice drills enhance obstetrical readiness and communication for all team members, particularly in high acuity/low frequency events such as shoulder dystocia. Simulation training has been shown to increase the evidence-based management of shoulder dystocia and decrease the rate of neonatal brachial plexus injury. Mnemonics are often used to plan a step-wise approach to managing shoulder dystocia. One such mnemonic is *ALARMER*:

A—Ask for help (assistant, anaesthesia, neonatology)
L—Lift legs (McRoberts)
A—Anterior shoulder delivery (suprapubic pressure)
R—Rotate (Wood's screw maneuver)
M—Manual removal of the posterior arm and shoulder
E—Episiotomy
R—Repeat steps above

CONCLUSION

Shoulder dystocia is an unpredictable and usually unpreventable obstetric event. Several factors have been identified in the literature as contributing to this condition, but these factors in isolation have poor predictive value for shoulder dystocia. However, they help raise awareness of the possibility of shoulder dystocia and readiness of the health care provider. All delivering personnel need to have a uniform and organized approach to handling this emergency in order to minimize risks to the mother and infant.

SELECTED READING

Acker DB, Sachs BP, Friedman EA: Risk factors for shoulder dystocia. Obstet Gynecol 66:762, 1985

American College of Obstetricians and Gynecologists: ACOG Practice Bulletin Number 178. Shoulder Dystocia. May 2017. Obstet Gynecol 129:e123-e133, 2017

Al Hadi M, Geary M, Byrne P, et al: Shoulder dystocia: Risk factors and maternal and perinatal outcome. J Obstet Gynaecol 21:352, 2001

Bahar AM: Risk factors and fetal outcome in cases of shoulder dystocia compared with normal deliveries of a similar birth weight. Br J Obstet Gynaecol 103:868, 1996

Baskett TF, Allen AC: Perinatal implications of shoulder dystocia. Obstet Gynecol 86:14, 1995

Boulvain M, Irion O, Dowswell T, Thornton J: Induction of labour at or near term for suspected fetal macrosomia. Cochrane Database Syst Rev 5, 2016

Ecker JL, Greenberg JA, Norwitz ER, et al: Birth weight as a predictor of brachial plexus injury. Obstet Gynecol 1997; 89:643, 1997

Fuchs F: Prevention of shoulder dystocia risk factors before delivery. J Gynecol Obstet Biol Reprod (Paris). 44:1248-1260, 2015

Gherman RB: Persistent brachial plexus injury: The outcome of concern among patients with suspected fetal macrosomia. Am J Obstet Gynecol 178:195, 1998

Gherman RB: Shoulder dystocia: An evidence-based evaluation of the obstetrical nightmare. Clinic Obstet Gynecol 45:345, 2002

Gherman RB, Goodwin TM, Souter I, Neumann K, Ouzounian JG, Paul RH: The McRoberts' maneuver for the alleviation of shoulder dystocia: How successful is it? Am J Obstet Gynecol 176:656, 1997

Ginsberg NA, Moisidis C: How to predict recurrent shoulder dystocia. Am J Obstet Gynecol 184:1427, 2001

Grobman WA, Hornbogen A, Burke C, Costello R: Development and implementation of a team-centered shoulder dystocia protocol. Simul Healthc 5:199, 2010

Gross TL, Sokol RJ, Williams T, et al: Shoulder dystocia: A fetal-physician risk. Am J Obstet Gynaecol 156:1408, 1987

Hoffman MK, Bailit JL, Branch DW, et al: A comparison of obstetric maneuvers for the acute management of shoulder dystocia. Obstet Gynecol 117:1272, 2011

McFarland MB, Langer O, Piper JM, Berkus MD: Perinatal outcome and the type and number of manoeuvres in shoulder dystocia. Int J Gynecol Obstet 55:219, 1996

Morris WIC: Shoulder dystocia. J Obstet Gynaecol 62:302, 1955

Ouzounian JG, Korst LM, Ahn MO, et al: Shoulder dystocia and neonatal brain injury: Significance of the head-shoulder interval. Am J Obstet Gynecol 178:S76, 1998

Paris AE, Greenberg JA, Ecker JL, McElrath TF: Is an episiotomy necessary with a shoulder dystocia? Am J Obstet Gynecol 205:e1, 2011

Resnik R: Management of shoulder girdle dystocia. Clin Obstet Gynecol 23:559, 1980

Rozenberg P: In case of fetal macrosomia, the best strategy is induction of labor at 38 weeks gestation. J Gynecol Obstet Biol Reprod (Paris) 45:1037-1044, 2016

Sentiilhes L, Sénat M, Boulonge A-I, et al: Shoulder dystocia: Guidelines for clinical practice from the French College of Gynecologists and Obstetricians (CNGOF). Eur J Obstet Gynecol Reprod Biol 203:156-61, 2016

Sheiner E, Levy A, Menes TS, et al: Maternal obesity as an independent risk factor for caesarean delivery. Paediatr Perinat Epidemiol 18:196, 2004

Smith RB, Lane C, Pearson JF: Shoulder dystocia: What happens at the next delivery? Br J Obstetric Gynecol 101:713, 1994

Society of Obstetricians and Gynaecologists of Canada: MORE[OB]: Shoulder Dystocia and Umbilical Cord Prolapse. http://www.moreob.com, 2010

Stallings SP, Edwards RK, Johnson JWC: Correlation of head-to-body delivery intervals in shoulder dystocia and umbilical artery acidosis. Am J Obstet Gynecol 185:268, 2001

Wood C, Ng KH, Hounslaw D, et al: Time: An important variable in normal delivery. J Obstet Gynaecol Br Commonw 80:295, 1973

PART IV

Third Stage of Labor

Delivery of the Placenta, Retained Placenta, and Placenta Accreta Spectrum Disorder

Lawrence Oppenheimer
Sukhbir S. Singh

NORMAL PLACENTA

Size and Shape

The placenta is a round or oval disk, 20 × 15 cm in size and 1.5 to 2.0 cm thick. The weight, usually 20 percent of that of the fetus, is between 425 and 550 g.

Organization

On the uterine side, there are eight or more maternal cotyledons separated by fissures. The term *fetal cotyledon* refers to the part of the placenta that is supplied by a mainstem villus and its branches. The maternal surface is covered by a layer of decidua and fibrin, which comes away with the placenta at delivery. The fetal side is covered by membranes.

Location

Normally, the placenta is implanted in the upper part of the uterus or fundus. Occasionally, it is placed in the lower segment, and sometimes it lies over the cervix. The latter condition is termed *placenta previa* and is a cause of bleeding in the third trimester.

ABNORMALITIES OF THE PLACENTA

Succenturiate Lobe

This is an accessory lobe that is placed at some distance from the main placenta. The blood vessels that supply this lobe run over the intervening membranes and may be torn when the latter rupture or during delivery. A succenturiate lobe may be retained after birth and cause postpartum hemorrhage (PPH).

Circumvallate Placenta

The membranes are folded back on the fetal surface and insert inward on themselves. The placenta is situated outside of the chorion.

Amnion Nodosum

This is a yellow nodule, 3 to 4 cm in diameter, situated on the fetal surface of the amnion. It contains vernix, fibrin, desquamated cells, and lanugo hairs. It may form a cyst. This condition is associated with oligohydramnios.

Infarcts

Localized infarcts are common. The clinical significance is not known, but if the condition is excessive, the functional capacity of the placenta may be reduced.

Discoloration

Red staining is associated with hemorrhage. Green color is caused by meconium and may be an indication of fetal hypoxia.

Twin Placenta

In monochorionic twins, the placenta forms one mass, whereas in dichorionic twins, the placentas may be fused or separate.

Weight

Placentas weighing more than 600 g or less than 400 g are usually associated with an abnormal pregnancy.

DELIVERY OF THE PLACENTA

Delivery of the placenta occurs in two stages: (1) separation of the placenta from the wall of the uterus and into the lower uterine segment and/or the vagina, and (2) actual expulsion of the placenta out of the birth canal. There are two approaches to delivery of the placenta: active management and physiological management. These have been compared in a number of trials, and active management is recommended because it reduces the incidence of PPH (blood loss >1000 mL) and shortens the third stage.

Active management consists of:

- Use of uterotonics
- Early cord clamping or cutting
- Controlled cord traction

Oxytocin (10 international units [IU]) should be given by intramuscular injection, preferably after delivery of the fetal head or after delivery of the body. An equally effective alternative is oxytocin 5 IU plus ergot alkaloid (called Syntometrine as used commonly in the United Kingdom), although there is a higher incidence of nausea with this combination.

Separation of the Placenta

Placental separation takes place, as a rule, within 5 minutes of the end of the second stage. Signs suggesting that detachment has taken place include:

1. Gush of blood from the vagina
2. Lengthening of the umbilical cord outside the vulva
3. Rising of the uterine fundus in the abdomen as the placenta passes from the uterus into the vagina
4. Uterus becoming firm and globular

Expulsion of the Placenta

When these signs have appeared, the placenta is ready for expression. This is achieved by the Brandt-Andrews maneuver. This procedure involves exerting gentle traction on the cord by one hand while the other hand applies upward counterpressure on the uterus above the symphysis pubis. It is wise to avoid rough manipulations of the uterus before placental separation has taken place. Such actions do not hasten delivery of the placenta and may lead to excessive bleeding (Fig. 19-1). The average blood loss during the third stage is 250 to 500 mL.

Physiological Management

Women at low risk of PPH who request physiological management of the third stage should be supported in their choice. Physiological management consists of:

- No routine use of uterotonic drugs
- No clamping of the cord until pulsation has ceased
- Delivery of the placenta by maternal effort

If there is hemorrhage, failure to deliver within 1 hour of physiological management, or increased risk of PPH, then active management should be implemented. Women at higher risk of PPH include those with: (1) an overdistended uterus (multiple pregnancy, polyhydramnios); (2) high parity; (3) history of previous PPH; (4) prolonged labor, especially when associated with ineffective uterine contractions; (5) deep general anesthesia; (6) difficult operative delivery; and (7) induction or augmentation of labor by oxytocin. They should be managed actively.

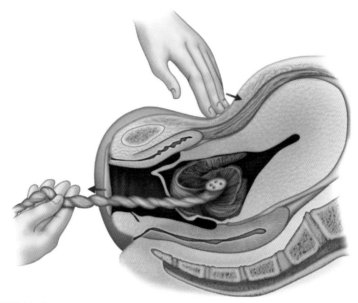

FIGURE 19-1. Expulsion of the placenta.

Delayed Cord Clamping

Early cord clamping as part of active management is associated with a reduction in PPH. Delaying clamping of the cord by at least 3 minutes or until it has stopped pulsating has been shown to reduce the incidence of anemia in the baby by giving an infusion of blood from the placenta. This benefit is particularly seen in lower-income countries.

There is limited medium-level evidence from trials in high-income countries showing that delayed cord clamping reduced the incidence of anemia and increases in hyperbilirubinemia in the baby. Other longer-term outcomes are reported variably. There is high-level evidence from low- to middle-income countries that delayed cord clamping reduces the incidence of anemia in the baby.

Delivery of the Membranes

In most cases, as the placenta is born, the membranes peel off from the endometrium and are delivered spontaneously. Occasionally, this does not take place, and the membranes are removed by gentle traction with forceps (Fig. 19-2). Retention of small bits of membrane does not usually seem to lead to any untoward effects.

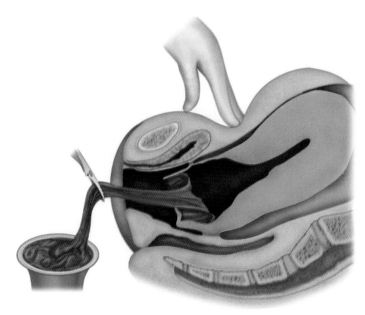

FIGURE 19-2. Delivery of the membranes.

Examination of the Delivered Placenta

Examination of the delivered placenta is performed to see that no parts are missing (i.e., left in the uterus). Torn blood vessels along the edge suggest that an accessory lobe may have remained in the uterus. Some obstetricians believe that examination of the placenta does not ensure that fragments have not been left behind, and they explore the uterine cavity manually after each delivery. Even with the best efforts, retained products, usually manifested by delayed PPH, will occur in about 1 percent.

Delayed Separation and Delivery of the Placenta

The third stage of labor is diagnosed as prolonged if not completed within 30 minutes of the birth of the baby with active management and 60 minutes with physiological management.

Retention of the placenta in utero falls into four groups:

1. *Separated but retained:* There is failure of the forces that normally expel the placenta
2. *Separated but incarcerated:* An hourglass constriction of the uterus, or cervical spasm, traps the placenta in the uterus

3. *Adherent but separable:* In this situation, the placenta fails to separate from the uterine wall. The causes include failure of the normal contraction and retraction of the third stage, an anatomic defect in the uterus, and an abnormality of the decidua, which prevents formation of the normal decidual plane of cleavage
4. *Adherent and inseparable:* Here are the varying degrees of placenta accreta spectrum disorders. The normal decidua is absent, and the chorionic villi are attached directly to and through the myometrium (see later in this chapter)

Manual Removal of the Placenta

Current practice is to remove the placenta manually if it does not deliver within 30 to 60 minutes after the birth of the baby, provided bleeding is not excessive. If hemorrhage is profuse, the placenta must be removed immediately. An intravenous infusion is set up and blood is made available; anesthesia may be necessary. The procedure is carried out under aseptic conditions.

The uterus is steadied by one hand holding the fundus through the maternal abdomen and applying downward counterpressure (Fig. 19-3). The other hand is inserted into the vagina and through the cervix into the uterine cavity. The placenta is reached by following the umbilical cord. If the placenta has separated, it is grasped and removed. The uterus is then explored to be sure that nothing has been left.

If the placenta is still adherent to the uterine wall, it must be separated. First some part of the margin of attachment is identified and the fingers inserted between the placenta and the wall of the uterus. The back of the hand is kept in contact with the uterine wall. The fingers are forced gently between the placenta and uterus, and as progress is made, they are spread apart. In this way, the line of cleavage is extended, the placenta is separated from the uterine wall, and it is then extracted. Oxytocics are given to ensure good uterine contraction and retraction.

Manual Exploration of the Uterus

Manual exploration of the uterus for tears or retained products is required if there is PPH not responsive to therapy. Lacerations of the uterus and cervix should also be excluded by careful inspection.

Placenta Previa

Placenta previa should be suspected antenatally in women with a history of vaginal and/or an unstable lie. Ultrasound should preferably be

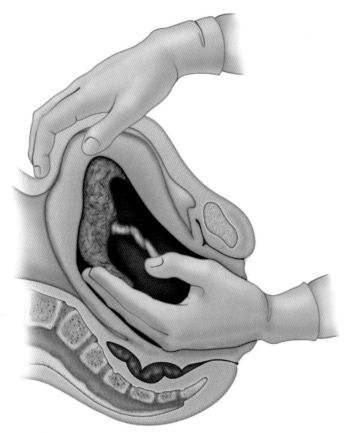

FIGURE 19-3. Manual removal of the placenta.

performed in late pregnancy to confirm location. Where available, transvaginal sonography is the preferred modality and the distance from the placental edge to the internal os should be measured. In women where the placental edge overlaps the internal os after 36 weeks' gestation [placenta previa], cesarean section is indicated. Where the placenta is low-lying but does not overlap the internal os, patients can be divided into 2 groups: those with the placental edge ≤10 mm from the cervical os versus 11 to 20 mm from the cervical os. The risk of antepartum hemorrhage is 29 versus 3 percent, respectively, and the likelihood of a vaginal delivery is 9 to 38 percent versus 57 to 93 percent, respectively, with 75 to 80 percent of deliveries occurring at term. A trial of labor is recommended in women with the placental edge 11 to 20 mm from the cervical os; a trial of labor can also be considered in carefully selected women with the placental edge ≤10 mm from the cervical os and without risk factors for significant hemorrhage.

These include recurrent antepartum hemorrhage, thick placental edge greater than 1 cm, short cervical length less than 2 cm with low-lying placenta, previous cesarean delivery, and evidence of invasive placentation.

PLACENTA ACCRETA SPECTRUM

Placenta accreta spectrum (PAS) disorders is the term used to describe the abnormally adherent or abnormally invasive placenta. Classically, placenta accreta is defined as the abnormal adherence, either in whole or in part, of the afterbirth to the underlying uterine wall. The placental villi may adhere to, invade into, or penetrate through the myometrium.

Pathology

Normally, the decidua basalis lies between the myometrium and the placenta (Fig. 19-4A). The plane of cleavage for placental separation is in the spongy layer of the decidua basalis. In placenta accreta, the decidua basalis is partially or completely absent (Fig. 19-4B), so that the placenta is attached directly to the myometrium. The villi may remain superficial to the uterine muscle or may penetrate it deeply. This condition is caused by a defect in the decidua rather than by any abnormal invasive properties of the trophoblast.

In the superficial area of the myometrium, a large number of venous channels develop just beneath the placenta. Rupture of these sinuses by forceful extraction of the placenta is the source of the profuse hemorrhage that occurs.

The FIGO Placenta Accreta Spectrum Disorders Diagnosis and Management Expert Consensus Panel have suggested an international classification to assist with standardization in reporting. A simplified summary is provided here for the reader.

FIGO Classification of Placenta Accreta Spectrum (PAS)

Grade 1: Placenta Accreta, adherenta or creta (Abnormally adherent placenta)
• The placenta is adherent to the superficial myometrium. There is no line of cleavage
Grade 2: Increta (Abnormally invasive placenta)
• The villi penetrate the uterine muscle but not its full thickness (Fig. 19-4C)

Grade 3: Percreta (Abnormally invasive placenta)

- The villi penetrate the wall of the uterus and perforate the serosa (Fig. 19-4D). Intraperitoneal bleeding occurs frequently. Occasionally, the uterus is ruptured. The villi may grow into the cavity of the bladder and cause gross hematuria
- Grade 3a: Limited to the uterine serosa
- Grade 3b: With urinary bladder invasion
- Grade 3c: With invasion of other pelvic tissue/organs

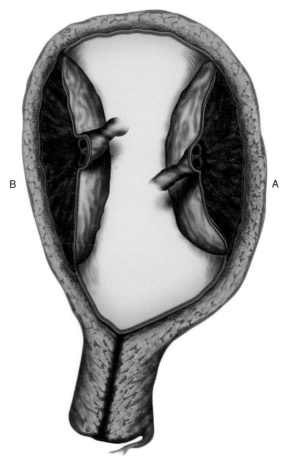

FIGURE 19-4. Uteroplacental relationships. A. Normal: decidua separates the placenta from the myometrium. **B.** Placenta accreta: absence of the decidua. **C.** Placenta increta: villi penetrate the myometrium. **D.** Placenta percreta: villi extend through the uterine wall.

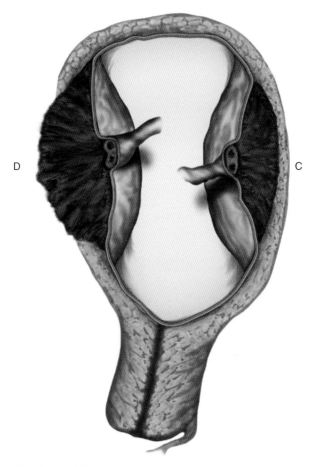

D   C

FIGURE 19-4. (*Continued*)

Incidence

The prevalence of incidence of PAS is directly related to an increase in cesarean delivery rates in middle- and high-income countries. Previous estimates of PAS (1980s) reported an incidence of approximately one in 2000; however, contemporary data suggest that one in 500 pregnancies may be complicated by PAS disorders. The morbidity and mortality of PAS is dependent on many factors including access to an experienced tertiary level care, blood products, and timing of diagnosis and level of invasion. This disorder must be seen as one of the most complex and difficult obstetrical issues faced by health care practitioners and their patients. As such, local and regional planning to optimize care are essential; however, this will be out of scope for this text.

Risk Factors for PAS

Risk factors for PAS include the following:

- Maternal age ≥35 years
- In vitro fertilization
- Placenta previa
- Cesarean section (risk increases with number of previous cesarean sections)
- Previous minor uterine surgery (e.g., dilation and curettage, hysteroscopic surgery)
- Other reported: myomectomy, fibroid embolization, intrauterine adhesions

Etiology

By far, the most important predisposing factors are the combination of placenta previa and previous cesarean section. Because the decidua of the lower segment is less abundant than that in the fundus, a placenta implanted near the cervix may be abnormally adherent, especially where there has been disruption of the lower segment by previous surgery. In this situation, there is an 11 percent risk of accreta with one, 40 percent with two, and up 60 percent with three prior cesarean section(s). A history of any uterine surgery, curettage, or previous manual removal of placenta or cornual pregnancy is significant. PAS is less common in primigravidas.

The underlying condition that appears to be common to all causal conditions is a deficiency of the endometrium and the decidua:

1. The decidua overlying the scar of a previous cesarean section is often deficient
2. In women who have placenta previa, the decidua of the lower uterine segment is relatively poorly developed
3. The decidua of the uterine cornu is usually hypoplastic
4. With increasing age and parity, there is, in many women, a progressive inadequacy of decidua
5. Previous curettage or manual removal of placenta may not be an etiologic factor so much as an indication that an abnormal adherence of the placenta was the reason for the procedure being necessary

Prenatal Diagnosis

Diagnosis prior to labor is the ideal for cases of PAS disorders because this allows for preoperative optimization and mobilizing an experienced team. The "ideal" team for PAS disorders would have the experience in dealing with these cases and have an established local approach. The team often includes, but is not limited to, obstetrician or maternal fetal medicine specialists, pelvic surgeons, urologists, interventional radiologists, anesthesiologists, general surgeons, and neonatologists. Preestablished checklists, guidelines, and regional centers of excellence will all facilitate the best outcome for these difficult cases.

Ultrasonography is reasonably accurate at diagnosing PAS, although it is highly dependent on operator experience. The ultrasonic features include multiple placental lakes or vascular lacunae and a loss of the normal hypolucent zone between the placenta and uterine wall. A lack of ultrasonic features of PAS does not exclude the diagnosis with certainty, especially with a high-risk situation of previa and a prior cesarean section. Magnetic resonance imaging may be a useful adjunct for prenatal diagnosis.

If PAS is suspected, delivery may be planned accordingly and often planned between 34 and 36 weeks' gestational age in confirmed cases to avoid the possibility of spontaneous labor and urgent delivery after hours.

Clinical Picture

Unexpected PAS after Vaginal Delivery

1. *Retained placenta*: This is the main and presenting feature. Manual attempts to remove the placenta may demonstrate no plane of cleavage between the placenta and the uterus
2. *PPH*: The amount of bleeding depends on the degree of placental attachment. In complete placenta accreta, there may be no bleeding. In the partial variety, bleeding takes place from the uterine vessels underlying the detached area, and the adherent portion prevents the uterus from retracting properly. Often the bleeding is precipitated by the obstetrician as they attempt manual removal of the placenta. Blood loss with attempted removal of placenta accreta can be extreme
3. *Uterine inversion*: This is a rare but serious complication. This may occur spontaneously but is more often the result of attempts to remove the placenta
4. *Rupture of the uterus*: This may occur during too vigorous attempts to extract the afterbirth

Placenta Previa and PAS

The presence of placenta previa significantly increases the risk of placenta accreta, particularly with a prior cesarean section as discussed earlier. PAS may be suspected during cesarean section for previa because of the presence of abnormal vascularity on the surface of the uterus, or with percreta, there may be visible placental tissue extruding through the uterus. If abnormal placentation is suspected, it is best to avoid incising the lower segment by performing a classical cesarean section. Once the baby has been delivered, the placenta should be left undisturbed and the situation assessed.

Management Options

National and international (FIGO) guidance are being constantly updated due to the increasing incidence of PAS disorders. It is recommended that each local provider review their specific guidance on the management of PAS.

Hysterectomy

This is generally preferred by patients in whom further childbearing is not desired, or in unstable patients where there is ongoing bleeding. Blood should be available and expertise in tying off the internal iliac arteries in the most difficult cases. Unless there is doubt about the diagnosis, no attempt should be made to remove the placenta because profuse hemorrhage can result. If there is extensive invasion of the lower segment (increta or percreta), one strategy in deciding whether to embark on a challenging hysterectomy in stable patients is to attempt to reflect the bladder. If this proves very difficult because of abnormal vascularity, conservative management can still be followed. If bladder involvement is suspected preoperatively, cystoscopy may be helpful in planning.

Conservative Management

This may be indicated in patients who do not have significant bleeding from the placental site and in whom preservation of fertility is preferred or when the surgical expertise to perform a difficult hysterectomy is not available. The umbilical cord is trimmed and ligated, and the whole placenta left in situ (or any retained pieces where a partial removal of placenta has been performed). In a stable patient, transfer to a larger center may be indicated when the placenta has been left in situ. Methotrexate is not recommended any longer for conservative management cases. Uterine artery embolization (UAE), if available, may be a useful adjunct to prevent hemorrhage. In about 80 percent of cases, conservative management with uterine preservation will be successful. The placenta takes up to 6 months or more to be completely reabsorbed. Pregnancies after both conservative management and UAE have been reported; however, there is a significant risk of PAS disorder and/or other complications of pregnancy.

SELECTED READING

American College of Obstetricians and Gynecologists, Society for Maternal-Fetal Medicine: Obstetric care consensus No. 7: Placenta accreta spectrum. Obstet Gynecol 132:e259-e275, 2018

Geary M, ed. Themed issue: Placenta accreta spectrum disorders. Int J Gynecol Obstetr 140:e1-e4, 259-380, 2018

Hobson SR, Kingdom JC, Murji A, Windrim RC, Carvalho JCA, Singh SS, Ziegler C, et al: No. 383-Screening, diagnosis, and management of placenta accreta spectrum disorders. J Obstet Gynaecol Can 41:1035-1049, 2019

Jain V, Bos H, Bujold E: Guideline No. 402: Diagnosis and management of placenta previa. J Obstet Gynaecol Can 42:906-917.e1, 2020

Leduc D, Senikas V, Lalonde AB: No. 235-Active management of the third stage of labour: Prevention and treatment of postpartum hemorrhage. J Obstet Gynaecol Can 40:e841-e855, 2018

Mavrides E, Allard S, Chandraharan E, Collins P, Green L, Hunt BJ, Riris S, et al: on behalf of the Royal College of Obstetricians and Gynaecologists: Prevention and management of postpartum haemorrhage. BJOG 124:e106-e149, 2016

Timmermans S, van Hof AC, Duvekot JJ: Conservative management of abnormally invasive placentation. Obstet Gynecol Surv 62:529-539, 2007

CHAPTER 20

Postpartum Hemorrhage

Glenn D. Posner

The term *postpartum hemorrhage* (PPH), in its wider meaning, includes all bleeding after the birth of a baby—before, during, and after the delivery of the placenta. By definition, loss of more than 500 mL of blood during the first 24 hours constitutes PPH. After 24 hours, it is called late PPH. The incidence of PPH worldwide is about 5 percent and is a major contributor to maternal mortality.

During normal delivery, an average of 200 mL of blood is lost. Episiotomy raises this figure by 100 mL and sometimes more. Pregnant women have an increased blood volume, enabling the healthy patient to lose 500 mL without serious effect. To a patient with anemia, however, an even smaller amount of bleeding can be dangerous.

CLINICAL FEATURES

Clinical Picture

The clinical picture is one of continuing bleeding and gradual deterioration. The pulse becomes rapid and weak; the blood pressure falls; the patient turns pale and cold; there is shortness of breath, air hunger, sweating, and finally coma and death. A treacherous feature of the situation is that because of compensatory vascular mechanisms, the pulse and blood pressure may show only moderate changes for some time. Then suddenly the compensatory function can no longer be maintained, the pulse rises quickly, the blood pressure drops suddenly, and the patient is in hypovolemic shock. The uterine cavity can fill up with a considerable amount of blood, which is lost to the patient even though the external hemorrhage may not be immediately apparent or visibly alarming.

Danger of Postpartum Hemorrhage

The danger of PPH is twofold. First, the resultant anemia weakens the patient, lowers her resistance, and predisposes to puerperal infection. Second, if the loss of blood is not arrested, death will be the final result.

Studies of Maternal Deaths

Studies of maternal deaths show that women have died from continuous bleeding of amounts that at the time were not alarming. It is not the sudden gush that kills, but the steady trickle. In a large series of cases, Beacham found that the average interval between delivery and death was 5 hours,

20 minutes. No woman died within 1 hour, 30 minutes of giving birth. This suggests that there is adequate time for effective therapy if the patient has been observed carefully, the diagnosis made early, and proper treatment instituted.

ETIOLOGY

The causes of PPH fall into four main groups:

Uterine Atony

The control of postpartum bleeding is by contraction and retraction of the myometrial fibers. This causes kinking of the blood vessels, cutting off flow to the placental site. Failure of this mechanism, resulting from disordered myometrial function, is called *uterine atony* and is the main cause of PPH. Although the occasional case of postpartum uterine atony is completely unexpected, in many instances, the presence of predisposing factors alerts the observant accoucheur to the possibility of trouble.

1. *Uterine dysfunction*: Primary uterine atony is an intrinsic dysfunction of the uterus
2. *Mismanagement of the placental stage*: The most common error is to try to hurry the third stage. Kneading and squeezing the uterus interfere with the physiologic mechanism of placental detachment and may cause partial placental separation with resultant bleeding
3. *Anesthesia*: Deep and prolonged inhalation anesthesia can cause uterine atony. There is excessive relaxation of the myometrium and failure of contraction and retraction, resulting in uterine atony and PPH
4. *Ineffective uterine action*: Ineffective uterine action during the first two stages of labor is likely to be followed by poor contraction and retraction during the third stage
5. *Overdistention of the uterus*: A uterus that has been overdistended by conditions such as a large baby, multiple pregnancy, and polyhydramnios has a tendency to contract poorly
6. *Exhaustion from prolonged labor*: Not only is a tired uterus likely to contract weakly after delivery of the baby, but a severely fatigued mother is less able to tolerate loss of blood
7. *Grandmultiparity*: A uterus that has borne many children is prone to inefficient action during all stages of labor

8. *Myomas of the uterus*: By interfering with proper contraction and retraction, uterine myomas predispose to hemorrhage
9. *Operative deliveries*: These include operative procedures such as ventouse and forceps deliveries, especially those that involve version and extraction

Trauma and Lacerations

Considerable bleeding can take place from tears sustained during normal and operative deliveries. The birth canal should be inspected after each delivery so that the sources of bleeding can be controlled.

Sites of hemorrhage include:

1. Episiotomy: Blood loss may reach 200 mL. When arterioles or large varicose veins are cut or torn, the amount of blood lost can be considerably more. Hence, bleeding vessels should be clamped immediately to conserve blood
2. Vulva, vagina, and cervix
3. Ruptured uterus
4. Uterine inversion
5. Puerperal hematomas

In addition, other factors operate to cause an excessive loss of blood where there is trauma to the birth canal. These include:

1. Prolonged interval between performance of the episiotomy and delivery of the child
2. Undue delay from birth of the baby to repair of the episiotomy
3. Failure to secure a bleeding vessel at the apex of the episiotomy
4. Neglecting to inspect the upper vagina and cervix
5. Failure to appreciate the possibility of multiple sites of injury
6. Undue reliance on oxytocic agents accompanied by too long a delay in exploring the uterus

Retained Placenta

Retention in the uterus of part or the entire placenta interferes with contraction and retraction, keeps the blood sinuses open, and leads to PPH. Once part of the placenta has separated from the uterine wall, there is bleeding from that area. The part of the placenta that is still attached prevents proper retraction, and bleeding continues until the rest of the organ has separated and is expelled.

Retention of the whole placenta, part of it, a succenturiate lobe, a single cotyledon, or a fragment of placenta can cause postpartum bleeding. In some cases, there is placenta accreta. There is no correlation between the amount of placenta retained and the severity of the hemorrhage. The important consideration is the degree of adherence.

Bleeding Disorders

Any of the hemorrhagic diseases (blood dyscrasias) can affect pregnant women and occasionally are responsible for PPH.

Disseminated intravascular coagulation (DIC) may follow abruptio placentae, prolonged retention in utero of a dead fetus, and amniotic fluid embolism. One etiologic theory postulates that thromboplastic material arising from the degeneration and autolysis of the decidua and placenta may enter the maternal circulation and give rise to intravascular coagulation and loss of circulating fibrinogen. The condition, a failure of the clotting mechanism, causes bleeding that cannot be arrested by the measures usually used to control hemorrhage.

INVESTIGATION

1. To obtain a reasonable idea of the amount of blood lost, an estimate is made and the figure doubled
2. The uterine fundus is palpated frequently to make certain it is not filling up with blood
3. The uterine cavity is explored both for placental remnants and for uterine rupture
4. The vulva, vagina, and cervix are examined carefully for lacerations
5. The pulse and blood pressure are measured and recorded
6. A sample of blood is observed for clotting, and blood work is sent for a complete blood count as well as a type and screen

TREATMENT

Prophylaxis

1. Every pregnant woman's blood group and Rh status should be known
2. Antepartum anemia is treated using iron supplementation or even iron transfusion, if necessary

3. Certain patients are susceptible to and certain conditions predispose to PPH. These include:
   a. Multiparity
   b. History of PPH or manual removal of the placenta
   c. Abruptio placentae
   d. Placenta previa
   e. Multiple pregnancy
   f. Polyhydramnios
   g. Intrauterine death with prolonged retention of a dead fetus
   h. Prolonged labor
   i. Difficult operative vaginal delivery
   j. Version and extraction
   k. Breech extraction
   l. Cesarean section
4. When uterine atony is anticipated, an intravenous infusion is set up before the delivery, and oxytocin is added to ensure good uterine contractions. This is continued for at least 1 hour postpartum
5. Excessive and prolonged inhalatory anesthesia should be avoided
6. As long as the fetus is in good condition and there is no need for rapid extraction, the body is delivered slowly. This facilitates placental separation and permits the uterus to retract sufficiently to control bleeding from the placental site
7. Once the placenta has separated, it should be expelled
8. Squeezing or kneading the uterus before the placenta has separated can be traumatic and harmful
9. Careful postpartum observation of the patient is made, and the uterine fundus is palpated to prevent its filling with blood. The patient remains in the delivery room for at least 1 hour postpartum
10. Fibrinogen studies are done in cases of placental abruption and retained dead fetus
11. When hemorrhage is anticipated, adequate amounts of blood should be cross-matched and available

Supportive Measures

1. The key to successful treatment is the transfusion of blood. The amount must be adequate to replace at least the amount lost. Usually a minimum of 1 unit is needed, and it is given quickly. When response to

blood replacement is not satisfactory, the following conditions must be considered:

   a. Continued unappreciated ooze
   b. Bleeding into an atonic uterus
   c. Silent filling of the vagina
   d. Bleeding behind and into a uterine pack or tamponade balloon
   e. Hematoma formation
   f. Intraperitoneal bleeding as with ruptured uterus
   g. DIC
2. Until blood is available, plasma expanders are used
3. If the blood pressure is falling, the foot of the table is elevated
4. General anesthesia should be discontinued and oxygen given by facemask
5. Warmth is provided by blankets or intraoperative warming units (e.g., Bair Hugger)
6. If bleeding continues, the coagulation factors of the blood must be measured and deficiencies corrected

Placental Bleeding

Active management of the third stage of labor is recommended. This includes any interventions designed to assist in expulsion of the placenta and the prevention of excessive blood loss. In the presence of excessive bleeding associated with the third stage, no time should be wasted. Manual removal of the placenta is carried out immediately and oxytocics given. The uterus should not be manhandled in efforts to squeeze out the placenta.

Uterine Atony

Uterine Massage
The uterine fundus is massaged through the abdomen.

Uterine Exploration
Manual exploration of the uterus is carried out, and blood clots and fragments of placenta and membrane are removed. Examination under anesthesia along with dilatation and curettage in the operating room may be necessary.

Lacerations
The cervix, vagina, and vulva are examined for lacerations.

Uterine Compression
Bimanual compression of the uterus (Fig. 20-1) is a valuable method of controlling uterine atonic bleeding. One hand is placed in the vagina against the anterior wall of the uterus. Pressure is exerted against the posterior aspect of the uterus by the other hand through the abdomen. With a rotatory motion, the uterus is compressed and massaged between the two hands. This provides twice the amount of uterine stimulation that can be achieved by abdominal massage alone. In addition, compression of the venous sinuses can be effected and the flow of blood reduced. As part of this procedure, the atonic uterus is elevated, anteverted, and anteflexed.

Oxytocin
Oxytocin can be given intramuscularly, and 10 units IM is the recommended dose and route for uncomplicated vaginal deliveries. Alternatively,

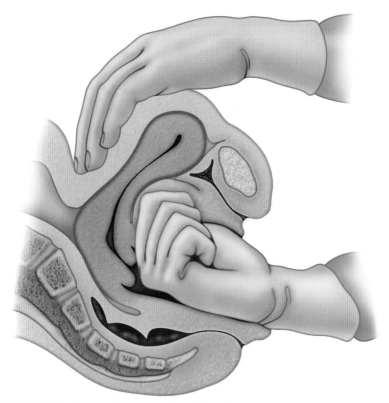

FIGURE 20-1. Bimanual compression of the uterus.

an intravenous drip containing 20 to 40 units of oxytocin in 1 L of fluid can be run at a speed sufficient to keep the uterus contracted, often 150 to 500 cc/hr. Oxytocin can also be given as an intravenous bolus of 5 to 10 units over 1 to 2 minutes. Rapid infusions of high doses of oxytocin should be avoided in hypotensive patients.

Carbetocin
Carbetocin is a long-acting oxytocin that has been shown to decrease the need for uterine massage for uterine atony. The recommended dose of carbetocin is 100 μg given either intravenously or intramuscularly slowly (over 1 minute). The use of carbetocin for prevention of PPH after uneventful low-risk vaginal delivery is not warranted, but its use has been advocated to reduce blood loss at the time of elective cesarean section or in patients with risk factors for PPH.

When first-line therapy with oxytocics is insufficient, there are several more pharmacologic interventions in the armamentarium.

Ergometrine
The first pure ergot alkaloid, ergotamine, was isolated in 1920. Later, another active alkaloid was discovered and named ergometrine (ergonovine). Only the latter is used in obstetrics. It has no adrenergic blocking action, and the emetic and cardiovascular effects are less than those of ergotamine. These are powerful ecbolic agents, exciting a tonic contraction of the myometrium. The maximum effect is during labor and the puerperium. They are never used during the first and second stages of labor. Ergometrine 0.125 or 0.25 mg is given intravenously and/or 0.5 mg intramuscularly.

Undesirable effects include hypertension, tachycardia, headache, and nausea and vomiting. The ergot alkaloids should not be used in hypertensive patients, in women with cardiac disease, and in HIV-positive patients taking protease inhibitors.

Prostaglandin
Prostaglandins are 20-carbon carboxylic acids that are formed enzymatically from polyunsaturated essential fatty acids. Most organs are capable of synthesizing prostaglandins, as well as metabolizing them to less-active compounds. On the basis of their structure, prostaglandins are divided into four groups: E, F, A, and B. Three of the E group and three of the F group are primary compounds. The other eight are metabolites of the parent six. Thirteen of the 14 known prostaglandins occur in humans.

First isolated from the seminal fluid, these substances are distributed widely in all mammalian tissues. Their exact mode of action is not known, but prostaglandins are thought to be part of the mechanism that controls transmission in the sympathetic nervous system. Two generalized activities are apparent: (1) alteration of smooth muscle contractility and (2) modulation of hormonal activity. How an organ will respond depends on the (1) specific prostaglandin, (2) dose, (3) route of administration, and (4) hormonal or drug environment. Prostaglandins are metabolized rapidly, and their systemic effects are of short duration.

Prostaglandins produce a wide variety of physiologic responses. Both E and F have profoundly stimulating effects on the myometrium. In adequate dosage, they can initiate labor at any stage of pregnancy. Prostaglandins can be given intravenously, intramuscularly, intravaginally, and directly into the myometrium. The latter technique will control PPH when other methods fail.

Adverse reactions include:

1. Gastrointestinal symptoms, including nausea, vomiting, and diarrhea occur in half of patients. In most cases, these effects are short in duration and not severe
2. A syndrome of bronchial constriction (asthma) with tachycardia, vasovagal effects, and alterations in blood pressure may take place. If this occurs, the drug is discontinued and supportive therapy instituted. The vital signs return to normal within a few minutes, probably because the drug is metabolized rapidly
3. Hyperpyrexia occurs occasionally

Contraindications to prostaglandins include asthma, cardiovascular disease, and hypertension.

Prostaglandins appear to be involved in postpartum hemostasis by means of their versatile biologic properties, including the function of platelets; vasoactive effects; and, especially, myometrial stimulation. These drugs have a powerful effect on uterine contractility. PPH resulting from uterine atony has been treated by intramuscular injections of prostaglandin $F_{2\alpha}$ (PGF$_{2\alpha}$; Carboprost or Hemabate) and direct intramyometrial injection of PGF$_{2\alpha}$. The latter technique is the most effective. The dose is 1 mg administered transabdominally into the myometrium (1 cc of Hemabate diluted in 9 cc of sterile saline can be injected suprapubically after emptying the bladder) (Fig. 20-2). A transvaginal approach has also been used using the same dose. A sustained uterine contraction develops rapidly, and bleeding is reduced within 2 to 3 minutes. Side effects include nausea and hypertension, both of which are controlled easily. Care must be

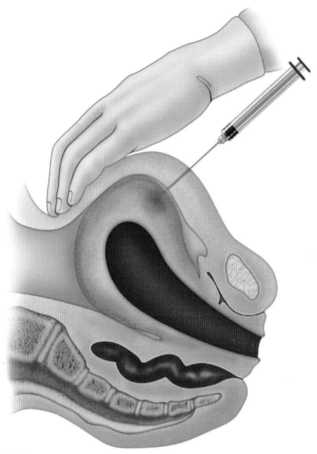

FIGURE 20-2. Transabdominal intramyometrial injection of prostaglandin.

taken to avoid direct intravenous injection. In patients who have asthma or hypertension, a test dose of 0.25 mg should be tried before giving the full amount. Misoprostol or Cytotec is a synthetic prostaglandin E1 (PGE1) analogue that has been studied and used for labor induction as well as both prevention and treatment of PPH. Misoprostol is a tablet that can be administered orally, sublingually, vaginally, or rectally. The typical dose is 600 to 800 μg orally, sublingually, or rectally. Misoprostol is especially suited to management of the third stage of labor when other medications are not available for reasons of cost, storage, or difficulty of administration.

Tranexamic Acid

Tranexamic acid (TXA), or Cyklokapron, is an antifibrinolytic that inhibits the breakdown of fibrin, acting as a hemostatic agent. The use of TXA in obstetrics has increased over the last few years and it has become an important agent in our armamentarium. TXA can be used intraoperatively at the time of cesarean section, or can be used in situations where there is ongoing trickling of blood that must be controlled. It can be used proactively prior to vaginal or cesarean delivery in patients who are at high risk of hemorrhage. TXA can be given both orally or intravenously, but the dose and route for PPH is 1g IV (or 10 mg/kg) and this can be repeated in 30 minutes if bleeding persists. TXA is well tolerated with minimal side effects, the most common being nausea and vomiting, but disturbances in color vision can occur as an indication of toxicity. The only absolute contraindications are renal failure, active venous thromboembolic disease, active subarachnoid hemorrhage, and color blindness. TXA has not been shown to be of any benefit when administered more than 3 hours after delivery.

When PPH is refractory to medical management, compressive techniques and surgical intervention become necessary.

Uterine Packing

Packing the uterine cavity is a controversial subject (Fig. 20-3). Most authorities condemn its use because the procedure is unphysiologic.

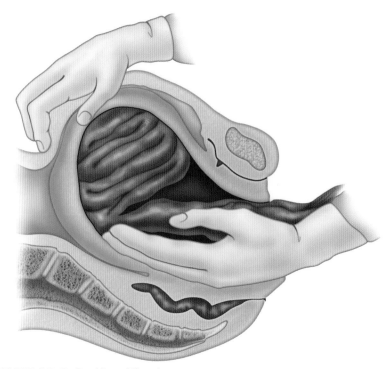

FIGURE 20-3. Packing of the uterus.

Up to this point, attempts had been made to empty the uterus; now it is to be filled. It is unlikely that a uterus that does not respond to powerful oxytocic drugs will be stimulated to contract by a gauze pack. It is impossible to pack an atonic uterus so tightly that the blood sinuses are closed off. The uterus simply balloons and fills up with more blood. Thus, the packing not only does no good but is also dangerous in that it leads to a false sense of security by obscuring the flow of blood. Ten yards of 3-inch packing gauze absorbs 1000 mL of blood. Furthermore, packing favors infection.

Despite these antipacking arguments, many obstetricians believe that it is worth trying to control bleeding by this method before more radical measures are used. The patient must be observed carefully. Deterioration of the vital signs, ballooning of the uterus, and continuation of the bleeding are signs that the pack is ineffective and must be removed. Packing must be done properly. One or two 5- or 10-yard rolls of gauze are needed. With one hand on the abdomen, the operator steadies the uterine fundus while the pack is pushed through the cervix and into the cavity of the uterus with the fingers of the other hand. The gauze is placed first into one corner of the uterus and then the other, coming down the cavity from side to side. The uterus must be packed tightly. Then the vagina is packed. A large, firm pad is placed on the abdomen above the uterus, and a tight abdominal and perineal binder is applied. The gauze packing is removed in 12 hours.

Beyond the use of gauze, internal uterine compression using tamponade balloons (Bakri SOS tamponade balloon catheter) have become popular (Fig. 20-4). Several commercially available silicon models are on the market, although regular Foley catheters and Sengstaken-Blakemore tubes can be used as well. Essentially, the balloon is inserted into the uterus and inflated with a large volume of water or saline (250-500 cc). The balloon is kept in place by packing the vagina with gauze and slowly deflated 8 to 48 hours later. The use of a device with a secondary port that drains any blood accumulating above the balloon allows caregivers to monitor ongoing bleeding. Of note, the Bakri balloon can also be inserted at the time of a cesarean section in situations of uterine atony or to tamponade the lower uterine segment in the case of bleeding from a low placental implantation site. When inserted at the time of laparotomy, the inflation channel is pushed into the vagina from above.

Uterine Compression Sutures

When uterine atony is the culprit and laparotomy is performed to control the hemorrhage, consideration can be given to external compression sutures, as popularized by B-lynch and Cho. In these uterus-sparing techniques, relatively large, braided, absorbable sutures (such as #2 Polysorb or

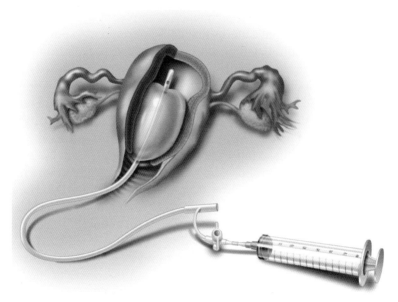

FIGURE 20-4. The Bakri SOS tamponade balloon catheter deployed within the uterus.

Vicryl) are used to bind the uterus and force compression of the bleeding sinuses. In the B-lynch technique, the goal is to create a pair of "overalls" for the uterus to compress it (Fig. 20-5). In the Cho or "square-suture" technique, areas of posterior and anterior myometrium are sutured together to force compression (Fig. 20-6).

If neither external nor internal compression is adequate to control hemorrhage, techniques aimed at reducing the blood flow to the uterus are next in the algorithm.

Compression of the Aorta
In thin women, compression of the aorta against the spine may slow down the bleeding.

Embolization of Pelvic Arteries
This technique can be used instead of, or after failure of, hysterectomy or ligation of the internal iliac artery for the treatment of pelvic hemorrhage. Under radiologic angiographic control, a polyethylene catheter is introduced into the aorta via the right femoral artery. Each internal iliac artery is catheterized and occluded with small (2-3 mm) fragments of Gelfoam. In situations of pelvic hemorrhage other than that caused by uterine atony,

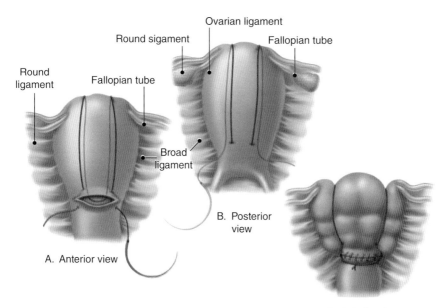

FIGURE 20-5. B-Lynch technique for uterine compression sutures.

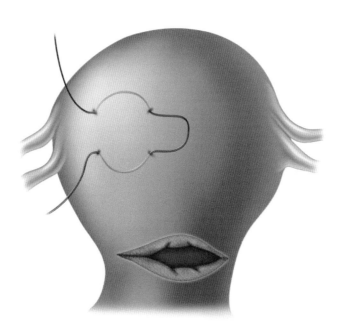

FIGURE 20-6. Cho technique for uterine compression sutures.

the specific bleeding vessel can be identified and selectively embolized. The procedure can be carried out in less than 2 hours and imposes little additional morbidity and no mortality. An advantage over internal iliac ligation is that the distal blood vessels are occluded, so that bleeding from reconstituted distal vessels is rare. In addition, the uterus is preserved, and further childbearing is possible.

Ligation of Uterine Arteries

Since most of the uterine blood is supplied by the uterine arteries, their ligation can control PPH. The collateral supply is sufficient to maintain the viability of the organ. The abdomen is opened, the uterus is elevated by the surgeon's hand, and the area of the uterine vessels is exposed. Using a large needle and absorbable suture (#1 Vicryl/Polysorb or Chromic Catgut), the suture is placed through the myometrium of the lower segment of the uterus 2 to 3 cm medial to the vessels. It is brought out through the avascular area of the broad ligament. A substantial amount of myometrium is included in the suture to occlude some of the inferior coronary branches of the uterine artery. In most cases, the uterine vein is also ligated, but the hypertrophied ovarian veins drain the uterus adequately. The vessels are ligated but not divided. Recanalization will take place in most cases. The uterus becomes blanched with a pink hue, and bleeding subsides. Subsequent menstruation and pregnancy are unaffected. Transvaginal ligation of the uterine arteries is a blind and hazardous procedure that is not recommended. Subsequent pregnancy has been successful after uterine artery ligation.

Ligation of Internal Iliac Arteries

This procedure may be performed in any situation associated with uncontrollable pelvic bleeding (Fig. 20-7). The collateral circulation is so extensive that the pelvic arterial system is never deprived of blood, and no necrosis of any of the pelvic tissue takes place. Entry into the abdomen is made by a midline or transverse incision. First the common iliac artery and its bifurcation into the external and internal iliac arteries is palpated and visualized through the posterior peritoneum. The bifurcation feels like the letter Y. The branch coming off at right angles is the internal iliac artery; it courses medially and posteriorly. The continuing branch is the external iliac artery. It is essential that these two branches be identified positively. If the external iliac artery is ligated by accident, loss of the lower limb may result. The ureter lies anterior to the vessels and crosses the common iliac artery from lateral to medial at a point just proximal to the bifurcation. It must be identified to prevent it being damaged.

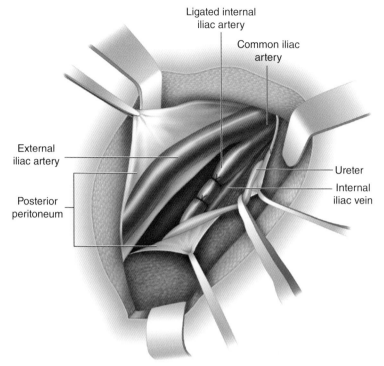

FIGURE 20-7. **Ligation of the internal iliac artery.**

The posterior peritoneum is tented and incised in a longitudinal direction, beginning proximal to the bifurcation of the common iliac artery and extending caudad for 4 to 6 cm. The incision is lateral to the ureter. The ureter is located on the medial peritoneal flap and usually remains attached to it. The external and internal iliac arteries must be re-identified to avoid any error. Care is taken to avoid injury to the veins. The internal iliac artery is elevated from the vein gently and with care to avoid damage to the vein. Two no. 2-0 silk sutures are placed beneath the artery and tied firmly but gently. The artery is not transected. If possible, identification and ligation of only the anterior branch of the internal iliac artery is ideal because it will spare potential devascularization of muscles supplied by the posterior branch. The peritoneum is closed with interrupted 3-0 catgut or similar suture; a continuous suture might kink the ureter. The procedure is repeated on the contralateral side.

Hysterectomy
If the bleeding continues, the abdomen must be opened and hysterectomy performed. Deaths after and during hysterectomy have been reported;

these resulted from delaying the operation until the patient was nearly moribund. Performed in time, hysterectomy is effective and lifesaving.

Lacerations

1. Rupture of the uterus necessitates laparotomy with either repair of the tear or hysterectomy
2. Lacerations of the cervix, vagina, and vulva are repaired and the bleeding controlled with figure-8 sutures
3. In some cases, the bleeding from the vaginal tears cannot be controlled with sutures. Where there are large varicosities, each passage of the needle through the tissue seems to provoke fresh bleeding. In such cases, the vagina should be packed firmly with gauze that is left in for 24 hours; TXA can be particularly useful in these cases

PITUITARY INSUFFICIENCY

The profound hypotension that may result from PPH has a particular effect on the blood supply to the anterior pituitary gland. In 1937, Sheehan described insufficiency of the anterior lobe of the pituitary gland in women of childbearing age. Symptoms include:

1. Mammary involution and failure to lactate
2. Weakness and lethargy
3. Hypersensitivity to cold
4. Diminished sweating
5. Excessive involution of the uterus
6. Atrophy of the external genitalia
7. Amenorrhea or oligomenorrhea
8. Loss of body hair, including the pubic area
9. Absence of menopausal symptoms
10. Later signs of failure of the thyroid and adrenal glands may appear

The condition is initiated by severe shock, the result of massive hemorrhage. The pituitary gland undergoes ischemia followed by necrosis. From 5 to 99 percent of the anterior lobe may be affected. As long as 10 percent of the gland is left in a functioning state, the patient will retain reasonably normal glandular function. In severe cases, death may occur. In less acute situations, the patient can live for years in a subnormal state, and the resulting immunocompromise may lead to infection.

The exact nature of the vascular disturbance is not known. Possible conditions include:

1. Arterial spasm
2. Interruption of the portal circulation of the pituitary
3. Coagulation in the capillaries
4. Venous thrombosis
5. DIC

LATE POSTPARTUM HEMORRHAGE

Late PPH is the loss of 500 mL of blood after the first 24 hours but within 6 weeks following delivery. Although most of these episodes occur by the 21st day, the majority take place between the fourth and ninth postpartum days. The incidence is around 1 percent.

Non-uterine Bleeding

In a few cases, the origin is the cervix, vagina, or vulva. Local infection leads to sloughing of sutures and dissolution of thrombi, with hemorrhage at the site of the episiotomy or lacerations. The amount of blood lost depends on the size of the vessels. Treatment includes cleaning out infected debris; suturing bleeding points; and if necessary, pressure packing the vagina. Blood transfusion is given as needed.

Uterine Bleeding

Etiology

1. Retained fragments of placenta
2. Intrauterine infection
3. Subinvolution of the uterus and the placental site
4. Uterine myoma, especially when submucosal

Mechanism of Bleeding

The exact sequence of events is not known, but some type of subinvolution is present. Three probable factors are: (1) late detachment of thrombi at the placental site with reopening of the vascular sinuses; (2) abnormalities in the separation of the decidua vera; and (3) intrauterine infection, leading to dissolution of the thromboses in the vessels. The basic mechanism is similar regardless of whether placental tissue has been retained.

Clinical Picture

The amount of bleeding varies. Some of these patients require hospitalization and blood transfusion; hemorrhagic shock can occur.

Treatment

1. Oxytocics are given
2. If bleeding continues, curettage is performed carefully, so as not to perforate the soft uterus. In many cases, no placental tissue is found, the histologic examination showing organized blood clot, decidual tissue, or fragments of muscle. The results of curettage are satisfactory regardless of whether placenta was present. Removal of the inflamed tissue with its superficial bleeding vessels permits the uterus to contract around the deeper, healthier vessels, thus producing more effective hemostasis
3. Blood is replaced by transfusion
4. Antibiotics are given to control infection
5. If all other treatment fails, hysterectomy may be required

ETIOLOGY OF SHOCK IN OBSTETRICS

Direct Obstetric Causes

Placental Site

1. Spontaneous abortion
2. Placenta previa
3. Abruptio placentae
4. Retained placenta
5. Postpartum uterine atony

Trauma

1. Lacerations of the vagina and vulva
2. Uterine rupture
3. Uterine inversion

Extraperitoneal

1. Broad ligament hematoma
2. Paravertebral hematoma

Intraperitoneal

1. Ectopic pregnancy

Related Obstetric Conditions

1. Embolism
   a. Thrombotic
   b. Amniotic
   c. Air
2. Eclampsia
3. Septic shock
4. Neurogenic shock
5. Anesthetic complications
   a. Aspiration of gastric fluid
   b. Extended spinal or regional block
6. Drug reactions

Nonobstetric Conditions

1. Cardiac (e.g., myocardial infarct)
2. Respiratory (e.g., spontaneous pneumothorax)
3. Cerebrovascular accidents
4. Abdominal causes
   a. Ruptured spleen
   b. Torsion or rupture of ovarian cyst
   c. Perforated peptic ulcer
   d. Acute pancreatitis

SELECTED READING

Ahmadzia HK, Phillips JM, Katler QS, James AH: Tranexamic acid for prevention and treatment of postpartum hemorrhage: An update on management and clinical outcomes. Obstet Gynecol Surv 73:587-594, 2018

American College of Obstetrics and Gynecology: Practice bulletin: Postpartum hemorrhage. Obstet Gynecol, 130:168–186, 2017

Bakri YN, Amri A, Abdul Jabbar F: Tamponade-balloon for obstetrical bleeding. Int J Gynaecol Obstet 74:139, 2001

B-Lynch C, Coker A, Lawal AH, Abu J, Cowen MJ: The B-Lynch surgical technique for the control of massive postpartum haemorrhage: An alternative to hysterectomy? Five cases reported. Br J Obstet Gynaecol 104:372, 1997

Cho JH, Jun HS, Lee CN: Hemostatic suturing technique for uterine bleeding during cesarean delivery. Obstet Gynecol 96:129, 2000

Leduc D, Senikas V, Lalonde AB, et al: Active management of the third stage of labour: Prevention and treatment of postpartum hemorrhage. J Obstet Gynaecol Can 40:e841-e855, 2018

O'Leary JL, O'Leary JA: Uterine artery ligation for control of post cesarean section hemorrhage. Obstet Gynecol 43:849, 1974

Pais SO, Glickman M, Schwartz P, et al: Embolization of pelvic arteries for control of postpartum hemorrhage. Obstet Gynecol 55:754, 1980

World Health Organization. WHO recommendations for the prevention and treatment of postpartum haemorrhage. http://www.who.int/reproductivehealth/publications/maternal_perinatal_health/9789241548502/en, 2012

World Health Organization. WHO recommendation on tranexamic acid for the treatment of postpartum haemorrhage. http://www.who.int/reproductivehealth/publications/tranexamic-acid-pph-treatment/en, 2017

CHAPTER 21

Episiotomy, Lacerations, Uterine Rupture, and Inversion

Aisling A. Clancy
Ramadan El Sugy

EPISIOTOMY

An episiotomy (perineotomy) is an incision into the perineum to enlarge the space at the outlet, thereby facilitating the birth.

Maternal Benefits

1. A straight cut incision may be simpler to repair
2. Protection of surrounding structures. The anal sphincter may be protected by directing the episiotomy laterally (mediolateral). By increasing the room available posteriorly, there is less stretching of and less damage to the anterior vaginal wall, bladder, urethra, and periclitoral tissues
3. The second stage of labor is shortened

Fetal Benefits

Proposed fetal benefits of episiotomy arising from a more expeditious delivery may provide cranial protection, reduced perinatal asphyxia, less fetal distress, better APGAR scores, and less fetal acidosis. Episiotomy may be useful to facilitate the management of shoulder dystocia by increasing room for manipulation.

Indications

1. Prophylactic: To preserve the integrity of the pelvic floor
2. Arrest of progress by a resistant perineum
   a. Thick and muscular tissue
   b. Operative scars (including previous episotomy)
3. To obviate uncontrolled tears, including extension into the rectum
   a. When the perineum is short with little room between the back of the vagina and the front of the rectum
   b. When large lacerations seem inevitable
4. Fetal reasons
   a. Premature and infirm babies
   b. Large infants

c. Abnormal positions such as occipitoposteriors, face presentations, and breeches

d. Fetal distress, where there is need for rapid delivery of the baby and dilatation of the perineum cannot be awaited

e. Operative vaginal delivery

f. Shoulder dystocia

Current data and clinical opinion suggest that there are insufficient objective evidence-based criteria to recommend routine use of episiotomy. Episiotomy (mediolateral) may aid in reducing the risk of obstetrical anal sphincter injury at the time of instrumental delivery. Clinical judgment remains the best guide for use of this procedure.

Timing of Episiotomy

There is a proper time to make the episiotomy. When made too late, the procedure fails to prevent lacerations and to protect the pelvic floor. When made too soon, the incision leads to unnecessary loss of blood. The episiotomy should be made when the perineum is bulging, when a 3- to 4-cm diameter of fetal scalp is visible during a contraction, and when the presenting part will be delivered with the next three or four contractions. In this way, lacerations are avoided, overstretching of the pelvic floor is prevented, and excessive bleeding is obviated.

There are a variety of techniques for episiotomy and a standardized terminology has been recommended (Table 21-1).

Midline Episiotomy

Technique

In making the incision, two fingers are placed in the vagina between the fetal head and the perineum. Outward pressure is made on the perineum, away from the fetus, to avoid injury to the baby. The scissors are placed so that one blade lies against the vaginal mucosa and the other on the skin. The incision is made in the midline from the fourchette to half the length of the perineum with care to avoid fibers of the external anal sphincter (EAS). The cut is in the central tendinous portion of the perineal body to which are attached the bulbocavernosus muscle in front, the superficial transverse perineal and part of the levator ani muscles at the sides, and the anal sphincter behind (Fig. 21-1).

TABLE 21-1: SUMMARY OF EPISIOTOMY TECHNIQUES

Episiotomy Type	Technique
Midline or median (1)	Begins at posterior fourchette and runs midline. Typically, half the length of the perineum.
Modified median (2)	Modification of the midline episiotomy with addition of two transverse incisions laterally above the level of the anal sphincter. Provides a greater enlargement of the vaginal outlet and reduces risk of anal sphincter injury compared to midline episiotomy.
J Shaped (3)	Midline incision until 2.5 cm above anus, then curved toward the ischial tuberosity
Mediolateral (4)	Incision starting at the midline in the posterior fourchette and directed at least 60 degrees away from the midline. Most commonly used technique.
Lateral (5)	Begins 1-2 cm lateral to the midline and directed toward the ischial tuberosity. Rarely used.
Radical lateral (Shuchardt incision) (6)	Lateral episiotomy carried down into the vaginal sulcus and part way around the rectum. Rarely used in obstetrics.
Anterior (7)	Anterior episiotomy, which is typically used for deinfibulation for women with type-III female genital cutting.

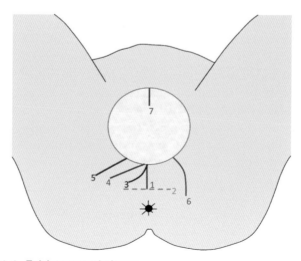

FIGURE 21-1. Episiotomy techniques.

Advantages

1. The muscle belly is not cut
2. It is easy to make and easy to repair
3. Bleeding is less than with other episiotomy incisions
4. Lower postoperative pain and lower rate soft dyspareunia compared to other episiotomy techniques
5. Healing is superior, and dehiscence is rare

Disadvantages

If there is extension of the incision as the head is being born, the anal sphincter can be torn and the rectum entered. Although most bowel injuries heal well if repaired properly, this complication should be avoided. Median episiotomies should be avoided in the following situations:

1. Short perineum
2. Large baby
3. Abnormal positions and presentations
4. Difficult operative deliveries

Repair

Since in most cases the third stage is completed soon after the birth of the child, the repair of the episiotomy is performed after the placenta is delivered, the uterus contracted, and the cervix and vagina found to be uninjured. Not only are intrauterine procedures, such as manual removal of the placenta, and intravaginal procedures more difficult to perform after the episiotomy has been closed, but the repair may be disrupted.

Except for the subcuticular layer, a medium, tapered needle is used. In the deep tissues, a cutting edge needle may lacerate a blood vessel and cause a hematoma. Our preference is for a minimally reactive, absorbable 2-0 or 3-0 polyglycolic acid suture. Prior to any repair a digital rectal examination should be completed to ensure the integrity of the anal sphincter complex and anal mucosa.

First, the vaginal mucosa is sewn together (Fig. 21-2A). The procedure is begun at the top of the incision, the first bite being taken a little above the apex to include any retracted blood vessel. The suture is tied. The edges of the wound are then approximated but not strangulated using a simple continuous or a lock stitch to assure hemostasis. Each bite includes the mucous membrane of the vagina and the tissue between the vagina and rectum. This reduces bleeding, eliminates dead space, and allows for better healing. The repair is carried just beyond the hymenal ring, and then carried through to the perineum. A crown stitch is completed to unite the

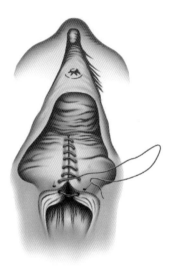

A. Closure of the vaginal mucosa
   by a continuous suture.

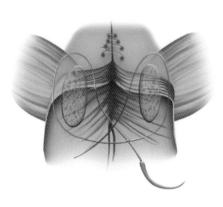

B. The crown suture, reuniting the
   divided bulbocavernous muscle.

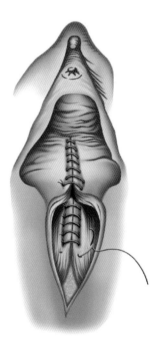

C. Drawing together the perineal muscles
   and fascia with interrupted sutures.

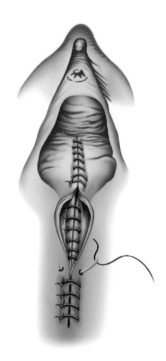

D. Approximation of the skin edges
   with interrupted sutures.

FIGURE 21-2. **Repair of a midline episiotomy.**

bulbocavernosus muscles (Fig. 21-2B). The needle passes under the skin deeply enough to catch and bring together the separated and retracted ends of the bulbocavernosus muscle and fascia. The crown suture is important: If these tissues are approximated too tightly, coitus is painful, and if too loose, the introitus gapes. The transverse perineal muscles, levator ani muscles and fascia can be reapproximated with interrupted sutures (Fig. 21-2C) or with a running length of suture in a continuous fashion.

Finally, the perineal skin incision is closed by one of several methods:

1. The skin edges are united by interrupted, or mattress, sutures that pass through the skin and subcutaneous tissue. These are tied loosely to prevent strangulation as postpartum swelling takes place (Fig. 21-2D)
2. The skin edges are approximated using a continuous subcuticular stitch on a small cutting needle, starting at the lower end of the incision. The first bite is taken in the subcuticular tissue just under but not through the skin, going from side to side until the base (upper end) of the wound is reached. There it is tied separately, or if the suture used to repair the vaginal mucosa has been left untied, this suture and the subcuticular are tied together. This completes the repair (Fig. 21-3D)

Aftercare

The perineum can be irrigated with warm water after each urination and bowel evacuation using a simple perineal irrigation bottle. Sitz baths can also be helpful for cleanliness and soothing of the area. Daily showers and cleaning the area with water is recommended, with care to avoid scrubbing. The incision can be patted dry after urination, bowel movements or showers. Use of ice packs and cold gel packs in the early postpartum period has been shown to reduce pain. We typically recommended acetaminophen and ibuprofen together for pain control. In addition, opioids medications can be offered but should be coupled with stool softeners or laxatives to minimize the potential for repair breakdown from straining during defecation. If a woman has excessive pain in the days after a repair, she should be examined in a timely fashion because pain is a frequent sign of infection in the perineal area.

Mediolateral Episiotomy

The mediolateral episiotomy is often preferred to minimize the risk of injury to the anal sphincter complex, and with a restricted approach to episiotomy, the mediolateral type is the most often performed. A mediolateral episiotomy may be particularly valuable for prevention of third- or fourth-degree extension in women with short perinea, contracted outlets, large babies, face-presentation deliveries, attitudes of extension, breech births, and forceps deliveries. Reported disadvantages of the mediolateral procedure include difficulty of repair, greater blood loss, and possibly more perineal pain and dyspareunia.

Technique

The incision is made from the midline of the posterior fourchette toward the ischial tuberosity, far enough laterally to avoid the anal sphincter. After the infant is delivered and the perineum is no longer bulging, the angle of the episiotomy appears closer to the midline. It is estimated that the healed angle is approximately 20 degrees closer to the midline than the angle cut. Therefore, with the bulging perineum, it is recommended that the episiotomy be cut at a 60 degrees angle from the midline (Fig. 21-1). The risk of sustaining an anal sphincter injury is lower if the healed angle is further from the midline (at least 15 degrees) and a longer episiotomy is cut. The average episiotomy is about 4 cm long and may even reach the fatty tissues of the ischiorectal fossa. Whether it is placed on the left or right side is unimportant.

The following structures are cut:

1. Skin and subcutaneous tissue
2. Bulbocavernosus muscle and fascia
3. Transverse perineal muscle
4. Levator ani muscle and fascia. The extent to which this structure is involved is determined by the length and depth of the incision.

Repair

The technique is essentially the same as for the median perineotomy but the tension on the wound may be higher. Prior to repair, digital rectal examination should be performed to confirm that the anal sphincter complex is intact. The vaginal epithelium is repaired starting at the apex and brings together the underlying supporting tissue (Fig. 21-3A). The crown suture is placed carefully (Fig. 21-3B).

The muscles and fascia that were cut are approximated with interrupted sutures to minimize tension on the closure (Fig. 21-3C). The tissues on the medial side tend to retract, and care must be taken not to enter the rectum. Some operators prefer to place these sutures, leaving them untied, before the vaginal mucosa is repaired. In many patients, a single layer of

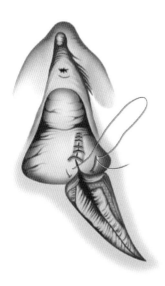

A. Closure of the vaginal mucosa
   by a continuous suture.

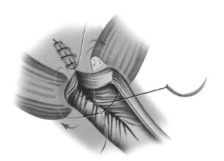

B. The crown suture.

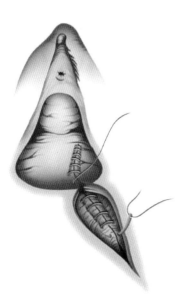

C. Drawing together the perineal
   muscles and fascia with interrupted
   sutures.

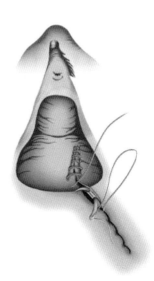

D. Approximation of the skin
   edges with a continuous
   subcuticular suture.

FIGURE 21-3. Repair of a left mediolateral episiotomy.

four or five stitches is sufficient. When the wound is deep or when there is much bleeding, two layers may be necessary, one in the muscles, and one to bring together the overlying fascia. The skin edges are joined by a subcuticular stitch beginning at the apex (Fig. 21-3D) or by interrupted sutures through skin and subcutaneous tissue.

Finally, after repair of any perineal laceration or episiotomy we perform a digital rectal exam to ensure there are no sutures passing into the rectal mucosa unintentionally. If identified, these must be removed, and the repair revised accordingly to minimize the risk of infection and fistula formation.

LACERATIONS OF THE PERINEUM

Over 50 percent of women sustain a laceration at the time of vaginal delivery and most of these are first- or second-degree lacerations. Only about 5 percent are more severe lacerations involving the anal sphincter complex. There is some evidence that perineal massage in the weeks preceding delivery and during labor, warm compresses in labor, and controlled delivery of the fetal head may be associated with some reduction in perineal injury. Birthing in a lateral position may confer some benefit in reduction of perineal trauma, whereas a standing/upright position seems to be associated with a higher risk of anal sphincter injury.

Maternal risk factors for more severe perineal injury (third or fourth degree) include:

1. Primiparity
2. Older age at birth
3. Asian race
4. Maternal diabetes
5. Infibulation

Delivery risk factors for severe perineal injury include:

1. Operative vaginal delivery (with forceps having a higher rate of injury compared to vacuum)
2. Midline episiotomy
3. Occiput posterior fetal position
4. Prolonged second stage
5. Precipitous, uncontrolled, or unattended delivery
6. Macrosomia

Evaluation of the Perineum Postpartum

The perineum should be carefully examined following delivery of the infant prior to suturing. It is important that adequate lighting and analgesia are available to allow a thorough evaluation. Obstetrical anal sphincter injuries require repair by an experienced provider and if missed, can lead to significant maternal morbidity. The perineum should be evaluated by inspection with parting of the labia. The provider should also assess the labia bilaterally and the vaginal walls in an organized way so as not to miss an upper vaginal sulcus tear or anterior laceration. A rectal examination should be performed prior to repair with the examiners index finger in the anus, and their thumb using a "pin-rolling" motion to assess the anal sphincter. For more severe injuries, transfer to the operating room for adequate lighting, surgical assistance and analgesia may be helpful to facilitate repair. The authors advocate for spinal anesthetic in cases of third- or fourth-degree perineal lacerations without epidural to facilitate approximation of the retracted EAS.

Classification of Perineal Lacerations

First-Degree Tear

First-degree tear involves the vaginal mucosa, the fourchette, or the skin of the perineum just below it.

Repair. These tears are small and are repaired as simply as possible. The aim is approximation of the divided tissue and hemostasis. In the average case, a few interrupted sutures through the vaginal mucosa, the fourchette, and the skin of the perineum are enough. If bleeding is profuse, figure-8 stitches may be used. Small lacerations that are not bleeding may not require suturing.

Second-Degree Tear

Second-degree lacerations are deeper. They are mainly in the midline and extend through the perineal body. Often the transverse perineal muscle is torn, and the rent may go down to but not through the anal sphincter. Usually, the tear extends upward along the vaginal mucosa and the submucosal tissue. This gives the laceration a doubly triangular appearance with the base at the fourchette, one apex in the vagina, and the other near the rectum.

Repair. Repair of second-degree lacerations is in layers:

1. Interrupted, continuous, or locked stitches are used to approximate the edges of the vaginal mucosa and submucosa (Fig. 21-4A)
2. The deep muscles of the perineal body are sewn together with interrupted sutures (Fig. 21-4B) or a running layer of suture
3. A running subcuticular suture or interrupted sutures, loosely tied, bring together the skin edges (Fig. 21-4C)

Third-Degree Tear

Third-degree tears extend through the perineal body, the transverse perineal muscle, and the anal sphincter. The anal sphincter is composed of the EAS and the internal anal sphincter (IAS). The EAS is comprised of striated muscle and appears as a ring of pink tissue but the ends can often retract if is torn. The IAS is a continuation of the circular smooth muscle of the rectum and appears as a pale tissue, which is often described as a "raw white fish" texture and appearance. Care should be taken to identify and repair the EAS and IAS separately because persistent IAS defects are associated with higher rate of postpartum accidental bowel leakage, particularly more passive bowel leakage. Third-degree tears are subclassified into 3a where less than 50 percent of the EAS thickness is torn, 3b where more than 50 percent of the EAS thickness is torn, and 3c where both the EAS and IAS are torn.

Repair. For third- or fourth-degree tears, a single dose of antibiotic prophylaxis is recommended. This can be a second- or third-generation cephalosporin (cefotetan or cefoxitin). We also cleanse the area with proviodine prior to repair to decrease the bacterial burden and give a dose of metronidazole in addition. Repair can be delayed by 8-12 hours if needed to allow access to a more experienced provider.

The IAS, if torn, should be repaired with interrupted sutures or mattress sutures. Separate repair of the IAS has been shown to lower risk of anal incontinence at 1-year postpartum. The authors prefer a 2-0 polygalactin (Vicryl) suture but a 3-0 polydioxanone (PDS) suture can also be used. Figure 21-5A shows a closure of the IAS with mattress sutures. Care should be taken to avoid passage of the suture into the underlying rectal mucosa and rectal exam should be completed after (or even during) approximation of the IAS.

The torn edges of the EAS should be grasped with Allis clamps to facilitate repair. It may be necessary to mobilize the torn ends by dissecting

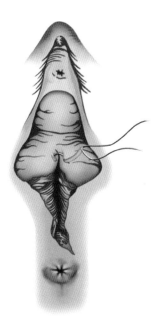

A. Closure of the rent in the vaginal
mucosa with a continuous suture.

B. Drawing together the perineal
muscles and fascia with
interrupted sutures.

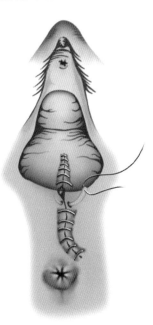

C. Closure of the skin edges with
interrupted sutures tied loosely.

FIGURE 21-4. **Repair of a second-degree perineal laceration.**

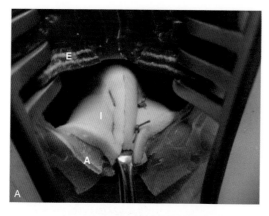

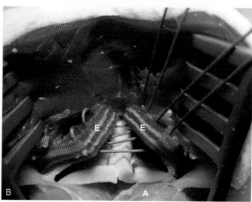

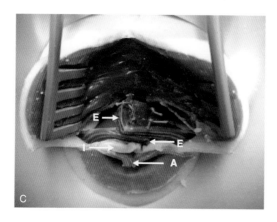

FIGURE 21-5. Repair of a third-degree laceration. A. IAS repair with mattress sutures. (Reproduced with permission from Abdul H. Sultan, Ranee Thakar and Dee E. Fenner: Perineal and Anal Sphincter Trauma: Diagnosis and Clinical Management. Springer Nuture 2009; (Fig. 4.3): p 40.) **B.** EAS repair using end-to-end technique with two mattress sutures. (Reproduced with permission from Abdul H. Sultan, Ranee Thakar and Dee E. Fenner: Perineal and Anal Sphincter Trauma: Diagnosis and Clinical Management. Springer Nuture 2009; (Fig. 4.6): p 40.) **C.** Overlapping repair technique of the EAS. The first suture is inserted about 1.5 cm from the edge of the muscle and carried through to within 0.5 cm of the edge of the other side of the EAS. A second row of sutures is used and the end result provides overlapping edges of the EAS. A, anal mucosa; I, internal anal sphincter (IAS); E, external anal sphincter (EAS). (Reproduced with permission from Abdul H. Sultan, Ranee Thakar, and Dee E. Fenner: Perineal and Anal Sphincter Trauma: Diagnosis and Clinical Management. Springer Nuture 2009; (Fig. 4.6): p 39.)

them out with Metzenbaum scissors. Care should be made to include the fascial sheath of the EAS for strength of the repair. Knots should be buried to avoid suture migration on the perineal side. A 2-0 polygalactin (Vicryl) suture or delayed absorbable suture such as a 3-0 polydioxanone (PDS) suture can be used. The authors use a delayed absorbable suture for at least part of the EAS repair for a longer lasting tensile strength, with care to ensure that the knots are covered by the overlying superficial perineal muscles.

There are two techniques for repair of the EAS: end-to-end repair or overlapping repair. The end-to-end technique involves placement of two or three mattress sutures to reapproximate the cut edges of the EAS. Figure-8 sutures or interrupted sutures can also be used. The overlapping technique is only used with 3b or more severe lacerations and may require additional dissection of the EAS retracted ends. The sutures are started 1.5 cm from the EAS edge on one side and brought through to the posterior side, then into the anterior EAS on the opposite side approximately 0.5 cm from the cut edge (Fig. 21-5B). The end result provides approximately 1 cm of overlap of the two EAS ends (Fig. 21-5C). There is some suggestion that the overlapping technique may be associated with lower rates of fecal urgency and fecal incontinence but there is heterogeneity in data comparing the two techniques. We typically choose an overlapping technique for full thickness 3c injuries of the IAS and an end-to-end approach for 3a and 3b tears.

After reapproximation of the IAS and EAS, the remaining closure is completed in the same technique as the second-degree tear.

Fourth-Degree Tear

Fourth degree lacerations involve injury to the anal sphincter complex (IAS and EAS) and anal epithelium. Injury to the vaginal epithelium and rectal mucosa with a preserved anal sphincter complex are separately classified as button-hole injuries because they are not associated with the same risk of accidental bowel leakage as fourth-degree lacerations.

Repair. Where the anal mucosa is injured, there are three options for repair:

1. Interrupted sutures with knots in the anal lumen
2. Interrupted sutures with knots external to the anal canal
3. Submucosal continuous unlocked suture

A 3-0 polygalactin suture should be used for repair. Interrupted sutures were widely recommended prior to availability of polygalactin, but given the lower tissue reactivity with polygalactin (compared to catgut), continuous sutures are often now used. The technique of knots in the anal canal was thought to lower the risk of tissue reaction and infection but there is no evidence to suggest a benefit of any repair technique over another. figure-8 sutures should be avoided because they may cause ischemia and poor wound healing.

Aftercare.   Aftercare of third- and fourth-degree tears includes:

1. General perineal asepsis
2. The use of sitz baths
3. An analgesic such as ibuprofen and/or longer acting intrathecal analgesia
4. Low-residue diet
5. Encouragement of soft bowel movements with mild laxatives
6. Evaluation for urinary retention which is common after third- and fourth-degree tears. We routinely place an indwelling Foley catheter for 12 hours postpartum.

LACERATIONS OF ANTERIOR VULVA AND LOWER ANTERIOR VAGINAL WALL

Various areas may be involved. Superficial tears are not serious, but with deep tears, the bleeding may be profuse.

Locations of Lacerations

1. Tissue on either side of the urethra
2. Labia minora
3. Lateral walls of the vagina
4. Area of the clitoris: With deep tears, the corpora cavernosa may be torn. Because of the general vascularity of this structure, as well as the presence of the deep and dorsal clitoral blood vessels, these lacerations are accompanied by severe bleeding
5. Urethra under the pubic arch
6. Bladder: The bladder is close to the anterior vaginal wall and may be damaged. Vesicovaginal fistula can occur. The main cause of vesicovaginal

fistula worldwide is prolonged obstructed labor with pressure necrosis of the wall of the bladder. Although rare, bladder injury can also be cause by instrumental damage during difficult deliveries

Repair of Lacerations

Superficial small lacerations do not require repair in many cases. When the legs are brought together, the torn edges are approximated and heal spontaneously. Larger tears should have the edges brought together with interrupted sutures to promote healing.

Deep lacerations must be repaired. Profuse bleeding is controlled best by figure-8 sutures placed to control bleeding vessels. In some cases, the lacerated area is the site of varicosities, and passage of the needle through the tissue provokes fresh bleeding. If sutures do not stop the bleeding, a firm pack should be applied against the bleeding site and the hemorrhage controlled by tamponade.

Often the area of bleeding is *near the urethra*, and when the periclitoral region is involved, the hemorrhage can be excessive. Repair is difficult because of the proximity of the urethra. To prevent damaging the urethra, a catheter should be inserted during the repair, and sutures directed away from the urethra (Fig. 21-6).

Tears of the *urethra and bladder* are repaired in three layers to approximate the bladder mucosa, bladder wall, and anterior wall of the vagina. An indwelling catheter should be inserted into the bladder for drainage.

LACERATIONS OF UPPER VAGINA AND CERVIX

These lacerations may take place during spontaneous delivery but are more common with operative deliveries and are associated with a variety of conditions. Predisposing factors include congenital anomalies of the vagina, narrow vagina, loss of tissue elasticity in older primigravidas, scar tissue, and lower genital edema.

Forceps rotation and extractions after deep transverse arrest, persistent occipitoposteriors, or face presentations often cause high vaginal tears or cervical tears. The fact that these malpositions are frequently associated with a small or android pelvis also increases the incidence and extent of the lacerations. During rotational forceps, the edge of the blades may shear off the vaginal mucosa. Improper traction tends to overstretch the tissues and

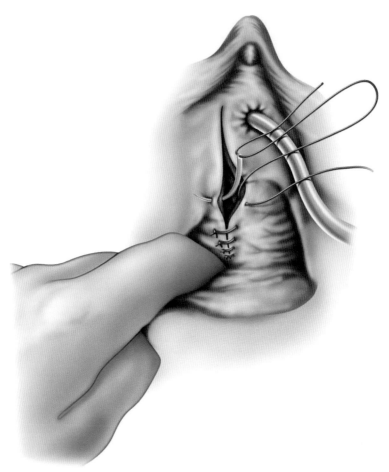

FIGURE 21-6. Anterior paraurethral laceration: placing of fine interrupted sutures. A catheter is in the urethra.

may result in a large tear. A large infant increases the danger of extensive lacerations.

Most high vaginal tears are longitudinal and extend in the sulci along the columns of the vagina. In many cases, the lacerations are bilateral. Following any delivery, but particularly instrumental delivery, it is important to assess the upper vagina and cervix for tearing. This is best done before repair of perineal laceration when exposure is easier. Deaver or right-angle retractors may be required to achieve adequate exposure for evaluation.

Technique of Repair

Lacerations of the upper vagina and cervix can bleed profusely; the bleeding must be controlled as soon as possible. Because the tear is often high and out of sight, good exposure, good light, and good assistance are essential. Bleeding from the uterus may obscure the field. The placenta should be removed and uterotonics given before the repair is begun. The operator must be certain that the apex of the tear is included in the suture or hemorrhage may take place from a vessel that has retracted. If the apex cannot be reached, several sutures are placed below it, and traction on these then expose the apex of the laceration (Fig. 21-7). Figure-8 sutures are preferable if bleeding is profuse, or a continuous lock stitch may be used.

In some instances, the sutures do not control the bleeding adequately. The vagina should be packed tightly with a 5-yard gauze. This reduces the oozing and helps prevent the formation of hematomas. The pack is removed after 24 hours.

LACERATIONS OF THE CERVIX

As a result of its dilatation, superficial lacerations of the cervix occur during almost every confinement. They are partly responsible for the bloody show. These small tears heal spontaneously and require no treatment.

Deep lacerations, on the other hand, can cause severe hemorrhage and shock to the extent of endangering the life of the patient. This is particularly so when the laceration extends into the lower uterine segment, where the large uterine vessels may be involved. The lacerations may be unilateral or bilateral. The most common sites are at the sides of the cervix, at 3 or 9 o'clock.

Etiology

The etiology of deep lacerations includes precipitate labor, a rigid or scarred cervix, the forceful delivery of the child through an incompletely dilated cervix, breech extraction, and a large baby.

Diagnosis

The diagnosis is made by careful inspection. We believe that the cervix and vagina should be inspected after every delivery. A full exam of the upper vagina and cervix is particularly important after all operative vaginal deliveries and

THIRD STAGE OF LABOR

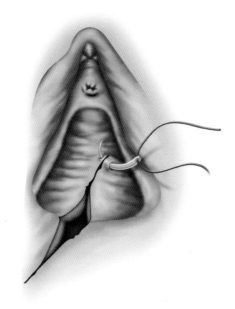

A. Introduction of first suture at highest point visible.

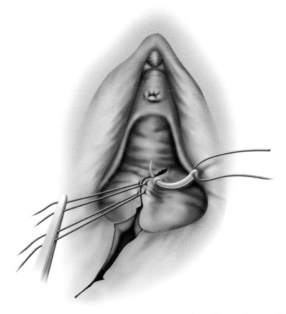

B. Traction on first suture exposes apex of the laceration and enables top suture to be placed. The remainder of the vaginal laceration is closed with continuous or interrupted sutures.

FIGURE 21-7. Right mediolateral episiotomy with a high left vaginal sulcus tear.

whenever bleeding is excessive. Ring forceps are used to grasp the lips of the cervix in a systematic way so that the whole circumference can be visualized.

Repair

Repair of cervical tears is important. The cervix is exposed with a vaginal speculum or with retractors. An assistant is invaluable. Ring forceps are placed on each side of the laceration. Interrupted or figure-8 sutures are placed starting at the apex and are tied just tightly enough to control the bleeding and to approximate the tissues. Care must be taken not to include the ring of the forceps in the stitch. It is important that the first stitch be placed a little above the apex (Fig. 21-8) to catch any vessel that may have retracted. If the tear is high, there is danger of injury to the ureter. When the tear has extended into

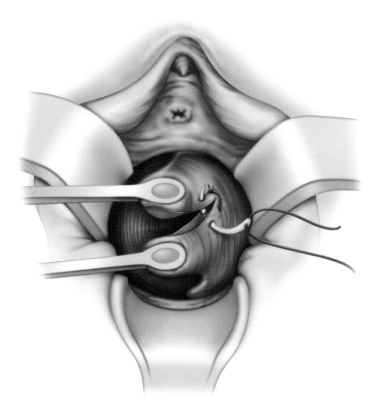

FIGURE 21-8. The uppermost suture is placed just above the apex of the tear. The laceration is being closed with interrupted sutures. Figure-8 sutures may be used.

the lower uterine segment or into the broad ligament, repair from below may be impossible and laparotomy necessary.

COMPLICATIONS OF PERINEAL TRAUMA

Infection

Etiology

Similar to incisions in other parts of the body, an episiotomy or perineal laceration may dehisce or become infected. Predisposing factors include:

1. Poor healing powers:
   a. Nutritional deficiencies
   b. Anemia
   c. Exhaustion after a long and difficult labor
   d. Avascular scarred tissue
2. Failure of technique:
   a. Careless approximation of the wound
   b. Incomplete hemostasis leading to hematoma formation
   c. Failure to obliterate dead space
3. Devitalization of tissue:
   a. Use of crushing instruments
   b. Strangulation of tissue by tying sutures too tightly
4. Infection:
   a. Infected lochia in endometritis
   b. Poor technique and neglect of aseptic standards
   c. Proximity of the rectum and/or postpartum contamination
   d. Passage of the needle through the bowel or extension of the incision into the bowel
   e. Infection of a hematoma

Clinical Course

Typically, the first sign of infection is extreme or worsening pain. Swelling, redness or induration can also be noted. The patient may or may not have fever and/or discharge from the incision. Rarely, the infection can extend into the ischiorectal fossa, presenting as buttock pain. Although most cases of infection occur within the first week of delivery, women can present later. In most cases, infections are localized and may resolve with perineal wound care. In rare cases, an abscess may form, which may require disruption of the repair to allow for evacuation of the abscess or may lead to spontaneous breakdown of the repair. In extreme cases, infections such as necrotizing fasciitis can cause maternal death if not effectively evaluated and treated.

Management

Supportive Management. The area is kept clean and free from irritating discharge and debris by warm sitz baths twice daily for 20 minutes. After this, the perineum is dried and open to the air. The wound granulates in and heals from the deep layers up. This expectant management with perineal care allows for spontaneous healing to occur over a period of several weeks. We typically reassess every 1 to 3 weeks during this time in an outpatient setting. As much as possible, care should be done in an outpatient setting to minimize disruption to mother-infant bonding. If there is concern for a larger infection extending to the surrounding tissues, deeper abscess or if there are signs of systemic infection, consideration should be made for further exploration, drainage of abscess, and/or tissue debridement.

Antibiotics. Following identification of perineal infection, if there are signs of cellulitis or abscess then systemic oral antibiotics should be initiated. Rapid progression of erythema, worsening symptoms after 48 hours of antibiotics, signs of systemic illness (such as fever), or inability to tolerate oral antibiotics are indications for parenteral therapy and/or admission. For mild perineal wound cellulitis, we typically initiate a course of cephalexin for 7-10 days, which is well tolerated and acceptable for breast feeding. For women with breakdown or infection after third- or fourth-degree laceration, anaerobic coverage should be considered.

Abscess Drainage and/or Wound Debridement. If an abscess is present, it should be opened and drained. This can often be achieved under local anesthetic. Drainage of a perineal wound abscess may require removal of some of the sutures but typically relieves some discomfort/pressure. If there is concern for extension of infection into the surrounding tissues or deeper wound, exploration and debridement may be needed. For large infections or abscesses, we prefer to do this in the operating room where anesthesia and lighting are optimal.

Secondary Repair. Although most wounds will heal well by secondary intention, there is some limited evidence that early secondary repair within the first two weeks postpartum may reduce perineal pain during the healing process, limit the need for delayed revision, and speed the healing process. Early secondary repair can be completed when there are no signs of infection, granulation tissue is starting to form, and the wound is free of exudate. The patient is anesthetized, the devitalized tissue debrided, and the episiotomy repaired with interrupted sutures.

Wound Separation

Occasionally, wound disruption can occur without infection and may be associated with pain, burning, new bleeding, a feeling of gaping at the introitus, or popping sensation. The peak time for wound disruption without infection is 1 to 2 weeks postpartum. In this case, the wound should be carefully examined for signs of infection and supportive management is typically sufficient but secondary repair can be considered.

VESICOVAGINAL FISTULA

A fistula is an epithelialized communication between two or more organs. One variety is formed between the vagina and the urinary tract—the urethra, bladder, or ureter. The classic clinical symptom of a urinary tract fistula is the painless and almost continuous loss of urine, usually from the vagina. A fistula may be confirmed by placing a tampon in the vagina and instilling a dilute solution of methylene blue dye into the urinary bladder.

Fistulas can result from complications of childbirth, surgery, trauma, infection or malignancy. Because of improved obstetrics, most fistulas in North America are associated with surgery, but can occur in association with parturition in the following ways:

1. During prolonged and obstructed labor, the bladder is trapped between the fetal head and the maternal pubic symphysis. The resulting ischemic necrosis and slough results in fistulas of varying sizes. The proximal urethra, vesical neck, and trigone are involved
2. Direct injury can occur during a difficult forceps delivery. Usually the trigone and urethra are damaged
3. During cesarean section, the bladder and ureter may be cut or torn

Management

As with most other postoperative complications, preventive medicine is paramount. Prevention of fistula formation include:

1. Optimum operative technique
2. Emptying of the urinary bladder
3. Adequate exposure of the site
4. Sharp dissection made along tissue planes with proper traction and countertraction
5. Adequate hemostasis

If the injury is recognized, an immediate two- or three-layer repair should be performed followed by continuous bladder drainage for 10 days. The principles for a successful operation include adequate exposure, dissection, and mobilization of each tissue layer; excision of the fistulous tract; closure of each layer without tension on the suture line; and excellent hemostasis with closure of the dead space.

When the damage is not recognized or if repair is not possible, continuous bladder drainage is instituted. Sometimes spontaneous closure of the fistula takes place. If the fistula has not closed within 4 weeks it is unlikely to do so without surgical intervention. If the fistula persists, active treatment is delayed for 2 to 3 months to allow the edema to subside, the slough to separate, and a new blood circulation to be established. Repair of the fistula can then be completed with the approach dependent on the location and size of the fistula. However, the loss of urine from the vagina causes considerable distress can be challenging to manage. If the initial attempt at repair is not successful, subsequent repair operations can be more challenging due to scarring and therefore, a surgeon with expertise in fistula repair should be involved in the assessment and repair.

RECTOVAGINAL FISTULA

This is an opening between the rectum and the vagina. The patient notices the passage of air from the vagina and an irritating vaginal discharge.

Most of these occur as the result of an unsuccessful repair of a third- or fourth-degree laceration and occur in the lower third of the vagina. The sphincter, or part of it, heals, but the area above the sphincter breaks down. Occasionally, a stitch from the laceration or episiotomy repair enters the rectum and can lead to formation of a fistula tract. Rectovaginal fistulas can often be identified by physical exam with careful vaginal exam and concurrent digital rectal exam. In addition, imaging, installation of fluid into the vagina and visualization of gas bubbles from the fistula site, or methylene blue installation into the rectum can be helpful in identifying the fistula location.

Surgical repair should be delayed until surrounding tissue edema and infection have resolved. Success of repair and approach to repair depends on the fistula site, fistula size and patient factors, and occasionally bowel diversion may be recommended. Fistulas in individuals with inflammatory bowel disease or previously radiation are more difficult to treat. Success rates of surgical repair are generally highest with the first attempt and thus an experienced surgeon should be involved.

HEMATOMAS

Vulva and Vagina

Puerperal Hematoma

1. *Vulvar*: The bleeding is limited to the vulvar tissue and is readily apparent
2. *Vulvovaginal*: The hematoma involves the paravaginal tissue and the vulva, perineum, or ischiorectal fossa. The extent of the bleeding is only partially revealed on inspection of the vulva
3. *Vaginal or concealed*: The hematoma is confined to the paravaginal tissue and is not visible externally
4. *Supravaginal or subperitoneal*: The bleeding occurs above the pelvic fascia and is retroperitoneal or intraligamentous

These result from rupture of the blood vessels, especially veins, under the skin of the external genitals and beneath the vaginal mucosa. The causal trauma occurs during delivery or repair. In rare cases, the accident takes place during pregnancy or early labor, in which case a large hematoma can obstruct progress. Damage to a blood vessel may lead to its necrosis, and the hematoma may not become manifest for several days.

Most hematomas are small and are located just beneath the skin of the perineum. Although they cause pain and skin discoloration, they are self-limited. Because the blood is absorbed spontaneously, no treatment is required beyond ordinary perineal care.

Rupture of the vessels under the vaginal mucosa is serious because large amounts of blood can collect in the loose submucosal tissues. Many vaginal hematomas contain more than 500 mL of blood by the time the diagnosis is made. The mass may be so large that it occludes the lumen of the vagina, and pressure on the rectum is intense. Bleeding can sometimes extend in the retroperitoneal space even as far as the kidneys.

Many hematomas occur after easy spontaneous deliveries as well as in association with traumatic deliveries. The hematoma often is located on the side opposite the episiotomy. Stretching of the deep tissues can result in rupture of a deep vessel without visible external bleeding. Varicosities play a predisposing role. The possibility of a coagulation defect must be considered. Failure to achieve perfect hemostasis is an important etiologic factor.

Diagnosis

The diagnosis is usually made within 12 hours of delivery. Classically, the patient's complaints of pain are dismissed as being part of the usual postpartum perineal discomfort. After a time, it is realized that the pain is out of proportion to that associated with the ordinary trauma of delivery. Sedatives and analgesics do not provide adequate pain relief. Careful examination of the vulva and vagina reveals the swelling, discoloration, extreme tenderness, rectal pressure, and large fluctuant mass palpable per rectum or vagina. When large amounts of blood have been lost from the general circulation, patients have pallor, tachycardia, hypotension, and even shock. If the hematoma is high and ruptures into the peritoneal cavity, sudden extreme shock may occur, and the patient may die.

Treatment

Active treatment is not needed for small hematomas and those that are not getting larger. The area should be kept clean; and since tissue necrosis may be followed by infection, antimicrobial agents can be prescribed.

Big hematomas and those that are enlarging require surgical therapy. The wound is opened; the blood clots are evacuated; and if bleeding points can be found, they are ligated. The area is packed with sterile gauze, and a pack is placed in the vagina. This is left in situ for 24 to 48 hours. Antibiotics are given, blood transfusion is used as needed, and the patient is observed carefully for fresh bleeding. An indwelling catheter should be placed as urinary retention is common.

Because there is a tendency for the bleeding to recur and the hematoma to reform, careful observation is necessary. Most patients do well, but several weeks pass before the wound heals and the perineum looks normal.

Broad Ligament

The danger of broad ligament hematomas is that they can rupture into the general peritoneal cavity and cause sudden and extreme shock.

Diagnosis
The diagnosis is made by vaginal examination. Rupture of the lower uterine segment must be ruled out. If the hematoma is large, the uterus is pushed to the opposite side.

Treatment
Treatment depends on the degree of bleeding. Conservative therapy consists of bed rest, antibiotics, blood transfusion, and observation. Serial hemoglobin and platelet counts are recommended.

In the event of continued bleeding or progressive anemia, surgical intervention is carried out. The abdomen is opened, and the blood clots are evacuated. When possible, the bleeding points are tied off, care being taken to avoid the ureter. A drain may be inserted to monitor for postoperative bleeding. In older women, hysterectomy is considered, and this operation may also be necessary in young women to control the situation.

Careful repair of the torn cervix is important, not only to control bleeding, but also as prophylaxis against scarring, erosions, and chronic ascending infections. Lacerations more than 1 cm in length warrant treatment.

DÜHRSSEN CERVICAL INCISIONS

Incisions of the cervix are used to facilitate immediate delivery when the cervix is fully effaced but not completely dilated. This procedure is used rarely today due to improved access to cesarean section and improved management of labor (particularly for infants in a breech presentation).

Indications

Dührssen incisions may be necessary to relieve cervical head entrapment in vaginal breech delivery. However, extension of the incision can occur into the lower segment of the uterus, and the operator must be equipped to deal with this complication.

Technique

The cervix is grasped with ring forceps, and the incisions are made between them at 2, 6, and 10 o'clock (Fig. 21-9). These are extended to the junction

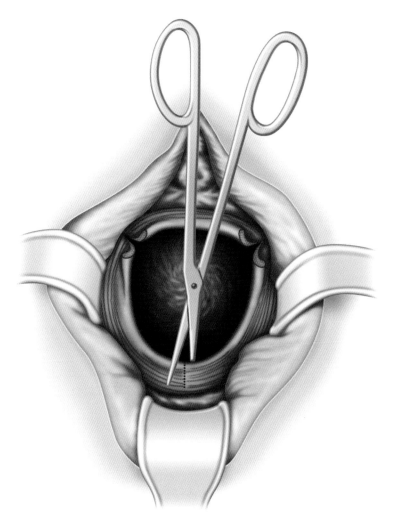

FIGURE 21-9. Dührssen cervical incisions at 2, 6, and 10 o'clock.

of the cervix and vaginal wall. When the three incisions have been made, the diameter of the cervix is equivalent to full dilatation.

Because the bladder is pulled upward as effacement takes place, its dissection from the anterior vaginal wall is not required.

Appropriate measures for delivery of the infant are then carried out. The incisions are repaired with continuous, interrupted, or figure-8 sutures in the same fashion as spontaneous cervical lacerations. Although there is rarely much bleeding, preparations to treat hemorrhage should be at hand. Most cervices heal well, and future pregnancies deliver normally.

ANNULAR DETACHMENT OF THE CERVIX

The anterior lip of the cervix may be compressed between the fetal head and the pubic symphysis. If this situation continues for a long time, edema, local anemia, anoxia, and even necrosis may develop. Rarely, an entire ring of cervix undergoes anoxic necrosis, and a section of the vaginal part of the cervix comes away. This is known as annular detachment of the cervix. Because the prolonged pressure has caused the blood vessels to thrombose, excessive bleeding from the cervix is unusual.

Etiology

1. Seventy-five percent of cases occur in primigravidas
2. Prolonged labor is almost always the rule
3. There is often a history of early rupture of the membranes
4. The fetal head is low in the pelvis
5. The cervix is well effaced and often quite thin. It is the external os that does not dilate. Several observers have reported that the cervix feels rigid to palpation during the first stage of labor
6. The uterine contractions are strong and efficient

Mechanism

The myometrial contractions press the presenting part against the thinned out, rigid external os; in addition, the retracting upper segment of the uterus pulls the cervix upward. This double action leads to poor circulation in the cervix, anoxia, and necrosis. A tear starts at the cervicovaginal junction, and a line of cleavage develops and continues until the separation is complete. The characteristic doughnut-shaped ring of tissue becomes detached when the cervix is about 3 to 5 cm dilated. Gross histologic examinations have revealed these cervices to be no different from the normal term organ.

Clinical Picture

The clinical picture is one of good labor obstructed by an unyielding external os. In almost every case, the fetus is delivered without difficulty once the cervical obstruction is overcome. Annular detachment is the result of true cervical dystocia.

Treatment

Because the vessels are thrombosed, serious bleeding from the stump is rare. No active treatment is needed. The rare maternal death occurs either from sepsis or from uterine bleeding associated with prolonged labor and postpartum uterine atony. Any hemorrhage that originates in the cervix must be controlled by figure-8 sutures.

Prevention

Prevention is achieved by recognizing the situation before the actual detachment takes place. Timely cesarean section for women who are not achieving adequate progress in labor is preventative.

Prognosis

Many women avoid future pregnancy. Stenosis and hematometra have been recorded. Several subsequent gestations have been delivered vaginally with no difficulty, and there is a risk for cervical incompetence in future pregnancies. As such, future pregnancies may require additional antenatal cervical length monitoring.

RUPTURE OF THE UTERUS

Rupture of the uterus is a dangerous complication of pregnancy. It is responsible for 5 percent of maternal deaths in the United States and Canada and is an even greater hazard in many low-income countries. *The most common cause of uterine rupture is separation of a previous cesarean section scar.*

Incidence

The reported incidence in Canada amongst women with a prior cesarean delivery is 0.3 percent but is higher for those women undergoing a trial of labor after cesarean section. A large Canadian study suggested that the baseline risk of uterine rupture for women undergoing a trial of labor after cesarean section is 0.47 percent.

Types of Rupture

1. *The rupture is complete* when all the layers of the uterus are involved and there is a direct communication between the uterine and abdominal cavities. This is the common variety

2. *An incomplete rupture* includes the whole myometrium; the peritoneum covering the uterus remains intact
3. *A third variety* may occur. In this instance, the serosa and part of the external myometrium are torn, but the laceration does not extend into the cavity. A severe intraperitoneal hemorrhage may take place without the condition being diagnosed. This situation should be suspected when there are signs of an intraabdominal catastrophe during or after labor but no uterine defect is detectable on manual exploration of the uterine cavity

Site and Time of Rupture

Tears that take place during pregnancy are more often in the upper segment of the uterus at the site of previous operation or injury. During labor, the rupture is usually in the lower segment. The longer the labor, the more thinned out the lower segment and the greater the danger of rupture. The tear may extend into the uterine vessels and cause profuse hemorrhage. Tears in the anterior or posterior walls of the uterus usually extend transversely or obliquely. In the region of the broad ligament, the laceration runs longitudinally up the sides of the uterus.

It may occur during pregnancy, normal labor, or difficult labor, or it may follow labor. Most ruptures take place at or near term. Those happening before the onset of labor are usually dehiscences of cesarean section scars.

Classification

Spontaneous Rupture of the Normal Uterus
These accidents occur during labor, are more common in the lower segment of the uterus, and are the result of mismanagement. Etiologic factors include:

1. Multiparity
2. Cephalopelvic disproportion
3. Abnormal presentation (brow, breech, transverse lie)
4. Improper use of oxytocin
5. Uterine anomalies

Traumatic Rupture
This is caused by ill-advised and poorly executed operative vaginal deliveries. The incidence is decreasing. Etiologic factors include:

1. Version and extraction
2. Difficult forceps operations
3. Forceful breech extraction
4. Craniotomy
5. Excessive manual pressure on the fundus of the uterus
6. Manual dilatation of the cervix

Postcesarean Rupture

This is the most common variety seen today. It may occur before or during labor. Upper segment scars rupture more often than lower segment incisions. There is no accurate way of predicting the behavior of a uterine scar. All cesarean section scars present a hazard. Factors that increase the risk of uterine rupture after cesarean section include:

1. Induction of labor with cervical ripening medications
2. Oxytocin use for augmentation or induction
3. Two or more previous cesarean sections
4. Short interpregnancy interval
5. Thin lower uterine segment
6. Classical, low vertical, or T-shaped uterine scar

Rupture After Trauma Other Than Cesarean

The danger is that often the damage is not recognized, and the accident comes as a surprise. Included in this group are:

1. Previous myomectomy
2. Overly vigorous curettage
3. Perforation during curettage
4. Cervical laceration
5. Manual removal of an adherent placenta
6. Placenta percreta
7. Endometritis and myometritis
8. Hydatidiform mole
9. Cornual resection for ectopic pregnancy
10. Hysterotomy
11. Amniocentesis during the pregnancy may lead to a weakened area in the myometrium

Silent Bloodless Dehiscence of a Previous Cesarean Scar

This is a complication of lower segment cesarean sections. The complete incision or only part of it may be involved. Usually the peritoneum over the scar is intact. Many of these windows are areas not of current rupture but of failure of the original incision to heal. This complication is in no way as serious as true uterine rupture. With improved ultrasound imaging, these are sometimes noted during pregnancy. Features of this complication include:

1. Usually diagnosed during repeat cesarean section, being unsuspected before operation
2. No hemorrhage at the site of dehiscence
3. No shock
4. Hysterectomy not necessary
5. No fetal death
6. No maternal mortality

Clinical Picture

The clinical picture of uterine rupture is variable in that it depends on many factors:

1. Time of occurrence (pregnancy, early or late labor)
2. Cause of the rupture
3. Degree of the rupture (complete or incomplete)
4. Position of the rupture
5. Extent of the rupture
6. Amount of intraperitoneal spill
7. Size of the blood vessels involved and the amount of bleeding
8. Complete or partial extrusion of the fetus and placenta from the uterus
9. Degree of retraction of the myometrium
10. General condition of the patient

On a clinical basis, rupture of the uterus may be divided into four groups.

1. *Silent or quiet rupture*: The accident occurs without (initially) the usual signs and symptoms. The diagnosis is difficult and often delayed. Nothing dramatic happens, but the observant attendant notices a rising pulse rate, pallor, and perhaps slight vaginal bleeding. The patient complains of some pain. The contractions may go on, but the cervix fails to dilate. This type is usually associated with the scar of a previous cesarean section

2. *Usual variety*: The picture develops over a period of a few hours. The signs and symptoms include abdominal pain, vomiting, faintness, vaginal bleeding, rapid pulse rate, pallor, tenderness on palpation, and absence of the fetal heart. These features may have arisen during pregnancy or labor. If the diagnosis is not made, hypotension and shock supervene

3. *Violent rupture*: It is apparent almost immediately that a serious accident has taken place. Usually a hard uterine contraction is followed by the sensation of something having given way and a sharp pain in the lower abdomen. Often the contractions cease, there is a change in the character of the pain, and the patient becomes anxious. The fetus can be palpated easily and feels close to the examining fingers. The presenting part is no longer at the pelvic brim and can be moved freely. Sometimes the uterus and fetus can be palpated in different parts of the abdomen. Fetal movements cease, and the fetal heart is not heard. The symptoms and signs of shock appear soon, and complete collapse may occur

4. *Rupture with delayed diagnosis*: Here the condition is not diagnosed until the patient is in a process of gradual deterioration. Unexplained anemia leads to careful investigation, a palpable hematoma develops in the broad ligament, signs of peritoneal irritation appear, or the patient goes into shock (either gradually or suddenly as when a hematoma in the broad ligament ruptures). Sometimes the diagnosis is made only at autopsy

Diagnosis

The diagnosis is made easily when the classic picture is present or when the rupture is catastrophic. In atypical cases, the diagnosis may be difficult. A high index of suspicion is important. The first sign of uterine rupture is typically abnormal fetal heart rate. Recurrent late decelerations can be a sign if impending uterine rupture. Prolonged bradycardia or complicated variable decelerations should also raise the suspicion for uterine rupture. The classic triad of abnormal fetal heart rate, abdominal pain, and bleeding is present in less than 10 percent of cases. Signs of uterine rupture include:

1. Vaginal bleeding
2. Scar pain or tenderness (often acute, and may be present even with epidural)
3. Hematuria
4. Maternal tachycardia, hypotension or hypovolemic shock

5. Easily palpable fetal parts on abdominal exam
6. Loss or higher station of the presenting fetal part on vaginal exam
7. Chest pain, shortness of breath and/or shoulder tip pain

In all difficult deliveries, whenever there is unexplained shock or postpartum bleeding, the interior of the cavity should be explored manually and the lower segment searched for tears.

Treatment

Treatment must be prompt and in keeping with the patient's condition. Laparotomy is performed, and the bleeding is controlled as quickly as possible. Aortic compression (by the hand or by using a special instrument) is useful in reducing the bleeding until the situation can be evaluated. Most patients are critically ill and are unable to stand prolonged surgery.

In many cases, hysterectomy may be required. If the patient is in poor condition, rapid subtotal hysterectomy may be performed. If, however, the tear has extended into the cervix, the bleeding will not be controlled by subtotal hysterectomy. In such cases, if it cannot be removed, the cervix must be sutured carefully to tie off all bleeding points.

In young women and in those who desire more children, treatment may be limited to repair of the tear. This should be done only when the uterine musculature can be so reconstituted as to ensure a reasonable degree of success and safety for a future pregnancy. In repairing the laceration, the edges of the wound are freshened and the tissues approximated carefully in two or three layers. As supportive treatment, blood must be replaced rapidly. Subsequent fertility is impaired, and the reported rate of recurrent rupture is between 4 and 19 percent.

Maternal Mortality

Maternal deaths from rupture are uncommon. In 2.5 million women who gave birth in Canada between 1991 and 2001, there were 1898 cases of uterine rupture, and four of these—0.2 percent—resulted in maternal death.

Spontaneous rupture of the uterus is responsible for the largest number of deaths followed by the traumatic variety. The amount of hemorrhage is greatest in these types. The lowest death rate is associated with postcesarean ruptures, probably because these patients are observed so carefully during labor.

The main causes of death are shock and blood loss (usually over 1000 mL). Sepsis and paralytic ileus are contributory factors.

The prognosis for the mother depends on: (1) prompt diagnosis and treatment, the interval between rupture and surgery being important; (2) the amount of hemorrhage and the availability of blood; (3) whether infection sets in; and (4) the type and site of the rupture.

The mortality rate is lower today because of:

1. Early diagnosis
2. Immediate laparotomy
3. Blood transfusion
4. Antibiotics
5. Reduction or elimination of traumatic vaginal operative deliveries
6. Better management of prolonged or obstructed labor

Fetal Mortality

Fetal mortality is high, ranging from 30 to 85 percent. Most fetuses die from separation of the placenta. There is a reduction of blood supply available to the fetus after the uterus has ruptured. The prolonged labor before rupture probably plays a part in causing fetal hypoxia. Many of these babies are premature. The highest mortality rate is associated with fundal rupture in which the fetus has been extruded into the abdominal cavity.

Pregnancy after Rupture of the Uterus

Ritchie reported 28 patients who had 36 pregnancies after repair of a ruptured uterus. Repeat rupture occurred in 13 percent, with two maternal deaths. The risk of repeat rupture is:

1. Least when the scar is confined to the lower segment
2. Greater if the scar extends into the upper segment
3. Greatest in women whose original rupture occurred after classic cesarean section

Management

In cases of pregnancy after uterine rupture, cesarean section should be performed before the scar is subjected to stress and this may require consideration of preterm delivery for some women, particularly those with upper uterine segment scars.

INVERSION OF THE UTERUS

Uterine inversion is a turning inside out of the uterus. In the extreme case, the doctor may see the purplish endometrium, with the placenta often still attached. In the severe situation, the patient may be bleeding profusely, hypotensive, and sometimes pulseless. The reported incidence ranges from one in 100,000 to one in 5000 deliveries. It occurs rarely in the nongravid uterus in association with a pedunculated submucous myoma. The rate of maternal mortality rate varies between 0 and 18 percent, depending on diagnosis and management.

Hippocrates (460-370 BC) recognized uterine inversion, and Avicenna (980-1037 AD) described uterine inversion and prolapse, but it is chiefly since the time of Ambroise Paré in the 16th century that a true understanding of uterine inversion exists.

Etiology

Uterine inversion is almost always the result of inappropriate management of the third stage of labor with cord traction prior to complete placenta separation. Some inversions are spontaneous and tend to recur at subsequent deliveries. Most cases occur in low-risk deliveries.

Predisposing Factors

1. Abnormalities of the uterus and its contents
   a. Adherent placenta
   b. Short umbilical cord
   c. Congenital anomalies
   d. Weakness of uterine wall at the placental site
   e. Fundal implantation of the placenta
   f. Neoplasm of the uterus
2. Functional conditions of the uterus
   a. Relaxation of the myometrium
   b. Disturbance of the contractile mechanism

Exciting Causes

1. Manual removal of the placenta
2. Increase in abdominal pressure

   a. Coughing
   b. Sneezing
3. Mismanagement of third stage of labor
   a. Improper fundal pressure
   b. Traction on the cord
   c. Injudicious use of oxytocics

Classification

Classification on the basis of stage is as follows:

1. *Acute*, occurring immediately after birth of the baby or placenta before there is contraction of the cervical ring
2. *Subacute,* beginning when contraction of the cervix becomes established
3. *Chronic*, present for more than 4 weeks

   Classification on the basis of degree includes three types:

1. *Incomplete*, when the fundus is not beyond the internal os of the cervix
2. *Complete*, when the fundus protrudes through the external os of the cervix
3. *Prolapse*, in which the fundus protrudes through the vulva

Pathology

The following sequence of events may take place, especially if the diagnosis is not made:

1. Acute inversion
2. Contraction of the cervical ring and lower segment of the uterus around the encircled portion of the uterus
3. Edema
4. Reduction of blood supply
5. Gangrene and necrosis
6. Sloughing

Clinical Picture

Sometimes, the symptoms are minor so the diagnosis is not made, or the condition is recognized but treatment is not carried out at the time.

These are the chronic inversions. Those that cause shock and require immediate therapy are the acute ones.

In the typical case, after the birth of the infant, traction on the cord, in an effort to deliver the placenta, leads to its advancement, but if the patient is awake, there is a good deal of pain. Finally, with continued traction on the cord, the placenta is delivered, but it is attached to a bluish-gray mass that fills the vaginal outlet. This is the interior of the uterine fundus. If the diagnosis is made and replacement accomplished quickly, the patient will remain in good condition and bleeding will not be excessive.

In a different situation, the placenta is delivered with some difficulty by fundal pressure and traction on the umbilical cord. As the episiotomy is being repaired, the physician notes that bleeding is profuse. The uterus cannot be felt by the nurse as he or she tries to massage it. On vaginal examination, the cervix cannot be located. Instead, a grayish mass, oozing blood, fills the vagina. Rapid diagnosis and de-inversion of the uterus will avoid blood loss, trauma, and shock. The latter will take place if the diagnosis is not made.

When the inversion is complete, the diagnosis is easy. Partial inversions may fool the observer. Classically, shock is greater than expected for the amount of bleeding. The extreme shock is probably caused by tension on the nerves of the broad ligament, which are drawn through the cervical ring, and by irritation of the peritoneum. Whenever shock is out of proportion to hemorrhage, the accoucheur should think of uterine inversion. The placenta may have separated or may remain attached. The hemorrhage may be excessive or minimal.

Diagnosis

1. High index of suspicion
2. Absence of uterine fundus on abdominal examination
3. Vaginal examination
4. Uterine rupture must be excluded

Prophylaxis

1. No attempt should be made to deliver the placenta until it has separated
2. To deliver the placenta, the Brandt maneuver is safer than the Credé method of expression by fundal pressure or by traction on the cord
3. Routine exploration of the postpartum uterus will detect a uterine inversion in its incomplete stage before it has descended through the vaginal introitus

Treatment of Acute Inversion

The aim of treatment is to replace the uterus as soon as possible. The patient should be cross-matched and blood given as necessary. Replacement of the uterus must not be delayed until shock has been treated because the latter may not be overcome as long as the uterus remains inverted.

In most cases, the placenta will have been delivered. If it is still attached, it can be removed manually or replaced with the fundus, whichever is easier. On the one hand, attempts to remove the placenta before the uterine replacement may lead to profuse bleeding. On the other hand, if the placenta has been removed, correction of the inversion will be easier because the mass that has to be replaced is smaller. In the acute setting uterotonics should he delayed until the uterine replacement has occurred or been attempted. General anesthetic may be required if uterine contraction has already occurred.

Technique of Replacement

The patient is anesthetized. In the first step of the procedure, the uterus is grasped so that the inverted fundus lies in the palm of the hand with the fingers placed near the uterocervical junction (Fig. 21-10A). As pressure is exerted on the uterus, it gradually returns into the vagina. In the second step (Fig. 21-10B), the uterus is lifted out of the pelvis and held in the abdominal cavity above the level of the umbilicus. This stretches and tautens the uterine ligaments. As the uterine ligaments are placed under tension, the resultant pressure widens the cervical ring and then pulls the fundus through it. In this way, the uterus is replaced to its normal position. Success may not be immediate, and it may take 3 to 5 minutes until the uterine fundus recedes from the palm of the hand. Care must be taken to avoid using too much pressure with fingertips, because uterine perforation can occur.

Treatment of Subacute Inversion

Once the cervix has contracted, immediate replacement of the uterus is no longer feasible.

1. The vagina is packed with 2-inch gauze without replacing the uterus, pushing the cervix into the abdominal cavity. A Foley catheter is inserted into the bladder
2. The patient is treated for shock, and blood transfusion is given in the amount lost
3. Antibiotics may be used

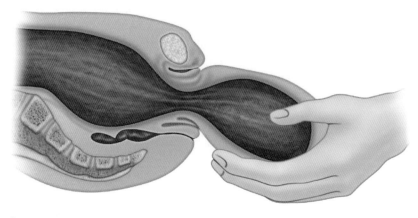

A

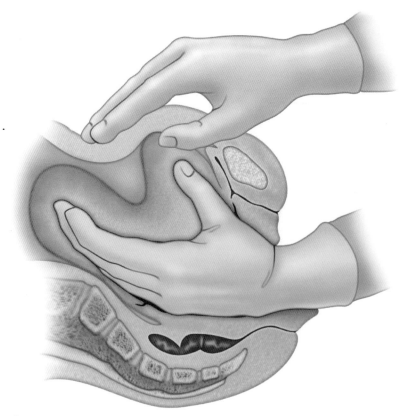

B

FIGURE 21-10. Replacement of the inverted uterus. A. Step 1. B. Step 2.

4. During the next 48 hours, fluids and electrolytes are infused in an attempt at restoring the patient to a condition suitable for surgery. At the same time, it is hoped that some uterine involution will take place
5. Laparotomy is carried out and the inversion corrected by a combined abdominovaginal operation, as for chronic inversion

Treatment of Chronic Inversion

Spinelli Procedure
Using the vaginal approach, the contracted cervical ring is incised anteriorly, so that the fundus of the uterus can be pushed back into place.

Haultain Procedure
Laparotomy is performed. The cervical ring is incised posteriorly, and the uterine fundus is drawn up.

Huntington Procedure
The approach is per abdominal incision. The surface of the uterus inside the crater is grasped with Allis forceps about 2 cm below the inversion cup on each side and upward traction exerted. As the uterus comes up through the ring, additional forceps are placed below the original ones and further traction is exerted. This procedure is continued until the inversion is completely reversed. Simultaneous pressure on the fundus through the vagina by an assistant may make the procedure easier.

Prognosis

The reported rate of recurrence is greater than 40 percent. Some authorities believe that further pregnancy should be avoided or that subsequent delivery should be by cesarean section. However, this does not obviate the problem entirely because inversion can occur even during cesarean section.

SEPARATION OF THE SYMPHYSIS PUBIS

During pregnancy, relaxation and weakening of the pelvic joints take place. This begins during the first half of pregnancy and reaches a maximum in the seventh month. Return to normal begins after delivery and is complete by the sixth month.

Incidence and Etiology

This varies from one in 250 to one in 30,000 confinements. Minor degrees of separation take place, but because the symptoms are minimal, the diagnosis is not made, and spontaneous correction follows. This accident may occur during labor or in the second half of pregnancy.

Rupture of the pubic symphysis occurs in patients with excessive relaxation of the pelvic joints. Precipitating factors include:

1. Tumultuous labor
2. Difficult forceps extractions
3. Cephalopelvic disproportion
4. Excessive abduction of the thighs at delivery
5. Any condition that might place sudden and excessive pressure on the pubic symphysis

Many cases occur after spontaneous delivery.

Pathology

There is an actual tear of the ligaments connecting the pubic bones. The rupture is usually incomplete, and a fibrocartilagenous bridge remains. Hemorrhage and edema are present. Arthritis and osteomyelitis are possible complications.

Clinical Picture and Diagnosis

The onset of symptoms is usually sudden but may not be noted until the patient tries to walk. At the time of rupture, the patient may experience a bursting feeling, or a cracking noise may be heard.

Motion of the symphysis (as by moving the legs) causes great pain. If the patient can walk, she does so with a waddling gait.

There is a marked tenderness of the pubic symphysis. Edema and ecchymosis are present frequently. A gaping defect in the joint is often palpable. Walking or pressure causes motion of the loose joint.

The diagnosis is made by the symptoms and signs. Radiography helps, but the degree of separation seen on radiologic study may not be proportional to the clinical manifestations. To be considered pathologic, the separation seen on radiographs should be greater than 1 cm.

Management of symptomatic separation must be directed at relieving the patient's discomfort and compensating for her disability. Treatment is governed by the severity of the condition. Analgesia is essential.

Some patients require prolonged bed rest, with a tight corset or peritrochanteric belt to keep the separated bones as nearly apposed as possible. The local injection of local anesthetic may help. While in hospital, the patient should sleep with a bed board under the mattress; she should also use assistive devices to pull herself to a sitting position so as not to strain her pelvis.

When the rupture is minor, early ambulation is permissible. When the problem is more severe, crutches should be used. Support is needed for 6 weeks. Physiotherapy can aid in technique for ambulation and transfers to avoid further strain to the symphysis.

Surgical intervention is indicated rarely. When necessary, fusions may be carried out, often supplemented by bone grafts, bolts, and crossed wires.

SELECTED READING

American College of Obstetricians and Gynecologists. ACOG Practice Bulletin, No. 71: Episiotomy. Obstet Gynecol 107:956-962, 2006

Bodner-Adler B, Bodner K, Kaider A, Wagenbichler P, Leodolter S, Husslein P, et al: Risk factors for third-degree perineal tears in vaginal delivery, with an analysis of episiotomy types. J Reprod Med 46:752, 2004

Dy J, DeMeester S, Lipworth H, Barrett J: No 382 Trial of labour after cesarean section. J Obstet Gynaecol Can 41: 992-1011, 2019

Harris BA: Acute puerperal inversion of the uterus. Clin Obstet Gynecol 27:134, 1984

Hartmann K, Viswanathan M, Palmieri R, Gartlehner G, Thorp J, Lohr KN: Outcomes of routine episiotomy: A systematic review. JAMA 293:2141, 2005

Harvey MA, Pierce M, Walter JE, Chou Q, Diamond P, Epp A, et al: Obstetrical anal sphincter injuries (OASIS): Prevention, recognition, and repair. J Obstet Gynaecol Can 37:1131-1148, 2015

Lee WK, Baggish MS, Lashgari M: Acute inversion of the uterus. Obstet Gynecol 51:144, 1978

Leeman L, Spearman M, Rogers R: Repair of obstetric perineal lacerations. Am Fam Physician 68:1585, 2003

Ritchie EA: Pregnancy after rupture of the pregnant uterus. J Obstet Gynecol Brit Commonw 78:642, 1971

Schrinsky DC, Benson RC: Rupture of the pregnant uterus: A review. Obstet Gynecol Surv 33:217, 1978

Shiono P, Klebanoff MA, Carey JC: Midline episiotomies: More harm than good? Obstet Gynecol 75:765, 1990

Spaulding LB, Gallup DG: Current concepts of management of rupture of the gravid uterus. Obstet Gynecol 54:437, 1979

Thacker SB, Banta HD: Benefits and risks of episiotomy: An interpretive view of the English language literature, 1860-1980. Obstet Gynecol Survey 38:322, 1983

Watson O, Besch N, Bowes WA: Management of acute and subacute puerperal inversion of the uterus. Obstet Gynecol 55:12, 1980

Complicated Labor

PART V

CHAPTER 22

Cesarean Section

Darine El-Chaâr

Cesarean section is an operation by which a child is delivered through an incision in the abdominal wall and the uterus. The first professional cesarean section was performed in the United States in 1827. Before 1800, cesarean section was performed rarely and was usually fatal. In London and Edinburgh in 1877, of 35 cesareans performed, 33 resulted in the death of the mother. By 1877, there had been 71 cesarean section operations in the United States. The mortality rate was 52 percent, mainly because of infection and hemorrhage.

FREQUENCY OF CESAREAN SECTION

The rate of cesarean section has risen steadily from an incidence of 3 to 4 percent, over 30 years ago, to the present rate 25 to 30 percent depending on region. Not only has the operation become safer for the mother, but the number of infants damaged by prolonged labor and traumatic vaginal operations has been reduced. In addition, concern for the quality of life and the intellectual development of the child has widened the indications for cesarean section.

The largest increase in the use of cesarean section is in those cases described as having "dystocia." Although conditions such as disproportion, malpresentation, and incoordinate uterine action are included in this group, in many instances, the exact diagnosis is not made, and the diagnosis of "dystocia" represents slow progress in labor from whatever cause. The use of cesarean section for these patients is part of a more aggressive management of poor progress in labor and the abandonment of difficult midforceps operations.

Although it appears clear that the replacement of high forceps and difficult midforceps operations by cesarean section has reduced the perinatal morbidity and mortality in this area, the available evidence does not support the contention that the great expansion in the rates of cesarean section for other indications has contributed significantly to the reduction in the rates of perinatal mortality in recent years. Certainly, the more frequent use of cesarean section has led to an increase in the rate of maternal morbidity. Higher rates of repeat cesarean sections are a cause for complications with placental anomalies in subsequent pregnancies.

INDICATIONS FOR CESAREAN SECTION

Indications for cesarean section are absolute or relative. Any condition that makes delivery via the birth canal impossible is an absolute indication for abdominal delivery. Among these are extreme degrees of pelvic contraction and neoplasms blocking the passage. With a relative indication, vaginal birth is possible, but the conditions are such that cesarean section is safer for the mother, the child, or both.

Pelvic Contraction and Dystocia

1. Fetopelvic disproportion
2. Malpresentation and malposition
3. Uterine dysfunction
4. Soft tissue dystocia
5. Neoplasms
6. Failure to progress
7. Previous shoulder dystocia

Previous Uterine Surgery

1. Cesarean section
2. Hysterotomy
3. Myomectomy
4. Cervical suture

Hemorrhage

1. Placenta previa or vasa previa
2. Abruptio placentae

Toxemia of Pregnancy

1. Preeclampsia and eclampsia
2. Hypertension
3. Renal disease

Fetal Indications

1. Fetal distress
2. Previous fetal death or damage
3. Prolapse of the umbilical cord
4. Placental insufficiency (IUGR)
5. Maternal diabetes
6. Rhesus incompatibility
7. Postmaternal death
8. Maternal genital herpes
9. Prevent vertical transmission of HIV infection

COMPLICATED LABOR

Miscellaneous

1. Advanced maternal age
2. Previous vaginal repair or pelvic surgery
3. Congenital uterine anomaly
4. Poor obstetric history
5. Failed forceps or vacuum
6. Elective cesarean: cesarean delivery on maternal request

Pelvic Contractions and Mechanical Dystocia

Fetopelvic Disproportion

Fetopelvic disproportion includes a contracted pelvis, an overgrown fetus, or a relative disparity between the size of the baby and that of the pelvis. Contributing to the problem of disproportion are the shape of the pelvis, the presentation of the fetus and its ability to mold and engage, the dilatability of the cervix, and the effectiveness of the uterine contractions.

Malposition and Malpresentation

These abnormalities may make cesarean section necessary when a baby in normal position could be born per vagina. A great part of the increased incidence of cesarean section in this group is associated with breech presentation. Today, more than half of babies in breech presentation are born by cesarean section. Revised guidelines have been encouraging breech delivery with specific criteria, and access to this is now more routinely implemented in some units with experienced breech delivery providers.

Uterine Dysfunction

Uterine dysfunction includes incoordinate uterine action, inertia, constriction ring, and inability of the cervix to dilate. Labor is prolonged, and progress may cease altogether. These conditions are often associated with disproportion and malpresentations.

Soft Tissue Dystocia

Soft tissue dystocia may prevent or make normal birth difficult. This includes such conditions as scars in the genital tract, cervical rigidity from injury or surgery, and atresia or stenosis of the vagina. Forceful vaginal delivery results in large lacerations and hemorrhage.

Neoplasms

Neoplasms that block the pelvis make normal delivery impossible. Invasive cancer of the cervix diagnosed during the 3rd trimester of pregnancy is treated by cesarean section followed by radiation therapy, radical surgery, or both. Benign growth such as fibroids could also pose a problem.

Failure to Progress

This group includes such conditions as cephalopelvic disproportion, ineffective uterine contractions, a poor pelvis, a large baby, and deflexion of the fetal head. Often an exact diagnosis cannot be made and is academic in any case. The decision in favor of cesarean section is made on the failure of the labor to achieve cervical dilatation and/or fetal descent regardless of the etiology.

Previous Uterine Surgery

Cesarean Section

In 1916, E.B. Cragin expressed the opinion that in women who had had a previous cesarean section, the risk of uterine rupture was so high and the consequences of such an accident so costly that a repeat cesarean section should be performed before the onset of labor. His dictum, "Once a cesarean, always a cesarean," has been observed for many years, but the concept is being reevaluated because of the increasing incidence of cesarean section, the high rate of maternal morbidity with abdominal delivery, and the lower risk of rupture when the original incision was transverse and confined to the lower segment of the uterus. Under certain conditions, a trial of labor is permissible for women who have had a cesarean section. When successful, maternal morbidity, length of stay in hospital, and period of convalescence are reduced. The faster recovery enables the woman to participate earlier in the care of the infant, herself, and her family. Recent data suggest that about half the women who have had a delivery by cesarean section can have a trial of labor in future pregnancies (see Chapter 23).

Hysterotomy

Pregnancy in a uterus in which a previous gestation was terminated by hysterotomy is attended by danger of uterine rupture. The risk is similar to that of classical cesarean section. Hysterotomy should be avoided whenever possible, keeping in mind that the next pregnancy might necessitate cesarean section.

COMPLICATED LABOR

Extensive Myomectomy

Myomectomy in the past is an indication for cesarean section only if the operation was extensive, the myometrium disorganized, and the incision extended into the endometrial cavity. The previous removal of peduncu-lated or subserous fibromyomas does not call for cesarean section.

Cervical Cerclage

In some cases when there has been a cervical suture or repair of an incom-petent os, cesarean section is necessary if the cerclage was performed abdominally, either by laparotomy or by a laparoscopic approach.

Hemorrhage

Placenta Previa

Cesarean section in all cases of central and many cases of marginal pla-centa previa has reduced both fetal and maternal mortality. Cesarean sec-tion is also indicated in suspected vasa previa in patients with a history of a low-lying placenta.

Abruptio Placentae

Abruptio placentae occurring before or during early labor may be treated by rupture of the membranes and oxytocin drip. When the hemorrhage is severe, the cervix hard and closed, or uteroplacental apoplexy suspected, cesarean section may be necessary to save the baby, control hemorrhage, prevent disseminated intravascular coagulation, and observe the condition of the uterus and its ability to contract and control the bleeding. In some cases, hysterectomy is necessary.

Toxemia of Pregnancy

These states must be considered:

1. Preeclampsia and eclampsia
2. Essential hypertension
3. Chronic nephritis

Toxemia of pregnancy may require termination of the pregnancy before term. In most cases, induction of labor is the method of choice. When the cervix is not ripe and induction would be difficult, cesarean sec-tion is sometimes preferable.

![Fetal Indications]

ABNORMAL FETAL HEART RATE (FHR) Fetal distress, severe bradycardia, irregularity of the FHR, or late patterns of deceleration sometimes necessitates emergency cesarean section. The rate of cesarean section is high in monitored patients. This is not surprising since the main indications for monitoring are those that predispose to fetal hypoxia. However, fetal distress is not the prime reason for increasing the rate of cesarean section. Problems associated with dystocia are the main indications for abdominal delivery. A new indication for cesarean section is described as fetal intolerance of labor. This is seen in patients who have desultory labors. Stimulation by oxytocin may result in abnormalities of the FHR. Often an emergency cesarean section is performed, but a normal baby with no evidence of asphyxia is delivered.

PREVIOUS FETAL DEATH OR DAMAGE Especially in older women who have had an intrapartum death or a child with birth injuries, cesarean section may be elected.

PROLAPSE OF THE UMBILICAL CORD Prolapse of the umbilical cord in the presence of an undilated cervix is managed best by cesarean section, provided the baby is in good condition.

PLACENTAL INSUFFICIENCY In cases of intrauterine growth restriction or postterm pregnancy, when clinical examinations and various tests suggest that the baby is in jeopardy, delivery may be necessary. If induction is not feasible or fails, cesarean section is indicated. There is an increased ability of pediatricians to resuscitate small babies and, when the need exists, cesarean section may offer these infants the best chance for survival and a good chance for normal development.

MATERNAL DIABETES Fetuses of diabetic mothers are inclined to be larger than normal, which can lead to difficult labor and delivery. Although these infants are large, they behave like premature infants and do not withstand well the rigors of a long labor. Death during labor and the postnatal period is common. In addition, there is an increased risk of stillbirth with maternal diabetes. Because of these dangers to the fetus and because a high proportion of pregnant women with diabetes develop toxemia, the pregnancy may require termination before term. When conditions are favorable and a rapid and easy labor is anticipated, induction of labor can be carried out. However, if there are urgent reasons for immediate delivery, if induction fails, or if good progress in labor is not made, cesarean section should be performed.

RHESUS INCOMPATIBILITY When a fetus is becoming progressively damaged by the antibodies of a sensitized Rh-negative mother and when

COMPLICATED LABOR

induction and delivery per vagina would be difficult, the pregnancy may be terminated by cesarean section in selected cases for fetal salvage.

POSTMORTEM CESAREAN SECTION Postmortem cesarean sections were performed in Rome as early as 715 BC, when Numa Pompilius decreed that if a pregnant woman died, the fetus was to be cut out of her abdomen. The intent of the decree was not to save the life of the infant but to obviate his or her being buried with the mother. In 237 BC, the first reported infant who survived postmortem cesarean section was Scipio Africanus. He grew up to become the Roman General who defeated Hannibal. Some 15 percent of infants born in these circumstances are in good condition. Their survival depends on how soon they are delivered, their maturity, the nature and duration of the maternal illness, the performance of cardiopulmonary resuscitation on the mother, and the availability of neonatal intensive care.

HERPES VIRUS INFECTION OF THE GENITAL TRACT This is a cause of serious, often fatal, infection of the newborn infant. When genital herpes infection is present at term, the risk of clinically apparent infection in the infant delivered per vagina has been estimated at being between 40 and 60 percent. In about half of these, the infection will be severe or fatal. Herpes infection in the newborn is almost always acquired from the mother's infected birth canal, either as an ascending infection after the membranes have ruptured or during passage through the vagina. In the latter situation, there is contamination of the child's eyes, scalp, skin, umbilical cord, and upper respiratory tract. The possibility of transplacental transmission is small, certainly far less important than direct contact during labor and delivery. The greatest hazard to the baby exists when the primary genital infection occurred 2 to 4 weeks before delivery. The risk of fetal infection at term is greater during primary genital herpes infection than during recurrent genital herpes. Often it is difficult to distinguish between these two. Fetuses at risk receive some maternal antibodies transplacentally, and this may play some part in limiting infection.

All women with known recurrent genital HSV infection should be offered acyclovir or valacyclovir suppression at 36 weeks' gestation to decrease the risk of clinical lesions and viral shedding at the time of delivery and therefore decrease the need for cesarean section.

Cesarean section is indicated for women with prodrome symptoms or clinically suspicious cases of genital herpes infection at the time of labor. Although the risk of fetal infection is higher when the membranes have been ruptured for 4 to 6 hours, cesarean section should be performed in all cases of proven or strongly suspicious cases of herpes infection regardless of the duration of labor or the length of time that the membranes have been ruptured.

Breast feeding by infected mothers is permissible, provided that direct contact between the infant and infected areas in the mother is avoided. Nursing is prohibited when herpetic lesions are present on the breast.

HIV INFECTION The available evidence regarding the prophylactic role of cesarean section in preventing vertical transmission of HIV to the neonate applies only to women who have not received optimal antiretroviral therapy.

Miscellaneous

LATE MATERNAL AGE Late maternal age in a primigravida patient is difficult to define. Although the age varies from 35 to 40 years, other factors are equally important. These include the presence or absence of a good lower uterine segment, elasticity or rigidity of the cervix and the soft tissues of the birth canal, ease of becoming pregnant, number of abortions, fetal presentation, and coordination of the uterine powers. When all of these points are favorable, vaginal delivery should be considered. When the adverse factors are present, cesarean section may be the wiser and safer procedure, therefore it can be offered as a delivery option.

PREVIOUS VAGINAL REPAIR Fear that vaginal delivery will cause a recurrence of cystocele, rectocele, and uterine prolapse may lead to an elective cesarean section. A history of pelvic surgery for fistulas because of inflammatory bowel disease may be an indication for cesarean section.

CONGENITAL UTERINE ANOMALY Not only does an abnormal uterus often function badly, but in the case of anomalies such as a bicornuate uterus, one horn may block the passage of the baby from the other. In such cases, cesarean section must be performed.

POOR OBSTETRIC HISTORY When a previous delivery has been difficult and traumatic with extensive injury to the cervix, vagina, and perineum or when the baby has been injured, cesarean section may be selected for subsequent births.

FAILED INSTRUMENTAL ASSISTED VAGINAL DELIVERY Failed forceps or failed vacuum delivery is an indication for cesarean section. It is wiser to turn to abdominal delivery than to drag a baby through the pelvis by force.

COMPLICATED LABOR

ELECTIVE CESAREAN SECTION OR CESAREAN DELIVERY ON MATERNAL REQUEST (CDMR) This is a controversial topic where some women prefer a cesarean delivery. The reasons for this include avoiding pelvic floor injury, fear of labor, convenience, and perceived reduced risk to the fetus. Challenges in characterizing cesarean delivery on maternal request epidemiology include a lack of internationally accepted case definitions and inconsistencies in documentation that hinder meaningful comparisons across jurisdictions. In Canada, CDMR has been estimated at 2 percent of cesarean deliveries, but robust contemporary data are lacking. Professional organizations in the United States, Canada, and Europe have adopted a precautionary approach and do not recommend CDMR over vaginal delivery, but to allow patient autonomy with patient counselling. Patient counseling is recommended to inform patients of pain management options, and potential benefits and harms related to cesarean deliveries. The conclusions drawn to date are that more research is required in this area and that cesarean section should be performed after 39 weeks of gestation and should be avoided in women desiring several children because of the risk of placental invasion in future pregnancies.

TYPES OF CESAREAN SECTION

Position of the Patient on the Operating Table

The practice of placing a wedge under the patient's right hip to tilt her to her left side at the time of cesarean section is well established. This permits the uterus and its contents to fall away from the inferior vena cava and the aorta. The return circulation from the patient's lower extremities to the right heart is improved, supine hypotension is prevented, and good placental perfusion is maintained. When difficult delivery of an impacted head (e.g., after failed forceps or vacuum or after prolonged second stage) or excessive bleeding is anticipated (e.g., placenta previa or accreta), the legs may be placed in Yellofin stirrups to allow for abduction and enhanced surgical site access to the lower pelvis and vagina.

Skin Incisions

Vertical Incision
The skin incision used for cesarean section in an acute emergency is the midline, vertical, hypogastric incision, extending from the symphysis pubis

to the umbilicus and above the umbilicus when necessary. The advantages of this approach are that it provides excellent exposure, and entry into the abdominal cavity can be made rapidly. In cases of acute fetal distress, when time is of paramount importance, the vertical incision is the one of choice.

Transverse Incision

The Pfannenstiel transverse suprasymphyseal incision is the most commonly used. The incision in the skin is semilunar just above the pubic hairline, the angles inclined slightly upward toward the anteriorsuperior iliac crests. This incision has several advantages. The cosmetic result is far better than the vertical incision, and the scar is narrow and often is partly hidden by the hair on the mons pubis. The abdominal wall, postoperatively, is stronger because of the perpendicular relationship between the incisions in the fascia, the muscles, and the peritoneum and because there is less side-to-side tension on the scar. Postoperative pain is reduced, and the patient can be active much sooner. The risk of dehiscence is low. The disadvantages of the Pfannenstiel incision are that the exposure may not be as good as with a vertical incision and the fact that the procedure is time consuming and should not be used when an acute emergency exists.

Uterine Incisions

Lower Segment of Uterus: Transverse Incision

Because it permits safe abdominal delivery even when performed late in labor and even when the uterine cavity is infected, the lower segment transverse incision (Fig. 22-1A) has revolutionized obstetric practice in the following respects:

1. It has resulted in the concepts of trial of labor, trial of oxytocin stimulation, and trial forceps
2. The need for traumatic forceps delivery has been virtually eliminated
3. The indications for cesarean section have been widened
4. Maternal morbidity and mortality rates are lower than with upper segment procedures
5. The uterus is left with a stronger scar

The lower uterine segment transverse incision is the procedure of choice. The abdomen is opened and the uterus exposed. The vesicouterine fold of peritoneum (bladder flap), which lies near the junction of the upper and lower uterine segments, is identified and incised transversely;

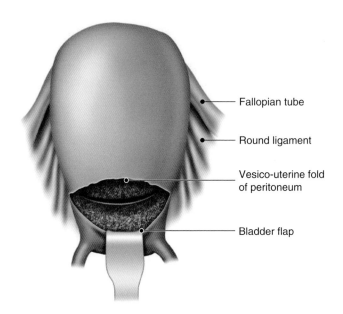

Fallopian tube

Round ligament

Vesico-uterine fold
of peritoneum

Bladder flap

A. Lower segment transverse incision.

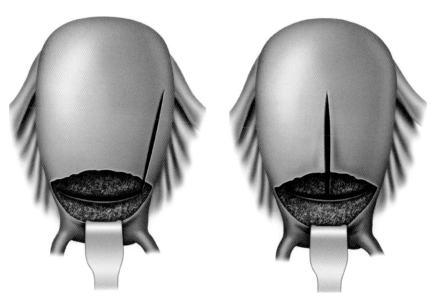

B. J incision.

C. T incision.

FIGURE 22-1. Cesarean section incisions.

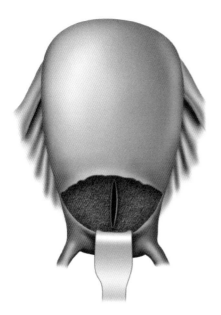 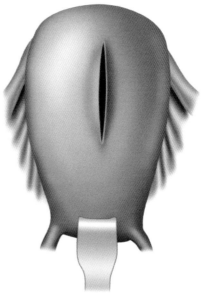

D. Lower segment vertical incision.   E. Classical (upper segment vertical) incision.

FIGURE 22-1. (*Continued*)

it is dissected off the lower segment and, with the bladder, is pushed downward and retracted out of the way. A small transverse incision is made in the lower segment of the uterus and is extended laterally with the fingers or with bandage scissors, stopping short of the area of the uterine vessels. It is important to make a higher incision on the uterus in women with advanced or complete cervical dilatation in order to minimize lateral extension and to avoid bladder injury because it can be higher and, in some cases, almost to the level of the umbilicus. To avoid injury to the fetus by the sharp blade of the scalpel, this incision can be made easily by the scalpel handle. The fetal head, which in most cases lies under the incision, is extracted or expressed, followed by the body and then the placenta and membranes. The head is delivered by gently elevating it and directing it through the incision; this is assisted with transabdominal fundal pressure. In some cases, a vacuum or forceps device may be used to assist in delivery of the head.

Fundal pressure should be initiated after delivery to reduce bleeding and to aid in delivery of the placenta. The uterine incision should be clamped with ring forceps or Green-Armytage clamps to reduce vigorous bleeding until the incision is closed. The transverse incision is closed with a single or double layer of continuous #0 or #1 absorbable suture. Traditionally, the bladder flap of peritoneum is sewn back to the wall of the uterus above the incision so that this area is covered completely and isolated from the general peritoneal cavity. Many trials have suggested that omission of this step causes no further complications postoperatively and is not associated with increased adhesion formation. The abdomen is closed in layers after proper inspection to control bleeding. The closure of parietal peritoneum is not necessary because it has not shown to be of added benefit. The subcutaneous tissue is closed if it is more than 2 cm in thickness to prevent wound disruption; studies have found this to be superior to placing a subcutaneous drain (see Chapter 24).

Advantages

1. The incision is in the lower segment of the uterus. However, one must be certain it is in the thin lower segment and not in the inferior part of the muscular upper segment
2. The muscle is split laterally instead of being cut; this leads to less bleeding
3. Incision into the placenta is rare
4. The head is usually under the incision and is extracted easily
5. The thin muscle layer of the lower segment is easier to reapproximate than the thick upper segment
6. Rupture of the transverse scar in a subsequent pregnancy poses only a small threat to the mother and fetus
   a. The incidence of rupture is lower
   b. This accident occurs rarely before term. Hence, the patient is in the hospital under close observation at the onset of active labor
   c. The loss of blood from the less vascular lower segment is less than from the corpus
   d. Rupture of the low transverse incision is followed only rarely by expulsion of the fetus or by a separation of the placenta, so that there is a chance to save the baby

Disadvantages

1. If the incision extends too far laterally, as may occur if the baby is very big, the uterine vessels can be torn, causing profuse hemorrhage
2. The procedure is not advisable when there is an abnormality in the lower segment, such as fibroids or extensive varicosities

3. Previous surgery or dense adhesions that prevent easy access to the lower segment make the operation tedious
4. When the lower segment is not well formed, the transverse operation is difficult to perform
5. Sometimes, the bladder is adherent to a previous scar, and it may be injured
6. On rare occasions, because of a narrow lower uterine segment or a large baby, the infant cannot be delivered through the transverse incision. To make more room, a J-shaped (Fig. 22-1B) or a T-shaped (Fig. 22-1C) extension is necessary. These should be avoided if possible because they have a weakening effect on the uterus. Future deliveries should be by repeat cesarean section

Lower Segment of Uterus: Vertical Incision

The exposure is the same as with the transverse incision. The vertical incision (Fig. 22-1D) is made with the scalpel and is enlarged with blunt scissors to avoid injury to the baby.

The vertical incision has an advantage in that it can be carried upward when necessary. This may be needed when the baby is large, when the lower segment is poorly formed such as in extreme prematurity, when there is a fetal malposition such as transverse lie, or when there is fetal anomaly such as conjoined twins. Some obstetricians prefer this incision for placenta previa.

One of the main disadvantages is that because the muscle is cut, there is increased bleeding from the incised edges of the thicker muscle in this part of the uterus. The uterus is usually closed in two to three layers to obtain excellent hemostasis; often, too, the incision extends inadvertently into the upper segment, and the value of a completely retroperitoneal closure is lost. Future deliveries should be by repeat cesarean section as the vertical incision weakens the uterine muscle and the risk of uterine rupture is increased compared to that of a transverse incision.

Classical Cesarean Section: Upper Segment of Uterus

A longitudinal midline incision (Fig. 22-1E) is made with the scalpel into the anterior wall of the uterus and is enlarged upward and downward with blunt-nosed scissors. A classical upper segment vertical uterine incision is performed for the same indications as a lower segment vertical incision, but a larger opening is required. Technical difficulty in exposing the lower segment or wanting to avoid the lower segment due to placenta accreta or previa are other indications for the upper segment procedure. The fetus and placenta are removed, and the uterus is closed in three layers.

In modern times, a classical incision is rarely indicated. Future deliveries should be by repeat cesarean section because the vertical incision weakens the uterine muscle and the risk of uterine rupture is increased compared to that of a transverse incision.

Indications

1. Difficulty in exposing the lower uterine segment
   a. Large blood vessels on the anterior wall
   b. High and adherent bladder
   c. Myoma in the lower segment
2. Impacted transverse lie (back down transverse)
3. Some cases of anterior placenta previa or accreta
4. Certain uterine malformations
5. Massive maternal obesity
6. Preterm infant with underdeveloped lower uterine segment

Disadvantages

1. Thick myometrium is cut, large sinuses are opened, and bleeding is profuse
2. The baby is often extracted as a breech with greater aspiration of amniotic fluid
3. If the placenta is attached to the anterior wall of the uterus, the incision cuts into it and may lead to dangerous loss of blood from the fetal circulation
4. The incision lies uncovered in the general peritoneal cavity, and there is greater chance of seepage of infected uterine contents with resultant peritonitis
5. There is a higher incidence of adhesion formation of abdominal contents to the line of closure in the uterus
6. There is a higher incidence of uterine rupture in subsequent pregnancies

MORTALITY AND MORBIDITY AFTER CESAREAN SECTION

Maternal Mortality

The maternal mortality rate from cesarean section in the Western world continues to drop steadily. In 2008, the mortality rate for cesarean sections in the United States was 2.2 per 100,000 cesarean deliveries. It is misleading to directly compare the mortality rates of vaginal and cesarean deliveries.

Women with adverse medical conditions, or higher risk pregnancies, often require a cesarean section, which can alter the mortality rates.

Factors That Add to the Risk

1. Maternal age older than 35 years
2. Grand multiparity
3. Obesity, body mass index (BMI) >30
4. Prolonged labor
5. Prolonged period of ruptured membranes
6. Numerous vaginal examinations
7. Low socioeconomic status

Causes of Maternal Death

1. Hemorrhage
2. Infection
3. Anesthesia
4. Pulmonary embolism
5. Renal failure after prolonged hypotension
6. Intestinal obstruction and paralytic ileus
7. Heart failure
8. Preeclampsia
9. Rupture of uterine scar
10. Miscellaneous causes not related to the operation (e.g., cancer)

Reasons for a Decline in Mortality Rate

1. Adequate blood transfusion
2. Use of antimicrobial drugs
3. Improved surgical methods
4. Better anesthetic techniques and specially trained anesthesiologists
5. The realization that patients with heart disease do better with vaginal delivery than with cesarean section
6. Basic treatment of preeclampsia by medical rather than by surgical methods
7. Alternative medical treatment of massive hemorrhage

Maternal Morbidity

Cesarean section can be associated with significant maternal morbidity. Patients undergoing cesarean section develop operative and/or postoperative complications, some of which are serious and potentially lethal. It must be accepted that cesarean section is a major operation with the attendant risks.

COMPLICATED LABOR

Serious Complications

1. *Hemorrhage from*
   a. Uterine atony
   b. Extension of uterine incision
   c. Difficulty removing the placenta
   d. Hematoma of the broad ligament
2. *Infection*
   a. Genital tract (endometritis)
   b. Incision
   c. Urinary tract
   d. Lungs and upper respiratory tract
   e. Pelvic abscess
3. *Venous thromboembolic events and thrombophlebitis*
4. *Damage to the urinary tract,* with or without the formation of a fistula, occurs in less than 1 percent of cesarean sections. Most important is the recognition of the injury at the time it happens. Those that are discovered during the operation can be repaired immediately, and the return of normal function is likely. Late diagnosis necessitates a second operation and considerable discomfort in the interim. Postoperative pain in the flank after a difficult cesarean section with much bleeding calls for an intravenous pyelogram
   a. Bladder injury is caused mainly during the development of the bladder flap over the lower uterine segment and the displacement of the bladder caudally. In repeat cesarean section, adhesions and scar tissue from the previous operation may make the dissection difficult. Defects in the bladder caused by accidental entry are repaired with a double layer of 3-0 absorbable or delayed-absorbable suture. Drainage of the bladder is continued for 7 to 10 days. In most of these cases, when the injury is recognized and repaired, healing takes place.

      A rare complication of cesarean section is a vesicouterine fistula. This condition occurs during the performance of a low cesarean section when unrecognized injury to the bladder takes place or the bladder is included in the closure of the uterine incision. The fistula is between the bladder and the uterus at the site of the incision for the cesarean section. These patients have incontinence, the urine passing from the bladder into the uterus and thence through the cervix into the vagina. Urinary infection may develop. Investigation: (1) Methylene blue dye instilled in the bladder enters the vagina. (2) Cystoscopy reveals the site of the fistula and determines the relationship of the fistula to the ureteral orifices. (3) An intravenous or a retrograde pyelogram will evaluate the upper urinary tract.

Because a number of these conditions will undergo spontaneous closure, a trial of conservative management is reasonable. This consists of continuous drainage of the bladder by urethral catheter and antibiotics to prevent infection. If this management fails, surgical closure of the fistula is performed. An abdominal approach is preferred. Early repair has been carried out successfully. It is probably advisable to wait, however, until uterine involution has taken place

b. Ureteral injury is caused by extension of the transverse incision in the lower uterine segment or the vagina and during attempts to control profuse bleeding in the broad ligament. The ureter may be cut, crushed, tied, or devitalized. If there is suspicion that a ureter has been injured, the bladder may be opened and the ureteral orifices inspected. One way of diagnosis is to inject 10 mL of indigo carmine intravenously and observe the efflux of blue urine from the ureters, indicating that they are intact. Or the dye may be seen in the surrounding tissue, suggesting that the ureter has been cut. If recognized, repair should be carried out immediately

5. *Intestinal complications*

a. Lacerations should be repaired immediately by a double-layer of 3-0 absorbable or delayed-absorbable suture. A general surgeon should be consulted for the injury subject to availability

b. Obstruction may be paralytic or mechanical. Volvulus accounts for some 25 percent of intestinal obstruction associated with pregnancy. The sigmoid is the most common site. Volvulus of the transverse colon, the small bowel, or the cecum occurs less frequently. The diagnosis of intestinal obstruction in post–cesarean section patients is difficult and is often delayed. The treatment is surgical

6. *Inadvertent vaginal incision* during cesarean section. The patient at risk is a parturient whose cervix is fully dilated and who has been pushing in the second stage of labor for some time. The operator, thinking he or she is making the incision in the thinned-out lower uterine segment, makes the incision into the vagina. Possible complications include injury to the bladder or ureter, vesical fistula, laceration of adjacent ligamentous structures, and hemorrhage. Management requires meticulous hemostasis, careful search for tears in the bladder, and anatomic

COMPLICATED LABOR

closure of the vagina. The problem can be avoided by making the incision in the lower uterine segment above the reflection of the vesicouterine peritoneum.

Prevention of Infection

Along with the rise in the rates of cesarean section there has been an increase in the incidence of maternal febrile morbidity, infections of the endometrium and wound, and prolonged hospitalization. Maternal febrile morbidity is defined as a temperature of 100.4°F (38°C) or above occurring on any 2 of the first 10 days postpartum, exclusive of the first 24 hours. It is more common after cesarean section than after normal delivery, the incidence being anywhere between 5 and 20 percent. Antimicrobials, blood transfusions, better surgical technique, use of the lower segment operation, and improved anesthesia have all contributed to the significant decrease in post–cesarean section maternal morbidity. Preoperative administration of a broad-spectrum antibiotic 30 minutes before the skin incision has been consistently shown to significantly reduce the risk of maternal postoperative infection. This is true for both high-risk laboring patients and for patients undergoing elective cesarean delivery. There is no evidence to support the delay of antibiotics until delivery of the infant.

Antibiotic of Choice. When used prophylactically, a single antibiotic with broad-spectrum coverage against most pelvic pathogens appears to be as effective as a combination of two or more drugs and would be associated with fewer side effects. The most commonly used antibiotic is a single dose of 1 to 2 g (based on BMI) of a beta-lactam drug, either cephalosporin or extended-spectrum penicillin. Some recent studies are also suggesting to add azithromycin for patients at higher risk of infections such as cases of elevated BMI.

Fetal Mortality

Fetal mortality associated with cesarean section is higher than that of vaginal delivery. Some of the reasons follow are related to the indication of cesarean delivery.

1. Conditions such as toxemia of pregnancy, erythroblastosis, and placenta previa that require treatment by cesarean section result in premature, small infants
2. Iatrogenic prematurity. On occasion, the performance of an elective cesarean section on a date determined entirely by the menstrual

history has led to the birth of a premature infant. In some cases, respiratory distress syndrome developed, and occasionally the baby died. It is important, therefore, that an accurate assessment of fetal gestational age be made before the pregnancy is terminated. Elective cesarean delivery in uncomplicated pregnancies should be scheduled at or after 39 weeks of gestational age to reduce the complications of iatrogenic prematurity. Certain situations may be exempted from this rule based on examination of risks and benefits

Methods of achieving assessment of gestational age include:

a. Clinical parameters, including the date of the onset of the last menstrual period, uterine size at the first prenatal visit, date of quickening, date when the fetal heart tones were first heard using an ordinary fetal stethoscope, and date of an early positive pregnancy test result, taken in combination, correlate well with the gestational age of the fetus

b. Ultrasonography. Measurement of the crown–rump length between the 8th and 14th weeks of gestation permits dating to within ±5 days, and by measurement of the biparietal diameter between 15 and 25 weeks, dating is possible to ±10 days. Serial ultrasonic scans will narrow the spread

c. Amniocentesis with measurement of the lecithin–sphingomyelin (L/S) ratio in the amniotic fluid is an accurate way of determining fetal pulmonary maturity. It is, however, an invasive technique and carries a small risk. For this reason, many physicians restrict its use to situations in which other methods of determining the maturity of the fetus leave serious doubt

3. Although respiratory complications such as atelectasis and hyaline membrane disease and the respiratory distress syndrome are more common in premature infants, the incidence is higher when the premature baby is born by cesarean section

4. Conditions such as placenta previa, abruptio placentae, diabetes, preeclampsia, eclampsia, essential hypertension, chronic nephritis, and prolapse of the umbilical cord result in babies whose general condition and powers of resistance and recuperation are low. When these conditions need treatment by cesarean section, fetal mortality is increased

There has been a decline in the mortality rate of infants born both by cesarean section and by vaginal delivery. The great majority of fetal deaths are associated with prematurity. On the one hand, cesarean section has reduced the number of babies damaged by traumatic vaginal procedures. On the other hand, a number of babies are born alive who have congenital defects incompatible with continuing a reasonable existence.

COMPLICATED LABOR

Cesarean Hysterectomy

This is the performance of a cesarean section followed by removal of the uterus. Whenever possible, total hysterectomy should be performed. However, because the subtotal operation is easier and can be done more quickly, it is the procedure of choice when there has been profuse hemorrhage and the patient is in shock or when she is in poor condition for other reasons. In such cases, the aim is to finish the operation as rapidly as possible. The incidence of peripartum hysterectomy is about 0.4 to 0.8 percent of all deliveries.

Indications

1. Hemorrhage from uterine atony after failure of conservative therapy
2. Uncontrollable hemorrhage in certain cases of placenta previa and abruptio placentae
3. Placenta accreta
4. Gross multiple fibromyomas
5. Certain cases of cancer of the cervix or ovary
6. Rupture of the uterus that is not repairable
7. Severe chorioamnionitis. There is danger of the peritoneal cavity becoming infected both when the uterus is incised and from the seepage through the incision after it has been repaired. In such cases, and especially if future childbearing is not an issue, it may be safer to remove the infected uterus *if adequate antimicrobial therapy cannot be given*
8. Defective uterine scar
9. Extension of incision into the uterine vessels resulting in bleeding that cannot be stopped by ligature

Complications

1. Morbidity rate of 20 percent
2. Increased loss of blood and higher rate of blood transfusion
3. The incidence of damage to the urinary tract and the intestines is higher than with cesarean section or hysterectomy alone
4. Psychological trauma because of the loss of the uterus
5. Maternal mortality. If the conditions that create the need for cesarean hysterectomy are eliminated, the mortality rate is not higher than that from cesarean section or hysterectomy alone
6. Postoperative hemorrhage. There is a significant danger of this complication occurring. About 1 percent of patients require reoperation in the immediate postoperative period for the control of intraperitoneal bleeding

SELECTED READING

Alinovi V, Herzberg FP, Yannopoulos D, et al: Cecal volvulus following cesarean section. Obstet Gynecol 55:131, 1980

American College of Obstetricians and Gynecologists: Use of prophylactic antibiotics in labor and delivery. Washington, DC: American College of Obstetricians and Gynecologists. ACOG Practice Bulletin no. 120, 2011

Bryan B, Strickler RC: Inadvertent primary vaginal incision during cesarean section. Can J Surg 23:581, 1980

Buckspan MB, Simha S, Klotz PG: Vesicouterine fistula: A rare complication of cesarean section. Obstet Gynecol 62:645, 1983

Chervenak FA, Shamsi HH: Is amniocentesis necessary before elective repeat cesarean section? Obstet Gynecol 60:305, 1982

Cunningham FG, Gant NF, Leveno KJ, et al: Cesarean delivery and peripartum hysterectomy. In: *Williams Obstetrics*, 23rd ed. New York: McGraw-Hill, 2009

DePace NL, Betesh JS, Kotler MN: "Postmortem" cesarean section with recovery of both mother and offspring. JAMA 248:971, 1982

Eisenkop SM, Richman R, Platt LD, et al: Urinary tract injury during cesarean section. Obstet Gynecol 60:591, 1982

Guo Y, Murphy MSQ, Erwin E, Fakhraei R, Corsi DJ, White RR, Harvey ALJ, et al: Birth outcomes following cesarean delivery on maternal request: A population-based cohort study. CMAJ 193:E634-E644, 2021

Lavin JP, Stephens RJ, Miodovnik M: Vaginal delivery in patients with a prior cesarean section. Obstet Gynecol 59:135, 1982

Ledger WJ: Management of postpartum cesarean section morbidity. Clin Obstet Gynecol 23:621, 1980

O'Driscoll K, Foley M: Correlation of decrease in perinatal mortality and increase in cesarean section rates. Obstet Gynecol 61:1, 1983

Park RC, Duff WP: Role of cesarean hysterectomy in modern obstetric practice. Clin Obstet Gynecol 23:601, 1980

Perkins RP: Role of extraperitoneal cesarean section. Clin Obstet Gynecol 23:583, 1980

Rayburn, WF: Prophylactic antibiotics during cesarean section: An overview of prior clinical investigations. Clin Perinatol 10:461, 1983

Society of Obstetricians and Gynaecologists of Canada: Antibiotic Prophylaxis in Obstetric Procedures. Clinical Practice Guideline No. 247. Ottawa, ON: Society of Obstetricians and Gynaecologists of Canada, September 2010.

Sullivan SA, Smith T, Chang E, Hulsey T, Vandorsten JP, Soper D: Administration of cefazolin prior to skin incision is superior to cefazolin at cord clamping in preventing post-cesarean infectious morbidity: A randomized, controlled trial. Am J Obstet Gynecol 196:455.e 1–5, 2007

Wallace RL, Eglinton GS, Yonekura ML, Wallace TM: Extraperitoneal cesarean section: A surgical form of infection prevention? Am J Obstet Gynecol 148:172, 1984

COMPLICATED LABOR

CHAPTER 23

Trial of Labor After Previous Cesarean Section

Nika Alavi-Tabari
Amanda Black

Trial of labor after cesarean delivery (TOLAC) refers to a planned attempt for a vaginal delivery by someone who has had a previous cesarean delivery, with the goal of having a successful vaginal birth after cesarean delivery (VBAC).

VBAC was first reported in 1923. Between 1970 and 2016, cesarean section rates in the United States increased from 5 to 31.9 percent due to several practice changes including the use of electronic fetal monitoring (EFM) and decreased operative and breech vaginal deliveries. TOLAC was reconsidered in the 1970s and supported as a reasonable approach in select pregnancies, which increased VBAC rates from approximately 5 percent in 1985 to 28.3 percent by 1996.

TOLAC should be considered for all women with one previous cesarean section presenting for prenatal care, provided there are no contraindications to TOLAC. In particular, women who are planning more than two children may be more motivated to consider TOLAC after their first cesarean due to the increased maternal risks associated with having three or more cesarean sections. Care providers and their patients should discuss the risks and benefits of both TOLAC and elective repeat cesarean section (ERCS) in a shared decision-making process while planning the birth. This discussion should be well documented in the prenatal record. TOLAC may be contraindicated in some situations and in those cases, a repeat cesarean section would be advised.

SUCCESS RATE

The success rate of TOLAC ranges from 50 to 85 percent. Factors that increase the likelihood of a VBAC include:

1. Previous vaginal birth and/or previous VBAC
2. Nonrecurring indication for the previous cesarean section such as malpresentation
3. Spontaneous labor
4. Favourable cervix on admission to the birthing unit (cervical dilation ≥4 cm)
5. No history of dystocia
6. Epidural use
7. Birthweight less than 4000 g

Although some factors decrease the likelihood of a VBAC, TOLAC may still be considered. However, these patients should be informed that they have a lower chance of VBAC and an increased risk of requiring a cesarean section and other complications. Factors that decrease the likelihood of a VBAC:

1. Increasing maternal age
2. High maternal BMI (>30 kg/m^2)
3. Previous dystocia
4. Induction of labor
5. Delivery more than 40 weeks' gestation
6. Birthweight more than 4000 g

Decision aids and prediction models for TOLAC success have been developed and can be used in antenatal counselling and shared decision-making. Prediction models have high predictive values for predicting VBAC but are poorer at predicting unsuccessful TOLAC.

PREREQUISITES FOR TOLAC

1. Patient understands and accepts the risks
2. Undertaken in an institution capable of performing an emergency cesarean section

Although it is ideal to have in-house obstetrics, anaesthesia, and surgical staff to optimize timely access to surgical management, this may not be a possibility in all birthing units. However, immediate mobilization of a surgical team is necessary when risk factors or signs of uterine rupture are identified. The woman and her care provider must be aware of the availability of obstetrics, anesthesia, pediatrics, and operating room staff at the center where she chooses to deliver and the center must have a plan for managing obstetrical emergencies, including a uterine rupture.

CONTRAINDICATIONS TO TOLAC

1. Previous fundal, classical, inverted T, or low vertical uterine incision
2. Previous major uterine reconstruction (e.g., full-thickness repair for myomectomy, repair of Mullerian anomaly, cornual resection)
3. Previous uterine rupture
4. Unknown previous uterine incision
5. Advice against TOLAC after prior cesarean section
6. Any other obstetrical contraindications for vaginal delivery

7. Unavailable timely access to the operating room for emergency cesarean section
8. Patient requests ERCS and declines TOLAC

RISKS OF TOLAC

The benefits and risks of TOLAC versus ERCS must be presented to the patient. The balance of risks and the chances of VBAC must be acceptable to the patient. The overall risk of a TOLAC resulting in a VBAC are lower than the risks of surgery associated with an ERCS; however, TOLAC has the chance of resulting in an emergency cesarean section, and a chance of uterine rupture with their associated increase in maternal morbidity and mortality. Although the risk of maternal mortality, uterine rupture, and serious maternal morbidity is higher in TOLAC, the absolute risks of these outcomes are low. Similarly, the relative risk of perinatal morbidity and mortality and serious morbidity is higher for TOLAC compared to ERCS but the absolute risk is low.

Uterine Rupture

Uterine rupture is defined as a full thickness disruption of the myometrium and overlying serosa. Uterine "dehiscence" is an incomplete disruption (or uterine window) that does not include the serosa. The risk of uterine rupture with TOLAC and a history of one prior low transverse cesarean section is approximately 0.47 percent. Management of uterine rupture includes stabilizing hemodynamically unstable patients with fluids and blood transfusions as required and urgent cesarean delivery. The choice of a midline or Pfannenstiel incision will depend on the clinical scenario and provider preference. Repair of the uterine defect at the time of laparotomy after delivery may be possible but depends on the extent of the rupture, maternal hemodynamic stabilty, and the surgeon. Uterine rupture is associated with an increased risk of hysterectomy (14-33%), particularly if the rupture is lateral or very large. The overall risk of perinatal mortality related to uterine rupture is 6.2 percent, although reports range from 5 to 26 percent.

Factors That Increase the Risk of Uterine Rupture

- Previous uterine rupture
- Previous fundal, classical, inverted T, or low vertical uterine incision; previous myomectomy
- Induction of labor (IOL) with pharmacologic cervical ripening agents, for example, prostaglandins

- Oxytocin for IOL or augmentation
- Two or more previous cesarean sections
- Short interpregnancy interval, especially less than 18 months
- Thin lower uterine segment (although there is no agreed upon threshold value to use to predict the risk of uterine rupture)
- Longer second stage

A prior vaginal delivery either before or after the prior cesarean delivery significantly reduces the risk of uterine rupture with TOLAC but does not eliminate it.

TOLAC MANAGEMENT GUIDELINES

I. Preadmission

1. The risks and benefits of TOLAC versus ERCS should be discussed prior to the onset of labor. The discussion is part of a shared decision-making process and should be documented in the patient chart
2. Patient should present to hospital immediately for:
   a. Suspected labor
   b. Suspected rupture of the membranes
   c. Vaginal bleeding
   d. Any other obstetrical concerns

II. Evaluation

1. Evaluation of maternal status:
   a. Physical examination
   b. Cervical assessment
   c. Initiation of intravenous line and infusion
   d. Bloodwork for complete blood count, type, and screen
2. Evaluation of fetal status:
   a. EFM
   b. Fetal presentation: vaginal examination and/or ultrasound

III. Intrapartum

1. Monitoring of fetal well-being: Continuous EFM is recommended because it is the best marker of uterine rupture. FHR tracing

abnormalities, especially complicated variable or late decelerations, are the most commonly observed signs of uterine rupture and may present up to 1 hour prior to rupture

2. Monitoring of maternal well-being. Maternal mobility does not need to be restricted (telemetry can be used)
3. Intravenous access: Recommended in case of cesarean section or blood product administrations
4. Monitoring of labor progress: usual uterine contraction pattern does not change in TOLAC, and usual standards should be used to assess labor progress. Lack of progress in 2 to 3 hours in the presence of adequate contractions requires reassessment of the method of delivery
5. Epidural or other pain management as normally indicated. These are not expected to mask signs or symptoms of uterine rupture, because the most common sign of rupture is fetal heart tracing abnormalities

IV. Postpartum. Exploration of the uterine cavity is not routinely indicated unless there are concerning signs or symptoms

INDUCTION OF LABOR

Delivery prior to the onset of spontaneous labor may be required for medical reasons in women with a previous cesarean section. IOL is not contraindicated for women wanting a TOLAC, but IOL has implications for the chance of a VBAC and the risk of uterine rupture.

1. Uterine rupture rates increase with IOL (0.7-2.7%). The highest risk is more than 40 weeks' gestation (3.2%). Uterine rupture risks differ with the type of induction method used
2. With IOL, vaginal birth rates with TOLAC are lower and cesarean section rates are higher
3. Mechanical induction with a balloon (Foley) catheter is not contraindicated. It is associated with VBAC rates of 54 to 58 percent
4. Oxytocin is not contraindicated for either induction or augmentation. It is associated with an increased risk of uterine rupture (1.1%, approximately double that of baseline risk)
5. Women induced with either artificial rupture of membranes (ARM) or oxytocin with a favourable cervix have VBAC rates similar to spontaneous labor (74%)
6. Prostaglandin E_2 (dinoprostone) is not recommended. It is associated with increased risk of uterine rupture (2%)

7. Prostaglandin E$_1$ (misoprostol) is contraindicated and is associated with a high risk of uterine rupture (6-19%)

UTERINE RUPTURE

Early recognition of uterine rupture and a facility that can provide rapid intervention are essential components of TOLAC. Failure of either of these may result in poor outcomes.

SIGNS AND SYMPTOMS OF UTERINE RUPTURE

1. Abnormal fetal heart rate (most common sign)
2. Abdominal pain
3. Vaginal bleeding
4. Acute onset of scar pain or tenderness
5. Hematuria
6. Maternal tachycardia, hypotension, or hypovolemic shock
7. Palpation of fetal parts abdominally
8. Elevation of the presenting part unexpectedly (i.e., loss of station)
9. Chest pain, shoulder tip pain, and/or sudden shortness of breath
10. A change in uterine activity (decrease or increase) may occur but no consistent change has been identified

There is no single sign that reliably indicates a uterine rupture has occurred. FHR abnormalities (uncomplicated or complicated variable decelerations, late decelerations), persistent abdominal pain, and tachsystole may be an indicator of the initiation of uterine scar separation and frequently precede uterine rupture during TOLAC. When confronted with significant FHR abnormalities and a birth that is not imminent, a cesarean section should be considered to avoid a terminal bradycardia. The classic triad—abdominal pain, vaginal bleeding, and abnormal fetal heart rate—is seen only in 9 percent of the cases.

When a uterine rupture is suspected, an emergency cesarean section should be performed immediately in order to decrease maternal and neonatal morbidity and mortality. Maternal and fetal outcomes worsen as the interval between decision to delivery increases and every minute counts. Centers that offer TOLAC should have a plan for managing obstetrical emergencies, including urgent cesarean sections.

COMPLICATED LABOR

OTHER CONSIDERATIONS

1. TOLAC success rates in patients with more than one previous cesarean are similar to women with only one previous cesarean section; however, they have a higher risk of uterine rupture (1.1-1.6%), blood transfusion, and hysterectomy

2. External cephalic version (ECV) is not contraindicated with previous cesarean section

3. Multiple gestation, diabetes, or fetal macrosomia are not contraindications for TOLAC

4. Interdelivery intervals do not appear to affect VBAC rates. However, the risk of uterine rupture increases with shorter interdelivery intervals. An interval of less than 18 months between deliveries is associated with an increased risk of uterine rupture for TOLAC. The best estimate of the uterine rupture rate for an interval of less than 12 months is 4.8 percent, while estimates of rates of rupture between 18 and 24 months and more than 24 months are 1.9 and 1.3 percent, respectively

5. Breech presentation is not an absolute contraindication for TOLAC; however, there is insufficient data to inform the discussion about possible additional risks

6. A single-layer locked uterine closure may increase the risk of uterine rupture with TOLAC compared to a double-layer closure of the uterus (3.1% vs. 0.5%)

7. Lower uterine thickness and uterine rupture are related; however, there is no clear cutoff for consideration of safe TOLAC. Routine ultrasound measurement of the lower uterine segment is not indicated for planning TOLAC

8. Previous operative reports should be obtained when possible to determine the type of prior uterine incision. If the information cannot be obtained but there is a high likelihood of a previous lower segment transverse uterine incision based on history and clinical circumstances of the previous surgery, a TOLAC may be offered

9. A maternal BMI >30 is associated with lower rates of VBAC, an increased risk of uterine rupture, increased maternal morbidity (compared to an ERCS), and possibly a longer decision-to delivery time. This should be addressed when considering TOLAC

10. There is a lack of data regarding previous uterine extensions, postpartum fever after prior cesarean section, Müllerian anomalies, and type of suture material used at surgery to make recommendations for risks/safety in TOLAC

11. The risk of placenta previa and placenta accreta, and their associated maternal morbidities, increases as the number of cesarean sections that a woman has had increases

SELECTED READING

American College of Obstetricians and Gynecologists: ACOG Practice Bulletin No. 205: Vaginal birth after cesarean delivery. Obstet Gynecol 33:e110-e127, 2019

Cahill A, Stamilio DM, Paré E, Peipert JP, Stevens EJ, Nelson DB, et al: Vaginal birth after cesarean (VBAC) attempt in twin pregnancies: is it safe? Am J Obstet Gynecol 193:1050, 2005

Chauhan SP, Martin JN Jr, Henrichs CE, Morrison JC, Magann EF: Maternal and perinatal complications with uterine rupture in 142,075 patients who attempted vaginal birth after cesarean delivery: A review of the literature. Am J Obstet Gynecol 189:408, 2003

Dy J, DeMeester S, Lipworth H, Barrett J. SOGC Clinical Practice Guideline No. 382: Trial of labor after caesarean. J Obstet Gynaecol Can 41:992-1011, 2019

Gupta JK, Smith GCS, Chodankar RR. Birth after previous caesarean birth (Green-top Guideline No.45). Royal College of Obstetricians & Gynaecologists. https://www.rcog.org.uk/en/guidelines-research-services/guidelines/gtg45/, 2015

Macones GA, Peipert J, Nelson DB, Odibo A, Stevens EJ, Stamilio DM, et al: Maternal complications with vaginal birth after cesarean delivery: a multicenter study. Am J Obstet Gynecol 193:1656, 2005

Maternal-Fetal Medicine Units Network: VBAC Calculator Tool. https://mfmunetwork.bsc.gwu.edu/web/mfmunetwork/vaginal-birth-after-cesarean-calculator

COMPLICATED LABOR

CHAPTER 24

Obesity in
Pregnancy

Darine El-Chaâr

Rates of obesity are continuing to rise dramatically in developed countries, including an increased prevalence of morbid obesity (body mass index [BMI] >35). This trend has led to a concurrent increase in health concerns for women of reproductive age, and it is now well established that weight gain and obesity cause major comorbidities in pregnancy that contribute to adverse maternal and neonatal outcomes.

DEFINITION OF OBESITY

The Institute of Medicine recommends use of BMI to classify maternal weight groups, using prepregnancy height and weight. According to the classification by the World Health Organization, obesity is defined as a BMI above 29 kg/m^2. Other definitions of obesity found in the literature include women who are 110 to 120 percent of their ideal body weight or weigh more than 91 kg (200 lb).

WEIGHT GAIN IN PREGNANCY

To reduce risk and complications of weight gain in pregnancy, women should set pregnancy weight goals according to Table 24-1.

If obesity is seen in prepregnancy counseling, recommendations are made about diet and lifestyle modifications. Bariatric surgery is also recommended in prepregnancy counseling because it has been shown to result in significant weight loss, which can improve pregnancy outcomes.

TABLE 24-1: PREGNANCY WEIGHT GAIN ACCORDING TO BMI

	BMI (kg/m^2)	Weight Gain (kg)	Weight Gain (lb)
Underweight	<18.5	12.5-18	28-40
Normal weight	18.5-24.9	11.5-16	25-35
Overweight	25.0-34.9	7-11.5	15-25
Obese	>30	5-9	11-20

BMI, body mass index.

Adapted from: Weight Gain During Pregnancy: Re-examining the Guidelines. Institute of Medicine (US) and National Research Council (US) Committee to Reexamine IOM Pregnancy Weight Guidelines, Rasmussen KM, Yaktine AL (Eds), National Academies Press (US), 2009.

Studies have shown that bariatric surgery also reduces hypertension, preeclampsia, and macrosomia.

ABNORMALITIES OF LABOR

Obese mothers have an increased incidence of medical complications, such as hypertension, diabetes mellitus, and obstructive sleep apnea. Obese mothers also have a higher rate of predisposing medical issues, which is what contributes to a higher rate of labor induction in this group or operative delivery.

There is still conflicting and limited studies on labor characteristics in obese gravid women. The best evidence suggests that obese women have longer labors. In a cohort study of nulliparous women, as maternal weight increased, the rate of cervical dilatation decreased, and the induction to delivery interval was longer. Increased duration of labor does not seem to be due to maternal poor expulsive efforts. A recent study showed that obese nulliparous women were found to have a higher rate of cesarean section in the first but not the second stage of labor. Therefore, pushing out the baby is not the issue, but getting to the second stage is.

Furthermore, numerous studies have associated obesity in pregnancy with higher rates of cesarean sections. The underlying mechanism leading to increased cesarean delivery rates in obese patients remains unclear. However, data suggest that decreased uterine contractility and higher induction rates in obese women may contribute to this phenomenon. There is also an increased rate of elective cesarean section because of adverse maternal outcomes, fetal macrosomia, or a scheduled repeat surgery given history of previous cesarean. Observational research has consistently reported that vaginal birth after cesarean section is decreased in obese pregnant women. Obstetricians may also be reluctant to perform operative vaginal delivery on obese patients given the increased risk of shoulder dystocia caused by macrosomia, which is often seen in infants of obese mothers.

FETAL GROWTH AND NEONATAL OUTCOME

The mean birthweight of infants born to obese mothers is greater. The incidence of macrosomia (>4000 g) in obese women is almost twice that of nonobese women. Fetal macrosomia is associated with an increased risk of shoulder dystocia, malpresentation, and hemorrhage and higher degree perineal and vaginal lacerations. The incidence of low birthweight babies (<2500 g) in obese women is reduced by half.

Maternal obesity has been associated with an increase in congenital anomalies, specifically neural tube defects, cardiac anomalies, anal atresia, and limb reduction anomalies. This may be related to the reduced sensitivity of ultrasound due to adiposity, therefore it is recommended to perform a screening anatomy ultrasound at a minimum of 20 weeks in obese patients. Perinatal outcomes are also affected, with an increased risk in stillbirth with a higher prepregnancy BMI.

It is recommended to perform serial growth assessment in the third trimester, with weekly fetal surveillance weekly after 37 weeks' gestation.

TIMING OF DELIVERY

Given some of the increased adverse perinatal outcomes, guidelines recommend that induction of labor should be considered at 39 to 40 weeks' gestation in women with a BMI over 40. Studies have not shown an increased rate of caesarian section rate in this population with induction of labor.

CESAREAN SECTION IN OBESE WOMEN

Meta-analysis studies have shown that obesity increases the risk of both elective and emergency cesarean delivery. Major surgery of any type in the obese patient is associated with an increase of intra- and postoperative complications. In pregnancy, there are special concerns, such as emergency delivery, prolonged operative time, increased blood loss, wound infection and endomyometritis, and thromboembolism. The procedure should be performed without delay if obstetric indications are present.

Care of the Skin

Preoperative care of the skin including cleansing and local therapy of intertrigo is important.

Prophylactic Antibiotics

The incidence of wound infection is high. Obesity increases the risk of serious maternal sepsis after cesarean section. Hence, prophylactic antibiotics should be prescribed for these patients in higher dose according to their current weight, and newer studies include broader coverage with additional antibiotics and at least 30 minutes prior to skin incision.

Thromboprophylaxis

The incidence of thrombosis and embolism is higher in obese patients. Reasons for this include prolonged operative time and the postoperative period of immobilization. Low-dose heparin may reduce the danger of thrombus formation and is indicated in massively obese women who undergo cesarean section. Subcutaneous injection of heparin, low-molecular-weight heparin, or dalteparin in appropriate doses are among the choices available based on institution preference; they should be administered until the patient is fully ambulatory. This prophylactic dose is not associated with increased maternal bleeding.

Anesthesia

Because of the increased incidence of medical problems including chronic hypertension, preeclampsia, coronary artery disease, diabetes mellitus, and pulmonary insufficiency, anesthesia in obese patients may be difficult. Consultation with the anesthetist should, when possible, be obtained well before the operation.

Respiratory Function

In obese women, total respiratory compliance is reduced because of a heavy chest wall and increased abdominal pressure on the diaphragm. The amount of work needed to breathe is increased. The residual volume and functional residual capacity are lower.

Choice of Anesthesia

Emergency Cesarean Section. In this situation, general anesthesia may be best given time involvement in regional anesthesia.

Nonemergency Cesarean Section. Because of the reduction in respiratory function, regional anesthesia does offer certain advantages and is the preferred choice, even though placing the catheter may be difficult in obese women. Techniques to improve successful regional anesthesia in obese women are being developed using ultrasound guidance.

COMPLICATED LABOR

Abdominal Wall Incisions

It is recommended to consider using a commercial retractor to improve exposure during surgery, such as a Mobius or Alexis-O retractor.

A: Pfannenstiel (Transverse) Incision

The transverse incision is demanded by patients because of the cosmetic result. It is performed after the panniculus has been retracted cephalad.

Advantages

1. Once the panniculus has been retracted, the amount of subcutaneous adipose tissue is less than in nonobese patients
2. The closure is more secure because the abdominal muscles tend to pull together the sides of the incision
3. Postoperative pain is less than with the vertical incision, and this facilitates early mobility and deep breathing
4. As a rule, transverse incisions heal well

Disadvantages

1. The area of the transverse incision is warm and moist, is difficult to clean, there is a high growth of bacteria, and intertrigo is common
2. Delivery of a large baby may be difficult
3. The vertical incision can be enlarged to make more room; the transverse incision cannot
4. Retraction of the panniculus may have an adverse effect on maternal cardiovascular functions. However, there is no clear evidence of this
5. The transverse incision takes longer

B: Vertical Incision

1. Low
2. High, periumbilical

These carry the same advantages and disadvantages except that in the upper abdomen, the layer of subcutaneous tissue that has to be cut is much less. The lower uterine segment can be reached with either incision.

Advantages. Speed: It takes less time to enter the abdominal cavity.

Disadvantages

1. There is an increased risk of dehiscence compared with the transverse incision
2. There is more pain
3. The patient is less mobile

C: High Transverse Skin Incision

Since the panniculus is voluminous, the projection of the lower uterine segments is thus above the umbilicus. Therefore, the incision may be either supraumbilical or subumbilical. The subcutaneous tissue is cut where the adipose tissue is thinnest, which reduces the risk of parietal complications.

This approach facilitates the access to the lower uterine segment and consequently facilitates the extraction of the fetus.

Closure of the Incision

Special attention is needed in obese patients.

Transverse Incision. The standard layered closure is adequate.

Midline Vertical Incision. Some surgeons advocate a layered closure with the addition of through-and-through retention sutures. Others prefer the use of internal retention sutures of the Smead-Jones variety (Fig. 24-1).

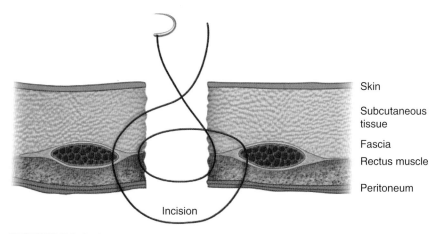

Skin

Subcutaneous tissue

Fascia

Rectus muscle

Peritoneum

Incision

FIGURE 24-1. Smead-Jones closure.

COMPLICATED LABOR

Subcutaneous Tissue. The placing of surgical drains at the time of closure is sometimes important in obese patients. This can be accomplished by a Hemovac drain placed through a small puncture wound lateral to the incision and extending the suction catheter the entire length of the incision above the fascia. Another method is to lay a small Penrose drain in the subcutaneous layer, making it exit through one end of the incision, and removing it in 24 hours. This ensures that serum and liquefied adipose tissue, good culture media, are removed from the wound. Studies looking at the benefit of a drain have not found an improvement in wound infections and complications. However, recent studies have also initiated the practice of closing the subcutaneous tissue, when it is thicker than 2 cm, with interrupted absorbable sutures to reduce the risk of seromas and hematomas. This has been shown to improve outcomes.

Postoperative Complications

1. Longer postoperative recovery period
2. Wound infection
3. Wound dehiscence
4. Atelectasis
5. Pulmonary embolism or deep venous thrombosis
6. Increased maternal morbidity and mortality rates

SELECTED READING

Chauhan SP, Magann EF, Carroll CS, Barrilleaux PS, Scardo JA, Martin JN Jr: Mode of delivery for the morbidly obese with prior cesarean delivery: Vaginal versus repeat cesarean section. Am J Obstet Gynecol 185:349, 2001

Crane JM, White J, Murphy P, Burrage L, Hutchens D: The effect of gestational weight gain by body mass index on maternal and neonatal outcomes. J Obstet Gynaecol 31:28, 2009

Davies GA, Maxwell C, McLeod L, Gagnon R, Basso M, Bos H, et al: SOGC Clinical Practice Guidelines: Obesity in pregnancy. Int J Gynaecol Obstet 110:167, 2010

Fyfe EM, Anderson NH, North RA, Chan EH, Taylor RS, Dekker GA, McCowan LM: Risk of first-stage and second-stage cesarean delivery by maternal body mass index among nulliparous women in labor at term. Obstet Gynecol 117:1315, 2011

Gross TL: Operative considerations in the obese pregnant patient. Clin Perinatol 10:411, 1983

Institute of Medicine, National Research Council: Weight Gain During Pregnancy: Reexamining the Guidelines. Washington, DC: National Academies Press, 2009

Kore S, Vyavaharkar M, Akolekar R, Toke A, Ambiye V: Comparison of closure of subcutaneous tissue versus non-closure in relation to wound disruption after abdominal hysterectomy in obese patients. J Postgrad Med 46:26, 2000

Robinson HE, O'Connell CM, Joseph KS, McLeod NL: Maternal outcomes in pregnancies complicated by obesity. Obstet Gynecol 106:1357, 2005

Tixier H, Thouvenot S, Coulange L, Peyronel C, Filipuzzi L, Sagot P, Douvier S: Cesarean section in morbidly obese women: supra or subumbilical transverse incision? Acta Obstet Gynecol Scand 88:1049-1052, 2019

Vahratian A, Zhang J, Troendle JF, Sciscione AC, Hoffman MK: Labor progression and risk of cesarean delivery in electively induced nulliparas. Obstet Gynecol 105:698, 2005

Weiss JL, Malone FD, Emig D, Ball RH, Nyberg DA, Comstock CH, Saade G, et al: Obesity, obstetric complications and cesarean delivery rate—a population-based screening study. Am J Obstet Gynecol 190:1091, 2004

World Health Organization: Obesity and Overweight. https://www.who.int/health-topics/obesity#tab=tab_1

COMPLICATED LABOR

Breech Presentation

Tamer Elfazari
Darine El-Chaâr

CHAPTER 25

GENERAL CONSIDERATIONS

Definition

Breech presentation is a longitudinal lie with a variation in polarity. The fetal pelvis is the leading pole. The denominator is the sacrum. A right sacrum anterior (RSA) is a breech presentation where the fetal sacrum is in the right anterior quadrant of the mother's pelvis and the bitrochanteric diameter of the fetus is in the right oblique diameter of the pelvis (Fig. 25-1).

Incidence

Breech presentation at delivery occurs in 3 to 4 percent of pregnancies. However, before 28 weeks of gestation, the incidence is about 25 percent. As term gestation approaches, the incidence decreases. In most cases, the fetus converts to the cephalic presentation by 34 weeks of gestation.

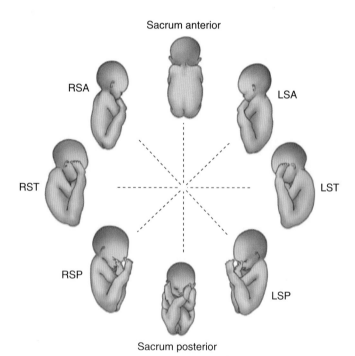

FIGURE 25-1. Positions of breech presentation. LSA, left sacrum anterior; LSP, left sacrum posterior; LST, left sacrum transverse; RSA, right sacrum anterior; RSP, right sacrum posterior; RST, right sacrum transverse.

Etiology

As term approaches, the uterine cavity, in most cases, accommodates the fetus best in a longitudinal lie with a cephalic presentation. In many cases of breech presentation, no reason for the malpresentation can be found and, by exclusion, the cause is attributed to chance. Some women deliver all their infants as breeches, suggesting that the pelvis is so shaped that the breech fits better than the head, and predisposed to this presentation.

Breech presentation is more common at the end of the second trimester than near term; hence, fetal prematurity is associated frequently with this presentation.

Maternal Factors

Factors that influence the occurrence of breech presentation include: (1) the uterine relaxation associated with high parity; (2) polyhydramnios, in which the excessive amount of amniotic fluid makes it easier for the fetus to change position; (3) oligohydramnios, in which, because of the small amount of fluid, the fetus is trapped in the position assumed in the second trimester; (4) uterine anomalies; (5) neoplasms or uterine masses, such as leiomyoma of the myometrium; and (6) while contracted pelvis is an uncommon cause of breech presentation, anything that interferes with the entry of the fetal head into the pelvis may play a part in the etiology of breech presentation.

Placental Factors

Placental site: There is some evidence that implantation of the placenta in either cornual-fundal region tends to promote breech presentation. There is a positive association of breech with placenta previa.

Fetal Factors

Fetal factors that influence the occurrence of breech presentation include multiple pregnancy, hydrocephaly, anencephaly, chromosomal anomalies, and intrauterine fetal death.

Notes and Comments

1. The patient commonly feels fetal movements in the lower abdomen and may complain of painful kicking against the rectum, vagina, and bladder
2. Engagement before the onset of labor is uncommon. The patient rarely experiences lightening

COMPLICATED LABOR

3. The uneven fit of breech to pelvis predisposes to early rupture of the membranes, with a danger of umbilical cord prolapse. The incidence of the latter, which is 4 to 5 percent, is higher with footling breeches. It is wise, therefore, when there is rupture of membranes, to perform a sterile vaginal examination to determine the exact state of the cervix and to make certain that the cord has not prolapsed

4. In theory, the breech is a poor dilator in comparison with the well-flexed head, and labor, descent, and cervical dilatation are believed to take longer. Although this is true in some cases, the mean duration of labor of 9.2 hours in primigravidas and 6.1 hours in multiparas suggests that in most cases, labor is not prolonged

5. In frank breeches, the baby's lower limbs, which are flexed at the hips and extended at the knees, lie anterior to and against the baby's abdomen. This has the effect of a splint and by decreasing the maneuverability of the baby may result in delay or arrest of progress

6. On the one hand, a frank breech has the disadvantage of a large and less maneuverable presenting part and may have difficulty passing through the pelvis. On the other hand, it dilates the soft parts to the greatest degree and makes the most room for the head. The small footling breech slips through the pelvis easily but makes less provision for the after-coming head

7. One of the dangers to a fetus in breech presentation is that the largest and least compressible diameter comes last

8. There is an added risk in premature infants because the head is relatively larger in proportion to the rest of the body than in full-term babies. Thus, although the small body slips through with no difficulty, it does not dilate the soft parts sufficiently to allow the head to pass easily

9. Because the posterior segment of the pelvis is roomier than the anterior segment, the posterior parts of the baby are usually born first

10. Because of the rapid passage of the head through the pelvis, there is no time for molding to take place. The fetal head is round and symmetrical

11. A baby that lies in utero as a frank breech lies with his or her hips flexed and the feet near his or her face for some time after birth

12. The external genitalia are edematous

13. The passage of meconium in a breech presentation does not have the same significance of fetal distress as in vertex presentation. The meconium is squeezed out of the intestine by the uterine contractions pressing the lower part of the baby's body against the pelvis

CLASSIFICATION

There are four types of breech presentation:

1. *Complete*: Flexion at the thighs and knees (Fig. 25-2A)
2. *Frank*: Flexion at the thighs; extension at the knees. This is the most common variety and includes almost two-thirds of breech presentations (Fig. 25-2B)
3. *Footling*: Single or double with extension at thighs and knees. The foot is the presenting part (Fig. 25-2C)

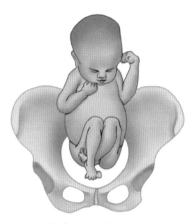

A. Complete breech.

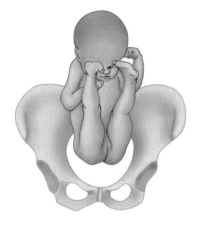

B. Frank breech.

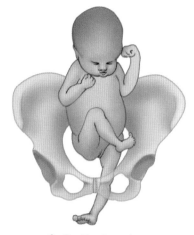

C. Footling breech.

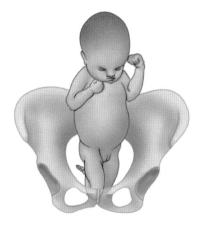

D. Kneeling breech.

FIGURE 25-2. Attitudes of breech presentation.

COMPLICATED LABOR

4. *Kneeling*: Single or double with extension at the thighs and flexion at the knees. The knee is the presenting part (Fig. 25-2D)

RIGHT SACRUM ANTERIOR

Diagnosis of Position

Abdominal Examination

1. The lie is longitudinal (Fig. 25-3A)
2. A soft, irregular mass lies over the pelvis and does not feel like the head. One therefore suspects a breech presentation. In a frank breech, the muscles of the thighs are drawn taut over the underlying bones, giving an impression of hardness not unlike the head and leading to diagnostic errors
3. The back is on the right near the midline. The small parts are on the left, away from the midline, and posterior
4. The head is felt in the fundus of the uterus. If the head is under the liver or the ribs, it may be difficult to palpate. The head is harder and more globular than the breech, and sometimes it can be balloted. Whenever a ballotable mass is felt in the fundus, a breech presentation should be suspected
5. There is no cephalic prominence, and the breech is not ballotable

Fetal Heart

The fetal heart tones are heard loudest at or above the umbilicus and on the same side as the back. In RSA the fetal heart is heard best in the right upper quadrant of the maternal abdomen. Sometimes the fetal heart is heard below the umbilicus; hence, the diagnosis made by palpation should not be changed because of the location of the fetal heart.

Vaginal Examination

1. The presenting part is high
2. The smooth, regular, hard head with its suture lines and fontanels is absent. This negative finding suggests a malpresentation
3. The presenting part is soft and irregular. The anal orifice and the ischial tuberosities are in a straight line (Fig. 25-3B). The breech may be confused with a face

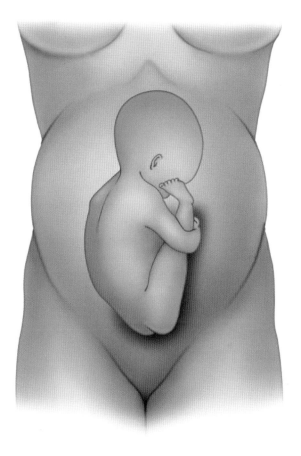

A. Abdominal view.

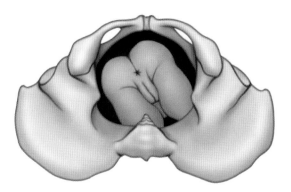

B. Vaginal view.

FIGURE 25-3. Right sacrum anterior.

4. Sometimes in frank breeches the sacrum is pulled down and is felt by the examining finger. It may be mistaken for the head because of its bony hardness
5. The sacrum is in the right anterior quadrant of the pelvis, and the bitrochanteric diameter is in the right oblique
6. Sometimes a foot is felt and must be distinguished from a hand

Ultrasonography

This is an important tool in the management of breech presentation, especially in the following areas: (1) confirmation of the clinical diagnosis; (2) diagnosis of hyperextension of the fetal head; (3) evaluation of the size of the fetal head; (4) estimation of fetal weight; and (5) diagnosis of major congenital anomalies, such as hydrocephaly, anencephaly, spina bifida. If ultrasound is not available, cesarean delivery is recommended because you are not able to confirm that it meets criteria to offer vaginal breech.

MECHANISMS OF LABOR: BREECH PRESENTATIONS

Cephalic and breech presentations are similar to triangles. When the head presents, the base of the triangle leads the way: The largest and most unyielding part of the baby comes first, and the parts that follow are progressively smaller. When the breech presents, on the other hand, the apex of the triangle comes first, and the succeeding parts are progressively bigger, with the relatively large head being last. In cases of cephalopelvic disproportion, by the time it is realized that the head is too big for the mother's pelvis, the rest of the baby has been born, and vaginal delivery must be carried on, with sad results for the baby.

In breech presentations, there are three mechanisms of labor: (1) the buttocks and lower limbs, (2) the shoulders and arms, and (3) the head.

Mechanism of Labor: RSA

Buttocks and Lower Limbs

Descent. Engagement has been achieved when the bitrochanteric diameter has passed through the inlet of the pelvis. In RSA, the sacrum is in

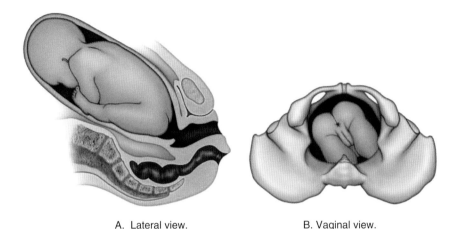

A. Lateral view.   B. Vaginal view.

FIGURE 25-4. **Right sacrum anterior: onset of labor.**

the right anterior quadrant of the maternal pelvis, and the bitrochanteric diameter is in the right oblique diameter of the pelvis (Figs. 25-4A and B). Because the breech is a less efficient dilator than the head, descent is slow, and the breech may remain high until labor has been in progress for some time. In many instances, the breech does not come down until the cervix is fully dilated and the membranes are ruptured.

Flexion. To facilitate passage of the breech through the pelvis, lateral flexion takes place at the waist. The anterior hip becomes the leading part. When the breech is frank, the baby's legs act as a splint along the body and, by reducing lateral flexion and maneuverability, may prevent descent into the pelvis.

Internal Rotation of Breech. The anterior hip meets the resistance of the pelvic floor and rotates forward, downward, and toward the midline (Figs. 25-5A and B). The bitrochanteric diameter rotates 45° from the right oblique diameter of the pelvis to the anteroposterior (AP). The sacrum turns away from the midline, from the right anterior quadrant to the right transverse (RSA to RST).

Birth of the Buttocks by Lateral Flexion. The anterior hip impinges under the pubic symphysis, lateral flexion occurs, and the posterior hip rises and is born over the perineum. The buttocks then fall toward the anus, and the anterior hip slips out under the symphysis (Fig. 25-6).

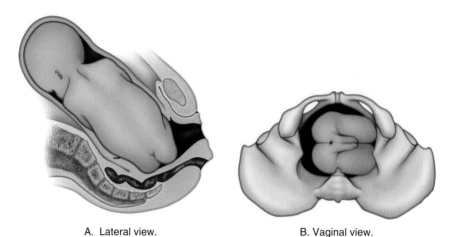

A. Lateral view. B. Vaginal view.

FIGURE 25-5. Descent and internal rotation of the buttocks.

Shoulders and Arms

Engagement. Engagement of the shoulders takes place in the right oblique diameter of the pelvis as the sacrum rotates RST to RSA (Fig. 25-7A).

Internal Rotation of the Shoulders. The anterior shoulder rotates under the symphysis, and the bisacromial diameter turns 45° from the right oblique to the AP diameter of the outlet. The sacrum goes along, RSA to RST (Fig. 25-7B).

Birth of Shoulders by Lateral Flexion. The anterior shoulder impinges under the symphysis, and the posterior shoulder and arm are born over the perineum as the baby's body is lifted upward (Fig. 25-7C). The baby is then lowered, and the anterior shoulder and arms pass out under the symphysis.

Head

Descent and Engagement. When the shoulders are at the outlet, the head is entering the pelvis (Fig. 25-8A). It enters the pelvis with the sagittal suture in the left oblique diameter. The occiput is in the right anterior quadrant of the pelvis.

Flexion. Flexion of the head takes place just as in any other presentation. It is important that flexion is maintained.

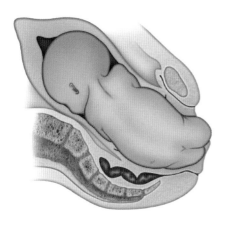

A. Breech crowning.

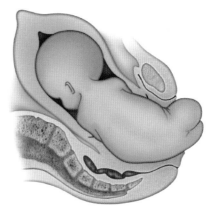

B. Birth of posterior buttock.

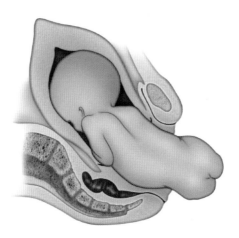

C. Birth of anterior buttock.

FIGURE 25-6. Birth of the buttocks.

Internal Rotation. The head strikes the pelvic floor and rotates internally so that it comes to the outlet with the sagittal suture in the AP diameter, the brow in the hollow of the sacrum, and the occiput under the symphysis (Fig. 25-8B). The sacrum rotates toward the pubis so that the back is anterior.

Birth of the Head by Flexion. The diameters are the same as in occipitoanterior positions but in reverse order. The nape of the neck pivots under the symphysis and the chin, mouth, nose, forehead, bregma, and occiput are born over the perineum by a movement of flexion (Fig. 25-8C).

COMPLICATED LABOR

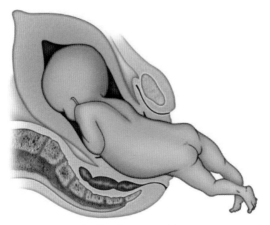

A. Feet born; shoulders engaging.

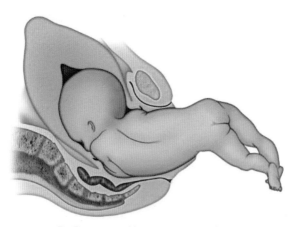

B. Descent and internal rotation of shoulders.

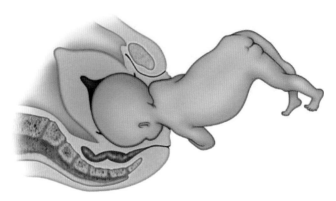

C. Posterior shoulder born; head has entered the pelvis.

FIGURE 25-7. Birth of the shoulders.

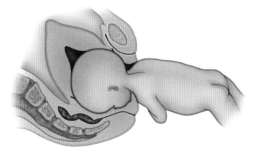

A. Anterior shoulder born, descent of head.

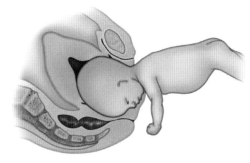

B. Internal rotation and beginning flexion of the head.

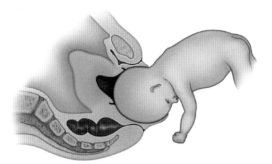

C. Flexion of the head complete.

FIGURE 25-8. **Birth of the head.**

Mechanism of Labor: Sacrum Directly Anterior

Descent
Engagement takes place with the bi-trochanteric diameter in the transverse diameter of the inlet. The sacrum is directly anterior behind the symphysis pubis (SA).

Flexion

Flexion is the same as in RSA.

Internal Rotation

The bitrochanteric diameter rotates 90° from the transverse diameter of the pelvis to the AP. The sacrum turns away from the midline to the transverse (SA to RST). The rest of the mechanism of labor is the same as in RSA.

Mechanism of Labor: Sacrum Posterior

In rare cases, the sacrum and head rotate posteriorly so that the occiput is in the hollow of the sacrum and the face is behind the pubis. If the head is flexed (Fig. 25-9A), delivery occurs with the occiput posterior. The nasion

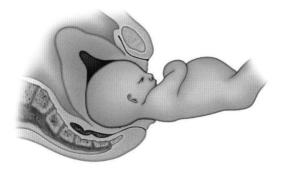

A. Head flexed.

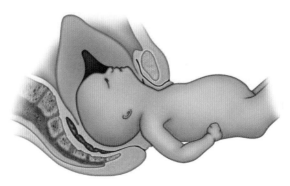

B. Head extended.

FIGURE 25-9. Arrest of the head: sacrum posterior.

pivots in the subpubic angle, and the nape of the neck, occiput, and vertex roll over the perineum. The face then emerges from behind the pubis. This method of delivery is helped by lifting up the fetus's body.

If the head is extended (Fig. 25-9B), the chin impinges behind the pubis and the submental area of the neck pivots in the subpubic angle. For delivery to take place, the infant's body must be raised by the accoucheur so that the occiput, vertex, and forehead can pass over the perineum in that order.

Delivery of the head from this position can be difficult. The best management of this complication lies in its prevention. Once the breech has been born, any tendency for the sacrum to rotate posteriorly must be restrained by the attendant and the breech encouraged to turn with the sacrum anteriorly toward the symphysis pubis.

Mechanism of Labor in Footling and Kneeling Breech

The mechanism of labor is the same as has been described in RSA with the difference being that in complete and frank breech presentations, the buttocks form the leading part. In footling presentations, it is one or both feet, and in kneeling breeches, it is the knees.

PROGNOSIS: BREECH PRESENTATIONS

Mother

When spontaneous delivery takes place, the maternal prognosis is good. Genital tract lacerations and hemorrhage may be caused by excessively rapid and forceful delivery of the baby through a pelvis that is too small or in which the soft parts have not been dilated sufficiently.

Fetus

In appropriately selected women, planned vaginal breech delivery is associated with greater short, but not long-term neonatal neurological morbidity. The risk is highest in double footling presentations and lowest with frank breech. Factors influencing perinatal mortality and morbidity include: (1) prematurity, (2) congenital abnormalities, (3) prolapse of the umbilical cord, (4) fetal asphyxia from other causes, and (5) fetal injury. Intracranial hemorrhage, more common with breech than with cephalic presentations, is a major cause of fetal mortality. Sometimes the unmolded head has to pass rapidly and with difficulty through a borderline pelvis.

Prolapse of the umbilical cord is more common than in cephalic presentation, especially when the presentation is footling and when the mother is multiparous. Frank breech has the lowest incidence.

The danger of injury is as great in multiparas as in primigravidas. Regardless of planned mode of delivery, cerebral palsy occurs in approximately 1.5 in 1000 breech births, and any abnormal neurological developments occur in approximately 3 in 1000. The fetal outcome is worse when the diagnosis is not made before the onset of labor.

Time of Death

About 15 percent of fetal deaths occur during labor. The remainder are divided more or less equally between fetal death in utero before the onset of labor, congenital anomalies incompatible with life, and neonatal death.

Causes of Death or Damage to the Baby

1. Prematurity is the major etiologic factor in the perinatal morbidity and mortality of infants presenting breech. The risk of death during labor is much higher for premature fetuses in breech than cephalic presentation
2. Congenital malformation. The incidence of anomalies among fetuses presenting by the breech is twice that seen in cephalic presentations, 6.3 versus 2.4 percent. Known fetal disorders associated with breech presentation include congenital dislocation of the hip, hydrocephaly, anencephaly, and meningomyelocele, as well as some less-common anomalies
3. Asphyxia
   a. Prolonged compression of the umbilical cord between the pelvis and the after-coming head
   b. Actual prolapse of the cord
   c. Aspiration of amniotic fluid and vaginal contents caused by active breathing before the head has been born
   d. Prolonged and hard labor
4. Injury to the brain and skull
   a. The after-coming head passes through the pelvis rapidly. Instead of gradual molding taking place over several hours, rapid and sometimes excessive compression and decompression occur within a few minutes. The ligaments of the brain are subjected to sudden and marked stretching, with the risk of laceration and intracranial hemorrhage. Injury to the brain may follow delivery through an

incompletely dilated cervix or through a pelvis whose adequacy has been estimated incorrectly

b. Minute hemorrhages

c. Fractures of the skull

d. Minimal brain dysfunction. One study has reported that the frequency of learning and motor defects is higher in infants delivered vaginally as breech presentations than in infants delivered as cephalic presentations. These include difficulties in reading and writing and disturbances in hearing, sight, and speech. It is not known whether the basic etiologic factor is anoxia or trauma. Unfortunately, this study has not matched a number of important variables, and a cause-and-effect relationship has not been proved. A study in the Netherlands of the neurologic status of infants born by vaginal delivery involving 256 cases and matched controls found that significant differences between the study and control groups existed only for minor neurologic dysfunctions. The conclusion reached was that the main danger of breech presentation lies in the associated complications of the pregnancy rather than the mode of delivery. Outcomes for children at 2-year follow-up in the Term Breech Trial published in 2004 showed that there was no difference between the planned cesarean delivery group and the planned vaginal delivery group

5. Damage resulting from difficult delivery

a. Fractures of the neck, humerus, clavicle, or femur

b. Cervical and brachial plexus paralyses

c. Rupture of the liver caused by grasping the baby too tightly around the abdomen while extracting him or her

d. Damage to fetal adrenal glands

e. Injury to the spinal cord

f. Traumatized pharynx caused by the obstetrician putting his or her finger in the baby's mouth to aid delivery

g. Damage to abdominal organs. The baby should be grasped by the hips and not the trunk

6. Size of the baby

a. Macrosomic babies, over 4000 g, may be too big for the mother's pelvis

b. Premature babies have small bodies in relation to their heads. A little breech is not a good dilator and fails to make room for the head. Fetal weight less than 2500 g is not recommended for trial of vaginal delivery

7. Rupture of membranes. It has been shown that the fetal mortality rate is significantly higher if the interval from rupture of the membranes to delivery is prolonged

INVESTIGATION OF BREECH PRESENTATION AT TERM

Ultrasound Examination

An ultrasound should be performed before the onset of labor in the setting of a breech presentation. If ultrasound is not available, cesarean section is recommended for confirmed breech presentations.

1. Confirm the presentation and diagnose the type of breech presentation—frank, complete, or footling
2. Diagnose any congenital fetal anomalies
3. Assess fetal attitude—flexion or extension. Rule out hyperextension of the fetal head
4. Estimate the fetal weight
5. Measure the biparietal diameter of the fetal head and the abdominal and thoracic girth
6. Compare the biparietal diameter of the fetal head and the measurements of the maternal pelvis
7. Localize the placenta and rule out placenta previa

MANAGEMENT OF BREECH PRESENTATION DURING LATE PREGNANCY

External Cephalic Version

Recent studies on outcomes of randomized controlled trials of external cephalic version (ECV) or no ECV have shown that there is a significant reduction of non-cephalic births and cesarean section. There was also no significant effect on perinatal mortality. It is therefore recommended that all women with a breech presentation should be offered an ECV. This should be performed at or beyond 36 weeks of gestation.

Timing

Delay of ECV to after 36 weeks of gestation has advantages: (1) fewer procedures are necessary because spontaneous version will occur in several cases, even in late pregnancy; (2) reversion to the original presentation is rare; (3) if fetal complications develop during the procedure that necessitate immediate delivery, the infant will be mature; and (4) contraindications to ECV, such as intrauterine growth restriction (IUGR), may become evident only in the later stage of the pregnancy.

In some circumstances, ECV can be offered in labor.

Prerequisites

1. Singleton pregnancy
2. No contraindication to labor and vaginal delivery
3. Normal fetal well-being
4. Normal amniotic fluid
5. Position confirmed before ECV
6. Facilities available for immediate cesarean section

Contraindications

1. Absolute
   a. Any contraindication to labor
   b. Antepartum hemorrhage
   c. Some major fetal anomalies
   d. Multiple gestation
   e. Ruptured membranes
2. Relative
   a. Oligohydramnios
   b. Hyperextension of the fetal head
   c. Two or more previous cesarean sections
   d. Morbid obesity
   e. Active labor
   f. Uterine anomalies

Procedure

1. Consent should be obtained from the patient before the procedure. The procedure is performed in a setting where immediate intervention, including a cesarean section, can be accessible
2. A nonstress test or biophysical profile are preformed before the procedure to ensure fetal well-being. An ultrasound is also performed to confirm position

3. The abdomen is usually lubricated to facilitate the version. The first attempt is usually made using the forward roll technique. With each hand on one of the fetal poles, the buttocks are elevated from the pelvis and moved laterally. The breech is then guided toward the fundus, with simultaneous direction of the head toward the pelvis. Another technique, if this unsuccessful, is the backward flip

4. In some cases, uterine relaxation is considered. Nitroglycerin, terbutaline, and ritodrine have been used in ECV in the same doses as for treating uterine hyperstimulation in labor

5. The procedure must be performed gently without excessive force because there is the risk of placental separation or damage to the fetus. Version may be unsuccessful, and the procedure abandoned. The procedure should also be abandoned if the patient is uncomfortable or if there are fetal heart rate (FHR) abnormalities. In cases in which the presentation has been changed to cephalic, most fetuses will remain in the new position, but in some instances, recurrence to the original presentation may take place

6. A nonstress test is performed for at least 20 minutes after attempted ECV, regardless if successful or not. It is important to administer Rh immunoglobulin in unsensitized Rh-negative women

Risks of External Cephalic Version

1. Abruption
2. Rupture of membrane and possibility of cord prolapse
3. Labor or preterm labor
4. FHR abnormalities
5. Alloimmunization or fetomaternal hemorrhage
6. Twofold increase in intrapartum cesarean delivery despite ECV

MANAGEMENT OF DELIVERY OF BREECH PRESENTATION

Classification of Breech Births

Vaginal Delivery

1. *Spontaneous breech delivery*: The entire infant is expelled by the natural forces of the mother with no assistance other than support of the baby as he or she is being born

2. *Assisted breech (or partial breech extraction)*: The infant is delivered by the natural forces as far as the umbilicus. The remainder of the baby is extracted by the attendant. In normal cases, we believe this to be the best method

3. *Total breech extraction*: The entire body of the infant is extracted by the attendant

Cesarean Section

It must be pointed out that delivery of a breech by cesarean section takes skill. Infants may be injured during the procedure. The incision must be adequate in length so there is no difficulty with the head. If the lower uterine segment is not well developed, as is often the case in preterm situations, a low vertical incision, which can be extended easily, may be preferable.

Elective Cesarean Section

The following factors are unfavorable for safe vaginal delivery, and cesarean section may be best:

1. Poor obstetrical histories, such as a difficult delivery or a damaged baby
2. Clinically inadequate maternal pelvis
3. Placenta previa of any degree
4. Prolapse of the umbilical cord, especially in footling breeches and/or cord presentation
5. Fetal growth restriction
6. Fetal macrosomia (estimated fetal weight >4000 g)
7. Hyperextension of the fetal head
8. Footling breech (one or both hip[s] extended). The limbs and pelvis of the footling breech deliver easily but do not dilate the maternal soft parts sufficiently to make room for the after-coming head. This may make delivery of the head difficult, especially in premature infants
9. Fetal anomaly likely to interfere with vaginal delivery

Because no clinical or ultrasonographic assessment can guarantee a safe and easy birth of the after-coming head, many obstetricians believe that all infants presenting in breech should be delivered by cesarean section. There are areas today where many infants in breech presentation are delivered abdominally without a trial of labor, however, there has been an increase in offering the option for breech vaginal delivery in appropriate cases.

Although maternal mortality due to cesarean delivery is rare, the overall morbidity associated with cesarean delivery is twofold higher compared

COMPLICATED LABOR

with vaginal delivery. Furthermore, definite proof of the superiority of cesarean section over vaginal delivery is difficult to obtain. The Term Breech Trial, published in 2000, was a multicenter trial in which women with a breech singleton pregnancy were randomized to a planned cesarean or a planned vaginal birth. The results of the trial showed the rate of perinatal or neonatal mortality or serious neonatal morbidity to be 1.6 percent in the planned cesarean group and 5 percent in the planned vaginal birth group.

The PREsentation et MODe d'Accouchement (PREMODA) study results were published in 2006 by Goffinet et al. Their study published prospective observational data from centers in France and Belgium for a total of 8105 women. A cesarean section was planned in 69 percent of these women, and a trial of labor was attempted in 31 percent of women. Of the 2526 women undergoing a trial of labor for breech presentation, 71 percent delivered vaginally. This study found no difference in perinatal or serious neonatal morbidity for either planned cesarean birth or trial of labor.

It is evident that, when the fetus is normal, cesarean section will reduce markedly, if not eliminate entirely, fetal death during delivery. At the same time, there is evidence that with proper selection of cases and meticulous management during labor and as long as indications for abdominal delivery are wide and include all unfavorable situations of even the mildest degree, many term breeches can be delivered vaginally and safely.

The controversy as to how to deliver breeches has not been settled.

Trial of Labor

Criteria. The criteria for consideration of vaginal delivery are:

1. Frank or complete breech
2. Term gestational age of 36 to 42 weeks
3. Estimated fetal weight between 2500 and 4000 g
4. Flexed or neutral fetal head
5. Adequate maternal pelvis
6. No maternal or fetal indication for cesarean section

Conditions. The trial of labor is carried out under the following conditions, with the understanding that any deviation from the normal is an indication for cesarean section.

1. The FHR is monitored continuously
2. The progress of labor is observed meticulously

3. Progressive cervical dilatation must take place
4. Adequate descent of the breech must occur
5. No heroic vaginal procedures are performed
6. The patient must be prepared and ready for cesarean section. The organization of the delivery room suite, the nurses, the anesthetist, and the obstetrician must allow the immediate performance of cesarean section if the need arises
7. Induction of labor is not recommended for breech presentation
8. A trained professional in neonatal resuscitation should be in attendance at time of delivery
9. An experienced obstetrician in vaginal breech delivery should be present at delivery

Management of Labor and Delivery in the Progressing Case

First Stage of Labor

1. Because most breech presentations that meet criteria for a trial of labor progress to successful vaginal delivery, observant expectancy, supportive therapy, and absence of interference are the procedures of choice
2. The patient may be ambulatory if the breech is well applied against the dilated cervix
3. It is best to maintain intact membranes until the cervical dilatation is far advanced. Too frequent vaginal or rectal examinations or any procedure that might contribute to premature rupture of the bag of waters should be avoided
4. When the membranes do rupture, vaginal examination is done to rule out prolapse of the umbilical cord and to determine the exact condition of the cervix
5. Meconium is no cause for alarm as long as the fetal heart is normal
6. An intravenous infusion of crystalloid solution (normal saline or Ringer lactate) should be instituted
7. Fetal well-being should be monitored using continuous electronic fetal monitoring
8. Progress of labor should be well documented. When progress is slow, oxytocin augmentation should be used with caution in cases of inadequate uterine contractions (e.g., caused by epidural anesthesia). If progress is less than 0.5 cm/hr or if there is no progress in 2 hours despite adequate uterine contractions, cesarean section should be performed

COMPLICATED LABOR

Second Stage of Labor

Once the cervix is fully dilated, the passive second stage may last up to 90 minutes. This allows the breech to descend into the lower pelvis. If delivery is not imminent after active pushing for 60 minutes, cesarean section should be performed.

When the breech begins to distend the perineum, the patient may be in a semi-supine or be in a hands and knees position to assist with the delivery. The semi-supine position is the best position in which to assist the birth and to handle complications. The patient's bladder should be emptied.

Assisted Breech. The fetal heart is checked frequently. As long as the baby is in good condition, spontaneous delivery is awaited. Fetal maneuvers should be used only after spontaneous delivery to the umbilicus. Premature traction on the baby, especially between contractions, must be avoided because it can lead to deflexion of the head and extension of the arms above or behind the head. It is important that the patient bear down with each contraction, and she must be encouraged to do so. Once the body has been born, the head is out of the upper contracting part of the uterus and in the lower segment, the cervix, or the upper vagina. Because these organs do not have the power to expel the head, its descent and delivery must be effected by the voluntary action of the abdominal muscles, with the attendant exerting suprapubic pressure.

Our experience has been that in normally progressing cases, the best results are obtained by a policy of:

1. No interference (except episiotomy) until the body is born to the umbilicus. This permits the cervix to become not only fully dilated but also paralyzed, an important factor in minimizing dystocia with the after-coming head
2. Hard bearing down and expulsive efforts by the mother during contractions
3. The maintenance of suprapubic pressure during descent to aid delivery and to keep the head in flexion

There are good reasons for using this technique:

1. It has proved successful
2. It is safe. There is less trauma to the baby
3. Flexion of the head is maintained

4. The danger of extension of the arms above the head is reduced
5. There is less chance of the cervix clamping down around the baby's head or neck

Anesthesia. A pudendal block or perineal infiltration permits episiotomy without pain and facilitates delivery by relaxing the muscles. In addition, with each contraction, the patient takes several breaths of an anesthetic vapor. This acts as an analgesic, eases the pain, and helps her to bear down more efficiently. Adequate anesthesia is best obtained by an epidural.

Necessary Equipment. The procedure requires that certain equipment be at hand.

1. A warm, dry towel to be wrapped around the baby's body as soon as he or she is sufficiently born. The purposes of this are:
   a. To reduce the stimulating effect of cold air on the baby in the hope that respiration does not begin while the head is in the pelvis, resulting in aspiration of amniotic fluid or vaginal contents
   b. To make it easier to hold the slippery baby
2. Piper forceps for the after-coming head if it does not deliver easily with assistance
3. Equipment for resuscitation of the infant ready for immediate use
4. Ability to perform an emergency cesarean section

Delivery of Breech

1. The patient is encouraged to bear down with the contractions but must rest between them
2. In instances where there is no fetal or maternal distress, spontaneous delivery to the umbilicus is awaited. Up to this point, there is no urgency, and the operator should not interfere
3. Once the umbilicus has been delivered, time becomes an important factor, and the remainder of the birth is expedited gently and skillfully. A free airway to the mouth should be available within 3 to 5 minutes to obviate anoxic brain damage
4. The legs usually deliver spontaneously, if not they are easily extracted. Do not extract the legs until the popliteal fossae are visible (Pinard's maneuver)
5. The baby is covered with a warm towel, and the body is supported

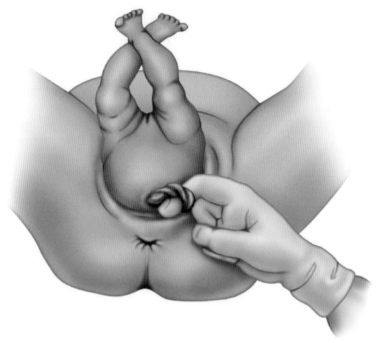

FIGURE 25-10. Delivery of the cord. Loop of umbilical cord being pulled down.

6. A loop of umbilical cord is pulled down (Fig. 25-10) to minimize traction on it in case it is caught between the head and the pelvic wall. At the same time, it is palpated for pulsations

Delivery of the Shoulders and Arms

1. The assistant exerts suprapubic pressure on the head to maintain its flexion
2. The operator depresses the buttocks and delivers the body to the anterior scapula so that the anterior shoulder comes under the symphysis
3. To deliver the anterior arm, the accoucheur passes his or her hand up the baby's back, over the shoulder, and down the chest, thus sweeping the arm and hand out under the pubis with his or her finger (Loveset maneuver; Fig. 25-11A)
4. The baby is raised so that the posterior scapula and then the posterior arm are born over the perineum by the same maneuver (Fig. 25-11B)
5. Some obstetricians deliver the posterior arm first

Delivery of the Head

1. In almost every case, the back turns anteriorly spontaneously. This must be encouraged so that the head rotates the occiput to the pubis

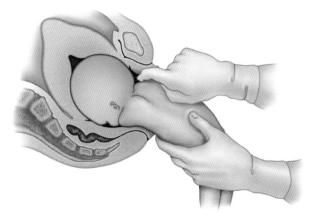

A. Extraction of anterior arm.

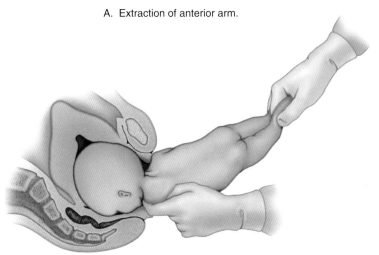

B. Extraction of posterior arm.

FIGURE 25-11. Delivery of the arms and shoulders.

and the face toward the sacrum. Rarely, there is a tendency for the back to turn posteriorly. The obstetrician must counteract this and rotate the back anteriorly to prevent the head's rotating face to pubis, a serious and always avoidable complication

2. Once the back has rotated anteriorly and the fetal head is in the AP diameter of the pelvis, the body is lowered so that the occiput appears under the symphysis and the nape of the neck pivots there (Fig. 25-12A)

3. At the same time, the assistant maintains suprapubic pressure to guide the head through the pelvis and to keep it flexed

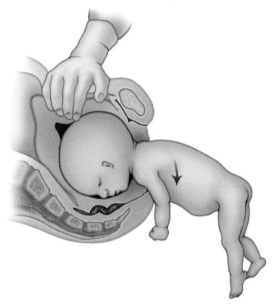

A. Body lowered so that nape of neck is in the subpubic angle.
   Assistant maintains flexion of the head.

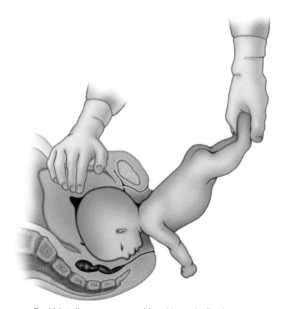

B. Kristellar maneuver; Head born in flexion.

FIGURE 25-12. Delivery of the head.

4. The body is then raised gently so that there is slight extension at the neck
5. Then by further suprapubic pressure (Kristellar maneuver, also known as Bracht maneuver) the head is delivered in flexion—the chin, mouth, nose, forehead, bregma, and vertex being born, in that order, over the perineum (Fig. 25-12B)
6. The speed of delivery of the after-coming head must be considered. The rapid passage of the head through the pelvis causes sudden compression and decompression of the cranial contents. In the extreme, the ligaments of the brain tear, leading to hemorrhage, cerebral damage, and death. On the other hand, too slow delivery of the head results in asphyxia, which may also be fatal. Experience teaches the middle road—slow enough to prevent injury to the brain and sufficiently rapid to avoid asphyxia

ARREST IN BREECH PRESENTATION

Most babies who present by the breech are born spontaneously or with the help of, but not interference from, the attendant. The Kristellar/Bracht maneuver (suprapubic pressure) is all that is needed to deliver the after-coming head. However, progress may cease, and active interference then becomes mandatory. Arrest may take place at the head, neck, shoulders and arms, or buttocks.

Arrest of the Head

Sometimes the body, shoulders, and arms are born, but the bearing-down efforts of the mother and the Kristellar/Bracht maneuver are not successful in delivering the head. When the head is arrested, several measures are available to extract it.

Wigand-Martin Maneuver

The body of the baby is placed on the arm of the operator with the middle finger of the hand of that arm placed in the baby's mouth and the index and ring fingers on the malar bones (Fig. 25-13A). The purpose of the finger in the mouth is not for traction but to encourage and maintain flexion. With the other hand, the obstetrician exerts suprapubic pressure on the head through the mother's abdomen.

COMPLICATED LABOR

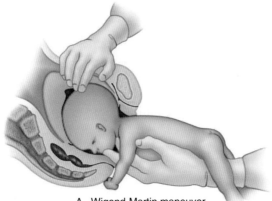

A. Wigand-Martin maneuver.

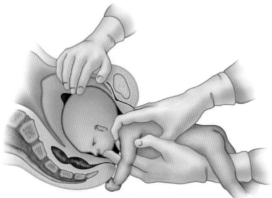

B. Mauriceau-Smellie-Veit maneuver.

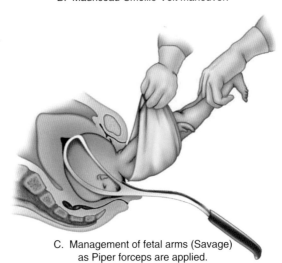

C. Management of fetal arms (Savage)
as Piper forceps are applied.

FIGURE 25-13. Different maneuvers for arrest of the head.

Mauriceau-Smellie-Veit Maneuver

The position is the same as the Wigand-Martin maneuver, with one finger in the baby's mouth and two on the malar bones. The difference is that the accoucheur places his or her other hand astride the baby's shoulders and produces traction in this way (Fig. 25-13B). The efficiency of this procedure is increased by an assistant's applying suprapubic pressure on the fetal head while the operator is performing the Mauriceau maneuver.

Piper Forceps on the After-Coming Head

With the exception of simple suprapubic pressure, the best method of delivering the after-coming head is by the use of the Piper forceps. In contrast to maneuvers in which traction on the head is applied through the neck, the forceps exert traction directly on the head, thereby avoiding damage to structures in the baby's neck.

Although any type of forceps can be used for this procedure, the Piper forceps, which was designed especially for this operation, is best. The handles are depressed below the arch of the shanks, the pelvic curve is reduced, and the shanks are long and curved. These features make this instrument easier to apply to the after-coming head.

Orientation

Vaginal Examination

1. The long axis of the head is in the AP diameter of the pelvis
2. The occiput is anterior
3. The face is posterior

Orientation and Desired Application

1. The cephalic application is biparietal and mento-occipital, with the front of the forceps (concave edges) toward the occiput and the convex edges toward the face
2. The pelvic application is good, with the diameter of the forceps in the transverse diameter of the pelvis, the concave edges pointing toward the pubis, and the convex edges toward the sacrum. The sides of the blades are next to the side walls of the pelvis

Application of Forceps

1. The baby's feet are grasped by an assistant, and the body is raised (Fig. 25-13C). Care must be taken not to elevate the body too much

for fear of damage to the sternomastoid muscles. The lower and upper limbs and the umbilical cord are kept out of the way. A good way to keep the arms out of the way is to use a folded towel as described by Savage

2. The handle of the left blade is grasped in the left hand
3. The right hand is introduced between the head and the left postero-lateral wall of the vagina
4. The left blade is then inserted between the head and the fingers into a mento-occipital application
5. The fingers are removed from the vagina, and the handle is steadied by an assistant
6. The handle of the right blade is grasped with the right hand
7. The left hand is introduced between the head and the right postero-lateral wall of the vagina
8. The right blade is introduced between the head and the fingers into a mento-occipital application
9. The fingers are removed from the vagina
10. The forceps are locked (Fig. 25-14), and vaginal examination is made to be certain that the application is correct

Extraction of the Head

1. Traction is outward and posterior until the nape of the neck is in the subpubic angle
2. The direction is then changed to outward and anterior, and the face and forehead are born over the perineum in flexion
3. An episiotomy should be used

Airway

When there is delay in delivery of the head and one is waiting for help or instruments, an ordinary vaginal retractor can be used temporarily to clear an airway in the vagina to the baby's mouth (Fig. 25-15). The retractor is placed in the vagina and pressure exerted posteriorly. The vaginal contents are sponged out so that air can get to the baby if he or she breathes.

Chin-to-Pubis Rotation

Anterior rotation of the chin is rare and occurs usually as part of posterior rotation of the back. The preferred management is as follows: (1) institute deep anesthesia, (2) cease all traction, (3) dislodge the chin from behind the pubis, (4) rotate the face posteriorly and the back anteriorly, (5) flex

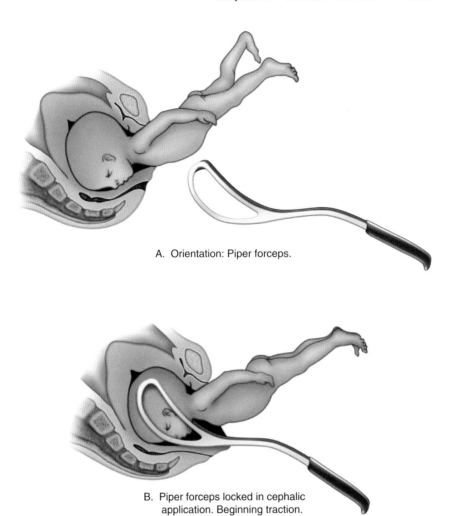

A. Orientation: Piper forceps.

B. Piper forceps locked in cephalic
application. Beginning traction.

FIGURE 25-14. Piper forceps for delivery of an after-coming head.

the chin, (6) effect engagement by suprapubic pressure, and (7) deliver the head with Piper forceps.

When this technique fails, the Prague maneuver (Fig. 25-16) may be used. Here, the fingers are placed over the shoulders, and outward and upward traction is made. The legs are grasped with the other hand, and the body is swung over the mother's abdomen. With this procedure, the occiput is born over the perineum. Because this method carries with it the danger of overstretching or breaking the infant's neck, it is used rarely.

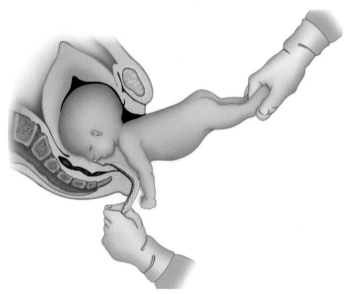

FIGURE 25-15. Vaginal retractor providing airway to the baby's mouth and nose.

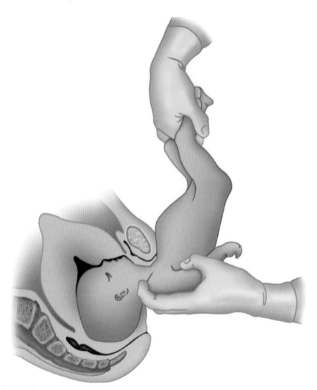

FIGURE 25-16. Prague maneuver.

Embryotomy

When delivery of the head is not accomplished within a reasonable time, the baby may die. If he or she does perish, the mother's welfare alone should be considered. To save her from needless injury, reduction of the size of the fetal head by perforation of the skull is preferable to extraction by brute force.

Arrest of the Neck

Occasionally, the cervix, which has opened sufficiently to allow the trunk and shoulders to be born, clamps down around the baby's neck, trapping the head in the uterus. The possibility of this happening is greater with premature delivery, when the body has not yet developed its adipose tissue and is a poor dilating wedge. This dangerous situation calls for rapid action to break the spasm of the previously dilated cervix. This is accomplished by a single bold incision of the cervix with the scissors. The resultant relaxation of the spasm permits the head to be born.

Arrest of the Shoulders and Arms

Extended Arms
The arms are simply extended over the baby's head (Fig. 25-17A).

Nuchal Arms
There is extension at the shoulder and flexion at the elbow so that the forearm is trapped behind the fetal head (Fig. 25-17B). One or both arms may be affected.

Prophylaxis
One method of reducing the incidence of this complication is to resist the temptation of pulling on the baby's legs to speed delivery, especially when the uterus is in a relaxed state.

Simple Extraction
When this problem occurs, an attempt should be made first to deliver the arms by sweeping them over the chest in the usual way. This succeeds in most cases of simple extension and in some instances of nuchal arms when the upper limb is not jammed tightly behind the head.

Rotation of the Body

If extraction fails in the case of a nuchal arm, the baby's body is rotated in the direction to which the hand is pointing (Fig. 25-17C). This dislodges the arm from behind the head, and its delivery is then usually possible as described above (Fig. 25-17D). If both arms are nuchal, the body is rotated in one direction to free the first arm, which is then extracted, and then in the opposite direction to free the other arm.

Fracture

In the rare instance when rotation fails, the humerus or clavicle must be fractured. This can be done directly, or it can be ensued by simply pulling

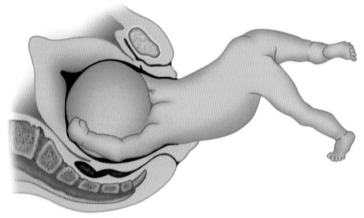

A. Arm extended above the head.

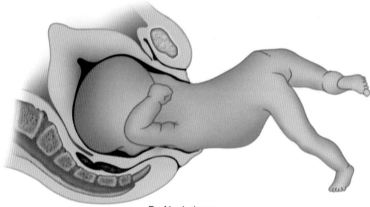

B. Nuchal arm.

FIGURE 25-17. Extended and nuchal arms.

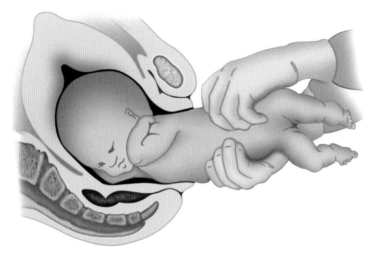

C. Nuchal arm: Rotation of the trunk of the child 90°
in the direction in which the hand is pointing.

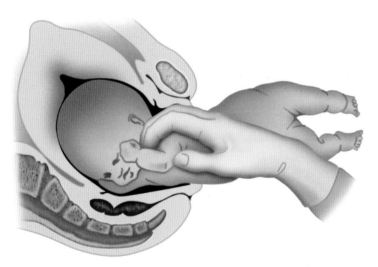

D. Nuchal arm: Hand introduced into the uterus to flex
and bring down the nuchal arm.

FIGURE 25-17. (*Continued*)

on the arm until it breaks. Once this occurs, delivery can be accomplished. Because the fracture usually heals rapidly and well and because the choice may be between a dead baby and a broken arm, extreme measures are justified.

COMPLICATED LABOR

Failure of Descent of the Breech

Etiology

In any situation, the size of the passenger, the capacity of the pelvis, the dilatability of the maternal soft tissues, and the character of the uterine contractions all play a part in determining whether spontaneous delivery takes place. In frank breech presentation, there is an added factor—the splinting effect of the baby's legs across its abdomen can reduce the maneuverability of the fetus to such an extent that progress is arrested.

Disproportion

In the presence of good uterine contractions, nondescent of the breech is an indication not for hasty interference but for the most careful reassessment. Keeping in mind the fact that one of the causes of breech presentation is a large head that cannot engage easily, the accoucheur must be assured not of the general capacity of the pelvis but of its adequacy with respect to that particular baby. When a breech fails to descend, despite good contractions, disproportion is present, and cesarean section should be performed.

Decomposition

Flexed Breech. If cesarean section cannot be performed, progress and descent can be expedited by reducing the bulk of the breech, an operation known as decomposition. This is done by bringing down the legs, both whenever possible. When there is flexion at the hips and the knees, the feet can be reached easily. The hand is placed in the uterus, the membranes are ruptured, and a foot is grasped and brought down (Fig. 25-18A). Be sure it is not a hand. The same is done with the other foot. The position has been changed to a footling breech, and labor proceeds.

Frank Breech: Pinard Maneuver. If the breech is frank (flexion at the hips and extension at the knees), it may be impossible to reach the feet because they are high in the uterus near the baby's face. In such a situation and when cesarean section cannot be carried out, the Pinard maneuver is performed under anesthesia (Figs. 25-18B and C). With a hand in the uterus, pressure is made by the fingers against the popliteal fossa in a backward and outward direction. This brings about sufficient flexion of the knee so that the foot can be grasped and delivered. When possible, both feet should be brought down. Unless there are urgent indications for immediate extraction of the infant, labor is allowed to carry on as for a footling breech.

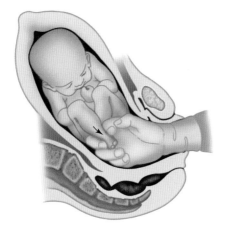

A. Decomposition of breech: Bringing down a foot and leg.

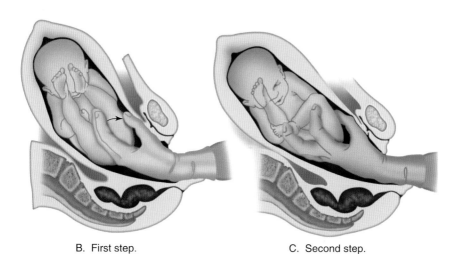

B. First step.

C. Second step.

FIGURE 25-18. Breaking up the breech.

BREECH EXTRACTION

This operation is the immediate vaginal extraction of the baby when signs of fetal distress demand delivery without delay and urgent cesarean section is not available. This is also used in delivery of a second twin in breech presentation. In general, total breech extraction in term singleton breech fetuses is *not* appropriate.

Prerequisites

Certain conditions must be present before this procedure may be performed: (1) the pelvis must be ample, with no disproportion; (2) the cervix must be fully dilated; (3) the bladder and rectum should be empty; (4) expert and deep anesthesia is essential; (5) good assistance is mandatory; and (6) neonatal resuscitation is ready.

Procedure

The patient is placed in the lithotomy position, the bladder catheterized, and anesthesia administered. As described in a previous section, the breech is decomposed, and the legs are brought down. The feet are pulled down if the breech is complete; the Pinard maneuver is used if the breech is frank. Instead of the patient going on to spontaneous delivery, the baby is extracted rapidly. Traction from below and fundal pressure from above are substituted for uterine contractions, but the maneuvers for delivery of the shoulders, arms, and head are those already set forth in the management of arrested cases.

HYPEREXTENSION OF THE FETAL HEAD

Hyperextension of the fetal head (Fig. 25-19) is most commonly seen in face presentation but also occurs with transverse lie and breech presentation. In the latter, it is a serious problem.

Etiology

1. Spasm or congenital shortening of the extensor muscles of the neck
2. Umbilical cord around the neck
3. Congenital tumors of the fetal neck
4. Fetal malformations
5. Uterine anomalies
6. Tumors in the placental site

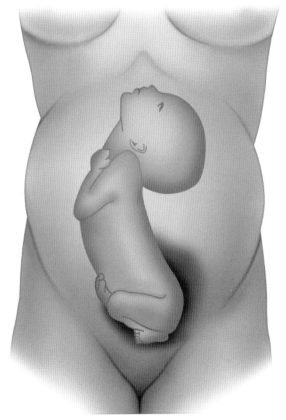

FIGURE 25-19. Hyperextension of the fetal head.

Diagnosis

The diagnosis is made by ultrasound examination; the appearance is characteristic. When the head presents, it is that of a face presentation. When the breech presents, the appearance has been described as a "star-gazing breech." In transverse lie, the condition is seen as a "flying fetus."

Fetal Danger

There is a definite risk of damage to the lower cervical spinal cord of the fetus during vaginal delivery. The mechanisms by which the injury is caused include: (1) excessive longitudinal stretching of the spinal cord, (2) extreme flexion of the neck during delivery, and (3) marked torsion. The resulting lesion is partial or complete laceration of the cervical spinal cord, occasional tears in the dura, and epidural hemorrhage. The latter is the most common manifestation and is associated with varying degrees of damage to the cord, brain stem, nerve roots, and meninges. Dislocation or fracture of the vertebrae is rare. In most cases, the injury is caused by the sudden flexion of the head as it descends through the vagina. However, occasionally, the damage may occur during pregnancy because of the malposition of the fetus.

Fetal Prognosis

In a collected series of 73 cases, the perinatal mortality rate was 13.7 percent in babies delivered vaginally in contrast to no deaths in those born by cesarean section. Medullary or vertebral injury occurred in 20.6 percent of babies born per vagina and in 5.7 percent delivered by cesarean section. Meningeal hemorrhage was found in 6.9 percent of children born vaginally, but none was noted after cesarean section. In another series of 814 breech presentations, there were 33 hyperextended heads, an incidence of 7.4 percent. All 33 infants survived. Follow-up for 2 to 4 years revealed neurologic sequelae in 5 of the 26 children born vaginally, but none in the 7 delivered by cesarean section.

A cesarean section should be performed when the fetal head is extended.

SELECTED READING

American College of Obstetricians and Gynecologists: ACOG Committee Opinion No. 745, Mode of term singleton breech delivery. Obstet Gynecol 108:235, 2018

Ben-Meir A, Erez Y, Sela HY, Shveiky D, Tsafrir A, Ezra Y: Prognostic parameters for successful external cephalic version. J Matern Fetal Neonatal Med 21:660, 2008

Collea JV: The intrapartum management of breech presentation. Clin Perinatol 8:173, 1981

Collea JV, Chein C, Quilligan EJ: The randomized management of term frank breech presentation: A study of 208 cases. Am J Obstet Gynecol 137:235, 1980

Cox C, Kendall AC, Hommers M: Changed prognosis of breech-presenting low birthweight infants. Br J Obstet Gynaecol 89:881, 1982

Cunningham FG, Gant NF, Leveno KJ, et al: Breech presentation and delivery. In: *Williams Obstetrics*, 23rd ed. New York: McGraw-Hill, 2009

Effer SB, Saigal S, Rand C, et al: Effect of delivery method on outcomes in the very low-birth weight breech infant: Is the improved survival related to cesarean section or other perinatal care maneuvers? Am J Obstet Gynecol 145:123, 1983

Faber-Nijholt R, Huisjes HJ, Touwen BCL, Fidler VJ: Neurological follow-up of 281 children born in breech presentation: A controlled study. Br Med J 286:9, 1983

Fall O, Nilsson BA: External cephalic version in breech presentation under tocolysis. Obstet Gynecol 53:712, 1979

Gimovsky ML, Wallace RL, Schiffrin BS, Paul RH: Randomized management of the non-frank breech presentation at term: A preliminary report. Am J Obstet Gynecol 146:34, 1983

Goffinet F, Carayol M, Foidart JM, Alexander S, Uzan S, Subtil D, et al: PREMODA Study Group. Is planned vaginal delivery for breech presentation at term still an option? Results of an observational prospective survey in France and Belgium. Am J Obstet Gynecol 194:1002, 2006

Green JE, McLean F, Smith LP, Usher R: Has an increased cesarean section rate for term breech delivery reduced the incidence of birth asphyxia, trauma, and death? Am J Obstet Gynecol 143:643, 1982

Hannah ME, Hannah WJ, Hewson SA, Hodnett ED, Saigal S, Willan AR, et al: Planned cesarean section versus planned vaginal birth for breech presentation at term: a randomised multicentre trial. Lancet 356:1375, 2000

Hofmeyr GJ: Effect of external cephalic version in late pregnancy on breech presentation and cesarean section: A controlled trial. Br J Obstet Gynaecol 90:392, 1983

Ridley WJ, Jackson P, Stewart JH, Boyle P: Role of antenatal radiography in the management of breech deliveries. Br J Obstet Gynaecol 89:342, 1982

Royal College of Obstetricians and Gynaecologists: RCOG Green Top Guidelines: The management of breech presentation. Guideline no. 20b. London: Royal College of Obstetricians and Gynaecologists, March 2017

Society of Obstetricians and Gynaecologists of Canada: Management of Breech Presentation at Term. Clinical Practice Guideline No. 384. Ottawa, ON: Society of Obstetricians and Gynaecologists of Canada, August 2019

Westgren M, Grundsell I, Ingemarsson A, et al: Hyperextension of the fetal head in breech presentation: A study with long-term follow-up. Br J Obstet Gynaecol 88:101, 1981

Whyte H, Hannah ME, Saigal S, Hannah W, Hewson S, Amankwah K, et al: Outcomes of children at 2 years after planned cesarean birth versus planned vaginal birth for breech presentation at term: The International Randomized Term Breech Trial. Am J Obstet Gynecol 191:864, 2004

CHAPTER 26

Transverse Lie

Roxanna Mohammed
George Tawagi

GENERAL CONSIDERATIONS

Definition

When the long axes of mother and fetus are at right angles to one another, a transverse lie is present. Because the shoulder is placed so frequently in the brim of the inlet, this malposition is often referred to as the shoulder presentation. The baby may lie directly across the maternal abdomen (Fig. 26-1) or may lie obliquely with the head or breech in the iliac fossa (Figs. 26-2A and B). Usually, the breech is at a higher level than the head. The denominator is the scapula (Sc); the situation of the head determines whether the position is left or right, and that of the back indicates whether it is anterior or posterior. Thus, LScP means that the lie is transverse, the head is on the mother's left side, and the baby's back is posterior. The part that actually lies over the pelvic brim may be the shoulder, back, abdomen, ribs, or flank. This is a serious malposition whose management must not be left to nature.

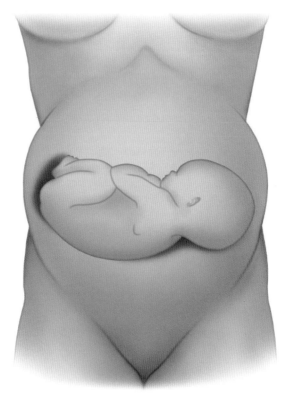

FIGURE 26-1. Transverse lie: LScP.

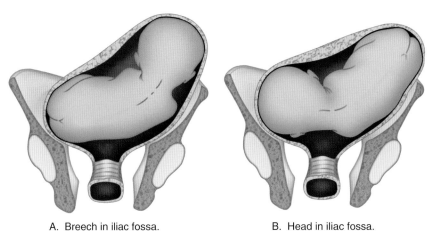

A. Breech in iliac fossa.   B. Head in iliac fossa.

FIGURE 26-2. Oblique lie.

Incidence

The incidence of transverse lie is around one in 300. The incidence is higher before term (as high as one in 50 at 32 weeks' gestation).

Etiology

This abnormality is more common in multiparas than primigravidas because of the laxness of the uterine and abdominal muscles. Similar conditions in which there is excess space for the fetus are polyhydramnios or prematurity. Other causes include anything that prevents engagement of the head or the breech, such as placenta previa; an obstructing neoplasm; multiple pregnancies; fetal anomalies; fetopelvic disproportion; contracted pelvis; and uterine abnormalities such as subseptate uterus, arcuate uterus, and bicornuate uterus. In many instances, no etiologic factor can be determined, and we assume that the malposition is accidental. The head happens to be out of the lower uterine segment when labor starts, and the shoulder is pushed into the pelvic brim.

DIAGNOSIS OF POSITION: TRANSVERSE LIE

Abdominal Examination

1. The appearance of the abdomen is asymmetrical
2. The long axis of the fetus is across the mother's abdomen

COMPLICATED LABOR

3. The uterine fundus is lower than expected for the period of gestation. It has been described as a squat uterus. Its upper limit is near the umbilicus, and it is wider than usual
4. Palpation of the upper and lower poles of the uterus reveals neither the head nor the breech
5. The head can be felt in one maternal flank. The buttocks are on the other side

Fetal Heart

The fetal heart is heard best below the umbilicus and has no diagnostic significance regarding position.

Vaginal Examination

The most important finding is a negative one—neither the head nor the breech can be felt by the examining finger. The presenting part is high. In some cases, one may feel the shoulder, a hand, the rib cage, or the back. Because of the poor fit of the presenting part to the pelvis, the bag of waters may hang into the vagina.

Ultrasonography

Ultrasonic examination will confirm the diagnosis and can detect certain abnormalities in the fetus or the presence of a maternal pelvic mass.

X-ray

When ultrasonography is unavailable, the fetal presentation can be established by a flat plate radiograph of the abdomen.

MECHANISM OF LABOR: TRANSVERSE LIE

Except in severely premature fetuses (in which a transverse lie may deliver vaginally), a persistent transverse lie cannot deliver spontaneously, and if uncorrected, impaction takes place (Fig. 26-3A). The shoulder is jammed into the pelvis, the head and breech stay above the inlet, the neck becomes stretched, and progress is arrested.

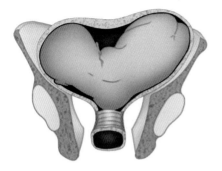
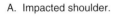

A. Impacted shoulder.

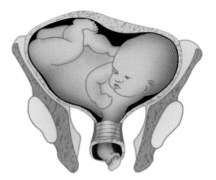

B. Prolapsed arm.

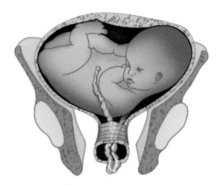

C. Prolapsed umbilical cord.

FIGURE 26-3. Complications.

Spontaneous Version

Spontaneous version takes place occasionally, more often with oblique than with transverse lies. Before or shortly after the onset of labor, the lie changes to a longitudinal one (cephalic or breech), and labor proceeds in the new position. Unfortunately, the chance of spontaneous version occurring is small, too small to warrant more than a very short delay in instituting corrective measures.

Neglected Transverse Lie

Neglected transverse lie results from misdiagnosis or improper treatment. At first, the contractions are of poor quality, and the cervix dilates slowly. Because of the irregularity of the presenting part, the membranes rupture early, and the amniotic fluid escapes rapidly. As the labor pains become stronger, the fetal shoulder is forced into the pelvis, the uterus molds itself

COMPLICATED LABOR

around the baby, a state of impaction ensues, and progress is halted. From this impasse, there is one of two outcomes:

1. *Uterine rupture:* Labor goes on. The upper part of the uterus becomes shorter and thicker, and the lower segment becomes progressively more stretched and thinned until it ruptures
2. *Uterine inertia:* The uterus becomes exhausted, and the contractions cease. Intrauterine sepsis sets in and may be followed by generalized infection

In either event, fetal death is certain and maternal mortality possible. Transverse lies must not be neglected!

Complications

Because the presenting part does not fill the inlet, the membranes tend to rupture early and may be followed by prolapse of a fetal arm or the umbilical cord (Figs. 26-3B and C). Both are serious complications necessitating immediate action.

PROGNOSIS: TRANSVERSE LIE

The prognosis depends on the management. With early diagnosis and proper treatment, the outcome is favorable. Neglect leads to the death of almost all infants and puts the mother in serious danger.

MANAGEMENT OF TRANSVERSE LIE

Management Before Labor

1. Careful abdominal, pelvic, ultrasonographic, and, if necessary, radiologic examinations are performed to confirm the diagnosis and to rule out fetal and pelvic abnormalities
2. Shoulder presentations that are diagnosed before term should be managed expectantly because there is a good chance that the malposition will correct itself. If the patient is not at term but the cervix is significantly dilated, hospitalization should be considered because of the incidence of cord prolapse if spontaneous rupture of membranes occurs
3. If the patient is at or near term, external version to a breech or preferably a cephalic presentation should be attempted

Management During Early Labor

In early labor, external version may also be attempted, and if successful, the new presentation is maintained by a tight abdominal binder until it is fixed in the pelvis.

Management of Patient in Advanced Labor

Cesarean section is the treatment of choice. It is safest for both mother and child. It is safest for the mother even in the case of a dead fetus. Because of the exceedingly high morbidity and mortality rates for both the mother and fetus, there is no role for internal podalic version and extraction in the management of transverse lie in singleton gestation. In some instances, extraction of the infant through a transverse lower segment incision may be difficult, and a vertical incision in the lower segment, which can be extended upward if necessary, is preferred by many obstetricians.

Management of Neglected Transverse Lie

This is an obstetric emergency. Typically, there has been prolonged labor. The lower uterine segment is very thin (or possibly ruptured). Fetal impaction has taken place. An intrauterine infection is present. The fetus is in distress or dead.

Management under these circumstances is difficult.

1. Cesarean section and intensive therapy with antibiotics are carried out even if the baby is dead
2. If infection is severe and widespread, hysterectomy may be necessary after the cesarean section
3. Internal podalic version and extraction or desperate destructive operations on the fetus should not be considered because they carry a grave risk of uterine rupture

CONCLUSION

Transverse lies at term after failure of external version are treated best by cesarean section. They must never be neglected or left to nature.

CHAPTER 27

Compound Presentations

Roxanna Mohammed
George Tawagi

PROLAPSE OF HAND AND ARM OR FOOT AND LEG

Definition

A presentation is compound when there is prolapse of one or more of the limbs along with the head or the breech, both entering the pelvis at the same time. Footling breech or shoulder presentations are not included in this group. Associated prolapse of the umbilical cord occurs in 15 to 20 percent of cases.

Incidence

Easily detectable compound presentations occur probably once in 500 to 1000 confinements. It is impossible to establish the exact incidence because:

1. Spontaneous correction occurs frequently, and examination late in labor cannot provide the diagnosis
2. Minor degrees of prolapse are detected only by early and careful vaginal examination

Classification of Compound Presentation

1. Cephalic presentation with prolapse of:
   a. Upper limb (arm–hand), one or both
   b. Lower limb (leg–foot), one or both
   c. Arm and leg together
2. Breech presentation with prolapse of the hand or arm

By far the most frequent combination is that of the head with the hand (Fig. 27-1) or arm. In contrast, the head–foot and breech–arm groups are uncommon, about equally so. Prolapse of both hand and foot alongside the head is rare. All combinations may be complicated by prolapse of the umbilical cord, which then becomes the major problem.

Etiology

The etiology of compound presentation includes all conditions that prevent complete filling and occlusion of the pelvic inlet by the presenting part. The most common causal factor is prematurity. Others include high presenting part with ruptured membranes, polyhydramnios, multiparity, a

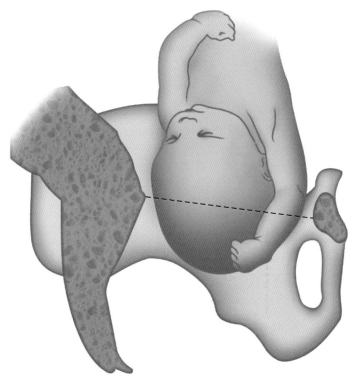

FIGURE 27-1. Compound presentation: head and hand.

contracted pelvis, pelvic masses, and twins. It is also more common with inductions of labor involving floating presenting parts. Another predisposing factor is external cephalic version. During the process of external version, a fetal limb (commonly the hand–arm, but occasionally the foot) can become "trapped" before the fetal head and thus become the presenting part when labor ensues.

Diagnosis

Diagnosis is made by vaginal examination, and in many cases, the condition is not noted until labor is well advanced and the cervix is fully dilated.

The condition is suspected when:

1. There is delay of progress in the active phase of labor
2. Engagement fails to occur
3. The fetal head remains high and deviated from the midline during labor, especially after the membranes rupture

Prognosis

In the absence of complications and with conservative management, the results should be no worse than with other presentations.

Mechanism of Labor

The mechanism of labor is that of the main presenting part. Because the diameter is increased, the chance of arrested progress is greater. In many cases, labor is not obstructed, and the leading part is brought down to the outlet. If dystocia occurs, the baby remains high, and operative treatment is needed.

MANAGEMENT OF COMPOUND PRESENTATIONS

The best treatment for compound presentations (in the absence of complications such as prolapse of the cord) is masterful inactivity.

Progressing Case

In most cases, as the cervix becomes fully dilated and the presenting part descends, the prolapsed arm or leg rises out of the pelvis, allowing labor to proceed normally. Rarely, the baby might also deliver with the arm or hand alongside the head. Hence, as long as progress is being made, there should be no interference.

Arrest of Progress

1. *Reposition of the prolapsed part*: In a normal pelvis, if progress is arrested, the arm or leg should be replaced, under anesthesia, and the head pushed into the pelvis. This is done by gently pushing the small part upward into the uterine cavity while simultaneously applying fundal pressure to effect descent of the vertex or breech. If the head is very low in the pelvis and the cervix is fully dilated, the use of a vacuum pump can be attempted
2. *Cesarean section*: If there is cephalopelvic disproportion, reposition is not feasible or is unsuccessful, or there is some other condition that militates against vaginal delivery, cesarean section should be performed

3. *Internal podalic version and extraction*: This procedure carries with it the danger of uterine rupture and fetal death. Hence, it should not be used in the management of compound presentations

Prolapse of the Cord

In 13 to 23 percent of cases, the compound presentation is complicated by prolapse of the umbilical cord. This then becomes the major and urgent problem, and treatment is directed primarily to it (see Chapter 28).

COMPLICATED LABOR

The Umbilical Cord

Hadeel Alenezi
Darine El-Chaâr

NORMAL UMBILICAL CORD

The umbilical cord is the lifeline that connects the fetus to the placenta providing life support through passage of nutrients, oxygen, and waste products to and from the fetus. It consists of three vessels, two arteries, and a vein, running in a spiral arrangement with a length of about 50 to 60 cm at term. It is lined on the inside with the thick myxomatous Wharton jelly and covered on the outside by a single layer of amnion providing protection to the cord from direct compression, kinking, and traction. The circulation in the umbilical cord is the reverse of the adult in that the vein carries the oxygenated blood to the fetus, and the arteries bring venous blood back to the placenta. Normally, the cord inserts into the center of the placenta.

Cords have been reported to measure as short as 0 cm and as long as 104 cm. It appears that the length of the umbilical cord is determined at least partly by the amount of amniotic fluid present in the first and second trimesters of pregnancy and on the mobility of the fetus. If there is oligohydramnios, amniotic bands, or limitation of fetal movement for any reason, the umbilical cord will not develop to an average length. A short cord may result in delay in descent of the fetus, fetal distress, and separation of the placenta from the wall of the uterus, inversion of the uterus, and rupture leading to hemorrhage and possible fetal exsanguination. On the other hand, a long cord is subject to entanglement, knotting, encirclement of the fetus, and prolapse.

When the cord is absent, the fetus is attached directly to the placenta at the umbilicus. Body stalk anomaly is seen accompanying the absent cord. Amniotic band syndrome is associated with the pathogenesis.

UMBILICAL CORD COILING ABNORMALITIES

Umbilical cord has characteristic screw-shaped coils with average of 11 loops or turns along its length. The coiling level can be objectively presented by the umbilical coiling index (UCI), which is the number of coils in the cord divided by cord length in cm. It is referred to as hypocoiled if the UCI is below the 10th percentile and hypercoiled if it is above 90th percentile. It is thought that cord coiling plays a role in protecting the umbilical cord from external pressure such as stretching, tension, and entanglement. There is a strong association between UCI and adverse pregnancy outcome including intrauterine growth restriction. Both hypocoiled and hypercoiled cords were associated with increased risk of preterm birth, need for intervention delivery for nonreassuring fetal heart rate, and meconium-stained amniotic fluid. There is a strong association between hypercoiled cord with intrauterine demise.

Single Umbilical Artery (SUA)

SUA is a variation in the umbilical cord anatomy in which there is only one umbilical artery. It is the most common abnormality of the umbilical cord and is found in 0.5 percent of pregnancies, and can be detected on ultrasound (Fig. 28-1). It may be an isolated finding or associated with chromosomal and structural abnormalities. It is more common in twin pregnancies with reported incidence of 1.7 percent of twins at 17 to 22 weeks of gestation. Risk factors associated with SUA include extreme of maternal age and maternal smoking, diabetes, hypertension, and seizure disorder. Fetuses with SUA are at increased risk of adverse pregnancy outcome such as preterm birth, perinatal mortality, and growth restriction. In isolated SUA, there is a fivefold increased risk of preterm birth and an 11-fold increased risk of fetal growth restriction. In nonisolated SUA, perinatal morbidity and mortality are increased and depend on the underlying anomalies.

Aneurysm and Varix

Aneurysm and varix are focal dilatation of the umbilical artery and vein, respectively. It is a rare complication that accounts for 4 percent of umbilical cord abnormalities. An umbilical vein varix is present if the vein measures more than 9 mm in diameter. This is usually seen in the intra-abdominal portion of the vein. Umbilical vein dilatation may be the first manifestation of increased venous pressure and should prompt a workup for other signs and possible etiologies. An umbilical artery aneurysm is seen near the placental end of the cord. Pulsed Doppler will confirm its arterial origin. If other anomalies are present, trisomy 18 is common. Both umbilical artery and vein aneurysms are associated with interruption of the umbilical cord flow, fetal compromise, and death. Venous compromise is a result of thrombosis. Umbilical artery aneurysms that expand can compress the umbilical vein, leading to hypoxia and death. Given the rarity of these lesions, the optimum management of affected pregnancies are unknown. Fetal surveillance with nonstress testing and ultrasound have been suggested because of reported risk of fetal demise.

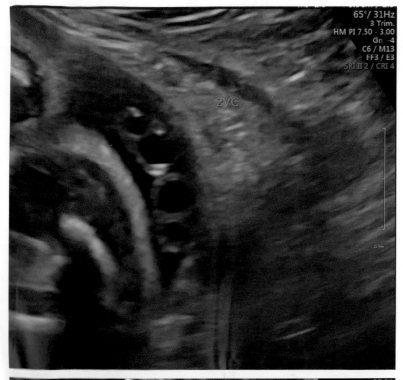

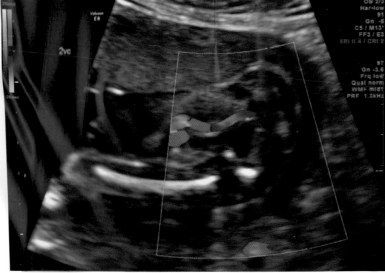

FIGURE 28-1. Two-vessel cord identified or single umbilical artery on ultrasound by 2-D views and colour Doppler.

Umbilical Cord Cyst

There is a 2 percent prevalence of umbilical cord cyst. They may be true cysts or pseudocysts. Most often these are transient finding in the first trimester. If they are transient, expectant management is appropriate because they have resolved and are not predictive of adverse pregnancy outcome. Pseudocysts in the second and third trimester are more common than true cysts. The detection of pseudocyst should prompt detailed anatomy ultrasound assessment and fetal chromosomal analysis. They may be associated with trisomy 13 and 18, and they have a poorer prognosis if they are multiple.

CORD INSERTION SITE ABNORMALITIES

Velamentous Cord Insertion

In this case, the vessels of the cord break up into branches before reaching the placenta so that the cord inserts into the membranes rather than the placental disc. The result is that large vessels course under the membrane and are unprotected by Wharton jelly. This is associated with fetal growth abnormalities, cord separation, and fetal bleeding, resulting in fetal death and retained placenta.

Vasa Previa

In this situation, the velamentous vessels lie over the cervix in front of the presenting part. Rupture happens when the membranes rupture during or before labor. This leads to fetal bleeding, which can be fatal within a few minutes. The diagnosis can be made by ultrasound. These patients do not have any symptoms; therefore, a high index of suspicion is required. Vasa previa is more common but not exclusive to low-lying placentas with velamentous cord insertion. Color Doppler can be used to demonstrate the umbilical vessels crossing the cervical os. When this diagnosis is made, preterm delivery by cesarean section is advised at about 34 weeks' gestation because of the high fetal death rate with rupture of membranes in this situation.

NUCHAL CORD

The most common variety of cord entanglement is the umbilical cord around the fetal neck. As many as nine loops of cord around the neck have been reported. A single loop of cord is present in 21 percent of deliveries.

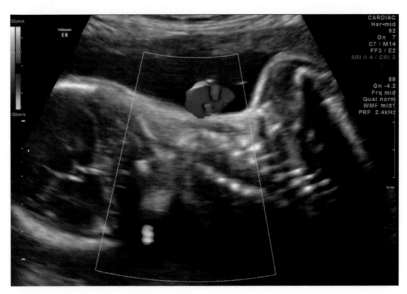

FIGURE 28-2. Nuchal cord on ultrasound.

The overall reported incidence of nuchal cord was 6 percent at 20 weeks of gestation and 29 percent at 42 weeks. The presence or absence of a nuchal cord can be determined by color Doppler ultrasound imaging (Fig. 28-2). It is unclear if nuchal cord is associated with a statistically increased risk of perinatal adverse outcome. A positive relationship has been found in some studies between nuchal cords and fetal demise, impaired fetal growth, meconium in the amniotic fluid, abnormal fetal heart rate, operative delivery, umbilical artery acidemia, and neurodevelopmental abnormalities.

CORD ENTANGLEMENT

Cord entanglement is most common in monoamniotic twins. The stillbirth rate is 50 percent. Delivery is recommended by cesarean section at 33 to 34 weeks' gestation.

KNOTS OF THE UMBILICAL CORD

True Knot

Occasionally, a true knot of the umbilical cord is noted after delivery. They occur in less than 1 percent and are generally single and loose.

This complication can occur when there is a long cord, large amounts of amniotic fluid, a small infant, or an overactive fetus or as a result of external version. In many instances, the knot is formed when a loop of cord is slipped over the infant's head or shoulders during delivery. Rarely is the knot pulled tightly enough to cause the death of the fetus from restriction of the circulation in the cord. The umbilical vessels, protected by the thick myxomatous Wharton jelly, are rarely occluded completely. The fetal mortality rate was reported to be more than fourfold higher in pregnancies complicated with true knot of the umbilical cord. In these cases, there is a flattening or dissipation of Wharton jelly and venous congestion distal to the knot, as well as partially or completely occlusive vascular thrombi.

False Knot

The blood vessels are longer than the cord. Often, they are folded on themselves and produce nodulations on the surface of the cord. These have been termed false knots and are not associated with adverse fetal outcome.

PROLAPSE OF THE UMBILICAL CORD

In this situation, the umbilical cord lies beside or below the presenting part. Although an infrequent complication (0.3-0.6%), its significance is disproportionately great because of the high fetal mortality rate. Compression of the umbilical cord between the presenting part and the maternal pelvis reduces or cuts off the blood supply to the fetus and, if uncorrected, leads to death of the fetus.

Classification of Prolapsed Cord

1. Umbilical cord presentation (funic presentation): The cord is seen on ultrasound or palpated on pelvic examination below the fetal presenting part. The fetal membranes are intact
2. Umbilical cord prolapse: The membranes are ruptured, and the cord is palpated below the fetal presenting part (Fig. 28-3)
3. Occult cord prolapse: The cord is not palpable but is being compressed by the presenting part. This diagnosis can only be made during cesarean section

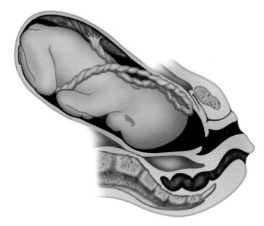

A. Cord prolapsed at the inlet.

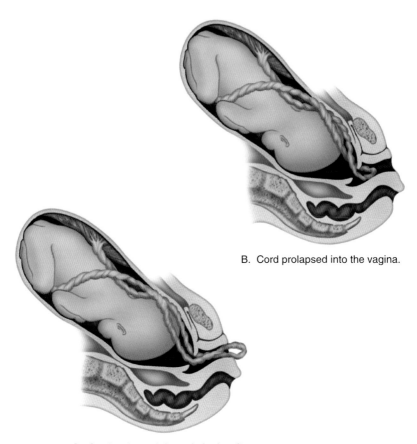

B. Cord prolapsed into the vagina.

C. Cord prolapsed through the introitus.

FIGURE 28-3. **Prolapsed umbilical cord.** (A) Inlet, (B) Vagina, (C) Introitus.

Risk Factors for Cord Prolapse

Malpresentation is the most commonly present risk factor for cord prolapse. Footling breech presentation is the presentation with the highest incidence of cord prolapse. Prematurity and the second twin are other fetal risk factors for cord prolapse. Maternal factors include a narrow pelvis, preventing descent of the fetal presenting part and multiparity. A long cord, a low-lying placenta, and polyhydramnios also increase the risk of cord prolapse. Many obstetric interventions can be associated with cord prolapse. The most common intervention is artificial rupture of membranes with a presenting part that is not fixed in the pelvis. Any intervention that could dislodge the presenting part, including insertion of a scalp electrode, insertion of an intrauterine pressure catheter, scalp pH sampling, manual fetal rotation, or vacuum or forceps delivery, may lead to cord prolapse if the presenting part is lifted from the pelvis.

Signs of Cord Prolapse

The first sign of cord prolapse is most often bradycardia or prolonged variable decelerations. When these occur, a digital examination should be performed to rule out cord prolapse. The only other presentation is feeling or seeing the cord in the vagina or protruding out of the introitus.

Management of Cord Prolapse

The outcome of cord prolapse is related to the length of time between the cord prolapse and delivery. In most cases, the safest and most rapid method of delivery is a cesarean section.

While preparing for a cesarean section, the following temporary measures may be appropriate:

1. Maternal Trendelenburg or knee–chest positioning and manual disimpaction of the fetal head by manual pressure in the maternal vagina
2. Replacing the cord above the fetal presenting part. This is often very difficult because the woman is usually in labor and there is a risk of further compromising the cord circulation
3. Tocolysis
4. Vaginal delivery may be an option if the cervix is fully dilated. This may particularly be an option for a second twin.

COMPLICATED LABOR

UMBILICAL CORD DOPPLER

Umbilical cord Doppler is a noninvasive test of fetal well-being with the most research to support its use. Abnormalities of the Doppler indices are strongly associated with fetal hypoxia, acidosis, and adverse perinatal outcome. It is most often found to be abnormal in fetus with IUGR in the early third trimester. Normally, there is forward flow in the umbilical artery throughout the fetal cardiac cycle. The ratio of the peak systolic flow to the diastolic flow of >3.0 or a resistance index (RI) >0.6 at ≥28 weeks of gestation is the threshold used to best identify pregnancies at high risk of adverse outcome. Absent end-diastolic flow (AEDF) and reverse end-diastolic flow (REDF) are associated with IUGR, oligohydramnios, and stillbirth. REDF in the umbilical artery is associated with fetal demise in 1 to 7 days. In pregnancies complicated by fetal growth restriction, delivery rather than expectant management in the setting of AEDF at ≥34 weeks' gestation and REDF at ≥32 weeks' gestation is recommended.

SELECTED READING

Clare NM, Hayashi R, Khodr G: Intrauterine death from umbilical cord hematoma. Arch Pathol Lab Med 103:46, 1979

Hasegawa J: Ultrasound screening of umbilical cord abnormalities and delivery management. Placenta 62:66-78, 2018

Hayes DJL, Warland J, Parast MM, et al: Umbilical cord characteristics and their association with adverse pregnancy outcomes: A systematic review and meta-analysis. PLoS One 15:e0239630, 2020

Katz Z, Lancet M, Borenstein R: Management of labor with umbilical cord prolapse. Am J Obstet Gynecol 142:239, 1982

CHAPTER 29

Multiple Gestation

Karen M. Fung-Kee-Fung
Hadeel Alenezi

INCIDENCE

Twin pregnancies account for 2 to 4 percent of total live births, with variable prevalence worldwide. The rate of twin gestation and higher-order multiples has dramatically increased over the last four decades in nearly all countries. In the United States, for example, the rate rose 76 percent from 1980 to 2009 (from 18.9 to 33.2 per 1000), was generally stable from 2009 through 2012, and then rose for 2013 and 2014; the 2014 rate of 33.9 was the highest ever reported. At the same time, a rise in twinning rate was also evident among other developed countries such as France, Germany, Japan, and South Korea. Of all countries, the highest rates were reported in Nigeria and the lowest in Japan. The significance of these trends in population statistics lies in the potential to negatively influence both perinatal morbidity and mortality rates. Fortunately, these demographics appear to be changing for the better with triplets and higher-order multiple births demonstrating a sharp decline of 52 percent from the 1998 peak (193.5 per 1000 live births). More recently, this declining trend is apparent in twin births as well. In 2018, a twin birth rate of 32.6 twins per 1000 births was noted, a 2 percent decline from the 2017 rate of 33.3 per 1000. A similar decline was also observed in the United Kingdom. This is undoubtedly related to improved control of reproductive cycles and advances in assistive reproductive technology (ART) techniques along with the increasing use of elective single embryo transfer. Although the precise etiology of multiple pregnancy is unknown in most cases, the rise in twinning rate has been attributed to the growing and liberal use of fertility-promoting treatments and technology and to delayed childbearing, implying an effect of advancing maternal age. Data from 2013 on ART showed that twin birth rates declined, with IVF accounting for no more than 16 percent. In contrast, methods other than IVF accounted for 20 percent of the twin birth rate. These methods include ovulation induction and intrauterine insemination (IUI) with superovulation. Variations are evident due to maternal age and ethnicity. In 2006, 20 percent of births to women 45 to 54 years were twins compared to 2 percent of births to women 20 to 24 years old.

The high twin birth rates carry a considerable resource implication on both the health care system and perinatal outcome. It has been estimated that the annual cost of caring for multiples born prematurely after ART is in excess of $1 billion annually or $52,000 per infant. Perinatal morbidity and mortality figures among multiples are also sobering. Population-based studies have reported stillbirth and neonatal mortality rates in twins in the order of 18 per 1000 births and 23 per 1000 birth, respectively, compared to 5 per 1000 births in singleton pregnancies (Table 29-1).

TABLE 29-1: RISK FOR TWINS AND HOM VERSUS SINGLETONS

	Singletons	Twins	HOM
Mortality Rate		5-7 times higher	10-12 times higher
GA at Delivery	39-40 weeks	35.8-36 weeks	32.5-34 weeks
RDS	60%	70%	15% higher (75%)
Cerebral Palsy	1.6%	7.4%	28%

HOM, higher order multiples; GA, gestational Age; RDS, respiratory distress syndrome

Shinwell ES et al; Neonatology 2008, Health Canada

Survival rates among multiples are also not uniformly distributed, and the effect of chorionicity on survival is profound (Table 29-2). Rates of fetal loss are substantially higher in monochorionic twins (44.4 in 1000 stillbirth rates) than in dichorionic twins (12.2 in 1000 births; relative risk [RR], 3.6) and neonatal losses (32.4 in 1000 monochorionic vs. 21.4 in 1000 dichorionic; RR, 1.5) in dichorionic twins. The prospective risk of stillbirth is higher in monochorionic twins at all gestational ages and highest before 28 weeks of gestation. Survival rates decline dramatically as the number of fetal occupants of the uterus rises, and triplet loss rates of 93-203 per 1000 live births have been reported.

TYPES OF TWINS

In common vernacular, the term "identical" twins is often used by the lay public to refer to twins who possess the same physical characteristics, are often indistinguishable, and are of the same sex. Conversely, the term

TABLE 29-2: EFFECT OF CHORIONICITY ON SURVIVAL

	Stillbirths/ 1000 births	Neonatal Deaths	Loss Rates <24 wks
Twins Overall	18	23	10.5%
Dichorionic Twins	12.2	21.4	2%
Monochorionic Twins	44.4	32.4	12%

Glinianaia SV, Obeysekera MA, Sturgiss S, Bell R: Stillbirth and neonatal mortality in monochorionic and dichorionic twins: A population-based study. Hum Reprod 26:2549-2557, 2011

Glinianaia SV, Rankin J, Wright C, Sturgiss SN, Renwick M: Northern Region Perinatal Mortality Survey Steering Group. A multiple pregnancy register in the north of England. Twin Res 5:436-439, 2002 "fraternal" twins are assumed to be dissimilar in appearance and may be of dissimilar or concordant sex. In modern usage and in the medical lexicon, the more precise, scientific terms "monozygotic" and "dizygotic" twins are generally used, referring to the mechanism of origin of the different types of twins and inferring the degree of genetic similarity between the individuals. Monozygotic twins develop when one ovum is fertilized by a single sperm and the developing embryo divides, resulting in two genetically identical individuals of the same sex. Dizygotic twins arise when two ova are fertilized by two separate sperm, which then implanted independently in the uterus. They share the same type of genetic relationship as non-twin siblings (Fig. 29-1).

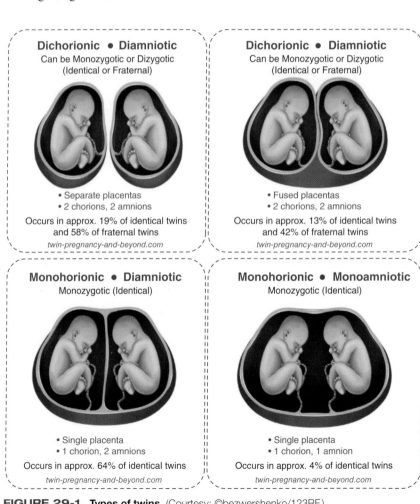

Dichorionic • Diamniotic
Can be Monozygotic or Dizygotic
(Identical or Fraternal)

• Separate placentas
• 2 chorions, 2 amnions
Occurs in approx. 19% of identical twins
and 58% of fraternal twins
twin-pregnancy-and-beyond.com

Dichorionic • Diamniotic
Can be Monozygotic or Dizygotic
(Identical or Fraternal)

• Fused placentas
• 2 chorions, 2 amnions
Occurs in approx. 13% of identical twins
and 42% of fraternal twins
twin-pregnancy-and-beyond.com

Monohorionic • Diamniotic
Monozygotic (Identical)

• Single placenta
• 1 chorion, 2 amnions
Occurs in approx. 64% of identical twins
twin-pregnancy-and-beyond.com

Monohorionic • Monoamniotic
Monozygotic (Identical)

• Single placenta
• 1 chorion, 1 amnion
Occurs in approx. 4% of identical twins
twin-pregnancy-and-beyond.com

FIGURE 29-1. Types of twins. (Courtesy: ©bezwershenko/123RF.)

The true incidence of zygosity can be established following careful assignment of sex, histological examination of the placenta and membranes, and detailed DNA analysis of the co-twins. This is beyond the scope of standard care offered in most institutions. In centers where the zygosity of twins was established by these methods, the frequency of dizygotic twins was found to be 71 percent and monozygotic twins was 29 percent. Dizygotic twins can occur due to increased concentrations of follicle stimulating hormone (FSH) and therefore it is influenced by maternal age (ovarian hyperstimulation due to increased gonadotropins between the age of 35 and 39 years old), ethnicity (black ethnicity), family history, parity, and use of ovulation-induction methods and ART. The frequency of monozygotic twinning remains independent of maternal age, ethnicity, family history, and parity and is constant over the world. Recent evidence suggests that use of ART may play a role in increasing monozygosity. This has been attributed to in vitro culture environment and extended culture duration and manipulation of zona pellucida in intracytoplasmic sperm injection (ICSI).

Confirmation of zygosity can be achieved through DNA and human leukocyte antigen testing of the fetuses, but this is rarely carried out in routine practice because the prospective knowledge of zygosity is unlikely to influence perinatal outcome. In same-sex twin pairs with dichorionic placentation, postnatal determination of zygosity can be of importance for future consideration of organ transplantation compatibility and to evaluate inheritance of specific disease states.

Dizygotic Twins. Two fetuses develop from the fertilization of two ova liberated during the same menstrual cycle. Each twin has his/her own placenta, chorion, and amniotic sac. When the ova are implanted near each other, the placenta may seem to be fused; however, the circulations remain completely separate. The offspring develop to become genetically distinct individuals. They may be of different sexes and sometimes look entirely dissimilar.

Monozygotic Twins. Two fetuses that have developed from fertilization of a single ovum by a single sperm with complete cleavage of blastodermic vesicle, therefore resulting into two individuals arising from the same germ plasm. The offspring are of same sex and appearance and are genetically identical.

CHORIONICITY

Chorionicity denotes the type of placentation. Twin placentae can be broadly classified into monochorionic (one placenta) and dichorionic (two placentae) (see Figure 29-2). The timing of the cleavage of the zygote or inner cell mass influences placentation and ultimately morbidity in twins. Factors that may influence timing are unknown. One remarkable aspect of ART is that, for yet unknown reasons, blastocysts/embryos often duplicate to form monochorionic twins.

Chorionicity of Dizygotic Twins

By virtue of their separate placental masses, dizygous twins exhibit obligate dichorionic placentation with two amions (dichorionic, diamniotic).

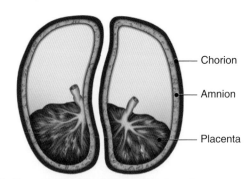

Chorion

Amnion

Placenta

A. Separate dichorionic diamniotic placentae.

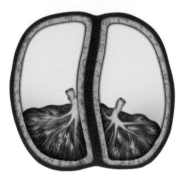

B. Fused dichorionic diamniotic placentae.

FIGURE 29-2. **Types of twin chorionicity.**

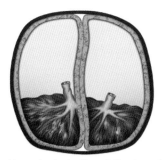

C. Monochorionic diamniotic placentae.

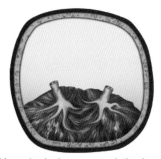

D. Monochorionic monoamniotic placentae.

FIGURE 29-2. (*Continued*)

Chorionicity of Monozygotic Twins

Chorionicity of monozygotic twins is determined by the timing of cleavage of the zygote. The exact mechanism underlying cleavage process is yet to be understood. Placental and vascular sharing in monozygous twins contributes to the high morbidity figures seen compared to dichorionic twins.

Dichorionic/Diamniotic
This occurs in 70 percent of all monozygous twins. The division of a single fertilized ovum occurs early in gestation, at the blastomere stage, 2 to 3 days after fertilization. Separate embryos develop, indistinguishable at birth from dizygous twins. Each twin has his/her own placenta, chorion, and amniotic sac. The latter may be separate or fused depending on the site of implantation.

Monochorionic/Diamniotic
This occurs in 25 percent of all monozygous twins. The division occurs at the blastocyst stage between day 4 and 6 after fertilization. The inner cell mass divides into two. The placenta has one chorion but two amnions. Each twin lies in his/her own amniotic sac.

Monochorionic/Monoamniotic

This occurs in 1 to 2 percent of all monozygous twins. The division occurs in the primitive germ disc at 7 to 13 days after fertilization. Both amnion and chorion were formed before cleavage. The twins lie in the same amniotic sac.

Conjoined Twins. A rare subset of monochorionic monoamniotic twins in which the division occurred later than day 13 postfertilization, after the primitive streak of the embryo has appeared and the cells of the germ disc have assumed an axial arrangement. Complete separation of the germ disc does not occur.

PRENATAL DIAGNOSIS OF MULTIPLE PREGNANCY

Ultrasound is a safe and reliable diagnostic modality for confirmation of twin pregnancy. Its role in the management of twin pregnancies from the first trimester to the delivery of the second twin is pervasive and indispensable. Established guidelines vary worldwide and are not uniformly followed. For example, the American College of Obstetricians and Gynecologists recommend ultrasound examination for all pregnant women at 18 to 22 weeks' gestation. In resource-limited geographical areas, a significant number of twin pregnancies may not be recognized until the third trimester or at the time of delivery.

Implementation of ultrasound in the care of women with twin pregnancies early in pregnancy is important for accurate determination of chorionicity and amniocity, which is critical in antenatal management. Most common clinical uses of ultrasound also include confirmation of gestational age, diagnosis of structural anomalies, as well as cervical length assessment to identify twins at significantly increased risk of preterm birth. Fetal growth and amniotic fluid assessment and screening for inter-twin discordance in growth or amniotic fluid (such as occurs in twin-to-twin transfusion syndrome), is important because studies have shown an association with increased mortality and morbidity. Ultrasound has proven reliable and accurate in identifying twins with these abnormalities, aiding in establishing the most appropriate management in terms of fetal surveillance or intervention. Fetal presentation and placental location affect the choice of delivery route and ultrasound confirmation of the presenting part and placental location during the antepartum and intrapartum periods is fundamental to appropriate delivery planning.

SPECIAL COMPLICATIONS OF MONOCHORIONIC TWINS

Gross examination of a single monochorionic placental disc will reveal vascular connections between the cord vessels of each fetus traveling on the surface of the placenta. These anastomoses can be arterio-venous (AV), areterio-aterial (AA) or veno-venous in nature. The specific arrangement of vascular sharing in monochorionic twins can give rise to several unique conditions and the clinical spectrum of these conditions is governed by the number, type, and caliber of these anastomoses. Fortunately, these vascular connections are usually balanced by bidirectional blood flow between the fetuses. The development of unbalanced, and often unidirectional anastomoses in some monochorionic twin pairs can give rise to hemodynamic derangements with unique clinical features and patterns that can adversely affect perinatal outcome in this subset of multiple gestations. Suspicion of any of these specialized conditions should prompt timely referral to a Fetal Medicine unit for definitive diagnosis and management.

Twin-to-Twin Transfusion Syndrome (TTTS)

This affects monochorionic twins, usually between 16- and 26-weeks' gestation. The basic pathophysiology is the existence of unbalanced, unidirectional anastomoses between the arteries of one twin (donor) and veins of the co-twin (recipient). Overtime, the donor twin becomes hypovolemic and oliguric, manifesting as oligohydramnios/anhydramnios ("stuck twin") on ultrasound. The co-twin, the recipient, responds to this by becoming progressively polyureic, manifesting polyhydramnios. This arrangement is coined "poly-oli syndrome" and is the hallmark of diagnosis of this condition on ultrasound (Fig. 29-3).

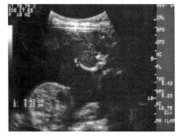

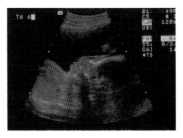

A. Twin pregnancy with poly-hydramnios in recipient twin (Lower Left of image) and oligohydramnios in donor twin (Upper Right) note: donor twin is suspended from anterior abdominal wall and not freely mobile due to low amniotic fluid.

B. Another case of TTTS in later pregnancy, demonstrating donor twin with oligohydramnios and amniotic membrane shrouding the fetal face (Stuck twin)

FIGURE 29-3. Poly-oli sequence "stuck twins."

COMPLICATED LABOR

This amniotic fluid discordance is defined as a deep vertical pocket (DVP) of >10 cm after 20 weeks, or >8 cm before 20 weeks, in the recipient twin and DVP <2 cm in the donor twin. Circulatory overload of the recipient twin can lead to cardiogenic compromise in the form of fetal hydrops, hypertrophic cardiomyopathy, or outflow tract obstruction. In contrast, prolonged oligo- or anhydramnios in the donor twin may be lethal due to the development of pulmonary hypoplasia. Risk of preterm labor is increased, usually secondary to overdistension of the uterus from the poly-hydramnios. The natural history of this disorder is known; perinatal loss of one or both fetuses may be as high as 80 to 90 percent after second trimester diagnosis, in the absence of fetal treatment.

Management strategies have included: (1) fetoscopic laser coagulation of anastomotic vessels, (2) serial amnioreduction, and (3) septostomy. Laser therapy is the preferred treatment because it directly addresses the pathophysiology behind this condition and has been found in randomized controlled trials to lead to improved short-term neurologic outcome in survivors. In a recent metanalysis, survival of at least one twin occurred in 87 percent of stage I, 85 percent of stage II, 81 percent of stage III, and 82 percent of stage IV TTTS. Studies evaluating neurodevelopmental outcome in cases treated with laser showed no significant difference in incidence of neurological morbidity at birth between donors and recipients with overall risk post-laser therapy not significantly different from the baseline risk in monochorionic twins without TTTS, matched for gestational age. In recent metanalysis assessing neurological outcome by stage of TTTS, the morbidity for stage I, II, III, and IV was 1.5, 5.2, 6.7, and 5.9 percent, respectively.

Twin Anemia-Polycythemia Sequence (TAPS)

The presence of arteriovenous anastomoses does not always commit the pregnancy to development of TTTS. Smaller AV connections within the placenta may, overtime, result in a net transfusion of blood between the fetuses such that one fetus manifests signs of severe anemia while the co-twin displays evidence of polycythemia (Fig. 29-4). This situation presents spontaneously in about 5 percent of monochorionic twins and up to 11 to 14 percent of monochorionic twins following laser therapy for TTTS. Diagnosis of this condition rests on interrogation of the peak systolic velocity in the middle cerebral artery on Doppler examination. Fetal anemia, with resulting hypoviscosity, results in increased velocity of blood through the middle cerebral artery during systole whereas hyperviscous blood with

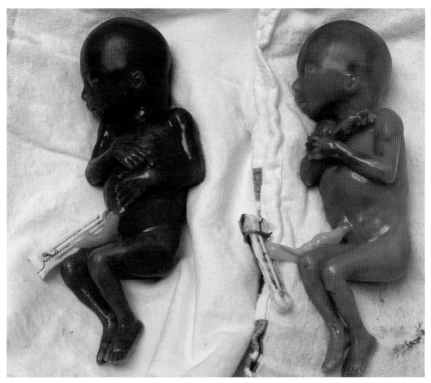

FIGURE 29-4. Monochorionic pregnancy complicated by TAPS: polycythemic fetus on left and anemic fetus on right.

higher hematocrit will travel at a slower velocity through this vessel. Doppler velocimetry can detect these disparities with a 12 percent false-positive rate. Diagnostic criteria for fetal anemia TAPS include peak systolic velocity of ≥1.5 multiples of the median (MoM) in the anemic fetus and <1.0 MOM in the polycythemic fetus or a delta MOM of 0.5 MOM, between the fetuses. On ultrasonography a differential placental appearance between the twins can also be seen with the anemic fetus demonstrating a more hyperechoic, "whitened" appearance and a hypoechoic appearance of the placental fraction dedicated to the polycythemic fetus (Fig. 29-5). Despite prenatal diagnosis of this condition, optimal management remains uncertain and various therapies, including expectant management, laser coagulation of small anastomotic vessels, intrauterine transfusion of the anemic fetus, and intrauterine transfusion with partial exchange transfusion of the polycythemic fetus, are therapeutic options.

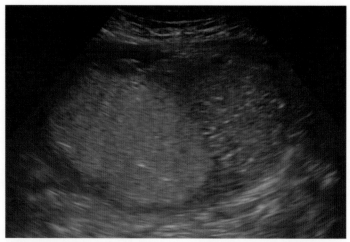

FIGURE 29-5. Sonographic appearance of TAPS placenta demonstrating placental fraction of anemic fetus on left ("whitened" appearance) and polycythemic fetus on the right (hypoechoic appearance).

Twin Reversed Arterial Perfusion (TRAP) Sequence

Twin reversed arterial perfusion (TRAP) sequence, or "acardiac twin" is a rare and complex malformation with a reported prevalence of at least one in 35,000 pregnancies. It occurs following early demise of one twin in the monochorionic pair and altered flow dynamics between the fetuses through a shared circulation. In this arrangement, the surviving twin (pump twin) maintains a normal fetal circulation but a portion of its cardiac output travels through one or more A-A anastomoses to the demised co-twin with retrograde perfusion via the umbilical arteries and into the systemic circulation of the acardiac twin. This retrograde perfusion of deoxygenated blood from umbilical artery of the normal "pump"/donor twin toward the "perfused"/anomalous twin contributes to the development of a broad spectrum of structural abnormalities in the anomalous, acardiac twin (Fig. 29-6).

The anomalous ("perfused") twin will have rudimentary or absent cardiac structures and is dependent on the pump twin's circulation. The lower half of the acardiac twin is believed to receive a preferential share from the pump twin's circulatory support resulting in a better development of lower structures in the fetus, such as abdomen, pelvis, and lower extremities which, nevertheless, often demonstrates various degrees of maldevelopment. Upper limb reduction defects in the perfused fetus are generally more severe (Fig. 29-7). The pump twin has to perfuse its own circulation

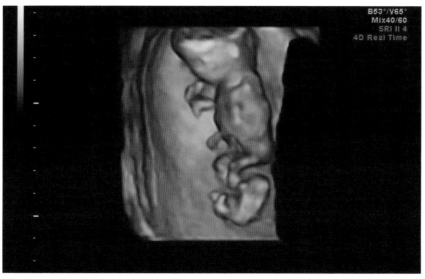

FIGURE 29-6. 3D sonographic image of TRAP pregnancy, illustrating larger pump twin and smaller parasitic perfused twin.

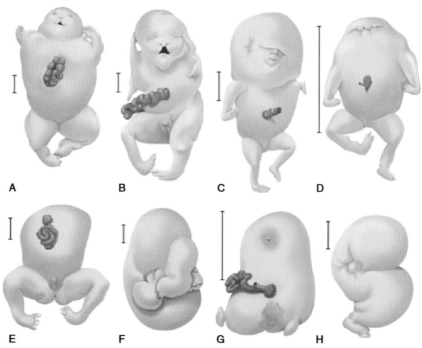

FIGURE 29-7. Spectrum of TRAP anomalies. (Reproduced with permission from Diana W. B, M. C Timothy, M E. D'Alton, F.D Malone, Fetology: Diagnosis and Management of the Fetal Patient, 2nd ed., McGraw Hill Education.)

as well as that of acardiac twin and this results in hemodynamic burden and increased risk for high-output heart failure. Fetal cardiac failure may manifest as cardiomegaly, polyhydramnios, ascites, hydrops fetalis, and preterm birth. Conservative management has been recommended when the perfused twin's fetal mass is <30 percent of the pump twin. Fetal therapy is offered when the perfused twin is larger or rapidly growing or has developed hydrops. Treatment involves interruptions of the vascular communication between twins, usually through cord occlusion or intrafetal radiofrequency ablation of blood flow to the perfused twin. In approximately 33 percent of cases, spontaneous death of the perfused twin will occur prior to the time of planned fetal intervention at 16 to 18 weeks. The mortality rate for the perfused twin is 100 percent, and mortality figures suggest that up to 50 percent of the normal "pump" twins survive. Neurodevelopmental disability has been reported in survivors. Recent evidence suggests that treatment prior to 16 weeks' gestation was associated with a significantly lower rate of adverse outcome. A multicentered clinical trial, the "TRAPIST Trial," is ongoing, addressing the question of whether early, first trimester intervention in TRAP sequence of this condition improves outcome over later therapy (16-19 weeks).

Selective Intrauterine Growth Restriction (sIUGR)

"Fetal growth restriction (FGR)" is a term used to describe a fetus that has not reached its growth potential either due to fetal, placental, or maternal factors. Affected fetuses are at increased risk of adverse perinatal outcome. In twin pregnancy, a large inter-twin growth discordance and low fetal weight in one member of a twin pair is known as "selective" intrauterine growth restriction (sIUGR) or sFGR. Approximately 10 to 15 percent of monochorionic twins manifest this growth pattern, likely as a consequence of unequal placental sharing. The consequence of concern in sIUGR in monochorionic twins is the possibility of intrauterine fetal death of the smaller fetus, leading to either fetal demise of both twins (12% after in utero death of one twin in the monochorionic twin pair) or the concomitant risk of ischemic brain damage in the survivor (30%), secondary to hypovolemia and decreased brain perfusion following exsanguination into the dead or dying fetus through functional vascular anastomoses within the shared placenta. Dichorionic twins, by virtue of their separate placental circulations, may exhibit disparate fetal growth patterns; however, the consequences for these fetuses remain comparable to those of fetal growth restriction in singleton pregnancies.

Despite its recognition as a clinical condition, controversy exists with respect to the definition and diagnostic criteria of sIUGR. In an attempt to unify diagnostic criteria for sIUGR, recent expert consensus, using the Delphi procedure, concluded that in both monochorionic and diamniotic twins, estimated fetal weight (EFW) <3rd centile in one twin is sufficient to classify the pregnancy as having sIUGR. Additionally, diamniotic twins meet the diagnostic criteria if two of the contributory parameters are met (EFW <10th centile, EFW discordance >25% or umbilical artery pulsitility index [UA-PI] >95th centile) and in a monochorionic twin, a diagnosis is met if two of the four contributory parameters were met (EFW< 10th centile, abdominal circumference <10th centile, EFW discordance >25% or UA-PI >95th centile).

Following diagnosis of this condition, three types of sIUGR have been identified, characterized by the pattern of arterial flow in the umbilical cord of the smaller fetus on Doppler ultrasound examination. Type-I displays normal forward flow in the umbilical artery of the affected twin throughout systole and diastole, Type-II shows persistently absent or reversed umbilical artery flow, and Type-III demonstrates intermittently absent end diastolic flow. Fetal outcome deteriorates with increasing type. Fetal therapy by cord occlusion or laser photocoagulation of communicating vessels is reserved for advanced disease (Type I or III), and delivery is usually accomplished before term. Type-1 sIUGR has generally good outcome with a progression rate of up to 26 percent, Type-II sIUGR has the least favorable outcome with progression rate as high as 90 percent. Type-III sIUGR has higher risk of sudden intrauterine demise or acute TTTS due to variable A-A anastomoses. Recent meta-analysis compared outcome following expectant management, fetoscopic laser photocoagulation, and selective termination. In Type-I sIUGR, the risk of co-twin demise is 3.1, 16.7, and 1 percent following expectant management, laser therapy, and selective termination, respectively. In Type-II, 16.6, 44.3, and 5 percent of co-twins, respectively, experienced in utero death following these treatments. On the other hand, in Type-III sIUGR, the risk of co-twin demise after these treatments was 13.2, 32.9, and 0 percent, respectively. There are no randomized control trials to guide the timing of delivery. Detailed and though counseling, taking into account the risk of still birth and co-twin morbidity, should guide the decision. Consider early delivery after a course of steroid after 26 weeks' gestation in cases of severe sIUGR.

Monoamniotic Twins

Monoamniotic twins occur in approximately 1-2 percent of monochorionic twins. Because the fetuses are not separated by membranes, this

COMPLICATED LABOR

environment carries with it the possibility of knotting, tangling, or strangulation of the umbilical cords. The resultant anoxia may lead to fetal death. In the absence of prenatal diagnosis of this condition and intense fetal surveillance, the prognosis for monoamniotic twins has been historically poor, with only 50 percent double survival of both twins. The high mortality rate was previously attributed to cord entanglement and strangulation; however, most recent evidence suggests other conditions, such as acute feto-fetal transfusion and congenital anomalies may contribute to the high loss rate. Routine use of antenatal ultrasound has led to earlier diagnosis of this condition, allowing for more informed parental counseling and management planning, including intensive fetal monitoring and early, elective delivery and with that, improved outcomes. The finding of entangled umbilical cords is the sine que non, of diagnosis, found in almost all cases on antenatal ultrasound. Fetal surveillance remains problematic, however, because entangled cords may strangulate at any time during the pregnancy. Modern management of this condition consists of intense, multimodality methods of fetal assessment, including (1) biophysical profile testing on ultrasound, and (2) frequent use of nonstress testing to rule out signs of cord compression and fetal compromise. Early delivery by cesarean section is carried out ($\geq$32 weeks) after priming of the immature fetal lungs by administration of maternal glucocorticoids to accelerate lung maturity. With a policy of aggressive fetal surveillance and early operative delivery by cesarean section at 32 to 33 weeks, the survival rates in this condition have been improved above that usually quoted in early literature (from 70% to less than 15%). In a recent retrospective series study by Van Mieghem et al, with close fetal surveillance starting from 26 to 28 weeks of gestation, the reported risk of intrauterine fetal death before 33 weeks' gestation was extremely low and risk of neonatal death resulting from prematurity was less than 2 percent.

CONJOINED TWINS

Conjoined twins are a rare type of monoamniotic twinning in which the embryonic disc has failed to split completely resulting in two fetuses with complex fusion anomalies with shared organs and structures (Fig. 29-8). It is estimated to occur in one in 50,000 to 100,000 births. Approximately 70 percent are female. The precise etiology is not known, but the same influences are responsible as those that cause monozygotic twinning. The basic defect is thought to be an incomplete, delayed fission of the inner cell mass, which takes place after the 14 days after fertilization.

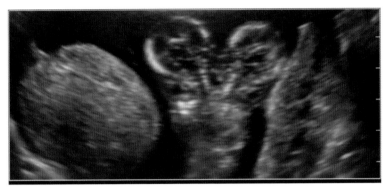

FIGURE 29-8. Dicephalus conjoined twins.

Classification

Classification of conjoined twins is based on the site of fusion between body parts. The numerous phenotypes fall into two main categories: (1) diplopagus (duplicatas completa) where there is equal or nearly equal and symmetrical duplication of structures, and (2) heteropagus (duplicatas incompleta). In this group, only part of the anatomic structure of the fetus is duplicated.

Diagnosis

Before the use of ultrasonography in routine obstetric care, it was rare for conjoined twins to be discovered before the time of delivery. Most cases were diagnosed only in the second stage of labor, when obstructed labor was encountered had taken place. Grayscale and color Doppler ultrasound has changed that. Antenatal diagnosis of conjoined twins has been made as early as 7 weeks by endovaginal sonography. False-positive diagnoses are possible before 10 weeks because monoamniotic twins in a single sac can falsely appear conjoined.

The diagnosis should be suspected in the first trimester monoamniotic twin pregnancy when:

- Fetal poles are closely associated and do not change position with respect to each other
- Presence of single cardiac activity
- Inseparable fetal parts with no sign of separate movements

Early diagnosis with first trimester ultrasound is now the norm in developed countries with access to routine first trimester ultrasound.

This allows for more informed counselling. Given the low survival rates, significant morbidity and complex nature of this rare twin condition with need for radical surgical intervention required to separate these infants with shared body organs, most parents are offered, and often opt for, termination of pregnancy. Late diagnosis presents controversies in management. Successful vaginal delivery has been reported; however, it is associated with high risk of labor dystocia, uterine rupture, and fetal demise. For ongoing, prenatally diagnosed cases, delivery by elective cesarean section is carried out. Detailed ultrasound (with or without MRI) and assessment of these pregnancies in a fetal medicine center with expertise in postnatal medical and surgical management is standard of care.

Twins Discordant for Fetal Structural or Chromosomal Anomaly

Twin gestations are at higher risk of aneuploidy and structural anomalies compared to singleton pregnancies. Structural anomalies in monochorionic twins are twice as high as their dichorionic twin counterparts, especially for cardiac defects, neural tube and brain defects, and gastrointestinal and abdominal wall defects. Both members of the twin pair, whether monochorionic or dichorionic twins, may not be concordant for the anomaly. Along with twins that are discordant for structural anomalies, genetic or chromosomal discordance between twins can also occur. Several postzygotic events may arise in the early embryonic period that may give rise to both subtle differences, even among a monochorionic twin pair, such as "mirror image" differences or lateral asymmetry between the fetuses or major anomalies that are not shared by both fetuses. Even karyotypically identical monochorionic twins may have, on occasion, different phenotypes because of differences in allocation of blastomeres or other genetic or epigenetic phenomena. Selective reduction of the anomalous co-twin may be offered based on patient preference and local regulations and practices. Appropriate methodology relies on accurate assignment of chorionicity. Intracardiac administration of potassium chloride (KCl) or lidocaine is offered only in dichorionic twins, resulting in cardiac asystole in the anomalous fetus. This approach is contraindicated in monochorionic twin gestations because of the intertwin vascular anastomoses within the single placental bed, which could lead to passage of the feticidal agent into the unaffected fetus or exsanguination of the survivor into the dying, anomalous fetus. In these single-placental pregnancies, a surgical approach is often taken to completely occlude the umbilical cord vessels of the affected fetus, often using bipolar cord cauterization, laser cord coagulation, radiofrequency ablation, or fetoscopic cord occlusion. With these options, survival of the unaffected fetus of the twin pair after selective reduction in monochorionic twins is in the order of 70 to 80 percent.

OTHER PREGNANCY COMPLICATIONS SPECIFIC TO TWINS

Vanishing Twins

Early pregnancy loss or miscarriage is higher in multiple gestation compared to singleton pregnancies, with reported incidence as high as 21 percent. Vanishing twin is a phenomenon that refers to spontaneous loss of one twin early in pregnancy. Studies of twin pregnancy resulting from ART demonstrate that approximately 10 to 15 percent of singleton births begin as twin gestations. Early first-trimester loss of one twin may result in vaginal bleeding and symptoms of spontaneous abortion without significant maternal morbidity. Second-trimester death of one fetus in the twin pair can lead to compression and resorption of the fetus with the development of a "fetus papyraceus." The dead fetus becomes wafer-thin, blanches, and resembles old parchment (papyrus). The diagnosis of fetus papyraceus is usually evident at delivery when examination of the placenta reveals the outline of the pale, paper-like fetus on the fetal surface of the placenta between the membrane layers.

In Utero Demise of Co-twin

The reported risk of fetal demise among twin pregnancies before 34 weeks is approximately 3 percent, and loss of both fetuses happens in 0.6 percent of twin gestations. Generally, despite enhanced fetal surveillance, the prospective rate of unexpected fetal death is higher among monochorionic twins, reaching one in 23 in some large series. In many cases, the etiology is unknown, although late-onset twin–twin transfusion has been implicated in some cases. The median gestational age of intrauterine fetal death of a co-twin is around 34 weeks. Based on recent data, the rate of single fetal demise was 3 percent in diamniotic twins and 15 percent in monochorionic twins. The impact on the surviving co-twin differs, depending on the chorionicity. In monochorionic twins, because of presence of placental vascular anastomoses, acute exsanguination of the surviving twin into the demised twin's circulation causes acute hypotension, decreased brain perfusion, severe fetal anemia, and/or ischemia in the co-twin leading to morbidity or death of the co-twin. A meta-analysis demonstrated that in monochorionic twins, single demise will result in a double death in about 15 percent, and neurodevelopmental impairment in another 26 percent due to acute perimortem exsanguination. In addition, a 68 percent risk of preterm birth is encountered, compared to a 3 percent risk of double death, 2 percent risk of neurological impairment, and 54 percent risk of preterm birth in diamniotic twins suffering single fetal demise. Hypoxic brain lesions, including porencephalic cysts, periventricular leukomalacia, and cerebral and cerebellar infarcts, may result. Thrombotic or ischemic events may occur elsewhere in the survivor after death of a co-twin, leading to renal cortical necrosis, bowel atresia, or aplasia cutis (Fig. 29-9).

The timing of the in utero demise is inversely related to the gestational age at delivery. First-trimester loss of a co-twin usually carries a

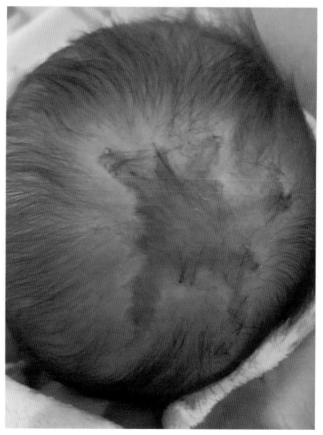

FIGURE 29-9. Aplasia cutis. Surviving twin, following in utero death of the monochorionic co-twin at 15 weeks gestation.

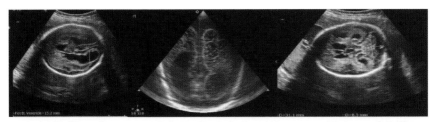

A. Ventriculomegaly | B. Periventricular Leukomalacia | C. Porencephalic Cysts

FIGURE 29-10. Sonographic consequences of in utero death of monochorionic co-twin.

more favorable prognosis than demise occurring in the second or third trimesters. In cases of twin–twin transfusion syndrome, in utero death of a recipient twin is associated with a higher rate of intracranial lesions in the surviving donor than if the donor had in utero loss.

Antenatal detection of destructive brain lesions in twins may not be obvious until several weeks after in utero demise of a co-twin. Ultrasonography remains less sensitive than MRI in detecting subtle, early ischemic changes in the brain. Ventriculomegaly may be the only sonographic sign of underlying damage (Fig. 29-10).

Because of the immediacy of damage caused by hypoperfusion of the brain of the surviving fetus, a better perinatal outcome is not assured by shortening the interval between death of one twin and delivery of the other.

Preventive strategies such as early delivery of monochorionic twins between 32 and 34 weeks of gestation has been proposed to reduce the risk of in utero death of a co-twin (after administration of antenatal steroids to accelerate lung maturity); however, it must be balanced against risk of iatrogenic prematurity and adverse neonatal outcomes.

ANTENATAL MANAGEMENT OF TWIN GESTATION

Principles of antepartum management of twin pregnancy include the following:

1. **Early diagnosis of multiple pregnancy and establishment of chorionicity** facilitates appropriate counseling of the parents regarding risks of multiples, directs obstetrical care to the appropriate caregiver, and ascertains the appropriate venue for delivery. Establishment of chorionicity in the first trimester, preferably, is a crucial component of risk

COMPLICATED LABOR

stratification and compilation of a chorionicity-specific surveillance protocol to aid in early detection of chorionicity-specific complications, such as TTTS, TAPS, sIUGR, etc.

2. **Consideration of aneuploidy screening,** as directed by parental choice
3. **Prevention of pre-eclampsia** (low-dose ASA in at-risk mothers)
4. **Optimization of maternal nutritional status** (prenatal vitamin, iron supplementation, appropriate weight gain, etc.)
5. **Enhanced maternal surveillance** for early detection of preterm labor, preeclampsia, etc.
6. **Detailed fetal structural survey (especially in monochorionic twins) and serial functional assessment of fetal health** (monochorionic twins, rule out TTTS, TAPS, sIUGR, etc.)

Maternal Complications

Women carrying twins are at higher rates of adverse maternal outcome compared to singleton pregnancies; the chorionicity and amnionicity do not appear to influence this risk. Hypertension, preeclampsia, and gestational diabetes are among the most common complications. Other maternal complications include increased incidence of iron deficiency anemia, hyperemesis gravidarum, gastroesophageal reflux, thromboembolism, and intrahepatic cholestasis of pregnancy. Prevention strategies to minimize risks of preeclampsia, such as administration of low-dose aspirin (80-150 mg ASA, at bedtime, starting before 16 weeks of pregnancy), have been proven to reduce risks in up to 56 percent in mothers at high risk of preeclampsia. Several clinical practice guidelines have extrapolated this evidence to twin pregnancies; although to date, data for similar efficacy in moderate-risk multiple pregnancies is not as convincing.

DELIVERY OF MULTIPLES

When planning for delivery of multiples, several intrapartum considerations in management arise, include: timing, presentation (Fig. 29-11), route of delivery, required resources for delivery, appropriate venue, mechanics of delivery, chorionicity-related considerations, the possibility of delayed interval delivery, and appropriateness of delayed cord clamping.

These considerations are aimed at reducing the intrapartum risks, especially to the second twin, whom by virtue of its position in the uterine

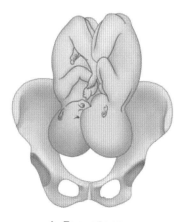

A. Two vertexes.

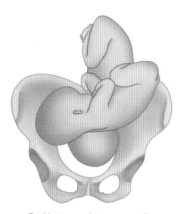

D. Vertex and transverse lie.

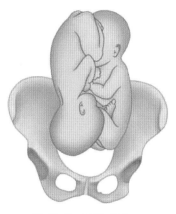

B. Vertex and breech.

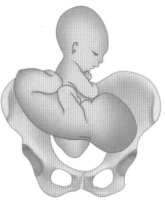

E. Breech and transverse lie.

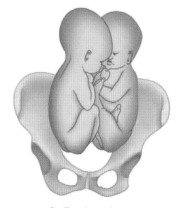

C. Two breeches.

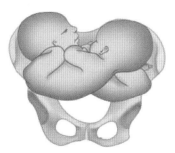

F. Two transverse lies.

FIGURE 29-11. Twin presentation.

COMPLICATED LABOR

TABLE 29-3: RISK TO SECOND TWIN

- ■ Low birth weight
- ■ ⇑ Malpresentation
- ■ ⇑ Operative delivery
- ■ Decreased uterine capacity with altered placental hemodynamics
- ■ ⇑Risk of hypoxia (velamentous, marginal cord insertion)
- ■ Difficulties in monitoring fetal status
- ■ ⇑ Risk of cord prolapse, abruption, etc.

cavity and birth order, is at increased risk of hypoxia, cord prolapse, abruption, malpresentation, and operative delivery (Table 29-3).

The optimum time to deliver uncomplicated twins depends on the chorionicity and amnionicity. Recommendations on timing of delivery are based on review of available data in regard to risk of late stillbirth and risk of neonatal mortality and morbidity with delivery. A 2014 Cochrane Review examined two randomized trials investigating risks to mothers associated with elective delivery of twins from 37 weeks versus expectant management and found no differences in maternal morbidity, maternal deaths, cesarean section rates, and so on.

Intrapartum risks are increased in twin pregnancies, and the delivery setting, and capabilities should be assessed in planning twin birth. Appropriate personnel and obstetric staff with appropriate training should be available at the time of birth, especially if breech extraction or internal or external version of the second twin is a possibility. Factors influencing the mode of delivery in twins are multiple and include presentation, estimated fetal weight, gestational age, skill of the operator, previous operative delivery, and maternal choice. With this multitude of influences, it is not surprising that planned vaginal delivery of viable twins occurs in less than 50 percent of all twins in developed countries. The Twin Birth Study (Barrett et al, 2013) is the best available evidence to date that elective, planned cesarean delivery does not significantly improve neonatal or early childhood outcomes. Overall, when trial of labor is offered to twins, it can be expected to be successful in approximately 56.2 percent of cases based on one recent randomized trial.

Various clinical practice guidelines have suggested that estimated fetal weight be used to plan mode of delivery in twins. When fetal weight is estimated to be less than 1500 grams, a liberal policy of cesarean section is suggested even when both fetuses are in vertex presentation.

Rates of combined delivery, that is, emergency delivery of the second twin by cesarean section after successful vaginal delivery of the presenting twin, appear to be highly influenced by fetal weight as well. Cesarean section rates of approximately 5.7 percent have been reported in larger second twins (>2500 grams) in contrast to rates of about 11.3 percent in second twins weighing less than 1500 grams. In the randomized Twin Birth Study by Barrett et al (twins ≥34 weeks' gestation) for women randomly assigned to planned vaginal delivery, 4.2 percent had combined vaginal-cesarean delivery and >40 percent had cesarean section for both twins. Among the factors that influenced the mode of delivery included the presentation at time of delivery; the non-cephalic second twin had a vaginal birth rate of 36 percent, and gestational age at delivery of the first twin. The highest rate of vaginal delivery of first twin was at 37 to 38 weeks' gestation. The frequency of fetal and neonatal death did not differ significantly in planned elective cesarean delivery (2.2%) compared to planned vaginal delivery (1.9%). The only factor significantly influencing the fetal and neonatal mortality rate was the gestational age (odds ratio of 1.25 for 32 weeks' gestation compared to 0.3 for 37 weeks' gestation).

Neonatal respiratory morbidity rates are lowest when elective delivery is completed at or beyond 37 completed weeks. Controversy stems from reports of increased stillbirth and early neonatal death rates when twin pregnancy is prolonged. In Australia, the lowest composite neonatal mortality and morbidity rates are seen when twin delivery is accomplished at 37 weeks and increases thereafter, but Canada and Japan report lowest rates of perinatal death in twins delivered at 38 weeks. The prospective risk of perinatal death in twins is such that it is reasonable to consider delivery of twins by 38 weeks. These figures do not take into consideration the influence of chorionicity on twin outcome. The risks of late fetal loss in monochorionic twin gestations are such that perinatal centers in the United Kingdom advocate elective delivery of these twins at 36 to 37 weeks and delivery of dichorionic twins approximately 1 to 2 weeks later. The recommendation is based on a systemic review of the prospective risk of stillbirth and neonatal complications in twin pregnancies which observed a trend toward higher risk of stillbirth than neonatal death beyond 36^{+0} to 36^{+6} in monochorionic/diamniotic twin pregnancies. It must be remembered, however, that if elective cesarean section of twins is performed at 35 weeks or later but before 37 weeks, respiratory morbidity is in the order of 5 percent, and patients should be counseled regarding the risks with consideration of optimization of fetal lung condition with antenatal steroids.

COMPLICATED LABOR

Intrapartum Management

Management of labor is generally similar to singleton pregnancies; however, it is well advised to plan the delivery in an operating room where urgent cesarean delivery can be performed, if required. Support from the anesthesia service during delivery is well-advised, to ensure maternal comfort, especially if manipulation of the second twin is anticipated. With multiples, challenges in monitoring of fetal status exist, especially for the more vulnerable second twin, yet reliable discrimination of heart rates of the mother and both fetuses is imperative for early diagnosis of fetal distress. Ideally a portable ultrasound should be available to confirm fetal presentation following delivery of the first twin and visualize the second fetus during internal podalic version or breech extraction if needed. Other considerations include anticipation of postpartum hemorrhage due to uterine atony, a common occurrence following delivery of multiples, with ready availability of uterotonics.

The first baby is delivered in the usual way as if it were a single pregnancy. Careful examination is made to determine the position and station of the second baby. Only if the vertex or breech is in or over the inlet and the uterus is contracting, should the membranes be ruptured artificially, because overzealous artificial rupture of the membranes in an unengaged fetal presenting part can result in cord prolapse. If uterine inertia has set in, an oxytocin drip may be commenced to reestablish uterine contractions; when this has been achieved, amniotomy can be safely performed. The presenting part is guided into the pelvis by the vaginal hand. If necessary, pressure is made on the fundus with the other hand. Because the first baby has already dilated the birth canal, the second one descends rapidly to the pelvic floor. Once the presenting part is on the perineum, it is delivered spontaneously or by simple operative measures. Delivery of the second, nonvertex twin can be accomplished spontaneously, if aligned longitudinally in breech presentation or assisted by breech extraction or external cephalic version. On occasion, the operator must be prepared to expedite the delivery of the vertex-presenting, nonengaged second twin by internal podalic version, particularly if acute fetal compromise is suspected.

The goal of intrapartum management of twins is to reduce acidosis in the second twin, which is reported to increase by 1 percent with each elapsing minute between delivery of the siblings. Fortunately, 68 percent of twins deliver within 30 minutes of each other with a median twin–twin delivery time of 19 minutes, according to one Swedish study. A higher pH in the second twin is noted when an inter-twin delivery time of <30 minutes is accomplished; although, the upper limit of time between twins remains unknown. In that study of 527 twin births, neither acidosis, low Apgar score <4, nor perinatal mortality was observed when the twin–twin delivery time was 19 minutes or less.

Despite careful planning and informed parental counselling, the realities of twin births are such that intrapartum events that potentially influence the timing and conduct of delivery of the second twin may arise, and the birth attendant needs to anticipate these and have at his/her fingertips a management strategy to deal with these occurrences. Uterine inertia may slow the progress of labor or lead to regression of cervical dilatation, prompting delayed delivery of the second twin. Sudden decompression of the uterus may occur with rupture of the second twin's membranes, precipitating abruptio placenta or cord prolapse, leading to acute fetal distress. While augmentation of labor with uterotonics may resolve uterine inertia, expeditious delivery of the second twin may be required in the latter circumstances and the operator should be skilled in breech extraction and internal podalic version. Detailed technical descriptions of these procedures can be found in standard obstetrical texts.

Cesarean section is not routinely advocated for the sole indication of twins but is reserved for twins with comorbidity such as severe preeclampsia, placenta previa and abruption placentae, breech or transverse lie of presenting twin, or prolapse of the umbilical cord. Despite evidence from large, multicentered, randomized trials to suggest planned cesarean section does not reduce the risk of fetal or neonatal death or serious neonatal morbidity over planned vaginal delivery in vertex-presenting twin at 32 weeks and above, cesarean section rates in twins vary widely internationally (Fig. 29-12).

Europe			Canada (2010–2011)
BJOG Online, March 2015			*Kelly et al, ADGC, March 2013*
	Twins	**Singletons**	
Iceland	31.1	14.8	
Netherlands	43.9	33.1	
Norway	47.4	17.1	
Finland	49.4	16.8	
Sweden	53.6	17.5	
France	54.8	21.0	
Denmark	59.6	22.1	
England	62.6	24.6	
Ireland	63.6	27.0	
Scotland	73.3	27.8	
Germany	74.8	31.3	
Switzerland	77.5	33.1	
Italy	85.6	38.0	Twins — 63% Singletons — 28%
Malta	98.6	33.1	

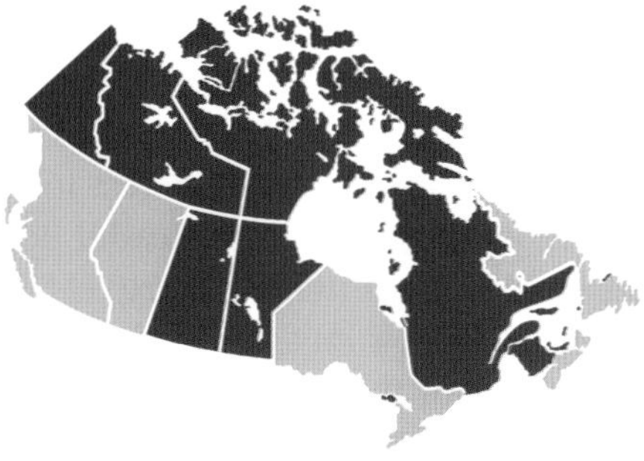

FIGURE 29-12. Cesarean section rates: European versus Canada.

COMPLICATED LABOR

Twin pregnancy does not impose a special threat to the integrity of a preexisting low transverse cesarean scar and a trial of labor is not contraindicated in those cases in a vertex-presenting twin.

Among cephalic/cephalic twins undergoing a trial of labor, 12 percent of second twins were found to be in a non-cephalic presentation after delivery of the first twin. "Combined" delivery, that is, unplanned cesarean delivery of the second twin is the least desirable option for both mothers and delivering caregiver and yet occurs in approximately 4 to 10 percent of cases after vaginal delivery of the first twin. These situations usually arise when acute fetal distress is encountered and vaginal delivery of the second twin cannot be affected promptly. Included here are separation of the placenta, malpresentation, abnormal fetal heart rate pattern, contracted cervix, prolapse of the umbilical cord, and failure to progress. This circumstance occurs more often in nulliparous women and is associated with higher rates of fetal or neonatal death (13.6% vs. 2%, $p < .001$). It is estimated that approximately two-thirds of combined deliveries may be avoidable. Following delivery of multiples, postpartum hemorrhage can be encountered, often due to uterine atony, and aggressive management of the third stage of labor, including use of various parental and intramuscular uterotonics, may help limit blood loss.

OTHER INTRAPARTUM CONSIDERATIONS

Delayed Interval Delivery of Twins

Delayed delivery of the second twin is a rare practice that aims to prolong gestation until viability in cases of delivery of a previable first twin. In 1880, the first published report of a prolonged delivery interval between premature birth of co-twins at 27 and 32 weeks of gestation appeared in the medical literature, with survival of the second twin. Since the late 1970s, there has been renewed interest in this management strategy, with several reports of cases of successful delayed interval deliveries of multiples reported in both twins and triplets. Interval delays in delivery have been reported from 1 day to 153 days in attempted cases. The relative statistical rarity of this approach has precluded attempts at prospective trials addressing outcome. Much of the published work in this area originates from case reports and small retrospective case series. Lack of published experience utilizing a structured, standardized approach to management, coupled with concerns over potential reporting bias in the literature makes informed patient counseling challenging. Published case series have suggested an improved success rate when the first fetus has delivered at a previable stage (i.e., less than 24 weeks). Most recent reported data from a multicenter trial in France confirms an improved survival rate of the second twin if the delivery of the first twin occurred before limit of viability.

There remains a lack of comprehensive evidence on optimal management on delayed interval delivery of twins. A reasonable approach would be ligating the cord as high as possible (need to say with which type of ligature) without exerting cord traction and in cases of confirmed preterm premature rupture of the membranes (PPROM) starting antibiotics prophylactically, according to local protocols. Vaginal microbiology and testing for infective markers (e.g., WBC and CRP) are advisable, after delivery of the first twin. There is no consensus on use of tocolysis. A short course of tocolysis may reduce severity of neurological outcome and allow for acceleration of fetal lung maturation with betamethasone. The use of cervical cerclage after delivery of the first twin is controversial in the literature. Concerns of cerclage increasing risk of infection have limited its use, as reported in most studies. Some others proposed use of cerclage in cases of cervical dilatation. Longer intertwin intervals have been reported in a few studies. Potential maternal risks include chorioamnionitis, abruption, hemorrhage, and so on, and detailed maternal counseling is imperative.

Delayed Cord Clamping (DCC)

Delay in clamping of the umbilical cord for 30 to 60 seconds after birth or until the spontaneous cessation of pulsations in the cord after delivery has been associated with improved neonatal outcomes for both term infants (e.g., improved hemoglobin at birth and better iron stores in early infancy) and preterm infants (improved transitional circulation, decreased need for transfusion, lower incidence of necrotizing enterocolitis, and intraventricular hemorrhage). Data of efficacy and safety in multiple pregnancy has been less well studied. One randomized trial of 47 mothers and 101 infants suggested that DCC did not offer an advantage to immediate cord clamping (ICC) in terms of improved placental transfusion or systemic blood flow. All but two of these mothers were delivered by cesarean section and a significant increase in postpartum hemorrhage was noted in the group undergoing DCC. Limitations of this study include the lack of analysis of subgroups by chorionicity or birth order. These considerations are important, as the presence of inter-twin vascular anastomoses carry potential risks of acute, intrapartum fetal-fetal transfusion, especially to the second fetus, and these risks can be additive in the context of existing comorbidity with these special, monochorionic twin conditions. Similarly, evidence from other studies demonstrated that newborn hemoglobin in infants delivered vaginally were higher in second twins than first twins. Hemoglobin levels in cesarean-delivered twins, were generally higher for both twins than that of the firstborn twin born vaginally. Dichorionic twins, by virtue of their independent circulations may benefit from a delayed approach to cord clamping similar to that noted in singletons but further studies are required to determine the efficacy of DCC in monochorionic twins.

TRIPLET AND HIGHER-ORDER MULTIPLES

In the past, multiple pregnancy involving more than two infants was rare, but the widespread use of ovulation induction agents, such as clomiphene citrate and gonadotropins, as well as other ART, increased the incidence of higher-order plural births significantly, especially between the years 1980 and 1997 in the United States, when a 400 percent rise in triplet births was noted. Interestingly, from 1998 to 2005, a substantive drop (16%) in the birth of these higher-order multiples was witnessed. This dramatic change was likely multifactorial in nature, resulting from better control of the reproductive cycle, enhanced vigilance regarding the number of embryo transfers per cycle, and/or increased access to multi-fetal reduction of triplets to twins or singletons. A continued decline in the rate of triplets and higher-order multiples has been observed in the last two decades. Currently, the incidence of triplet pregnancy in the United States is one in 880 pregnancies, down from the all-time high of one in 515 in 1998 with spontaneous conception of triplets occurring in approximately one in 8000 pregnancies. Irrespective of the multiplicity of factors contributing of this decline, reduction in the number of higher-order multiples is welcome news because of the inherent risks of these plural births.

This list does not address the other confounder, chorionicity, which is an additional independent risk factor that influences morbidity and mortality for higher-order multiples just as it does in twin pregnancy.

In general, all the special issues and complications of twin pregnancy for mothers and fetuses are augmented in higher-order multiples. Fetal outcomes tend to decline with increasing plurality, with perinatal mortality rates about 10 to 12 times higher than those found in singletons. Early pregnancy loss is also more common and spontaneous loss rates of >50 percent of one or more fetuses before 12 weeks has been reported when diagnosis of triplets is made in the early first trimester, at 6 weeks or less.

The prime cause of high fetal loss after viability is preterm labor, often preceded by spontaneous rupture of the membranes. The mean gestational age at delivery is 32.5 to 34 weeks. To date, no benefit has been established in the use of progesterone therapy (IV or IM), elective cerclage, bed rest, home monitoring for contractions or tocolytics for the purposes of reducing the incidence of preterm birth in triplets and higher-order multiples. Of particular concern in these higher-order multiples is the cerebral palsy rate, which is more than 15 times greater than in singleton pregnancies and often associated with preterm birth. Spastic diplegia and bilateral cerebral palsy are more common in this group. Neonatal risks are also high, with a reported threefold risk of infant death of one or more babies.

Given the additive, substantial risks of triplet and high order pregnancies on perinatal outcome, multifetal pregnancy reduction is an essential component of comprehensive counselling of these patients. Reduction of a triplet pregnancy to twins is associated with an increased gestational age at delivery (60-70% reduction in extreme premature delivery), increased birthweight, and decreased neonatal mortality. Loss rates prior to 24 weeks are not increased following pregnancy reduction. In addition, maternal risks such as hypertensive disorders of pregnancy and gestational diabetes are also decreased. Techniques of multifetal pregnancy reduction will be dependent on chorionicity with feticidal agents, such as intracardiac potassium chloride or lidocaine, limited to fetuses with dichorionic placentation, while ablative techniques, such as radiofrequency ablation, are reserved for multiples with monochorionic placentation.

Management

As in twins, modern clinical management of ongoing triplet pregnancies includes: (1) early diagnosis with assessment of chorionicity; (2) preventative strategies to decrease risk of preeclampsia (low-dose ASA 162 mg at bedtime); (3) enhanced maternal nutrition for optimal weight gain (~54 lbs. for mothers of normal BMI); (4) enhanced fetal surveillance for structural anomalies (especially if monochorionicity is present), fetal growth restriction or discordance, or complications on monochorionicity (TTTS, etc.); (5) serial assessment of fetal well-being to reduce stillbirth; (6) prediction of preterm birth, including cervical assessment (digital or ultrasound assessment of cervical length; and (7) optimization of fetal condition if early preterm birth is anticipated (e.g., prophylactic steroids [betamethasone] to accelerate fetal lung maturity, magnesium sulphate for fetal neuroprotection prior to preterm delivery).

Mode of Delivery in Triplets

Routine use of cesarean section for delivery of these higher-order multiples is highly favored in developed countries, especially for those pregnancies where a gestational age compatible with neonatal survival is reached and is often indicated by malpresentation of the presenting fetus. The liberal use of operative delivery avoids intrauterine instrumentation and manipulation in an overdistended uterus and minimizes maternal trauma. It also mitigates technical challenges in intrapartum monitoring of all three fetuses continuously. However, cesarean delivery of triplets carries with it an increased risk of postpartum hemorrhage, blood transfusion, and cesarean hysterectomy. Vaginal delivery of triplets can be accomplished but is considered safest if the following conditions are met: gestational age of ≥32 weeks, estimated fetal weights >1500 grams, the presenting triplet in vertex presentation, trichorionic or dichorionic, triamniotic placentation, availability of 24-hour anesthesia support, no significant inter-triplet growth discordance, and importantly, informed patient counseling and consent. The attendance of a care provider experienced in vaginal breech delivery is also essential. Data from the Consortium for Safe Labour indicates that of those triplet pregnancies attempting vaginal delivery, only 16 percent accomplish successful vaginal birth. The NICE Clinical Guidelines suggest delivery of uncomplicated trichorionic triplets at 35 to 37 weeks' gestation with consideration of earlier delivery for those of other chorionicities.

The arrival of triplets can have a profound psychosocial and economic impact on families and counseling should include the augmented risk of postpartum depression in this cohort.

SELECTED READING

Ananth CV, Chauhan SP: Epidemiology of twinning in developed countries. Semin Perinatol 36:156-161, 2012

Barrett JF, Hannah ME, Hutton EK, Willan AR, Allen AC, Armson BA, Gafni A, et al: A randomized trial of planned cesarean or vaginal delivery for twin pregnancy. N Engl J Med 369:1295-1305, 2013 [Erratum in: N Engl J Med 369:2364, 2013]

Breathnach FM, Malone FD: Fetal growth disorders in twin gestations. Semin Perinatol 36:175-81, 2012. doi: 10.1053/j.semperi.2012.02.002. PMID: 22713498

D'Antonio F, Khalil A, Dias T, Thilaganathan B: Weight discordance and perinatal mortality in twins: The Stork Multiple Pregnancy Cohort. Ultrasound Obstet Gynecol 41: 643-648, 2013

D'Antonio F, Thilaganathan B, Dias T, Khalil A: Southwest Thames Obstetric Research Collaborative (STORK). Influence of chorionicity and gestational age at single fetal loss on risk of preterm birth in twin pregnancy: Analysis of STORK multiple pregnancy cohort. Ultrasound Obstet Gynecol 50:723-727, 2017

Di Mascio D, Khalil A, Rizzo G, et al: Risk of fetal loss following amniocentesis or chorionic villus sampling in twin pregnancy: Systematic review and meta-analysis. Ultrasound Obstet Gynecol 56:647-655, 2020

Glinianaia SV, Obeysekera MA, Sturgiss S, Bell R: Stillbirth and neonatal mortality in monochorionic and dichorionic twins: A population-based study. Hum Reprod 26:2549-2557, 2011

Glinianaia SV, Rankin J, Wright C, Sturgiss SN, Renwick M: Northern Region Perinatal Mortality Survey Steering Group. A multiple pregnancy register in the north of England. Twin Res 5:436-439, 2002

Gratacós E, Lewi L, Muñoz B, et al. A classification system for selective intrauterine growth restriction in monochorionic pregnancies according to umbilical artery Doppler flow in the smaller twin. Ultrasound Obstet Gynecol 30:28-34, 2007

Kaufman MH: The embryology of conjoined twins. Childs Nerv Syst 20:508-525, 2004

Khalil A, Liu B: Controversies in the management of twin pregnancy. Ultrasound Obstet Gynecol 57:888-902, 2021

Khalil A, Beune I, Hecher K, et al: Consensus definition and essential reporting parameters of selective fetal growth restriction in twin pregnancy: A Delphi procedure. Ultrasound Obstet Gynecol 53(1):47-54, 2019 [Erratum in: Ultrasound Obstet Gynecol 56:967, 2020]

Khalil A, Rodgers M, Baschat A, et al: ISUOG Practice Guidelines: Role of ultrasound in twin pregnancy. Ultrasound Obstet Gynecol 47:247-263, 2016 [Erratum in: Ultrasound Obstet Gynecol 52:140, 2018]

Louchet M, Dussaux C, Luton D, Goffinet F, Bounan S, Mandelbrot L: Delayed-interval delivery of twins in 13 pregnancies. J Gynecol Obstet Hum Reprod 49:101660, 2020

Mackie FL, Rigby A, Morris RK, Kilby MD: Prognosis of the co-twin following spontaneous single intrauterine fetal death in twin pregnancies: A systematic review and meta-analysis. BJOG 126:569-578, 2019

Martin JA, Hamilton BE, Osterman MJK, Driscoll AK: Births: Final Data for 2018. Natl Vital Stat Rep 68:1-47, 2019

Maruotti GM, Saccone G, Morlando M, Martinelli P: First-trimester ultrasound determination of chorionicity in twin gestations using the lambda sign: a systematic review and meta-analysis. Eur J Obstet Gynecol Reprod Biol 202:66-70, 2016

McNamara HC, Kane SC, Craig JM, Short RV, Umstad MP: A review of the mechanisms and evidence for typical and atypical twinning. Am J Obstet Gynecol 214:172-191, 2016

Monson M, Silver RM. Multifetal Gestation: Mode of delivery. Clin Obstet Gynecol. 58: 690-702, 2015

National Collaborating Centre for Women's and Children's Health (UK): Multiple Pregnancy: The Management of Twin and Triplet Pregnancies in the Antenatal Period. London: RCOG Press; 2011

Ruangkit C, Moroney V, Viswanathan S, Bhola M: Safety and efficacy of delayed umbilical cord clamping in multiple and singleton premature infants - A quality improvement study. J Neonatal Perinatal Med 8:393-402, 2015

COMPLICATED LABOR

Shinwell ES, Haklai T, Eventov-Friedman S: Outcomes of multiplets. Neonatology 95:6-14, 2009

Shub A, Walker SP: Planned early delivery versus expectant management for monoamniotic twins. Cochrane Database Syst Rev 2015:CD008820, 2015

Townsend R, D'Antonio F, Sileo FG, Kumbay H, Thilaganathan B, Khalil A: Perinatal outcome of monochorionic twin pregnancy complicated by selective fetal growth restriction according to management: Systematic review and meta-analysis. Ultrasound Obstet Gynecol 53:36-46, 2019

Van Mieghem T, De Heus R, Lewi L, et al: Prenatal management of monoamniotic twin pregnancies. Obstet Gynecol 124:498-506, 2014

Zheng XQ, Yan JY, Xu RL, Wang XC, Li LY, Lin Z. An analysis of the maternal and infant outcomes in the delayed interval delivery of twins. Taiwan J Obstet Gynecol 59: 361-365, 2020

PART VI

Other Issues

CHAPTER 30

Preterm Labor

Griffith D. Jones

DEFINITION

In pregnancy, *term* refers to the gestational period from 37^{+0} to 41^{+6} weeks. Preterm births occur between 24^{+0} and 36^{+6} weeks. Although births earlier than this are referred to as miscarriages, occasional survivors are seen after delivery at 22^{+0} to 23^{+6} weeks, which has become the "gray zone" for viability.

Early births occur either because delivery is believed to be in the best interests of the mother or baby (indicated deliveries) or because the mother develops spontaneous contractions or membrane rupture earlier than normal (spontaneous deliveries). The latter group has two subdivisions: spontaneous preterm labor (PTL) and preterm prelabor rupture of the membranes (PPROM). Indicated deliveries, PTL, and PPROM each account for approximately one-third of early births.

PREVALENCE

From 2012 to 2020, there were 1,120,959 livebirths between 23 and 42 weeks of gestation in Ontario (BORN Ontario). A total of 7 percent of these births were preterm, occurring before 37 weeks, but the percentage of very early births is much smaller (Fig. 30-1). Although similar data is seen from the United Kingdom, significantly higher rates of preterm birth of up to 12 percent are reported from the United States. Conversely, many Nordic countries with very reliable data collection quote rates around 5 percent. This must reflect, at least in part, differing socioeconomic and

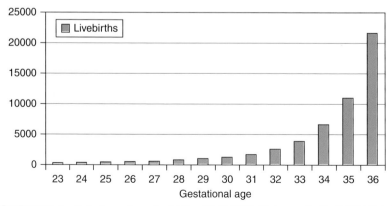

FIGURE 30-1. Ontario preterm livebirths, 2012-2020. (Data supplied by BORN Ontario.)

cultural factors. There is no evidence that the incidence of preterm birth is declining. National Perinatal Health Reports and Indicators from the Public Health Agency of Canada demonstrate that the preterm birth rate increased from 6.4 percent in 1985 to 8.2 percent in 2004 but has remained steady since then, with data up to 2014. Although just under 1 percent of singletons are delivered before 32 weeks, this rises to 8 percent for twins and nearly 40 percent for higher multiples.

Preterm births contribute significantly to perinatal mortality, half of which results from babies born before 32 weeks. The survival to discharge for very preterm infants admitted to Canadian neonatal intensive care units (NICUs) in 2019 is shown in Figure 30-2 (www.canadianneonatalnetwork. org). Predicted survival can be modified if accurate information concerning fetal sex, weight, and well-being is available. Parents are anxious about both survival rates and also the risks of later disability and handicap. These risks are especially significant before 26 weeks' gestation. The CNN data suggests that 60 percent of parents elect for neonatal palliative care only at 22 weeks falling to 28 percent at 23 weeks. When assessed at 6 years of age, nearly half the survivors at 23 to 25 weeks' gestation have a moderate or severe disability. Furthermore, many of these disabilities only become apparent after 2 to 3 years of age. Survival with no disability is only seen in 1, 3, and 8 percent of live births at less than 24, 24, and 25 weeks, respectively. There are other long-term worries after very preterm births, including subsequent growth, educational needs, and social behavior. There may also be influences on later adult health. Fortunately, both morbidity and mortality fall dramatically with increasing gestation.

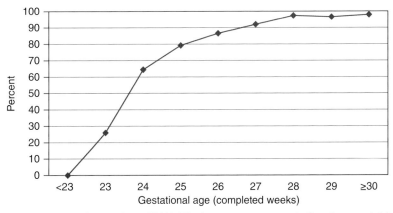

FIGURE 30-2. Survival to NICU Discharge versus gestational age at birth. (Reproduced with permission from the 2019 Canadian Neonatal Network (CNN) Annual Report. Canadian Neonatal Network; 2019.)

It is important to recognize the effect of denominator differences in survival figures, especially at the earliest gestations. If the figures are based on fetuses alive at the start of labor, the survival rates will be lower because there is an inherent risk of intrapartum death, greatest at the lowest gestational ages. If the figures are based on NICU admissions, the figures will be higher because some live births will succumb during initial resuscitation in the delivery room. At 25 weeks or less, such statistical manipulations may lead to a significant change in the quoted survival figures.

CLASSIFICATION

For reasons related to etiology, outcome, and recurrence risk, preterm births should be divided into three gestational periods: mildly preterm births at 32^{+0} to 36^{+6} weeks (incidence, 6.4%), very preterm births at 28^{+0} to 31^{+6} weeks (incidence, 0.7%), and extremely preterm births at 22^{+0} to 27^{+6} weeks (incidence, 0.4%).

ETIOLOGY

Labor at term and before term share a common pathway involving uterine contractility, cervical effacement and dilatation, and membrane rupture. At term, the activation of this pathway is physiologic. However, a variety of pathologies underlie labor remote from term. It has been suggested by some authors that preterm labor be considered a syndrome in order to emphasize its multifactorial nature.

Infection and Inflammation

Subclinical intrauterine infection and inflammation of the choriodecidual space and amniotic fluid is the most widely studied etiologic factor underlying spontaneous preterm births. The uterine cavity is normally sterile, but the vagina contains commensal bacteria. Depending on the bacterial load and cervical resistance, the bacteria may ascend through the cervix and reach the fetal membranes. This may activate the decidua, increase prostaglandin release, and trigger contractions. Alternatively, it may weaken the membranes, leading to rupture. Early-onset neonatal sepsis, maternal postpartum endometritis, and histologic chorioamnionitis are all significantly more common after preterm birth, particularly very early deliveries before 32 weeks.

Overdistension

The most common cause of uterine overdistension is multiple gestation. Polyhydramnios has a similar effect. Overstretching of the myometrium (and possibly the membranes) leads to increased contractile activity and premature shortening and opening of the cervix.

Vascular

Disturbance at the utero-placental interface may lead to intrauterine bleeding. The blood can track down behind the membranes to the cervix and be revealed. Alternatively, it may track away from the cervix and be concealed. Either way, the blood irritates the uterus, leading to contractions, and damages the membranes, leading to early rupture.

Surgical Procedures and Intercurrent Illness

Serious maternal infective illnesses such as pyelonephritis, appendicitis, and pneumonia are associated with preterm labor. In these cases, preterm labor is presumed to be caused by either direct blood-borne spread of infection to the uterine cavity or indirectly to chemical triggers, such as endotoxins or cytokines. Many other illnesses, such as cholestasis of pregnancy, and nonobstetric surgical procedures, are associated with preterm labor, although the mechanisms for this remain obscure.

Amniocentesis is a pregnancy-specific procedure associated with an increased risk of late miscarriage and early birth. It is most commonly performed at 15 to 18 weeks' gestation. It is associated with a 0.5 percent chance of subsequent pregnancy loss before viability. This may happen in the days after the procedure, but many losses occur several weeks later, and a small increased risk of preterm delivery persists after reaching viability.

Abnormal Uterine Cavity

A uterine cavity that is distorted by congenital malformation may be less able to accommodate a developing pregnancy. Associated abnormal placentation and cervical weakness may also contribute. Fibroids in a submucosal position may also lead to complications. However, fibroids are common, and most pregnancies are successful despite their presence.

OTHER ISSUES

Cervical Weakness

Because of previous surgical damage or a congenital defect, the cervix may shorten and open prematurely. The membranes then prolapse and may be damaged by stretching or by direct contact with vaginal pathogens. These same pathogens may ascend and trigger contractions. Often referred to as *cervical incompetence, weakness* may be a better term. The evidence suggests that gradations of deficiency exist, rather than an "all-or-nothing" phenomenon. It may also vary from one pregnancy to the next, depending upon the influence of other "variables."

This remains a notoriously difficult diagnosis to make, because dilatation of the cervix remains the final common pathway for all late miscarriages and early births. Reliably distinguishing between such dilatation being the primary event or secondary to other pathologies is challenging.

Idiopathic

In many cases, especially late preterm births between 34 and 36 weeks of gestation, no cause will be found. In these cases, the physiologic pathways to parturition may simply have been turned on too early.

RISK FACTORS

Nonmodifiable, Major

Last birth preterm: 20 percent risk
Last two births preterm: 40 percent risk
Twin pregnancy: 50 percent risk
Uterine abnormalities
Cervical anomalies:
- Cervical damage (cone biopsy, repeated dilatation, cesarean in advanced labor)
- Fibroids (cervical)

Factors in current pregnancy:
- Recurrent antepartum hemorrhage
- Intercurrent illness (e.g., sepsis)
- Any invasive procedure or surgery

Nonmodifiable, Minor

Teenagers having second or subsequent babies
Parity (0 or ≥5)

Ethnicity (black women)
Poor socioeconomic status
Education (not beyond secondary)
IVF pregnancies (independent of plurality)

Modifiable

Smoking: twofold increase of PPROM
Drugs of abuse: especially cocaine
Body mass index (BMI) <20: underweight women
Interpregnancy interval <1 year

When assessing symptomatic patients, the recognition of major risk factors in particular can help to modify an individual's actual risk of preterm delivery, especially in the absence of definitive signs.

CLINICAL FEATURES

History

Always check the dating of the pregnancy by reviewing the menstrual history and, if possible, any prior ultrasound examinations. This is critical at gestations near viability.

Fewer than 50 percent of all women presenting with symptoms suggesting a risk of early delivery will deliver within 7 days. Too much emphasis is often placed on the contraction frequency. In isolation, it correlates poorly with the risk of preterm birth. Markers of intensity, such as analgesic requirements or simple bedside clinical impression, may add refinement. Vague complaints such as increased discharge, pelvic pressure, or low backache are sometimes reported, with the latter two often showing a cyclical pattern. Nonetheless, the diagnosis of preterm labor remains notoriously difficult unless contractions are accompanied by advanced dilatation (>3 cm), ruptured membranes, or significant vaginal bleeding.

Examination

A brief general examination is important to assess overall health. This should include pulse, blood pressure, temperature, and state of hydration.

Abdominal examination may reveal the presence of uterine tenderness, suggesting abruption or chorioamnionitis. A careful speculum

OTHER ISSUES

examination by an experienced clinician may yield valuable information; pooling of amniotic fluid, blood, and/or abnormal discharge may be observed. A visual assessment of cervical dilatation is usually possible and has been shown to be as accurate as digital examination findings. Digital examinations should be limited because they are known to stimulate prostaglandin production and may introduce organisms into the cervical canal.

Differential Diagnosis

- Urinary tract infection (UTI)
- Red degeneration of fibroid
- Constipation
- Gastroenteritis

Investigations

Bedside Fibronectin

Fetal fibronectin (fFN) is a "gluelike" protein binding the choriodecidual membranes. It is rarely present in vaginal secretions between 23 and 34 weeks of gestation. Any disruption at the choriodecidual interface results in fFN release and possible detection in the cervicovaginal secretions. Its use is confined to symptomatic women who do not meet the major diagnostic criteria for preterm labor, namely advanced dilatation, PPROM, or significant bleeding.

Bedside fFN testing offers a rapid assessment of risk in symptomatic women with minimal cervical dilatation. If performed correctly, the test has a greater predictive value than digital examination. In one study, 30 percent of women with a positive fibronectin test result delivered within 7 days compared with only 10 percent of women who were 2 to 3 cm dilated. Only 1 percent of women who test negative for fFN deliver within 1 week. Aggressive intervention can be avoided in these women.

Cervical Length

Cervical length measurement by transvaginal ultrasound has also been shown to improve diagnostic accuracy. A normal cervix measures approximately 35 mm in length (Fig. 30-3A). Significant cervical shortening is often accompanied by dilatation and funneling of the membranes down the cervical canal (Fig. 30-3B). Although measurements can be repeated frequently, skilled ultrasonographers and suitable machines with transvaginal probes are required.

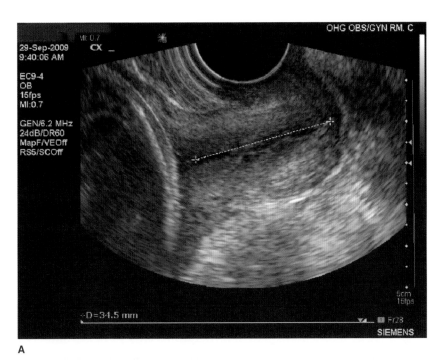

A

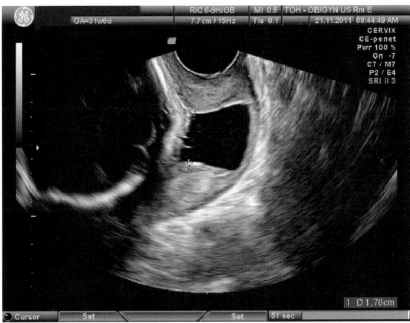

B

FIGURE 30-3. A. Normal cervical appearance on transvaginal scan. **B.** A shortened cervix with membrane funneling on transvaginal scan.

Repeat Vaginal Examination

Repeat vaginal examination in 1 to 4 hours should be considered essential in the absence of specialized tests. The interval between assessments should be guided by the severity of the symptoms.

CLINICAL FEATURES: PRETERM PRELABOR RUPTURE OF THE MEMBRANES

History

The most reliable diagnostic feature of PPROM from the history is the report of a "gush of fluid" vaginally, usually followed by a more or less continuous dribble. This "history" is as powerful as commonly relied upon tests, such as nitrazine swabs and ferning. This must be distinguished from leaking urine because incontinence or a UTI may present in a similar way. The presence of any vaginal discharge should be ascertained. Fetal movements may be reduced in strength or frequency after PPROM, and occasionally, uterine irritability or contractions may be reported.

Examination

Infection may lead to an increased pulse and temperature and a flushed appearance. Abdominal examination may reveal a clinical suspicion of oligohydramnios or uterine tenderness if chorioamnionitis is present. The definitive diagnosis of PPROM can only be made by performing a sterile speculum examination, preferably after the patient has been resting supine for 20 to 30 minutes. A pool of amniotic fluid in the posterior vagina is diagnostic. It is also important at this point to visualize the cervix. Fluid may be seen trickling through the external os, and dilatation can be visually assessed. Digital vaginal examinations should be avoided if possible in PPROM because they are associated with a significant reduction in the latent interval before labor. This reduction is most dramatic at the earliest gestations.

Differential Diagnosis

- Urine loss: Incontinence and UTIs are both more common in pregnancy
- Vaginal infection
- Leukorrhea: The cervical glands often become overactive during pregnancy

Investigations

Nitrazine Testing
Amniotic fluid is alkaline, whereas the vaginal secretions are usually acidic. An elevated pH turns a nitrazine stick black. Some units use nitrazine sticks to define the presence of amniotic fluid. Unfortunately, false-positives occur in 17 percent, with blood, semen, and even urine limiting its usefulness. However, the predictive value of a negative test result is very high.

Fern Testing
A drop of vaginal fluid from the posterior fornix is placed on a slide, allowed to dry, and examined under the high power of a microscope. Sodium chloride and proteins from the amniotic fluid, when allowed to dry on a clean slide, will crystallize and will show a characteristic fern pattern. Again, a sensitivity of 90 percent is achieved with a 6 percent false-positive rate.

Highly Specific Swab Tests
Highly specific markers for amniotic fluid can be detected using rapid bedside tests. These include immunoassays for insulin-like growth factor-binding protein-1 and of placental alpha-microglobulin-1 (Amni-Sure). The latter has a reported sensitivity of 98.9 percent for ruptured membranes, with 100 percent specificity. As always, cost is an issue.

Genital Tract Swabs
A high vaginal swab (HVS) may help to guide antibiotic therapy if subsequently required. Screening for group B streptococcus (GBS) can also be performed because there is a substantial risk of labor in the next few days.

Ultrasound
Ultrasound can give valuable information about the amniotic fluid volume. The presence or absence of oligohydramnios provides further diagnostic support. In established PPROM, there is a direct correlation between the amount of amniotic fluid remaining and the latency period. Unlike preterm labor, cervical length measurements have limited predictive ability in PPROM.

Amniocentesis
A sample of amniotic fluid can be sent for Gram stain, microscopy, and culture to establish whether an intrauterine infection (chorioamnionitis) is present. However, there is a risk of stimulating preterm labor by performing

an invasive test, and amniocentesis can be technically very difficult when there is little amniotic fluid.

Follow-up Monitoring

Maternal Well-Being
This should include regular assessment of the mother's blood pressure, pulse, and temperature. Blood tests, such as white cell (WBC) counts and C-reactive protein (CRP) are not diagnostic but should be used in combination with clinical assessment to arrive at a diagnosis of chorioamnionitis.

Fetal Well-Being
Serial antepartum cardiotocography is important after PPROM because a gradually increasing baseline heart rate or fetal tachycardia can be the first sign of intrauterine infection.

MANAGEMENT OF SYMPTOMATIC WOMEN

Communication and Support

A holistic approach to the situation is essential. Sympathy, explanations, and reassurance are mandatory. There are two vital areas of communication in the management of threatened preterm labor or PPROM. Communication with the woman and her family ensures that they have a full understanding of the risks involved and enables a clear management plan to be discussed. Communication with the neonatal unit staff ensures that adequate and appropriate resources are available at the time of delivery. Parents often also appreciate the opportunity to have discussed the care of their baby with the neonatology staff in advance of delivery.

Maternal Steroids

Current evidence shows that a single course of maternal steroids (two injections 12-24 hours apart) given between 24^{+0} and 34^{+6} weeks' gestation and received within 7 days of delivery results in markedly improved neonatal outcomes. This is primarily because of a reduction in neonatal respiratory distress syndrome (RDS). Maximum benefit from the injection is seen after 48 hours. Courses received less than 48 hours or more than 7 days before delivery still lead to benefit. Observational data suggests benefit at 23 weeks but evidence is weak for 22 weeks. Nonetheless, they are not indicated when palliative neonatal care is chosen or before viability. The steroids most commonly used are 12 mg of either betamethasone or dexamethasone.

There is considerable reassuring evidence about the long-term safety of single courses of maternal steroids, with pediatric follow-up into the teenage years. However, there have been concerns about adverse consequences of multiple dosing. Similar to antibiotics, steroids have the potential for harm in pregnancy and should be used carefully. Decisions about second courses of steroids should be made by senior clinicians and consider the gestational age, likelihood of delivery in the next 48 hours, interval since last course. A commonsense approach at present is to limit the number of courses to two with at least 4 weeks between the courses.

Tocolytics

The Canadian Preterm Labor Trial remains the most influential tocolytic trial to date. It concluded that ritodrine, a beta-agonist that relaxes smooth muscle, had no significant benefit on perinatal mortality or the prolongation of pregnancy to term. However, it was able to reduce the number of women delivering within 2 days by 40 percent. This 48-hour window of opportunity is the sole reason for using tocolytics. Beta-agonists have significant maternal side effects, and maternal deaths from acute cardiopulmonary compromise are described. Other smooth muscle relaxants used to treat preterm labor include nifedipine and glyceryl trinitrate. The former has become popular because it is inexpensive, is given orally, and has a low side effect profile. A common nifedipine dosing regime is 20 mg orally followed by 10 to 20 mg every 6 to 8 hours to a maximum daily dose of 60 mg. The oxytocin antagonist atosiban has a product license in some countries but not in North America. Although side effects are seen less frequently than with ritodrine, the cost is much higher. Because prostaglandins appear to be one of the pivotal chemicals involved in parturition, nonsteroidal anti-inflammatory drugs such as indomethacin have attracted considerable interest as tocolytics. They have been associated with significant fetal cardiovascular side effects, although these can be mitigated by limiting them to short-term use (<72 hours) and only at gestational ages less than 30 weeks.

Unfortunately, despite a multitude of pharmacologic approaches, no tocolytic medication has yet been conclusively shown to improve neonatal outcomes. Presently, the role for tocolysis is to allow a course of steroids for fetal lung maturation to be completed and to facilitate transfer of the

OTHER ISSUES

undelivered mother to a unit able to provide appropriate neonatal care if delivery occurs. They should be used with caution in the presence of ruptured membranes.

Neuroprotection

Magnesium sulphate has been shown to lead to a reduction in cerebral palsy after very preterm birth. Not surprisingly, it has the greatest benefit at the earliest gestations. The upper gestational age limit is suggested to be 33^{+6} weeks. A 4-gram loading dose is used followed by maintenance therapy for up to 24 hours. Treatment should only be initiated in patients at imminent risk of preterm birth, and there is currently no evidence to support repeat courses.

Antibiotics

Broad-spectrum antibiotics offering aerobic and anaerobic coverage are necessary in the presence of overt clinical infection, such as chorioamnionitis. The role of antibiotics in the absence of clinical signs of infection is much less clear.

The MRC Oracle Study initially concluded that the use of prophylactic antibiotics in uncomplicated preterm labor before 37 weeks with intact membranes did not confer any short-term neonatal benefit. Worryingly, subsequent long-term follow-up of survivors actually showed a significant increase in neurodevelopmental disability in those who received either erythromycin or co-amoxiclav.

In PPROM, the same study concluded that a 10-day course of erythromycin led to improved short-term neonatal outcomes. A much smaller U.S. study that only enrolled women below 32 weeks with PPROM also confirmed the benefit of antibiotics in the short term.

Most North American centers continue to give intrapartum antibiotics to women in preterm labor unless GBS status is known to be negative. For reasons that are unclear, the risk of early-onset neonatal disease appears much less in other countries, such as the United Kingdom.

Fetal Assessment

After 24 weeks, maternal steroid therapy can suppress both fetal activity and heart rate variability, although Doppler studies are not influenced. Whenever possible, the presentation in preterm labor should be confirmed by ultrasound, because clinical palpation is notoriously unreliable.

An estimated fetal weight, particularly before 28 weeks, can be helpful. Preterm infants have less reserve to tolerate the stress of labor, particularly in the presence of oligohydramnios. Therefore, continuous fetal monitoring may be required, although there may be considerable difficulties interpreting the fetal heart rate pattern in extremely preterm infants. At the extremes of viability, parents may decline intervention for suspected fetal compromise or aggressive resuscitation of the newborn. In these cases, continuous monitoring would be inappropriate.

In Utero Transfer

If local resources are unable to care for a viable neonate, in utero transfer to a unit with adequate neonatal facilities is recommended. It is generally accepted that this will improve the outcome for babies, particularly before 30 weeks of gestation. However, one must be careful not to convert a hospital delivery into a roadside one. A repeat assessment immediately before transfer is mandatory.

Modification of Activity

Randomized trials of social support in the United Kingdom failed to improve pregnancy outcomes, and in some studies, hospitalization for bed rest led to an increase in preterm birth. Roles for sexual abstinence and/or psychological support are no clearer. Patients should be informed that there is no evidence that their activity level influences outcome. The Society for Maternal-Fetal Medicine guidelines on activity restriction "recommend against the use of any type of activity restriction in pregnant women at risk of preterm birth." This should be tempered by the realization that there is a natural tendency to analyze the days leading up to a preterm birth, looking for triggers. Patients should be somewhat cautious and avoid overexertion or extreme stress, if only to minimize subsequent feelings of guilt, however misplaced.

Emergency Cervical Cerclage

When a patient presents with an open cervical os and bulging membranes before viability, the idea of closing the cervix by passing a stitch around it seems logical. However, the results of emergency cervical cerclage are poor and are related to the cervical dilatation at insertion. The procedure itself can be technically challenging. A dilatation of more than 3 cm with an effaced cervix poses extreme difficulties even for the most experienced operator. Every effort should be made to detect and treat other causes of the uterine instability. If persistent placental bleeding is leading to secondary opening of the cervix, suturing the cervix clearly does not address the primary issue and is unlikely to be successful. Bleeding, contractions, and infection are all contraindications to cerclage. Depending on the initial dilatation of the cervix, the chance of the pregnancy proceeding beyond 26 weeks may be less than 50 percent.

Induction or Augmentation

In some cases, it may be judged appropriate to hasten delivery because the maternal or fetal risks of continuing the pregnancy are judged too high. After 24 weeks, if there is no evidence of acute maternal or fetal compromise, induction with milder prostaglandins, such as Cervidil or conventional-dose oxytocin, can considered as an alternative to a planned cesarean section. Great care must be exercised if there is already clinical evidence of chorioamnionitis. In these cases, delay in ending the pregnancy may lead to worsening infection and consequent morbidity for both the mother and baby. Augmenting labor may be the most appropriate management. After extremely or very preterm PPROM, an initial period of conservative management is commonly undertaken. Close observation for evidence of clinical chorioamnionitis, such as maternal fever, uterine tenderness, and fetal tachycardia, is necessary. There is no evidence that serial WBC counts or CRP levels add to clinical examination. There is evidence appearing that supports active management after 33 completed weeks, particularly after a course of steroids has been completed.

Analgesia

For intrapartum analgesia, an epidural is frequently advocated. Postulated benefits include avoiding expulsive efforts before full dilatation or a precipitous delivery, a relaxed pelvic floor and perineum, and the ability to proceed quickly to abdominal delivery.

Mode of Delivery

Many clinicians believe that the combination of high fetal morbidity and mortality; difficulty in diagnosing intrapartum hypoxia or acidosis; and maternal risk of complications, both intraoperatively and in subsequent pregnancies, do not justify cesarean section for fetal indications before 24 weeks. As gestation advances, both neonatal outcomes and the ability to diagnose fetal compromise improve, and intervention for fetal reasons becomes appropriate. It is often appropriate to leave the membranes intact even if oxytocin is required. There is little risk of dystocia, and an intact gestation sac cushions both the fetal head and umbilical cord. The safety of preterm breech vaginal delivery between 26^{+0} and 36^{+6} weeks is often questioned. Cesarean section should be considered, although evidence to support this as a routine policy remains less than ideal.

Type of Cesarean Section

At the earliest gestations and in the presence of oligohydramnios, the lower segment is often poorly formed. Vertical uterine incisions may be necessary. This "classical" uterine incision carries an up to 5 percent risk of uterine rupture in subsequent pregnancies, some of which will occur before the onset of labor.

Timing of Cord Clamping

Ideally, delay cord clamping by around 60 seconds for preterm babies, if the mother and baby are stable. Ensure the baby is dried and kept warm during this interval.

SELECTED READING

National Institute for Health and Care Excellence: Preterm labour and birth. NICE Guideline NG25. http://www.nice.org.uk/guidance, 2019

Royal College of Obstetricians and Gynaecologists: Care of women presenting with suspected preterm premature rupture of the membranes from 24+0 weeks of gestation. Green-top Clinical Guideline No. 73. http://www.rcog.org.uk/guidelines, 2019

Society for Maternal-Fetal Medicine: The role of activity restriction in obstetric management. Consult Series #50. http://www.smfm.org, 2020

Society of Obstetricians and Gynaecologists of Canada: Clinical practice guideline – Antenatal corticosteroid therapy for improving neonatal outcomes. J Obstet Gynaecol Can 40:1219-1239, 2018

Society of Obstetricians and Gynaecologists of Canada: Clinical practice guideline – Magnesium sulphate for fetal neuroprotection. J Obstet Gynaecol Can 41:502-522, 2019

OTHER ISSUES

Antepartum Hemorrhage

Ana Werlang

CHAPTER 31

INTRODUCTION

Hemorrhage in the second half of pregnancy can pose a serious threat to the health of both mother and child. In the majority of cases, the exact cause will remain unknown antenatally. Rapid diagnosis and adequate management will determine the timing of delivery and outcomes. The principal causes associated with antepartum hemorrhage are:

1. Placenta previa
2. Abruptio placentae
3. Vasa previa
4. Early labor
5. Local lesions (e.g., cervical ectropion or polyp)
6. Unknown or idiopathic: no discoverable cause

PLACENTA PREVIA

In this condition, the placenta is implanted in the lower uterine segment and lies over or near the internal cervical os, below the presenting part of the fetus. The incidence is one in 350 pregnancies. It is responsible for about 10 percent of antepartum hemorrhages. The late development of the lower uterine segment after 28 weeks leads to the phenomenon of placental migration, in which an apparent placenta previa in early pregnancy moves away from the internal os toward term.

Etiology

The etiology is unknown. Risk factors include a previous pregnancy with placenta previa, number of previous cesarean sections, and advanced maternal age. Weaker risk factors include multiparity, endometrial trauma such as curettage, and cigarette smoking.

Classification

The clinical classification of placenta previa is now based on the ultrasound findings (Fig. 31-1).

Delineation of the location of the placental edge in relation to the cervical os is of paramount importance. The marginal sinus of the placenta should not be mistaken by the placental edge. However, a marginal sinus covering the internal os is clinically relevant due to the high risk of

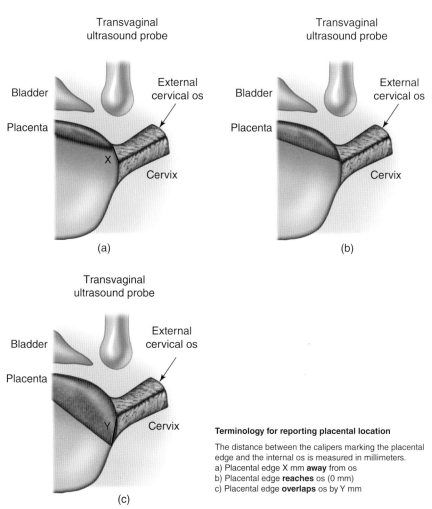

FIGURE 31-1. Modern approach to the ultrasonographic assessment of a low-lying placenta.

antepartum bleeding. In the case of complete placenta previa, the degree of overlap beyond the cervical os should be estimated. In the case of a low-lying placenta, the distance from the os should be documented. A simplified and clinically relevant classification is proposed:

1. Placenta previa (Fig. 31-2): when the placenta is covering or overlapping the cervical os. Complete previa (or central) defines a placenta that overlaps the internal os covering the anterior lower uterine segment.
2. Low-lying placenta: when the placental edge is within 2 cm of the cervical os

OTHER ISSUES

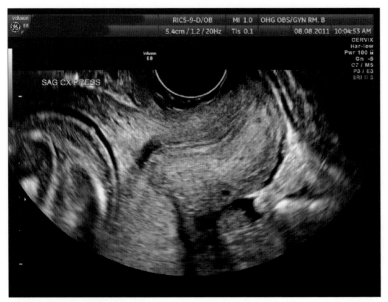

FIGURE 31-2. A posterior placenta with the lower edge just crossing the internal os on transvaginal ultrasound.

3. Normal placental location: when the placental edge is more than 2 cm away from the cervical os

In addition, the thickness of the placental edge should be assessed (see Fig. 31-3). The presence of a thick placental edge (>1 cm or 45°) is

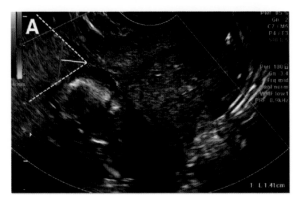

FIGURE 31-3. Measurement of the distance between internal os and the placental edge is L 1.41 cm (internal cervical os and placental edge are marked by calliper signs); measurement of placental edge thickness (red double arrow) in the low-lying placenta is performed within 1 cm (yellow line 1 cm); the angle (white dotted lines) between the basal and chorionic plate is >45°. These measurements must be undertaken by transvaginal scan. (Reprinted from Vintzileos A, et al. Am J Obstetr Gynecol 213;S70-77, 2015, with permission from Elsevier.)

associated with a higher risk of antepartum hemorrhage, cesarean delivery, and of occurrence of invasive placentation.

Clinical Manifestations

The classic symptom is painless vaginal bleeding. A feature of placenta previa is that the degree of anemia or shock is equivalent to the amount of blood loss. In most cases, the bleeding is unprovoked, but it may be preceded by injudicious trauma (e.g., digital vaginal exam or sexual intercourse). For some patients, it remains an ultrasound diagnosis that never leads to any symptoms. Other patients have a single bleed that leads to the diagnosis and never recurs. A worrying group is those patients with recurrent episodes of bleeding (so-called "warning bleeds"), who have a higher risk of presenting with significant hemorrhage.

Associated Findings

1. Failure of engagement of the presenting part
2. Abnormal presentations, such as breech and transverse lie, are more common
3. The uterus is soft and nontender
4. The fetal heart rate (FHR) pattern is often reassuring because the degree of placental separation is minimal, and there is little fetal compromise
5. Placenta accreta: The incidence is higher when the placenta implants in the upper segment of the uterus, especially if the placenta is anterior and the patient has had previous cesarean deliveries. The risk increases in line with the number of previous cesareans, with a 50 percent risk described for patients with four or more cesareans. The diagnosis and management of placenta accreta are covered in more detail in Chapter 19, "Delivery of the Placenta, Retained Placenta, and Placenta Accreta Spectrum Disorder."

Diagnosis

Placenta previa is a second-trimester diagnosis and should be confirmed by transvaginal ultrasound examination, the safest and most accurate tool currently available. When transvaginal probes are not available, transperineal or translabial scanning (using a transabdominal probe covered with gloves) is a reasonable alternative. Transabdominal imaging can be misleading in cases of a posterior placenta, or patients with challenging body habitus, or if performed with a full bladder, as it is associated with a higher

OTHER ISSUES

incidence of false positives. Once diagnosed, patients should be reassessed at 28 to 32 weeks of gestation, as the placenta tends typically to move up and away from the cervix. About 90 percent of low-lying placentas will be in normal location by 32 weeks of gestation. Because of the possibility of placental migration, final decisions regarding the mode of delivery in asymptomatic patients should only be based on the ultrasound appearance at 36 weeks.

Management of Asymptomatic Patients with Placenta Previa

1. Determine whether the previa resolves with increasing gestational age
2. Determine whether the placenta is also morbidly adherent (placenta accreta spectrum)
3. Reduce the risk of bleeding
4. Determine the optimal time for planned cesarean delivery if the previa persists

In the absence of risk factors, a final sonographic diagnosis should be made at 36 weeks.

- Low-lying placenta with tip between 10 and 20 mm from the internal os: a trial of labor may be considered if there are resources to promptly perform a cesarean in case of intrapartum hemorrhage
- Low-lying placenta with the tip less than 10 mm from the internal os: an elective cesarean section should be performed between 37^{+0} to 38^{+6} weeks if no history of bleeding
- If placenta previa (tip reaching or overlapping the os): an elective cesarean should be performed at 36^{+0} to 37^{+6} weeks. All risk factors should be considered in the decision-making regarding the time of delivery

Usually, most patients will be discharged after the first bleeding episode and can be monitored as outpatients. However, patient-specific risk factors need to be considered. Such factors may include short cervical length on transvaginal ultrasound examination (consider hospitalization if <15 mm), rapid cervical shortening, inability to get to the hospital promptly, and lack of home support in case of an emergency.

Generally, delivery is indicated when bleeding is heavy and persistent, or the patient goes into labor, or signs of fetal distress that do not respond to resuscitation measures (see "General Management of Third-Trimester Bleeding" at the end of this chapter).

Peripartum Care

It is important to know if placenta previa is located anterior or posteriorly in order to plan the hysterotomy type and location. Peripartum ultrasound can be performed with a transabdominal probe covered with sterile covers if delivery is nonemergent as an attempt to avoid placenta bulk when incising the uterus. A classical vertical incision may be necessary in some cases of anterior placenta with fetal malpresentation and in most cases if placenta accreta spectrum is present.

ABRUPTIO PLACENTAE

This condition, also known as premature placental separation, involves detachment of the placenta from the uterine wall. Its incidence rate is gestational-age specific, estimated at around 13 percent in the third trimester. Abruptio placentae is initiated by hemorrhage, leading to a variable degree of fetal and maternal morbidity depending on the degree of separation of the placenta.

In most cases, the bleeding progresses to the edge of the placenta. At this point, it may break through the membranes and enter the amniotic cavity or, more often, the blood tracks down between the chorion and the uterine wall until it exits via the cervix. Occasionally, there is extensive extravasation of blood into the myometrium; such condition is described as Couvelaire uterus.

Etiology

The cause of placental abruption is not known. Most abruptions seem to be related to a chronic underlying placental disease. Risk factors associated with this condition are:

1. History of a previous pregnancy complicated by an abruption increases 20 times the risk of recurrence
2. Other manifestations of placental dysfunction: Hypertensive disorders, intrauterine growth restriction, preeclampsia
3. Substance abuse: Smoking is associated with a 2.5-fold increased risk and is one of the few modifiable risk factors for abruption. Cocaine is one of the vasoconstrictors that leads to ischemia and placental abruption (higher risk in the third trimester). When smoking and cocaine are associated, risks are exponentially higher

OTHER ISSUES

4. Preterm premature rupture of the membranes (PPROM): There is a strong relationship between these two clinical entities, perhaps linked by infection because PPROM is associated with subclinical chorioamnionitis. A subchorionic blood collection is an ideal culture medium for bacteria leading to secondary chorioamnionitis and membrane weakening. Alternatively, when subclinical chorioamnionitis is the primary event leading to membrane rupture, the associated vasculitis may trigger an abruption.

5. Overdistention of the uterus: Multiple pregnancy or polyhydramnios, especially if there is an acute volume reduction (as seen after delivery of first twin or PPROM). Uterine anomalies also carry a small risk of placental mal-implantation and abruption.

6. Trauma: Most commonly, motor vehicle accidents

7. Iatrogenic: Although not common, abruption after manual external cephalic version or amnioreduction has been described

Classification

1. Revealed or *external* (Fig. 31-4A): The blood may be bright red or dark and clotted. The pain is mild to moderate unless the patient is in labor. The degree of anemia and shock is equivalent to the apparent blood

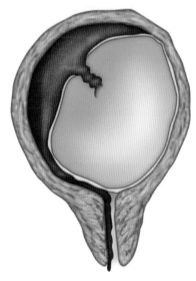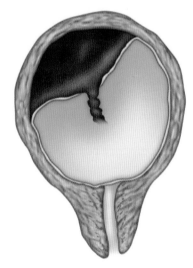

A. External or apparent.   B. Internal or concealed.

FIGURE 31-4. Revealed and concealed placental abruption.

loss; however, the degree of placental separation correlates poorly with the amount of vaginal bleeding and does not serve as a valuable marker of impending maternal or fetal risk

2. Concealed or *internal* (Fig. 31-4B): There is minor vaginal bleeding. The blood is trapped in the uterus. If it is a major abruption, the pain is severe, and the uterus is hard and tender. The degree of shock is more significant than expected for the amount of visible bleeding

3. *Mixed or combined:* A varying mixture of the above groups is seen

Placental abruption can be deceiving. Not only can some or all of the bleeding be hidden, but a seemingly normotensive woman may be profoundly hypovolemic if preeclampsia was the etiologic factor behind the abruption. In this circumstance, bladder catheterization will confirm significant proteinuria and document oliguria.

Clinical Manifestations

Clinical manifestations depend on the location of the blood (revealed or concealed) and the amount of blood lost. The latter may be relatively small or large enough to lead to hypovolemic shock and even maternal death. The classical clinical picture includes vaginal bleeding, abdominal pain, and uterine tenderness associated with fetal distress. Atypical back pain can be reported with a posterior placenta. The uterus may exhibit a "wood-like" rigidity and may enlarge as blood accumulates in the cavity. Often, the patient is in labor. The fetal heart rate may suggest significant compromise or may be absent. Abnormal maternal vital signs (orthostatic hypotension, reflex tachycardia, and tachypnea) are the earliest signs of shock and maternal compromise. When there is a loss of more than 40 percent of the volemia, hypotension and oliguria are ominous signs of shock. Severe abruptions involving more than 50 percent of the placental surface often can lead to disseminated intravascular coagulation and maternal death.

Associated Findings

1. Labor, especially preterm labor, can be triggered by abruption. It is probably caused by blood and coagulation products leading to myometrial contractility

2. Fetal distress is common; a nonreassuring FHR tracing is often seen with a major abruption involving more than 50 percent of the placenta. Fetal demise may occur. The perinatal mortality rate ranges from 25 to

50 percent. Perinatal asphyxia, intraventricular hemorrhage, periventricular leukomalacia, and cerebral palsy have been described as fetal outcomes of placental abruption.

Diagnosis

Abruptio placentae diagnosis is made on clinical grounds. Ultrasonography has a low sensitivity for abruption, detecting only 15 percent of cases. Therefore, prompt management should never be delayed while waiting for imaging. Ultrasound is used simply to rule out placenta previa. The Kleihauer-Betke test is of no diagnostic value but can guide WinRho or RhoGAM dosing in Rh-negative mothers. The diagnosis may only be confirmed at delivery when inspection of the placenta reveals an adherent retroplacental clot with disruption of the underlying tissue. However, subsequent pathologic examination of the placenta may be normal, especially in the setting of acute hemorrhage.

Differential Diagnosis

- Placenta previa
- Uterine rupture
- Subchorionic hematoma

Management of Hemodynamically Stable Patients with Reassuring Fetal Status

1. Below 34 weeks: admit for observation. Give steroids for lung maturation. Rule out differentials (placenta previa, uterine rupture, or others based on individual case). The goal is to deliver at 37 to 38 weeks if asymptomatic or earlier if any signs of fetal or maternal compromise or recurrent abruption
2. Between 34^{+0} to 36^{+6} weeks: delivery is indicated in cases of acute abruption. In cases of small abruption, light bleeding with no fetal or maternal compromise, delivery can be postponed as long as fetal monitoring is continuous and the patient remains asymptomatic
3. After 37^{+0} weeks: delivery is indicated. Cesarean is usually the mode of delivery when there is fetal compromise and an unfavorable cervix. If the abruption triggers labor, a trial of labor is acceptable, assuming adequate local resources permitting, including continuous fetal monitoring and the ability to promptly perform a cesarean section in case of maternal or fetal decompensation

VASA PREVIA

Vasa previa is a condition in which fetal vessels, unsupported by either the umbilical cord or placental tissue, are crossing or running close to the internal cervical os. The branching vessels run between the amnion and the chorion unprotected by Wharton jelly, vulnerable to compression or rupture, in which case fetal death by exsanguination can occur. In the vast majority of cases, the placenta is low lying or previa, and one of two clinical situations exists: (1) there is a velamentous insertion of the cord, or (2) there is a separate accessory placental lobe (bilobed or succenturiate) (Fig. 31-5).

Other risk factors for vasa previa include in vitro fertilization techniques and multiple pregnancies.

The overall incidence of vasa previa is estimated at approximately one in 3000. However, in association with known velamentous insertion of the cord, the incidence of vasa previa rises to one in 50.

Antenatal Diagnosis

Accurate prenatal diagnosis and timed preterm delivery are crucial to avoid premature rupture of the membranes (PROM) that can lead to vessel tearing and rapid fetal bleeding. No fetal death has been reported with antenatal diagnosis of vasa previa, hence the relevance of early and precise diagnosis. The presence of any risk factors should trigger targeted screening of the placental cord insertion. Antenatal diagnosis is possible by combining transabdominal and transvaginal ultrasound. Transabdominal ultrasound allows diagnosis of placental type, position and cord insertion. Mapping vessels transvaginally with color Doppler will demonstrate at least one vessel crossing or within 2 cm from the internal cervical os, with a detection rate of 99 percent. Power Doppler will confirm fetal pulse waveform and frequency. In the third trimester, when the fetal presentation may already be engaged, lifting the fetal parts with one hand and or tilting the patient to Trendelenburg position during transvaginal scan can improve visualization of the lower segment and internal os.

Intrapartum Diagnosis

In the absence of a prenatal diagnosis, this includes:

1. *FHR:* Vasa previa may be suspected when a relatively minor episode of painless vaginal bleeding is followed by a nonreassuring FHR tracing (fetal tachycardia followed by late decelerations, bradycardia, and sinusoidal pattern in the late stages precluding fetal demise)

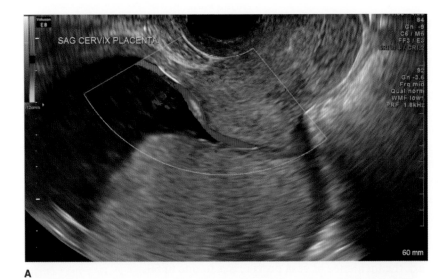

A

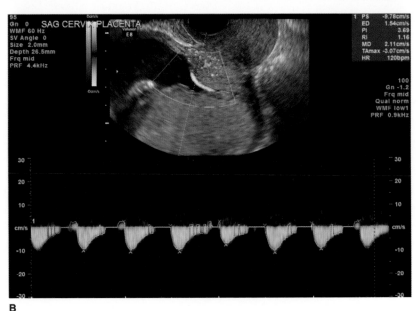

B

FIGURE 31-5. Transvaginal midsagittal view of the cervix and posterior placenta, **(A)** with Colour Doppler showing an unprotected velamentous vessel traveling from the placenta through the internal os of the cervix and **(B)** using PW Doppler to identify vessel origin, placing the gate within the vessel lumen. The fetal pulse is identified (FHR 120 bpm). All these features are diagnostic of vasa previa.

2. *Vaginal examination:* The examiner can feel the vessel or fetal pulse with the fingers. The condition may be confused with umbilical cord presentation
3. *Amnioscopy:* Visualization of the blood vessels within the membranes
4. *Apt test:* This acid-elution procedure demonstrates fetal red blood cells in the maternal plasma and establishes that the bleeding is of fetal origin

The resources and skills to perform amnioscopy or a bedside Apt test are unlikely to be available, therefore, not necessary for diagnosis.

Management

Conventional management of women diagnosed with vasa previa prenatally includes hospital admission sometime between 28 and 32 weeks and a planned cesarean delivery at 34 to 36 weeks. The rationale behind early admission is based on the impossibility to predict PPROM or early labor. If labor or membrane rupture occurs spontaneously before then, a prompt emergency cesarean section should be performed. Cervical length has been extensively evaluated and is a powerful predictor of spontaneous preterm birth in asymptomatic women and can minimize iatrogenic prematurity. If available, transvaginal ultrasound every 1 to 2 weeks should be done from 28 weeks onward to confirm the diagnosis, assess cervical length and assess the risk of preterm labor. If asymptomatic, maternal steroids and delivery before 34 weeks should be based on individualized risk. Immediate emergency cesarean section should be offered in case of PPROM and confirmed vasa previa.

EARLY LABOR

Some patients may present with a heavy "show" that is indistinguishable from an antepartum hemorrhage. However, most of these patients lack features associated with pathologic diagnoses. They do not have pain between contractions, and the FHR tracing remains normal. Over time, the cervix effaces and dilates. Often the bleeding abates as the presenting part descends and compresses veins within the cervix and lower segment.

LOCAL LESIONS

Although usually only associated with relatively minor bleeding episodes, cervical polyps or ectropion are readily detected on speculum examination. Chlamydial cervicitis can be diagnosed by swab. Rare cases of cervical cancer may also be diagnosed in these circumstances. Caution should be exercised in attributing bleeding to any local lesion before all other obstetric causes have been assessed as unlikely.

IDIOPATHIC

Frequently, no cause or reason for the bleeding is ever found. The bleeding is usually small in quantity, and there is no effect on the mother, fetus, or pregnancy. Treatment involves the ruling out of serious conditions followed by expectant management. Most patients go to term.

GENERAL MANAGEMENT OF THIRD-TRIMESTER BLEEDING

Initial Evaluation

1. Assess maternal hemodynamic status
   a. Check maternal vital signs and perform a clinical examination (cervical assessment by speculum examination only)
   b. Estimate prior blood loss from history and visual inspection
   c. Identify source of bleeding, determine ongoing blood loss, local lesions
2. Assess fetal well-being (initially by fetal heart rate monitor)
3. Placental localization: determine from previous ultrasound reports or by a bedside scan, if promptly available, whether a placenta previa exists
4. Confirm exact gestational age: management should always be guided by the risk to the mother and the risk to the fetus. To be put into the correct context, the gestational age must be taken into account.

Preliminary Management

In all but the minor episodes of bleeding, the following steps should be considered:

1. Establish an intravenous infusion with a large-bore catheter (14-16 gauge). A second IV line should be obtained if there are signs of hemodynamic instability. Crystalloids are the infusion of choice. Ringer's lactate is preferred over normal saline to avoid hyperchloremic acidosis

2. Blood is taken for a baseline blood count, creatinine, electrolytes, and type and screen. Cross-matching should be considered with more significant bleeds, especially in the presence of abnormal placentation. If the patient is rhesus negative, a Kleihauer-Betke test should be performed to ensure the correct dose of WinRho

3. The patient is admitted to the labor and delivery unit for observation. At preterm gestations, less than 34 weeks, maternal steroids for fetal lung maturity should be considered. When delivery is imminent but not emergent, magnesium sulphate for neuroprotection should be considered

4. Assistance from other health care team members, which may include an anesthetist, a second obstetrician, a critical care specialist, a hematologist, and experienced nursing staff, should be considered when appropriate and if available

Maternal or Fetal Compromise Suspected

Initial steps should be directed at stabilizing or resuscitating the mother. All obstetric units should have a multidisciplinary protocol in place to recognize and manage major obstetric hemorrhage.

Either immediately after or simultaneous with maternal resuscitation, steps should be taken toward emptying the uterus. In the presence of a major abruption, the cervix may be fully dilated rapidly, and artificial rupture of the membranes followed by vaginal delivery may be the best option. The fetal condition will influence decision-making. If the FHR pattern is preterminal or there has been prolonged severe bradycardia, the chance of fetal survival is slim, and the risks to the mother from surgery may be too high. Less severe degrees of suspected fetal compromise will push toward emergency cesarean delivery. In the presence of a significant previa (placental or vasa), delivery should be by emergency cesarean section.

No Maternal or Fetal Compromise Suspected

In the absence of any previa, if speculum examination reveals cervical dilatation and the gestation is suitably advanced, augmentation of labor may be appropriate. In other circumstances, expectant management is offered with a duration that will depend on many factors, including the placental site, the severity of blood loss, whether a recurrent problem is present, and the gestational age. Local resources should also be considered, particularly if specialized services such as interventional radiology are required at delivery. In general, the threshold for delivery is inversely related to the severity and frequency of bleeding and/or the gestational age.

OTHER ISSUES

Double Setup Examination

This procedure is carried out when the diagnosis is uncertain, and no ultrasound facilities exist locally. Although rarely, if ever, required in developed countries, it may still be necessary for under-resourced areas. The patient is taken to the operating room, where all preparations have been made for an immediate cesarean section. Under anesthesia, abdominal and vaginal examinations are performed to ascertain the fetal presentation, the condition of the cervix, and the location of the placenta. The vaginal examination begins in the fornices, assessing any soft tissue mass between the presenting parts and examining fingers. However, the vaginal examination may provoke heavy bleeding and is reserved for patients whose placenta previa is only suspected or whose vaginal bleeding is of unclear etiology. Only after a major previa is excluded should a cervical assessment be performed, gently feeling for a placental edge. Treatment is based on these findings.

SELECTED READING

Royal College of Obstetricians and Gynaecologists: Antepartum haemorrhage. Green-top Clinical Guideline No. 63. http://www.rcog.org.uk/guidelines, 2011

Royal College of Obstetricians and Gynaecologists: Placenta praevia, placenta praevia accrete and vasa previa: diagnosis and management. Green-top Clinical Guideline No. 27. http://www.rcog.org.uk/guidelines, 2011

Royal College of Obstetricians and Gynaecologists: Placenta praevia and placenta accreta: diagnosis and management. Green-top Clinical Guideline No. 27a. http://www.rcog.org.uk/guidelines, 2018

Royal College of Obstetricians and Gynaecologists: Vasa praevia: diagnosis and management. Green-top Clinical Guideline No. 27b. http://www.rcog.org.uk/guidelines, 2018

Royal College of Obstetricians and Gynaecologists: Maternal collapse in pregnancy and the puerperium. Green-top Clinical Guideline No. 56. http://www.rcog.org.uk/guidelines, 2019

Society of Obstetricians and Gynaecologists of Canada: Clinical Guideline No. 231: Guidelines for the management of vasa previa. J Obstet Gynaecol Can 39: e415-e421, 2017

Society of Obstetricians and Gynaecologists of Canada: Clinical Guideline No. 115: Hemorrhagic shock. J Obstet Gynaecol Can 40: e874-e882, 2018

Society of Obstetricians and Gynaecologists of Canada: Clinical Guideline No. 235: Active Management of the third stage of labor: Prevention and treatment of postpartum hemorrhage. J Obstet Gynaecol Can 40: e841-e855, 2018

Society of Obstetricians and Gynaecologists of Canada: Clinical Guideline No. 402: Diagnosis and management of placenta previa. J Obstet Gynaecol Can 42: 906-917, 2020

Vintzileos AM, Ananth CV, Smulian JC: Using ultrasound in the clinical management of placental implantation abnormalities. Am J Obstet Gynecol 213: S70-S77, 2015

CHAPTER 32

Maternal Complications in Labor

Julia Tai
Tammy Shaw

PREGESTATIONAL DIABETES

Diabetes is the leading endocrine condition complicating pregnancy, with rising incidence due to the obesity epidemic and advancing maternal age. It is estimated that 5 percent of pregnancies are complicated by diabetes, with the vast majority caused by gestational diabetes mellitus (GDM) followed by type 1 or type 2 diabetes mellitus (DM).

Physiologic Changes in Pregnancy

Pregnancy is associated with accelerated starvation, resulting in increased ketogenesis and lower fasting plasma glucose levels, most pronounced in the first trimester. The increased ketogenesis predisposes mothers to episodes of diabetic ketoacidosis. In early gestation, especially weeks 7 to 12, there may be a 10 to 20 percent drop in insulin requirements before insulin-resistant placental hormones rise. Impaired counterregulatory hormone responses (specifically epinephrine and growth hormone) also occur in pregnancy. This period is thus associated with an increased risk of hypoglycemic episodes without autonomic warning. Maternal hypoglycemia unawareness is an important risk factor for the development of severe hypoglycemia.

In mid-to-late pregnancy, increased levels of human placental lactogen (hPL), human placental growth hormone (hPGH), cortisol, and prolactin lead to an insulin-resistant state. This maternal insulin resistance at the level of skeletal muscle and adipose tissue facilitates metabolic fetal demands that are 80 percent derived from glucose. It is important to note that if insulin requirements decrease significantly late in gestation, it may be a sign of placental insufficiency. Changes in therapeutic requirements in patients with diabetes should be anticipated during this time by health care providers.

Important Comorbidities

Diabetes during pregnancy is associated with an increased risk of pre-eclampsia (15%-30%), polyhydramnios (15%-20%), and cesarean section or instrumental delivery (25%-40%).

Patients with diabetes also have important comorbidities that may need to be addressed during pregnancy, such as hypertension and obesity. There is also evidence of an increased risk of progression of retinopathy and nephropathy.

Ominous Signs

- Maternal hypoglycemia and unawareness
- Maternal acidosis

- Uncontrolled maternal hyperglycemia
- Severe fetal macrosomia
- Polyhydramnios and progressive growth restriction

Diabetic Ketoacidosis

Women with diabetes are at increased risk of diabetic ketoacidosis (DKA) during pregnancy due to increased ketogenesis, impaired buffering capacity of the chronically compensated respiratory alkalotic state, and maternal insulin resistance mid-to-late pregnancy. It is most often associated with type 1 DM; however, has been recognized in type 2 DM and GDM. Common triggers include protracted vomiting, hyperemesis gravidarum, infections, nonadherence to insulin or insulin pump failures, and use of corticosteroids for fetal lung maturation. DKA most commonly occurs in the second or third trimester. Although the presentation is similar to that in nonpregnant patients, glucose levels may be much lower, and the acidosis more pronounced. Ketones readily cross the placenta, and DKA is associated with high fetal mortality. Treatment is the same as in nonpregnant patients and requires prompt recognition, intravenous (IV) rehydration, electrolyte replacement, and IV insulin therapy. Identification and treatment of the triggering condition is crucial. Concise guidelines on the treatment of DKA in pregnancy are available.

Intrapartum Management of Diabetes

Timing and Mode of Delivery

Diabetes in itself is not an indication for cesarean section, and the route of delivery in women whose diabetes is well-controlled should be based on the same criteria that apply to nondiabetic patients. Timing of delivery varies but is generally believed to be best between the 38th and 40th weeks of gestation for uncomplicated well-controlled diabetes to reduce the risk of stillbirth. Earlier delivery should be considered based on other maternal or fetal factors, weighing the potential benefits against the risks of neonatal complications.

Glycemic Control During Labor and Delivery

Impaired counterregulatory hormone responses places patients at increased risk of hypoglycemia unawareness. Risk of neonatal hypoglycemia is also directly linked to maternal hyperglycemia. The goal of intrapartum

OTHER ISSUES

glycemic control is thus avoidance of maternal hypoglycemia and hyperglycemia for maternal and neonatal safety.

In early labor while the patient is still eating, subcutaneous insulin should be continued. Dose adjustment may be required based on oral intake. When the patient is in active labor and no longer eating, IV dextrose and insulin should be used. Target glycemic values between 4 and 7 mmol/L (72-126 mg/dL) are recommended.

In general, women with type 1 DM require 1 to 1.5 U/h, whereas women with type 2 DM or GDM may require higher doses due to progressive insulin resistance. Patients who are using an insulin pump may continue their basal infusion during labor although the rate may need to be reduced. Once the patient has delivered and is eating, IV insulin should be discontinued 2 hours after subcutaneous insulin resumed. Patients previously controlled on diet and/or oral agents can often resume their prepregnancy therapy with close monitoring.

Many local health centers have standardized orders that can be applied (Fig. 32-1).

Neonatal Considerations

Neonates should have frequent capillary glucose monitoring. The definition of clinically significant neonatal hypoglycemia has been difficult to define due to variability of glucose levels in the first hours of life and lack of clarity on which levels are linked to poor neurodevelopmental outcomes. Thresholds for intervention depend on age of infant and presence of symptoms where symptomatic or lower glucose levels require more aggressive interventions such as IV dextrose. Early breastfeeding has been shown to reduce the incidence of neonatal hypoglycemia. Institutions should carry protocols for neonatal hypoglycemia.

Postpartum

Immediately postpartum, insulin requirements decrease. In women with type 1 DM, a "honeymoon" period may occur 24 to 48 hours postpartum during which no insulin therapy is needed to maintain glycemic values at 6 to 10 mmol/L (108-180 mg/dL) following which reduced insulin doses are needed and typically return to prepregnancy doses over 6 to 8 weeks. It is recommended that one-half to two-thirds of the prepregnancy insulin requirements is an appropriate starting dose in the postpartum period.

Insulin, second-generation oral sulfonylureas, and metformin can be resumed postpartum while breastfeeding. No safety data are available for other oral agents. When indicated, the angiotensin-converting enzyme (ACE) inhibitors perindopril and captopril can be reintroduced during breastfeeding.

Breastfeeding is associated with lower risk of neonatal hypoglycemia, offspring obesity, or diabetes and therefore should be encouraged for a minimum of 4 months.

Pre-delivery diabetes orders ☐ Type 1 ☐ Type 2 ☐ Other

While patient is eating

1. BG testing: TID before meals, qhs and 3am
2. Insulin orders
   - ☐ Patient may self-manage (self-administer and adjust insulin)
   - ☐ Patient/family may continue insulin pump.
   - ☐ Nurse managed (or if patient unable to self-manage/continue with insulin pump)

> Option of self-management as per patient preference (if able)

☐ **Basal (long acting)**

☐ Humulin N/NPH	☐ QAM _____ units	
☐ Glargine (Lantus)	☐ QHS _____ units	
☐ Other _____	☐ Other _____ units	

☐ **Meal-time (short acting) + supplemental scale**

☐ Aspart (Novorapid)	☐ AC breakfast _____
☐ Glulisine (Apidra)	☐ AC lunch _____
☐ Other _____	☐ AC supper _____

Supplemental Scale

Blood glucose (mmol/L)	Short acting insulin (in addition to mealtime dose)
< 4	Give 175 ml juice or 25mL D50W IV. Retest in 15 min, call MD
4.1-8	0 additional units
8.1-10	Add ___units, retest in 4h. If BG > 8, start IV insulin protocol
>10	Start IV insulin protocol

Patient not eating/NPO

1. Start insulin IV protocol (or continue insulin pump)

> Option of continuous subcutaneous or IV insulin

Insulin IV protocol

1. IV D5W: Start at ☐ 100cc/h or ☐ 50cc/h
2. IV regular insulin 50 units/500ml 0.9% NS. Flush IV tubing with 50mL insulin infusion prior to starting drip and piggyback insulin into D5W.
3. BG testing:
   - q1h to start and with any insulin rate changes.
   - if BG 4-8 mmol/L x 2, check BG q2h

> BG monitoring frequency adjusted as needed

Blood glucose (mmol/L)	Insulin infusion rate (units/h).
< 4	Hold, give 25ml D50W and call MD for rate change
4.1-6	Decrease insulin by 0.5 units/h
6.1-8 (target)	No change
8.1-10	Increase insulin by 0.5 units/h
10.1-12	Increase by 0.75 units/h
12.1-14	Increase by 1 unit/h
>14	Increase by 1.25 units/h and call MD for new orders if 2 consecutive results of >14

> Target BG may vary slightly by institution: chosen to avoid maternal hypo- and hyperglycemia

Different rate adjustments can be offered based on patient's total daily dose (TDD) of insulin. TDD is a reflection of insulin sensitivity (eg, larger rate changes if higher TDD)

FIGURE 32-1. Example of peripartum orders with highlighted components.

OTHER ISSUES

Postpartum diabetes orders ☐ Type 1 ☐ Type 2 ☐ Other

1. BG testing:
   - TID before meals, qhs
   - 3am if on insulin postpartum

2. Diabetes Medications
   ☐ Stop all insulin
   ☐ Stop oral hypoglycemics
   ☐ Start _____ (oral hypoglycemic)
   ☐ Stop IV insulin and start SC insulin at next dose (see insulin orders below)
   ☐ Start SC insulin at next scheduled dose when eating well (see insulin orders below) and stop IV insulin 2 hours after SC insulin (injection or insulin pump) resumed
      - For injections, please call MD if next scheduled dose is short-acting (mealtime) dose or if patient was not starting on IV insulin

   > Ensure safe transition (for Type 1 diabetes)

3. Insulin Orders
   ☐ Patient may self-manage (self-administer and adjust insulin)
   ☐ Patient/family may continue insulin pump.
   ☐ Nurse managed (or if patient unable to self-manage/continue with insulin pump)

   > Option of self-management as per patient preference (if able)

   ☐ Basal (long acting)

☐ Humulin N/NPH	☐ QAM _____ units	
☐ Glargine (Lantus)	☐ QHS _____ units	
☐ Other _____	☐ Other _____ units	

   ☐ Meal-time (short acting) + supplemental scale

☐ Aspart (Novorapid)	☐ AC breakfast _____
☐ Glulisine (Apidra)	☐ AC lunch _____
☐ Other _____	☐ AC supper _____

   Supplemental Scale

Blood glucose (mmol/L)	Short acting insulin (in addition to mealtime dose)
< 4	Give 175 ml of juice or 25mL of D50W IV. Retest in 15 min, call MD
4.1-8	0 additional units
8.1-12	Add ___ units to mealtime dose
12.1-16	Add ___ units to mealtime dose
16.1-20	Add ___ units to mealtime dose
>20	Add ___ units to mealtime dose and call MD

FIGURE 32-1. (*Continued*)

HYPERTENSION

Hypertension is the most common chronic medical condition in pregnancy, with increasing incidence due to rising rates of obesity and advanced maternal age. It is estimated that up to 8 percent of all pregnancies are complicated by a hypertensive disorder.

During pregnancy, arterial blood pressure (BP) generally decreases by 10 to 15 mm Hg beginning in the first trimester and reaches a nadir mid-pregnancy, with a return to baseline during the third trimester. New onset hypertension after 20 weeks should prompt evaluation for preeclampsia. See Table 32-1 for the differential diagnosis of hypertension in pregnancy.

TABLE 32-1: DIFFERENTIAL DIAGNOSIS OF HYPERTENSION IN PREGNANCY

Condition	Definitions	Associated Conditions
Chronic hypertension	sBP ≥140 or dBP ≥90 mm Hg before 20 weeks' gestation or 12 weeks postpartum or patient already taking hypertensive medications at the onset of pregnancy	20% risk of developing preeclampsia; without preeclampsia, risk of IUGR or placental abruption likely <1%
Transient hypertension of pregnancy	Isolated BP sBP ≥140 or dBP ≥90 mm Hg	Hypertension resolves quickly and not reproducible at rest or subsequent readings
Whitecoat hypertension	sBP ≥140 or dBP ≥90 mm Hg on office readings but sBP ≤135 or dBP ≤85 mm Hg home or ambulatory readings	May be associated with increased risk of preeclampsia compared to consistently normotensives.
Masked hypertension	sBP ≤140 or dBP ≤90 mm Hg on office readings but sBP ≥135 or dBP ≥85 mm Hg home or ambulatory readings	May be associated with increased risk of preeclampsia and other complications compared to consistently normotensives
Resistant hypertension	BP control requiring ≥3 antihypertensives	
Severe hypertension in pregnancy	sBP ≥160 or dBP ≥110 mm Hg	sBP ≥160 mm Hg is associated with an increased risk of maternal stroke
Preeclampsia	Maternal hypertension complicated by end-organ damage after 20 weeks of gestation. May be superimposed on chronic or gestational hypertension	End-organ dysfunction includes neurologic, renal, hepatic, hematologic, and fetal complications (see section below)

BP, blood pressure; dBP, diastolic blood pressure; IUGR, intrauterine growth restriction; SBP, systolic blood pressure.

Preeclampsia

Preeclampsia affects up to 2 to 8 percent of all pregnancies globally and is the most common cause of pregnancy-associated mortality worldwide. Predisposing factors include extremes of age (younger than 20 or older than 40 years), elevated body mass index, underlying chronic hypertension, history of insulin resistance or diabetes, chronic kidney disease, antiphospholipid antibody syndrome, nulliparity, multifetal gestation, and previous preeclampsia.

The pathophysiology of preeclampsia is not fully understood but thought to be in part due to abnormal placentation with incomplete invasion of the embryo-derived cytotrophoblast into the decidua rather than tunica media of the maternal spiral arteries. The result causes increased systemic vascular resistance, endothelial cell dysfunction, activation of the coagulation cascade, and enhanced platelet aggregation, ultimately leading to numerous maternal and fetal complications.

Generally accepted diagnostic criteria include hypertension occurring after 20 weeks of gestation in a previously normotensive woman or resistant hypertension in a women with preexisting chronic hypertension and the presence of end-organ dysfunction including neurological (headaches, visual changes), cardiac (shortness of breath, chest pain), hepatic (epigastric or right upper quadrant pain, elevated transaminases), renal (elevated serum creatinine, elevated serum uric acid, or proteinuria defined as greater than 0.3 g/d or 30 g/mol Cr), hematologic (thrombocytopenia, coagulopathy), or fetal manifestations (IUGR, oligohydramnios, abnormal umbilical artery doppler velocimetry). Signs on clinical examination include hypertension, abdominal tenderness, and clonus. Serious manifestations are listed in Table 32-2.

TABLE 32-2: SERIOUS MANIFESTATIONS OF PREECLAMPSIA

Maternal	Fetal
Seizures (eclampsia)	Placental abruption
Stroke	Preterm delivery
Congestive heart failure	Fetal growth restriction
Acute renal impairment	Fetal hypoxia
HELLP syndrome	Perinatal death
DIC	
Hepatic infarction, hemorrhage, rupture	
Diabetes insipidus	

DIC, disseminated intravascular coagulation; HELLP, hemolysis, elevated liver enzymes, and low platelets.

Laboratory Investigation

If a diagnosis of preeclampsia is considered, fetal monitoring and the following laboratory investigations should be undertaken:

- Complete blood count (CBC): anemia, thrombocytopenia
- Blood film: red blood cell fragments
- Hemolysis screen: elevated lactate dehydrogenase (LDH) and bilirubin, low haptoglobin
- Coagulation studies if hemolysis suspected: elevated international normalized ratio (INR), elevated partial thromboplastin time (PTT), decreased fibrinogen
- Urinalysis: proteinuria screen
- Formal assessment of proteinuria by urine protein: creatinine ratio or 24-hour urine collection for protein
- Creatinine and urea: assess volume status and renal function
- Uric acid: commonly elevated in preeclampsia, indicator of renal dysfunction
- Liver enzymes: aspartate aminotransferase (AST) and alanine aminotransferase (ALT) elevation above two to three times normal is concerning for significant liver damage. Alkaline phosphatase (ALP) is produced by the placenta and may be slightly elevated in pregnancy

Intrapartum Hypertension Management

Timing and Mode of Delivery

If there is clear evidence of preeclampsia after 37 weeks of gestation, delivery should be advocated. At earlier gestational ages, evidence of severe fetal compromise or maternal risk should lead to consideration of delivery. Definitions of severe manifestations that may warrant preterm delivery vary; however, include seizures, acute onset of renal failure (Cr >88 umol/L (1.1 mg/dL) or doubling of creatinine in absence of underlying renal disease), severe hypertension, HELLP (hemolysis, elevated liver enzymes, low platelets) syndrome, retinal hemorrhage or papilledema, pulmonary edema, or evidence of significant fetal compromise. Timing of delivery should be balanced by the neonatal risks associated with prematurity. Corticosteroids should be given to promote fetal lung maturation if needed. Vaginal delivery should be considered unless another obstetrical reason exists for caesarean delivery.

Seizure Prophylaxis

All women with a firm diagnosis of preeclampsia requiring urgent delivery should be treated with magnesium sulfate for seizure prophylaxis. An IV bolus of 4 to 6 g followed by IV infusion of 1 to 2 g/hr is recommended, with caution in women with renal insufficiency, and continued for 24 hours after delivery. Signs of toxicity, such as hypotension, muscular weakness, and respiratory distress, can be reversed with administration of IV calcium gluconate. The management of eclampsia is described elsewhere.

Treatment of Hypertension

There is no consensus on blood pressure targets in pregnancy other than the need to treat severe hypertension defined as sBP ≥160 or dBP ≥110. Tighter control for women with preexisting comorbidities such as renal disease or diabetes, or end-organ damage is also generally recommended at <140/90. The Control of Hypertension in Pregnancy Study (CHIPS), a randomized controlled open multicenter international trial, compared "less-tight-control" (dBP 100) versus "tight-control" (dBP 85) and found similar outcomes in both the primary (pregnancy loss or high-level neonatal stay) and secondary arms (serious maternal complications). The application of these results remains under debate, with some societies recommending a dBP closer to 85, while others maintaining a wider range such as 130-155/80-105, balancing the need to avoid severe hypertension and its complications with the risk of placental hypoperfusion.

There is more consensus on agents to use in blood pressure management. Severe hypertension should be treated urgently with initial reduction of 25 percent then target of 140/150/90-100 to prevent loss of cerebral vasculature autoregulation. For urgent BP reduction, IV labetalol, oral immediate release nifedipine, or IV hydralazine are recommended:

- Labetalol: 10 to 20 mg IV then 20 to 80 mg every 10 to 30 minutes to maximum cumulative dose of 300 mg or continuous infusion of 0.5 to 2.0 mg/min
- Nifedipine: fast-acting capsules (bitten and swallowed) or immediate-release tablets given 5 to 20 mg orally with repeat in 20 to 30 minutes then 10 to 20 mg orally every 2 to 6 hours for maximum daily dose of 180 mg
- Hydralazine: 5 mg IV/IM then 5 to 10 mg IV every 20 to 40 minutes to maximum cumulative dose of 20 mg or infusion of 0.5 to 10 mg/hr

In cases of nonsevere hypertension with or without preeclampsia, methyldopa (250-500 mg orally twice to four times a day to maximum 2 g per day), labetalol (100-400 mg twice to three times a day to maximum 1200 mg per day), and nifedipine XL (20-60 mg orally daily to maximum 120 mg/day) are the most commonly used medications. ACE inhibitors and angiotensin receptor blockers (ARBs) are contraindicated. Atenolol and prazosin are also not recommended.

Management and Prevention of Complications

Judicious administration of fluids is suggested to avoid pulmonary edema. Acute treatment of pulmonary edema includes supplemental oxygen administration, diuretic use, and morphine if needed. In the setting of oliguria and rising creatinine, small IV boluses (250 cc) of saline can be used cautiously to try to improve urine output.

Postpartum Considerations

It is important to remember that both preeclampsia and eclampsia can present postpartum. Blood pressure from preeclampsia may remain elevated for 6 to 12 weeks postpartum even without underlying chronic hypertension. Platelets, liver function tests, and renal function must be closely monitored until results are normal. Antihypertensive agents acceptable for use in breastfeeding include nifedipine XL, labetalol, captopril, and enalapril. Preeclampsia is also associated with increased risk of premature cardiovascular risk, thus counseling and long-term monitoring of blood pressure and vascular risk factors are recommended.

ACUTE DYSPNEA IN PERIPARTUM PATIENTS

The degree and severity of dyspnea in pregnant patients can range from mild discomfort in keeping with the normal physiologic changes of pregnancy to severe, life-threatening respiratory distress and ultimately respiratory failure. Early recognition of ominous signs and symptoms is crucial in the successful management of critically ill patients. This chapter focuses on the identification, diagnosis, and management of severely ill patients in the peripartum period. Ominous signs are listed in Table 32-3.

Normal Respiratory Changes in Pregnancy

It is important for clinicians to have a fundamental understanding of the normal alterations in maternal respiratory physiology during pregnancy. Pregnancy-related increases in respiratory drive, oxygen consumption and basal metabolic rate lead to increased minute ventilation due to increased tidal volume without changes to respiratory rate. Minute ventilation

OTHER ISSUES

TABLE 32-3: OMINOUS SIGNS OF ACUTELY DYSPNEIC PATIENTS

Asterixis	May be observed with severe hypercapnia
Myoclonus and seizures	May occur with severe hypoxemia
Accessory muscle use	Indicates diaphragmatic fatigue
Cyanosis	Indicative of severe hypoxemia or intracardiac shunt
Tachypnea	(RR >30-40 breaths/min)
Difficulty speaking	(i.e., three- or four-word dyspnea)
Somnolence or alteration of mental status	May occur as a result of severe hypoxemia or hypercapnia
Crackles upon auscultation	May suggest pulmonary edema
Severe hypoxia refractory to oxygen therapy	(PaO_2/FiO_2 <200)
Hypercapnia or respiratory acidosis	PaO_2 >35 mm Hg; pH <7.35

FiO_2, fraction of inspired oxygen; PaO_2, partial pressure of oxygen in arterial blood; RR, respiratory rate.

changes ultimately reduce alveolar and arterial pCO_2. A normal arterial pCO_2 in pregnant patients is lower (28-30 mm Hg) than in their nonpregnant counterpart (35-40 mm Hg). Compensation through renal losses of bicarbonate ions leads to a chronic state of respiratory alkalosis with pH ranging 7.40 to 7.45 and bicarbonate 18 to 21 mEq/L (18-21 mmol/L). Maternal arterial pO_2 also increases to 100 to 105 mm Hg, likely related to increased cardiac output and improved ventilation-perfusion matching. These changes are important to keep in mind when interpreting arterial blood gas (ABG) values.

Pulmonary Function in Pregnancy

Pregnancy-associated increases in tidal volume (TV) comes at a mild decrease in residual volume (RV) and functional residual capacity (FRC). Forced vital capacity (FVC), forced expiratory volume in 1 second (FEV_1), and total lung capacity (TLC) remain unchanged. Increasing oxygen consumption paired with decreased FRC means overall oxygen reserve is decreased, thus pregnant patients are particularly at risk of rapidly worsening hypoxia due to hypoventilation or apnea.

General Management

Regardless of the etiology of dyspnea, the initial steps in management of the patient with respiratory distress are similar. Transfer to a high-dependency setting including continuous cardiac monitoring and pulse oximetry as well as appropriate monitoring for the fetus should be pursued immediately. Close attention to hemodynamic and respiratory changes should prompt more urgent intervention.

Supportive care including supplemental oxygen and IV access is also mandatory in this setting. The level of delivered oxygen depends largely on the extent of hypoxemia, and it is recommended that maternal oxyhemoglobin levels be kept above 95 percent, corresponding to a PaO_2 (partial pressure of oxygen in arterial blood) of approximately 70 mm Hg. If this level of oxygenation cannot be maintained, noninvasive or invasive positive-pressure ventilation should be considered.

General Investigations

Initial investigations must include a focused history and physical examination to narrow the differential diagnosis and to direct more specific testing. ABG analysis, chest radiograph, and an electrocardiogram should also be included in the initial workup. Further investigations will be case specific and will be addressed in more detail below.

PULMONARY EDEMA

Pulmonary edema occurs when there is a net movement of fluid from the pulmonary vasculature to the alveolar space and pulmonary interstitium. This process can occur in response to a variety of underlying conditions; however, for the purpose of this chapter, pulmonary edema can simply be classified into cardiogenic and noncardiogenic causes.

In pregnancy, a number of normal physiologic changes predispose patients to the development of pulmonary edema. These include an increased effective circulating volume (ECV), a relatively low oncotic pressure, and a decreased FRC, which promotes atelectasis and alveolar collapse. During labor and delivery, additional hemodynamic factors must be considered, including a sudden increase in both cardiac output and blood pressure secondary to the pain of uterine contractions and an abrupt increase in ECV from autotransfusion.

OTHER ISSUES

Diagnosis

The diagnosis can be made using a combination of clinical examination and radiographic investigations. Tachypnea and hypoxemia are important clinical clues of an underlying issue. The presence of new bilateral rales on pulmonary auscultation can be suggestive of pulmonary edema. A chest radiograph demonstrating bilateral airspace and interstitial infiltrates would further support the diagnosis. An elevated jugular venous pressure and increased cardiac silhouette may point to a cardiac cause. A transthoracic echocardiogram, if available, would also assist in identifying a cardiogenic etiology.

Cardiogenic Pulmonary Edema

Cardiogenic pulmonary edema can occur when left-sided cardiac filling pressures rise sufficiently to cause high pulmonary capillary pressure, resulting in extravasation of fluid from the pulmonary vasculature. A variety of mechanisms can account for left-sided filling pressures; the most common are presented below.

Arrhythmia

Although rarely a cause of pulmonary edema, acute supraventricular arrhythmias can compromise left ventricular filling in a patient with underlying cardiac dysfunction. More ominous ventricular arrhythmias can lead to hemodynamic instability and even death.

Valvular

Severe aortic stenosis and symptomatic aortic insufficiency and symptomatic mitral valve lesions (stenosis or regurgitation) represent the highest risk to pregnant patients.

Peripartum Cardiomyopathy

Peripartum cardiomyopathy (PPCM) is a condition that typically causes subacute dilatation of the myocardial tissue, resulting in left ventricular dysfunction and clinical heart failure. The prognosis for patients with peripartum cardiomyopathy is variable, with reported mortality rates ranging from 10 to 40 percent in some studies. A diagnosis of PPCM requires the following criteria:

1. An ejection fraction less than 45 percent by echocardiography
2. Clinical symptoms of heart failure

3. Development of cardiac failure toward the end of pregnancy and the months after delivery
4. Absence of another identifiable cause of cardiac failure or recognizable heart disorder before the last month of pregnancy

Ischemia and Infarction

Acute myocardial infarction in pregnant patients is a relatively uncommon problem although its incidence is gradually rising with advance maternal age, and is one of the leading causes of maternal mortality in the developed world. Both atherosclerotic and nonatherosclerotic (e.g., spontaneous coronary artery dissection, coronary thrombosis) mechanisms can contribute. Electrocardiographic and cardiac biomarkers (creatine kinase, troponin I) may assist in the diagnosis.

Noncardiogenic Pulmonary Edema

In contrast to cardiogenic pulmonary edema, noncardiogenic pulmonary edema occurs in the context of normal pulmonary capillary pressure. In this situation, the net movement of fluid into the alveolar and interstitial space can be accounted for by increased permeability of the pulmonary capillaries or low oncotic pressure.

Acute Respiratory Distress Syndrome

Acute respiratory distress syndrome (ARDS) is the most common cause of noncardiogenic pulmonary edema and can be seen in conditions such as pneumonia, sepsis, disseminated intravascular coagulation (DIC), and inhalation injury. In addition, there are a number of pregnancy-associated causes of ARDS, such as tocolysis, preeclampsia or eclampsia, massive hemorrhage and amniotic fluid embolism. The most common pregnancy-associated etiologies are discussed below.

Tocolysis

The use of tocolytic beta-adrenergic receptor agonists (e.g., ritodrine and terbutaline) to suppress preterm labor is associated with the development of ARDS. Although the mechanism remains unclear, it is postulated that prolonged exposure to beta-agonists may cause myocardial dysfunction. These drugs are also known to promote sodium and water retention.

Preeclampsia

Preeclampsia is also associated with the risk of developing ARDS. It is estimated that approximately 3 percent of patients with severe preeclampsia will develop pulmonary edema, with maternal mortality rates reported to be as high as 11 percent. As a result, judicious use of IV fluids is necessary in patients with preeclampsia.

Massive hemorrhage

Volume overload and decreased oncotic pressure from replacement of lost whole blood with packed red cells and crystalloids can lead to pulmonary edema following transfusions for massive antepartum or postpartum hemorrhage. Endothelial damage related to the systemic inflammatory response or transfusion reactions such as transfusion-related acute lung injury (TRALI) may also contribute.

Amniotic Fluid Embolism

Although amniotic fluid embolism (AFE) is a relatively rare condition, the diagnosis must be considered in any peripartum patient with acute dyspnea. Predisposing factors include prolonged labor, multiparity, advanced maternal age, and cesarean or instrumental delivery. Although AFE is a known cause of ARDS, the presentation is usually fulminant and is not limited to respiratory symptoms. Patients can present with profound hypotension and circulatory collapse, along with respiratory failure, and ultimately DIC. Treatment is largely supportive and is best managed in a critical care setting. Urgent cesarean delivery may be indicated if the patient is critically ill.

Medical Management

In a peripartum patient with pulmonary edema, management will not differ significantly from management of nonpregnant patients. Identification and treatment of the underlying cause is important and will guide definitive management and prevention of recurrence. However, treatment of symptoms and hypoxia is similar in most cases. In addition to the management discussed in the introduction, the following treatment is also recommended for acute pulmonary edema.

Diuretics

The use of diuretics is indicated in patients with pulmonary edema. Loop diuretics such as furosemide are generally preferred over thiazide diuretics, but either may be used. Loop diuretics have been shown to decrease jugular venous pressure and pulmonary congestion as well as improve cardiac function. Blood work monitoring is recommended as electrolyte abnormalities are common. Pregnant women usually have higher than normal glomerular filtration rates (GFRs), and often only low doses of diuretics are required to treat pulmonary edema and induce diuresis.

Nitrates

Nitrates are potent venodilators that are commonly used in acute decompensated heart failure. They rapidly decrease cardiac preload and have an effect on peripheral arterial tone. Nitrates can be safely used in pregnancy and can be administered sublingually, transdermally, or intravenously.

Special Considerations

Although ACE inhibitors, ARBs, and spironolactone are standard therapy in heart failure, they should generally be avoided in pregnant patients.

ACUTE PULMONARY EMBOLISM

Pregnancy is associated with an increased incidence of pulmonary embolism (PE). It is estimated that acute pulmonary embolism (PE) complicates 5 out of every 10,000 deliveries and is approximately 5 to 10 times more common in pregnant than in nonpregnant women. This is because pregnancy is associated with a number of changes that lead to increased hemostasis, endothelial damage, and a relatively hypercoagulable state.

Although PE can occur at any point throughout pregnancy, the highest incidence is in the postpartum period, with the risk decreasing after the first 6 weeks postpartum. Despite the low incidence of pregnancy-associated PE, it remains the most common cause of maternal morbidity and mortality in the developed world. Thus, prompt diagnosis and appropriate treatment are essential.

Diagnosis

There are multiple algorithms that can help clinicians diagnose a suspected PE in the pregnant patient. First, a combination of history and physical examination are used to develop a pretest probability of PE. A number of imaging modalities are subsequently used to establish the diagnosis.

History and Physical Examination
In addition to dyspnea, clinical features that suggest PE include pleuritic chest pain, tachycardia, hemoptysis, and/or signs and symptoms of

OTHER ISSUES

peripheral deep vein thrombosis (i.e., lower extremity tenderness, swelling and/or erythema). A personal or family history of VTE and a history of active malignancy also increase the pretest probability. Although clinical prediction tools are commonly used to calculate a patient's pretest probability of PE, they have not been validated for use in the pregnant population.

Imaging

Many imaging modalities exist to diagnose PE, each with its potential strengths and weaknesses. Initial testing should begin with bilateral lower extremity ultrasound examinations if leg symptoms exist and can be considered without leg symptoms (although of lower yield) because the diagnosis of PE can be assumed in patients with a confirmed DVT and clinical symptoms of PE. This approach would eliminate the need for further investigations and unnecessary radiation exposure to both the mother and fetus.

In patients with negative lower extremity ultrasounds and a normal chest radiograph, ventilation–perfusion (V/Q) scintigraphy is considered first-line imaging modality if available in the diagnosis of suspected PE. A low-probability test can confidently rule out the diagnosis, while a high-probability result confirms it. However, a potential downfall of this technique is that an indeterminate or moderate probability test would prompt further imaging, such as serial lower extremity ultrasound examinations in a patient with a low pretest probability, or a CT pulmonary angiography in a patient with high pretest probability of a PE.

Contrast-enhanced helical CT (CT pulmonary angiography) is another commonly used imaging modality to diagnose PE. It has a higher specificity than V/Q scintigraphy and can therefore be used to more accurately diagnose a PE in patients with an equivocal result. However, it involves administration of IV contrast and must be used with caution in patients with renal dysfunction.

With respect to radiation exposure, both tests fall well within the acceptable levels of fetal exposure to ionizing radiation and can be used in pregnancy. The level of radiation delivered to the fetus through V/Q scintigraphy is higher than through CT pulmonary angiography but can be reduced by performing the ventilation portion of the scan alone. In contrast, the amount of radiation delivered to the mother through CT pulmonary angiography is higher than through V/Q scintigraphy, creating a small increased lifetime risk of cancer to the radiation-sensitive maternal breasts. The potential risks of any imaging test must be weighed against its benefits.

D-Dimer

Due to the hypercoagulable state, D-dimer levels increase steadily in pregnancy and slowly return to normal in the puerperium. The use of D-dimer in the pregnant population to avoid need for further investigations, with trimester-specific cut-offs, cut-offs in combination with clinical symptoms (YEARS), or in combination with a modified Geneva risk score, has been examined but not yet universally recommended as part of the diagnostic approach. Further study is required.

Treatment

When a PE is suspected, treatment with IV unfractionated heparin (UFH) or low-molecular-weight heparin (LMWH) should be initiated immediately. LMWH is preferred because of its ease of administration and lower incidence of heparin-induced thrombocytopenia (HIT). Studies have also confirmed the safety and efficacy of LMWH in the pregnant population. Warfarin is not used for this indication in pregnancy due to its teratogenic effects, while the direct oral anticoagulants (DOACs) have not been studied in this population. Baseline CBC, coagulation profile, and creatinine are recommended.

One of the greatest challenges in treating pregnant women with acute PE is the management of anticoagulation during labor and delivery. In patients on therapeutic anticoagulation, a planned delivery is preferred, and anticoagulation should be held for 24 hours prior to neuraxial analgesia. If a patient goes into spontaneous labor, anticoagulation should be withheld immediately. Postpartum, some centers resume a lower dose of anticoagulation (e.g., prophylactic dose) on postpartum day 1 until hemostasis is achieved prior to restarting full dose anticoagulation. If a VTE was diagnosed within 4 weeks of delivery, consideration of IV UFH would be reasonable to minimize interruption of anticoagulation peripartum. For VTE diagnosed within 2 weeks of delivery, insertion of an inferior vena cava (IVC) filter in addition to IV UFH should be considered.

Pregnant women are treated with therapeutic anticoagulation for a minimum of 3 months. Although no studies have assessed the optimal duration of anticoagulant therapy, treatment is generally extended throughout pregnancy and for at least 6 weeks postpartum. Another option is to reduce the intensity of anticoagulation after 3 months to intermediate or prophylactic dosing for the remainder of pregnancy and for at least 6 weeks postpartum.

Warfarin can be used as an alternative to LMWH in breastfeeding and can be initiated following delivery. DOACs are an alternative option if the mother is not breastfeeding, because their safety and efficacy profile has not been established with lactation. Due to the potential teratogenic effects, patients started on treatment with warfarin or DOACs must be counseled on the importance of contraception. In particular, progestin only oral contraceptives, intrauterine devices (IUD), or surgical contraception should be considered because estrogen is a risk factor for developing venous thromboembolism.

Thrombolytic therapy is associated with severe bleeding and should be reserved for patients with severe hemodynamic instability in the context of confirmed PE. If thrombolysis is indicated, tissue plasminogen activator (tPA) at a dose of 200 mg administered IV over 2 hours is the recommended treatment.

PNEUMONIA

Community-acquired pneumonia (CAP) is a common cause of respiratory distress in both pregnant and nonpregnant patients. However, CAP seems to be more common in the pregnant population and can have a more severe course, suspected to be related to a high prevalence of gastroesophageal reflux disease and alterations in cell-mediated immunity. CAP may also be associated with preterm labor, small-for-gestational age, and intrauterine or neonatal death.

Diagnosis

Clinical features that may be useful in differentiating an infectious cause of dyspnea from other causes include general malaise fever; chills or rigors; a productive cough; and less frequently, pleuritic chest pain.

A chest radiograph is a safe imaging modality in pregnancy (especially with proper shielding) and may assist in diagnosis if there is evidence of airspace disease or consolidation. Concomitant peripheral leukocytosis would further support an infectious cause. Blood cultures may assist in narrowing antibiotic treatment.

Treatment

Treatment with antibiotics is indicated in any patient suspected to have bacterial pneumonia. In general, broad-spectrum empiric treatment is initiated to include coverage for typical and atypical bacterial infections. Initial treatment may include penicillins or azithromycin monotherapy in otherwise healthy patients who are not acutely unwell. In critically ill patients, a second- or third-generation cephalosporin in combination with azithromycin is preferred. Antibiotics such as clarithromycin, fluoroquinolones, and tetracyclines should be avoided.

Special consideration should also be given to viral pathogens, particularly influenza and varicella. Data from the 2009 H1N1 pandemic support the notion that pregnant women are more likely to have a severe course of illness with a higher risk of intensive care unit admission and death. Prompt recognition and treatment with an appropriate antiviral medication such as neuraminidase inhibitors (i.e., oseltamivir and zanamivir) should be considered because early treatment may diminish the severity of illness and decrease maternal mortality. Varicella pneumonia has also been associated with adverse pregnancy outcomes. Early treatment with acyclovir effectively improves outcomes. Finally, understanding of SARS-CoV-2 continues to grow. Thus far, analogous to other viral infections, pregnant women have similar presentation to their nonpregnant counterparts; however, they may be more susceptible to severe disease and increased preterm birth and cesarean delivery is likely related to more severe disease. Glucocorticoids as per indications in the nonpregnant population can be used, although the course may vary depending on whether dexamethasone for fetal lung maturity is also needed. Other agents being evaluated for SARS-CoV-2 management have limited data in pregnancy and their use needs to be discussed on a case-by-case basis.

ACUTE EXACERBATION OF ASTHMA

Asthma is a common chronic illness and an important consideration when assessing pregnant patients with dyspnea. In general, one-third of patients experience worsening asthma, and 20 to 36 percent have an acute asthma exacerbation during pregnancy. Uncontrolled asthma may be associated with poor fetal outcomes, including increased risk of preeclampsia, preterm delivery, and low birth weight.

Treatment

The treatment of acute asthma exacerbations in pregnancy is similar to the management in the nonpregnant patient. In addition to usual supportive care, the cornerstone of treatment in the acute setting is bronchodilator therapy. Concomitant treatment with both inhaled short-acting beta-adrenergic agonists (SABAs) and inhaled anticholinergic medication

(SAMAs) is warranted. Both agents can be delivered by metered-dose inhalers (MDIs) with aero-chambers or by nebulization and facemask.

For initial therapy, guidelines suggest three doses administered every 20 minutes. The frequency of further treatment will depend on the patient's response. In patients who do not respond or have severe airflow limitation (i.e., peak expiratory flow <60% of personal best or predicted value), continuous administration of inhaled beta-agonists may be more effective than intermittent administration.

In severe cases, the use of systemic corticosteroids may also be required to decrease airway inflammation. Steroids are generally recommended in all patients with moderate to severe airflow obstruction, as well as patients who do not respond to initial bronchodilator therapy. The dose of systemic corticosteroids in pregnancy is the same as those recommended for nonpregnant patients. For patients that do not respond to the above therapies, intravenous magnesium sulfate can be used as an adjunct.

Serial measurements of peak flow may be helpful in monitoring response to therapy. If signs of impending respiratory failure are present (see Table 32-3), prompt recognition and consultation with critical care specialists is recommended. Early intubation and mechanical ventilation are crucial, because respiratory failure can progress rapidly and can be difficult to reverse.

CARDIAC ARREST

Owing to a younger population with fewer comorbidities, cardiac arrest is rare in pregnancy, with an estimated incidence of one in 30,000 patients. However, approximately one in 12,000 admissions for delivery results in a maternal cardiac arrest. The most common causes are listed in Table 32-4.

TABLE 32-4: COMMON CAUSES OF CARDIAC ARREST IN PREGNANCY

VTE	Amniotic fluid embolus
Hypertensive disorders of pregnancy	Obstetric hemorrhage
Sepsis	Aspiration pneumonitis
Preexisting heart disease	Iatrogenic (medication allergies, anesthesia complications)

VTE, venous thromboembolism.

There are few changes to established protocols for cardiopulmonary resuscitation (CPR) and advanced cardiac lifesaving (ACLS) in pregnant patients who experience cardiac arrest. However, the following should be taken into consideration:

- Once the fetus is at or above the level of the umbilicus (approximately 20 weeks' gestation), manual left uterine displacement should be performed to relieve aortocaval compression. This maneuver has shown to improve venous return and may increase cardiac output by 25 to 30 percent. Previous wedge may interfere with the effectiveness of compressions
- Because pregnant patients are more susceptible to hypoxia, airway management should be prioritized and intubation should be performed as soon as possible to decrease the risk of maternal aspiration and fetal hypoxic brain injury
- Access (IV/IO) should be above the level of the diaphragm
- Fetal monitoring devices should be removed to prevent interference with maternal resuscitation
- Electrical synchronized cardioversion and defibrillation are safe in all phases of pregnancy, with no compromise in blood flow going to the fetus
- No drug should be withheld because of pregnancy if believed to be life-saving compared with an alternate choice
- Avoid vasopressin as an alternative to epinephrine in scenarios of pulseless ventricular tachycardia or ventricular fibrillation because the placenta produces vasopressinase, which may degrade the drug
- If return of spontaneous circulation (ROSC) is achieved, the fetus should be continuously monitored for bradycardia as the mother undergoes targeted temperature management

The key in maternal cardiac arrest is timely delivery of the fetus. Perimortem cesarean delivery (PMCD) should be considered in the latter half of pregnancy (20 weeks' gestational age or greater), ideally within 5 minutes of cardiac arrest. PMCD has been associated with both improved maternal and neonatal survival: 70 percent of infants who survive a PMCD were delivered within 5 minutes and 95 percent within 15 minutes. It is important that active maternal resuscitative efforts be continued through the delivery process. In specialized centers, maternal salvage may be attempted with extracorporeal cardiopulmonary resuscitation (ECMO).

In the rare and unfortunate instances in which maternal brain death occurs, there have been reported cases of somatic support until delivery. The longest reported duration of such support is 107 days. This issue raises a number of ethical and medical challenges and warrants in-depth discussion with the patient's family, the health care team, and possibly ethics committees.

THROMBOCYTOPENIA IN PREGNANCY

Thrombocytopenia is one of the most common hematological concerns in pregnancy second only to anemia. When defined as a platelet count less than 150,000/µl (150 × 10⁹/L), it occurs in 6 to 10 percent of all pregnancies, and less than 1 percent of pregnancies when defined as a platelet count of less than 100,000/µL (100 × 10⁹/L) as per the International Working Group. Normal pregnancy is associated with a physiologic fall in the platelet count that is characterized by a leftward shift in the platelet count distribution. Platelet counts usually remain within the normal range, but a 10 percent drop is deemed acceptable. The differential diagnosis of thrombocytopenia in pregnancy includes pregnancy- and nonpregnancy-specific conditions (Table 32-5).

Ominous Signs

- Diffuse petechia, ecchymoses, or purpura
- Spontaneous bleeding
- Platelet counts of less than 20,000/µL (20 × 10⁹/L)
- Postpartum hemorrhage
- Coagulopathy
- Association with hypertension, renal dysfunction, or liver dysfunction

Investigations

The diagnosis is made based on the platelet count on a CBC. When platelets are low, other investigations should include a blood film, coagulation studies including INR/PT, PTT, fibrinogen, D-dimer, liver function testing, electrolytes, creatinine, and urinalysis for proteinuria (Table 32-6).

General Guidelines for Management of Thrombocytopenia in Labor and Delivery

Maternal bleeding is uncommon unless the platelet count is below 20,000/µL (20 × 10⁹/L). Maternal hemorrhage most commonly occurs at the time of

TABLE 32-5: DIFFERENTIAL DIAGNOSIS OF THROMBOCYTOPENIA IN PREGNANCY

Gestational thrombocytopenia AFLP HELLP syndrome Preeclampsia or eclampsia	Decreased production Myelodysplasia Bone marrow infiltration Hematologic malignancy Chronic alcoholism Megaloblastic anemia (e.g., vitamin B_{12}, folate deficiency) Aplastic anemia Alcohol Chemotherapy

	Increased destruction/consumption:
	  Primary immune-mediated
	    ITP
	  Secondary immune-mediated
	    Infectious (viral: HIV, EBV, CMV, HCV)
	    Drug induced (e.g., heparin)
	    Autoimmune disorders (e.g., SLE)
	    Antiphospholipid antibodies
	    Posttransfusion purpura
	  Thrombotic microangiopathies
	    TTP
	    HUS
	  DIC
	  Sepsis
	  Liver failure
	  Drugs (e.g., antimicrobials, NSAIDs, antiepileptics)
	  Inherited thrombocytopenias
	  vWD Type 2b

	Splenic sequestration or hypersplenism

AFLP, acute fatty liver of pregnancy; CMV, cytomegalovirus; DIC, disseminated intravascular coagulation; EBV, Epstein-Barr virus; HCV, hepatitis C virus; HELLP, hemolysis, elevated liver enzymes, and low platelets; HUS, hemolytic uremic syndrome; ITP, immune thrombocytopenia; NSAID, nonsteroidal anti-inflammatory drug; SLE, systemic lupus erythematosus; TTP, thrombotic thrombocytopenic purpura; vWD, von Willebrand disease.

delivery. Generally, treatment is recommended in asymptomatic patients with platelet counts of less than 20,000/µL (20×10^9/L). Expert recommendations suggest that in anticipation of delivery, third trimester counts below 40,000 to 50,000/µL (40 to 50×10^9/L) should be treated. Patients who are actively bleeding should always be treated, and a hematologic consultation is recommended. Although platelet transfusions are generally the primary means of treatment, certain disease conditions require specific interventions, which are discussed below. Guidelines recommend a platelet count of at least 75,000/µL (75×10^9/L) for safe placement of an epidural catheter.

TABLE 32-6: LABORATORY INVESTIGATIONS TO DIFFERENTIATE CAUSES OF THROMBOCYTOPENIA

Condition	Hgb	Blood Film	Platelets	INR/PT	PTT	Fibrinogen	D-Dimer/FDP	Liver
Gestational	N	N	↓	N	N	N or ↑	N	N
ITP	N	Giant platelets	↓	N	N	N or ↑	N	N
TTP or HUS	↓	Fragments	↓	N	N	N or ↑	N or ↑	N
Preeclampsia	↓ or N	N or Fragments	↓	N	N	N or ↑	N or ↑	N
HELLP	↓	Fragments	↓	N	N	N or ↑	↑	↑
DIC	↓	Fragments	↓	↑	↑	N or ↓	↑	N

DIC, disseminated intravascular coagulation; FDP, fibrin degradation products; HELLP, hemolysis, elevated liver enzymes, low platelet syndrome; Hgb, hemoglobin; HUS, hemolytic uremic syndrome; INR, international normalized ratio; ITP, immune thrombocytopenia; N, normal; PT, prothrombin time; PTT, partial thromboplastin time; TTP, thrombotic thrombocytopenic purpura.

Specific Etiologies of Thrombocytopenia in Pregnancy

Gestational

Gestational thrombocytopenia accounts for approximately 70 to 80 percent of the causes of thrombocytopenia in pregnancy. It is a diagnosis of exclusion and generally reserved for cases of mild thrombocytopenia in the third trimester (usually counts >70,000/μL or 70×10^9/L) with no prior diagnosis, spontaneous resolution postpartum and no associated fetal thrombocytopenia or adverse outcomes. No specific treatment is required.

Preeclampsia

Preeclampsia is the leading cause of pregnancy-associated mortality worldwide. It is defined as hypertension diagnosed after 20 weeks of gestation with evidence of end-organ dysfunction.

The details regarding the diagnosis, presentation, and management of preeclampsia is described in the "Hypertension" section of this chapter. Thrombocytopenia occurs in approximately 20 percent of women with preeclampsia and may precede other manifestations of the disorder. The definitive treatment of preeclampsia is delivery.

HELLP Syndrome

HELLP is a syndrome of hemolysis, elevated liver enzymes, and low platelets. It affects 0.5 to 0.9 percent of all pregnancies, is most common in multiparous women, and develops in 10 percent of patients with preeclampsia. Up to 70 percent of cases occur before term, and the remainder usually occur within 48 hours of delivery, although thrombocytopenia and elevated LDH can last as long as several weeks postpartum.

Diagnosis rests on demonstrated evidence of microangiopathic hemolytic anemia, increased LDH, increased AST (usually no more than 400 IU/L), and thrombocytopenia. There are many associated features and overlap with preeclampsia. Up to 75 percent of patients have proteinuria, and 50 to 60 percent have hypertension. Symptoms include malaise, right upper quadrant pain (obstructed blood flow to hepatic sinusoids), nausea, and vomiting. Hypotension severe right upper quadrant pain or rapidly dropping hemoglobin should prompt consideration of a liver capsule hematoma or hepatic rupture, especially in the setting of transaminases above 500 IU/L.

There is a consensus that delivery is indicated beyond 34 weeks' gestation or earlier if there is evidence of multiorgan dysfunction, DIC, liver infarction or hemorrhage, renal failure, suspected abruptio placentae, or

OTHER ISSUES

nonreassuring fetal status. Corticosteroids used for fetal lung maturity may show temporary improvement in platelet count or liver enzymes; however, it has not been shown to change maternal morbidity or mortality. Patients with suspected liver rupture should undergo a CT scan or magnetic resonance imaging (MRI). Management of hepatic rupture requires surgical intervention, although hepatic artery embolization appears to be most effective.

Immune Thrombocytopenia

The prevalence of immune thrombocytopenia (ITP) is 1 to 10 in 10,000 pregnancies. Unlike other causes of thrombocytopenia, it may precede pregnancy or manifest at any time during pregnancy. Clinical features are easy bruising, mucosal bleeding, and petechiae. Only 30 percent of cases require therapy during pregnancy.

First-line therapy for treatment is IV immunoglobulin (IVIG), and/or corticosteroids. IVIG works rapidly (within 2-3 days) and lasts 2 to 3 weeks. There is no consensus on optimal dosing, but most centers recommend 1 g/kg/day for 2 days. Side effects include fever, headaches, chills, and chest pain. Corticosteroids are equally efficacious in pregnant women. The usual dose recommended is prednisone 1 mg/kg or high-dose pulse steroids (methylprednisolone 1 g/day for 2 days). The maximal effect is reached after 2 to 4 weeks. Corticosteroid use may be associated with premature rupture of membranes and placental abruption along with an increased risk of gestational diabetes and hypertension when used longer term. It is recommended to use corticosteroids sparingly and at the lowest effective dose. Women treated with long-term corticosteroids may have underlying adrenal suppression and should be considered for stress steroids dosing at the time of delivery.

Alternative treatments in patients who are actively bleeding include tranexamic acid, aminocaproic acid, and recombinant factor VIIa. Rarely, splenectomy can be performed during cesarean section in selected patients.

Of note, antiplatelet antibodies cross the placenta and may cause fetal thrombocytopenia, the degree of which does not correlate with maternal platelet levels. About 15 percent of the offspring of mothers with ITP will have platelet counts below 100×10^9/L (100,000/μL), 10 percent below 50×10^9/L (50,000/μL), and only 4 percent will have severe thrombocytopenia with counts below 20×10^9/L (20,000/μL). The incidence of neonatal intracranial hemorrhage is less than 1 percent. Studies have shown that most neonatal intracranial hemorrhage are not actually associated with the trauma of vaginal delivery; however, avoidance of procedures associated with increased hemorrhagic risk (e.g., forceps, vacuum, fetal scalp electrodes) is recommended.

Neonatal platelet counts should be determined in cord blood immediately on delivery and for the next 5 days because it may take several days to reach the nadir neonatal platelet count. Some centers recommend routine transcranial ultrasound, even in asymptomatic neonates, when the platelet count is below 50,000/μL (50×10^9/L).

Thrombotic Thrombocytopenic Purpura and Hemolytic Uremic Syndrome

Thrombotic thrombocytopenic purpura (TTP) and hemolytic uremic syndrome (HUS) are collectively referred to as thrombotic microangiopathies. Although they are not pregnancy specific, there is a slightly increased incidence of TTP in pregnancy. TTP is caused by a deficiency in ADAMTS-13, a metalloprotease that cleaves von Willebrand factor (vWF). This deficiency leads to ultra-large vWF multimers that promote platelet agglutination and microthrombotic events. It can be difficult to distinguish TTP from other disorders such as preeclampsia, HELLP syndrome, and acute fatty liver, which are commonly associated with microangiopathic hemolytic anemia (MAHA) and thrombocytopenia. TTP is classically associated with the pentad of MAHA, thrombocytopenia, fever, renal dysfunction, and neurologic impairment (confusion, headaches, seizures, coma). Of the nonhematologic manifestations, the neurologic changes are the most common. HUS is seen predominantly in children, and the renal impairment is typically the most important feature.

The management is the same as in the nonpregnant population, with plasma exchange yielding an 80 percent response rate. Although there are no randomized trials to support the use of corticosteroids in TTP, some authors recommend their use given the immune nature of the disorder. Importantly, unlike preeclampsia and the HELLP syndrome, delivery does not induce remission of TTP.

Disseminated Intravascular Coagulation

Disseminated intravascular coagulation (DIC) is the final common pathway resulting in overactivation of coagulation and/or fibrinolytic system that leads to unopposed production of thrombin, resulting in microvascular thrombotic obstruction and bleeding from a consumptive coagulopathy. Obstetric causes include placental abruption, amniotic fluid embolism, retained fetal products, massive obstetrical hemorrhage, preeclampsia or eclampsia, and uterine rupture. Nonpregnancy-related causes include trauma, hemolytic reactions, tissue damage, cancer, leukemia, and sepsis. The laboratory diagnosis rests on evidence of anemia and presence of red blood cell fragments (schistocytes), thrombocytopenia, increased PT or PTT, and increased fibrin degradation products or D-dimer. The fibrinogen level is normally elevated in pregnancy and may remain normal or decreased in severe cases.

Key management is to treat the underlying cause. Prompt evacuation of the uterus followed by hemodynamic and hemostatic support usually leads to complete reversal of the coagulopathy. Vaginal delivery is possible in the majority of cases, but local measures to reduce bleeding are crucial. With adequate fluid resuscitation, uterotonic medications, and hemostatic management, most patients have a spontaneous resolution of bleeding. Transfusions are indicated for ongoing bleeding. The American Society of Anesthesiologists suggests the following transfusion parameters:

- Platelet transfusion to maintain counts more than 50,000/μL (50×10^9/L)
- Fibrinogen concentrate or cryoprecipitate should be given to patients with levels less than 1.0 g/L. If available, fresh-frozen plasma (FFP) can be used, although is not as rich in fibrinogen
- FFP if INR greater than 1.5

In rare cases when severe bleeding persists, potential pharmacologic options include antithrombin, tissue factor pathway inhibitors, and activated protein C, although recent trials have shown no proven benefits. Recombinant factor VIIa may be potentially useful. Aminocaproic acid, a fibrinolysis inhibitor used in postoperative bleeding, should not be used because it may predispose to thrombotic events. Surgical interventions include selective pelvic arterial embolization.

ACUTE FATTY LIVER OF PREGNANCY

Acute fatty liver of pregnancy (AFLP) is a life-threatening condition that occurs in the third trimester. It is characterized by accumulation of microvascular fat within the liver parenchyma due to defects in fatty acid metabolism. Twenty percent of cases are secondary to a deficiency in long-chain 3-hydroxyacyl-CoA dehydrogenase (LCHAD) and can lead to severe hepatic failure. Risk factors for developing AFLP include multiple gestation, male fetal sex, and low body mass index (BMI <20 kg/m²). The differential diagnosis of liver diseases in pregnancy is presented in Table 32-7.

TABLE 32-7: DIFFERENTIAL DIAGNOSIS OF LIVER DISEASE IN PREGNANCY

Variable	Intrahepatic Cholestasis of Pregnancy	HELLP Syndrome	Hepatic Rupture	Hepatic Infarction	Acute Fatty Liver of Pregnancy
Timing	Late second to third trimester	≥20 weeks	≥20 weeks	≥20 weeks	Third trimester
Clinical signs	Pruritus (without rash)	Abdominal pain, preeclampsia	Abdominal swelling or tenderness, shock	Fever, abdominal pain	Abdominal pain, nausea, vomiting, jaundice, polydipsia, polyuria
Laboratory values	Elevated bile salts (fasting) +/− transaminases	Hemolysis, thrombocytopenia, elevated transaminases (>1000 U/L), unconjugated bilirubinemia	Anemia, second-degree bleeding	Anemia, elevated AST (>1000 IU/L)	Elevated transaminases (<500 IU/L), increased PTT, INR, decreased fibrinogen, hypoglycemia, conjugated bilirubinemia
Management	Ursodeoxycholic acid, rapid resolution after delivery	Delivery, treatment of preeclampsia	Surgical, hepatic artery embolization	Surgical, hepatic artery embolization; may require transplantation	Supportive, prompt delivery; may require transplant

AST, aspartate aminotransferase; INR, international normalized ratio; PTT, partial thromboplastin time.

Clinical Presentation

There is a wide spectrum of presentations for AFLP. Patients can range from being asymptomatic to having nonspecific symptoms such as nausea, vomiting, and abdominal pain and may be followed by jaundice, encephalopathy, and hepatic failure. Polydipsia and polyuria (central diabetes insipidus) may also occur. Preeclampsia is present in one-half of affected patients. Early recognition is important as untreated AFLP may lead to maternal and/or fetal demise. Diagnosis rests on a combination of clinical history and laboratory investigations. Aminotransferase and bilirubin levels are typically elevated, with evidence of hepatic failure, including coagulopathy, hypoglycemia, and hyperammonemia. The Swansea criteria, a combination of clinical and biochemical findings, can be used to help establish a diagnosis of AFLP in suspected patients.

Ominous Signs

- Encephalopathy
- Hypoglycemia
- Coagulopathy (hallmark features are increased PTT and decreased fibrinogen)

Intrapartum Management

The mainstay of treatment for AFLP is early recognition, prompt delivery, and supportive care. Continuous fetal monitoring should be undertaken. If initial serum glucose levels are normal, they can be monitored every 6 to 8 hours; however, more frequent monitoring is required if levels are trending downward. IV dextrose should be considered in the setting of refractory hypoglycemia. Lactulose can be administered for encephalopathy.

Once AFLP is diagnosed, prompt delivery should be planned. AFLP is not a contraindication to vaginal delivery, and induction of labor is reasonable if the patient will likely deliver within 24 hours. If this is not the case, or there is concern about deteriorating maternal or fetal status, a cesarean section should be attempted. In both cases, coagulation should be optimized and the same general principles as in DIC apply.

Postpartum Considerations

In mild cases, resolution of AFLP after delivery is prompt and is reflected by improvement in liver function tests and coagulation factors. In severe cases, patients may require ongoing support due to a variety of complications, including postpartum hemorrhage, renal failure, acute pancreatitis, and nephrogenic diabetes insipidus. Patients should be monitored in the hospital until signs of liver dysfunction have normalized. If patients do not rapidly improve, liver transplantation should be considered. All women with AFLP and their offspring should undergo molecular testing for LCHAD deficiency. Neonates affected by AFLP should also be monitored closely for clinical manifestations of the enzyme deficiency, including hypoglycemia and fatty liver disease.

SEIZURES IN PREGNANCY

Epilepsy

The most common cause of seizures in pregnancy is preexisting epilepsy. Although it is unclear if pregnancy increases the seizure frequency in patients with epilepsy, women that are seizure-free for at least 9 months prior to pregnancy have an 84 to 92 percent likelihood of remaining seizure-free during their pregnancy.

The management of pregnant patients with epilepsy is beyond the scope of this section. In general terms, monotherapy with antiepileptic drugs (AEDs) is preferred over polytherapy to reduce the risk of major congenital malformations and poor neurodevelopmental outcomes from fetal exposure of AED. Furthermore, valproic acid should be avoided to reduce the risk of major congenital malformations such as neural tube defects, facial clefts, and neurodevelopmental disorders. Finally, plasma volume expansion, induction of hepatic microsomal enzymes, increased renal clearance, and decreased volume of plasma proteins lead to changes in AED metabolism during pregnancy, thus therapeutic level monitoring should be considered.

Table 32-8 details a differential diagnosis of seizures in pregnancy.

Fetal monitoring of seizures during labor and delivery has demonstrated late decelerations and reduced variability. It is reported that a single brief generalized tonic-clonic seizure can be associated with fetal heart rate depression lasting more than 20 minutes.

Postpartum Considerations

Although breast milk has been found to have small levels of AEDs, the American Academy of Neurology continues to recommend breastfeeding.

TABLE 32-8: DIFFERENTIAL DIAGNOSIS OF SEIZURES IN PREGNANCY

Preexisting epilepsy	Cerebral arterial or venous thrombosis
Eclampsia	Metabolic abnormalities
Encephalitis or meningitis	Hypoglycemia
Intracranial lesion	Trauma
Hydrocephalus	Drug use or withdrawal
Postpartum pituitary hemorrhage	Posterior reversible encephalopathy syndrome (PRES)
Cavernous angioma	Stroke

Barbiturates, benzodiazepines, and primidone can cause excessive drowsiness in infants and should be reserved for refractory cases.

Eclampsia

Eclampsia refers to the development of new-onset, generalized, tonic-clonic seizures in patients with hypertensive disorders of pregnancy, such as preeclampsia, HELLP, or gestational hypertension. The pathophysiology of eclamptic seizures is not fully understood, but it is thought that profound hypertension can overwhelm the cerebral autoregulatory system and result in endothelial dysfunction, vasogenic edema, and ischemia. Preeclampsia, detailed in a previous section, can present with neurologic symptoms including headache, blurred vision, diplopia, hyperreflexia, agitation, or coma. The presence of seizures defines eclampsia; however, classic preeclamptic signs may be absent in patients at the onset of eclamptic seizures.

Eclampsia can occur in the antepartum, intrapartum, or postpartum period. In up to 15 percent of patients, eclamptic seizures occur postpartum, with reports of seizures occurring as late as 26 days. Although the incidence of eclampsia has decreased with early recognition and treatment of preeclampsia, it is associated with a 5 percent and up to 30 percent risk of maternal and perinatal mortality, respectively.

Diagnosis and Investigations

It is crucial to rule out other causes of acute seizures in pregnant women, because this will greatly dictate subsequent management. The differential diagnosis includes epilepsy, anatomic abnormalities, metabolic causes, toxins, infection, and head trauma.

Initial tests should include a basic chemistry panel to rule out metabolic abnormalities (electrolytes, magnesium, calcium, glucose, liver enzymes, thyroid-stimulating hormone), a CBC to rule out infection, AED levels in patients on chronic therapy, and a toxicology panel for potential substance abuse or withdrawal. If imaging is required, an MRI is preferred over CT.

Management of Acute Seizures

The first steps involve basic resuscitation. ABCs (airway, breathing, and circulation) should be prioritized. The patient should be placed in the left lateral decubitus position to prevent aspiration and supplemental oxygen should be applied. First-line therapy for terminating seizures is IV benzodiazepines. Lorazepam (1-2 mg IV bolus) and diazepam (5-10 mg IV bolus) are most commonly used. The drug of choice for eclamptic seizures is magnesium sulfate ($MgSO_4$). A landmark trial (MAGPIE study) revealed that $MgSO_4$ decreases the risk of recurrent eclamptic seizures by one-half to two-thirds, and the rate of maternal death by one-third. The recommended initial bolus is 4 to 6 g IV over 20 minutes, followed by a continuous infusion at 1 to 2 g/hr. Therapy should be continued for 24 to 48 hours postpartum. A repeat dose of 2 to 4 g IV over 5 to 10 minutes can be given for seizure recurrence.

Patients receiving $MgSO_4$ must be monitored for signs of toxicity, which include loss of deep tendon reflexes, decreased urine output, hypotension, bradycardia, and respiratory depression. Patients who exhibit signs of toxicity should be treated with IV calcium gluconate. The routine monitoring of magnesium levels is not recommended.

Up to 10 percent of patients with eclampsia are resistant to $MgSO_4$ and require additional treatment with AEDs. Phenobarbital and phenytoin can be given IV. It is important to note that other components of preeclampsia and eclampsia, such as hypertension, also need to be addressed to prevent recurrence. In patients with persistent seizure activity or focal neurological deficits, imaging should be pursued to rule out anatomic abnormalities and a neurology consultation should be considered.

Route of Delivery

Prompt delivery is the definitive treatment for eclampsia. After resolution of seizure activity, pregnant patients between 32 and 34 weeks' gestational age can be safely induced if delivery is expected to occur within 24 hours of induction. Cesarean section should be considered if the mother experiences frequent, uncontrolled generalized tonic-clonic seizures during labor or if she is unable to cooperate with labor because of absence seizures, complex partial seizures, or an altered level of consciousness.

SELECTED READING

American College of Obstetricians and Gynecologists: ACOG Practice Bulletin 190 Clinical management guidelines for obstetrician-gynecologists: Gestational Diabetes Mellitus. Obstet Gynecol 131:e49, 2018

American College of Obstetricians and Gynecologists: ACOG Practice Bulletin 201: Clinical management guidelines for obstetrician-gynecologists Pregestational Diabetes. Obstet Gynecol 132:e228, 2018

American College of Obstetricians and Gynecologists: ACOG Practice Bulletin Number 222: Gestation Hypertension and preeclampsia. Obstet Gynecol 135:e237, 2020

American Diabetes Association: Management of Diabetes in Pregnancy: Standards of Medical Care in Diabetes. Diabetes Care 43:S183, 2018

Bandi VD, Munnur U, Matthay MA: Acute lung injury and acute respiratory distress syndrome in pregnancy. Crit Care Clin 20:577, 2004

Bourjeily G, Paidas M, Khalil H, Rosene-Montella K, Rodger M: Pulmonary embolism in pregnancy. Lancet 375:500, 2010

Butalia S, Audibert F, Cote A-M, et al: Hypertension Canada's 2018 Guidelines for the Management of Hypertension in Pregnancy. Can J Cardiol 34:526, 2018

Camargo C, Rachelefsky G, Schatz M: Managing asthma exacerbations in the emergency department. Summary of the National Asthma Education and Prevention Program Expert Panel Report 3 Guidelines for the Management of Asthma Exacerbations. Proc Am Thorac Soc 6:357, 2009

Cohen SL, Feizullayeva CF, McCandlish JA, et al: Comparison of international societal guidelines for the diagnosis of suspected pulmonary embolism during pregnancy. Lancet 7:e247, 2020

Elkayam U: Pregnancy and cardiovascular disease. In: Zipes DP, Libby P, Bonow RO, Braunwald E, editors. Braunwald's Heart Disease: A Textbook of Cardiovascular Medicine, 7th ed. Philadelphia: Elsevier, 2005.

Feig DS, Berger H, Donovan L, et al: 2018 Clinical Practice Guidelines Diabetes and Pregnancy. Can J Diabetes 42:S255, 2018

Gernsheimer T, James AH, Stasi R: How I treat thrombocytopenia in pregnancy. Blood 121:38, 2013

Global Initiative for Asthma: Global Strategy for Asthma Management and Prevention https://ginasthma.org/wp-content/uploads/2019/06/GINA-2019-main-report-June-2019-wms.pdf, 2019

Harden CL, Hopp J, Ting TY, et al: Management issues for women with epilepsy-Focus on pregnancy (an evidence-based review): I. Obstetrical complications and change in seizure frequency: Report of the Quality Standards Subcommittee and Therapeutics and Technology Assessment Subcommittee of the American Academy of Neurology and the American Epilepsy Society. Epilepsia 50:1229, 2009

Harden CL, Meador KJ, Pennell WA, et al: Practice Parameter update: Management issues for women with epilepsy—Focus on pregnancy (an evidence-based review): Teratogenesis and perinatal outcomes: Report of the Quality Standards Subcommittee and Therapeutics and Technology Assessment Subcommittee of the American Academy of Neurology and American Epilepsy Society. Neurology 73:133, 2009

Harden CL, Pennell PB, Koppel BS, et al: Practice Parameter update: Management issues for women with epilepsy—Focus on pregnancy (an evidence-based review): Vitamin K, folic acid, blood levels, and breast feeding: Report of the Quality Standards Subcommittee and Therapeutics and Technology Assessment Subcommittee of the American Academy of Neurology and American. Epilepsy Society. Neurology 73:142, 2009

Lim W, Le Gal G, Bates SM, et al: American Society of Hematology 2018 guidelines for management of venous thromboembolism: diagnosis of venous thromboembolism. Blood Adv 2:3226, 2018

Magee LA, Pels A, Helewa M, et al: Diagnosis, evaluation, and management of the hypertensive disorders of pregnancy. Pregnancy Hypertens 4:105, 2014

Mallampalli A, Powner DJ, Gardner MO: Cardiopulmonary resuscitation and somatic support of the pregnant patient. Crit Care Clin 20:747, 2004

Marik PE, Plante LA: Venous thromboembolic disease and pregnancy. N Engl J Med 6;359:2025, 2008

McCrae KR: Thrombocytopenia in pregnancy. Hematol Am Soc Hematol Educ Program 2010;397-402, 2010

Murphy VE, Gibson P, Talbot PI, Clifton VL: Severe asthma exacerbations during pregnancy. Obstet Gynecol 106:1046, 2005

Nishimura RA, Otto CM, Sorajja P, et al: ACC/AHA 2014 guideline for the management of patients with valvular heart disease. JACC 63:e57, 2014

Panchal AR, Bartos JA, Cabanas JG, et al: Part 3: Adult Basic and Advanced Life Support: 2020 American Heart Association Guideliens for Cardiopulmonary Resuscitation and Emergency Cardiovascular Care. Circulation 142: Suppl 2, 2020

Parker JA, Conway DL: Diabetic ketoacidosis in pregnancy. Obstet Gynecol Clin North Am 34:533, 2007

Provan D, Arnold DM, Bussel JB, et al: Updated international consensus report on the investigation and management of primary immune thrombocytopenia. Blood Adv 3:3780, 2019

Sheffield JS, Cunningham FG: Community-acquired pneumonia in pregnancy. Obstet Gynecol 114:915, 2009

Sliwa K, Fett J, Elkayam U: Peripartum cardiomyopathy. Lancet 368:687, 2006

Tran T, Ahn J, Reau NS: ACG Clinical Guideline: Liver Disease and Pregnancy. Am J Gastroenterol 111:176, 2016

CHAPTER 33

Labor in the Presence of Fetal Complications

Felipe M. Moretti
Brigitte Bonin

FETAL GROWTH RESTRICTION

Background

Fetal growth restriction (FGR) occurs when the fetus is unable to achieve its full in utero growth potential, leading to increased risk for significant morbidity and mortality. This can be due to genetic or congenital malformations, placental conditions, congenital infections, and maternal medical conditions.

Maternal placental hypoperfusion accounts for 25 to 30 percent of all cases of FGR, while chromosomal disorders and congenital malformations are responsible for approximately 20 percent.

Pregnancies complicated by FGR have increased risk for adverse perinatal outcome including but not limited to preterm birth, stillbirth, neonatal morbidity, and mortality. Furthermore, those fetuses are at risk of long-term disabilities such as neurological (cognitive and learning disabilities), cardiovascular, and endocrine diseases.

FGR is classified as "early onset" when it occurs before 32 weeks and as "late onset" after 32 weeks' gestation.

Small for gestational age (SGA) is a terminology often *misused* to describe fetal growth restriction. It actually refers to neonatal birth weights below the 10th percentile, while FGR relates to the estimated fetal weight (EFW).

It is important to highlight that approximately 18 to 22 percent of FGR cases are healthy fetuses and considered constitutionally small at birth with a normal outcome.

Diagnostic Criteria

Differentiation between constitutional and pathological FGR remains a prenatal challenge for health care providers. There is a lack of agreement and broad consensus in the diagnostic criteria among different international guidelines from Canada, the United States, the United Kingdom, and International Societies such as the International Society of Ultrasound in Obstetrics and Gynecology (ISUOG).

Commonly, FGR would be defined as an EFW below the 10th percentile. This diagnostic criterion has high sensitivity but low specificity, including babies who are constitutionally SGA, but healthy and with normal perinatal outcomes.

The inclusion of other parameters such as abdominal circumference (AC) and Doppler improves the specificity of the diagnosis.

The Society of Obstetrics & Gynecology of Canada (SOGC) and The Society for Maternal Fetal Medicine in the United States (SMFM) both define FGR with an EFW or AC below the 10th percentile.

ISUOG Guidelines for defining FGR are based on the International Delphi Consensus using EFW and/or AC and may also include the fetal growth curve and maternal and fetal Doppler studies.

Differentiating between constitutional and pathological FGR has important impacts on antenatal surveillance, timing of delivery, and labor and delivery management (Fig. 33-1).

Antenatal Assessment

Fetuses with FGR should be investigated for genetic abnormalities, anatomical malformations, and congenital infections (TORCH).

Typically, early-onset FGR has a worse perinatal outcome and will demonstrate a pattern of fetal Doppler deterioration in cases of placental insufficiency. It is frequently associated with hypertensive disorders in pregnancy. When FGR is secondary to genetic abnormalities, anatomical malformations and amniotic fluid abnormalities are commonly present.

Late-onset FGR is usually less severe with lower perinatal morbidity and mortality. Frequently, the umbilical artery (UA) Doppler is normal but with an abnormal middle cerebral artery (MCA) resistance and/or low cerebral placental ratio (CPR).

Pregnant women presenting with FGR fetuses associated with genetic conditions and/or anatomical abnormalities should have multidisciplinary counseling with Maternal Fetal Medicine, Genetics, and Neonatology Specialists. The severity of conditions will impact timing and mode of delivery, fetal monitoring, and postnatal management planning.

Timing and Mode of Delivery

Currently, there is no consensus among International Societies on the timing of delivery for late-onset FGR. Early-onset FGR also has practice differences for fetal surveillance; some authors advocate for computerized cardiotocography (cCTG) in association with Doppler, and others include the biophysical profile (BPP).

Timing of delivery is driven by maternal and/or fetal factors. The commonest maternal factor is hypertensive disorders, whereas fetal factors taken into consideration include gestational age and risk of stillbirth and neonatal morbidity and mortality.

OTHER ISSUES

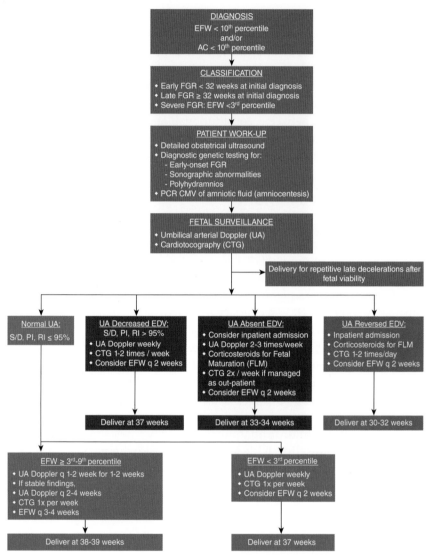

FIGURE 33-1. Algorithm for the diagnosis and management of fetal growth restriction **(FGR).** (Reproduced with permission from Society for Maternal-Fetal Medicine (SMFM). Electronic address: pubs@smfm.org, Martins JG, Biggio JR, Abuhamad A. Society for Maternal-Fetal Medicine Consult Series #52: Diagnosis and management of fetal growth restriction: (Replaces Clinical Guideline Number 3, April 2012). Am J Obstet Gynecol. 2020;223(4):B2-B17.)

Constitutional Small Fetuses

They are considered "healthy" fetuses, but constitutionally SGA. These fetuses have normal Doppler with an EFW or AC below the 10th percentile but not below the 3rd percentile. The SMFM and ISUOG recommend delivery at 38 to 39 weeks while the SOGC guideline suggests between 38 and 40 weeks. The mode of delivery is determined by obstetric indications. Continuous fetal monitoring is advised throughout the labor.

Late-onset FGR

These fetuses are pathologically growth restricted and close antenatal fetal surveillance is recommended. These fetuses have an increased risk for fetal distress in labor, operative vaginal delivery, emergency cesarean section, and neonatal intensive care admission. Fetal surveillance involves Doppler assessment, BPP, and CTG. If EFW less than 3rd percentile and/or abnormal Doppler, delivery is recommended at 37 weeks. Induction of labor may be performed in absence of contraindications. The Foley catheter balloon method of induction should be considered as a first choice, because it has been shown to have a higher success rates for vaginal delivery.

Early-Onset FGR

Gestational age is the most important independent predictor of neonatal outcome. In FGR with abnormal Doppler studies, neonatal survival rates increase from 13 percent at 24 weeks to 43 percent at 25 weeks and 58 percent at 26 weeks of gestation. Furthermore, intact survival rates improve from 0 percent at 24 weeks to 6 to 31 percent at 26 weeks. For extreme preterm deliveries below 26 weeks, an in-depth consultation with Maternal Fetal Medicine and Neonatology should discuss management options ranging from full-resuscitation to palliative care of the newborn. These women must be followed in a Tertiary Care Center. Ultrasound for Doppler, BPP, and cCTG or CTG are used for fetal assessment to determine timing of delivery. Maternal complications such as severe preeclampsia and HELLP require delivery regardless of gestational age.

Pregnant women at risk of preterm delivery less than 34 weeks should be offered corticosteroids. Magnesium sulfate ($MgSO_4$) prophylaxis for neuroprotection is also suggested for patients who will delivery prior 34 weeks, ideally be started at least 4 hours prior to delivery.

The threshold of 26 weeks and/or 500 grams has been suggested for delivery in cases of severe early onset FGR, based on the high morbidity and mortality below this cutoff.

Delivery criteria may vary within guidelines and local protocols; however, timing is usually determined by the degree of abnormal Doppler studies and the fetal heart rate pattern. From 26^{+0} to 28^{+6} weeks, delivery should be considered for an abnormal Ductus Venosus Doppler or repeated or persistent unprovoked decelerations. Delivery is suggested for reversed end diastolic flow in the umbilical artery Doppler from 32^{+0} weeks in the IUSOG Guideline and from 30 to 32 weeks in the SMFM Guideline. In the presence of absent end diastolic flow in the umbilical artery Doppler, the ISUOG Guideline suggests delivery from 34 weeks with the SMFM Guideline recommending 33 to 34 weeks.

The mode of delivery depends on several factors, although early-onset FGR has higher probability of cesarean section due to poor fetal tolerance of labor.

CONGENITAL ANOMALIES

The coauthors would like to acknowledge that a significant portion of this section was extracted from the prior chapter written by Dr. Laura Gaudet published in the 6th edition of this book in 2013. It has been updated and enhanced with new knowledge as deemed appropriate.

Background

A congenital anomaly is defined as any unusual variation or abnormality in the shape, structure, and/or function of an organ, tissue, or body part that occurs during intrauterine development and can be identified prenatally, at birth or later in life. Congenital anomalies can be classified in several ways: internal versus external, single (isolated) or multiple, and major or minor. They develop through four major pathways as detailed in Table 33-1.

TABLE 33-1: PATHOGENESIS OF CONGENITAL ANOMALIES

	Mechanism	Example
Malformation	Intrinsically dysfunctional developmental process	Anencephaly
Deformation	Mechanical forces on the embryo or fetus	Potter's sequence secondary to prolonged, early oligo/anhydramnios
Disruption	Extrinsic factor that disrupts normal development	Limb amputation from amniotic bands
Dysplasia	Abnormal organization of cells in a tissue	Abnormal cartilage formation in achondroplasia

They can be part of an identifiable syndrome or known sequence, related to an underlying genetic condition or maternal disease (e.g., poorly controlled diabetes or epilepsy) or due to environmental factors. However, in 65 percent of cases, their actual etiology remains unclear.

A European population-based registry of congenital anomalies from 22 countries (EUROCAT), covering 1.5 million births annually, recorded a total prevalence of major congenital anomalies of 23.9 in 1000 between 2003 and 2007. Of the infants with congenital anomalies, 80 percent were live born and 2.5 percent were stillborn (after 20 weeks' gestation). A further 17.6 percent of infants with congenital anomalies underwent termination of pregnancy after prenatal diagnosis, of which nearly half had associated aneuploidy.

The most common congenital anomalies among chromosomally normal fetuses were congenital heart defects (6.5 in 1000 births), limb defects (3.8 in 1000 births), anomalies of the urinary tract (3.1 in 1000 births), and nervous system (2.3 in 1000 births). For the purpose of this discussion, issues surrounding fetuses with life limiting conditions will be addressed separately from those with other types of congenital anomalies.

Fetuses with Prenatally Diagnosed Congenital Anomalies

First and foremost, it is important to ensure that these babies are born in a facility that can best accommodate the infant's condition while allowing for close family involvement. This may require delivery at a center with an advanced neonatal intensive care unit, access to medical subspecialists (e.g., pediatric surgeons, otolaryngologists, cardiologists) and paramedical support (e.g., lactation consultants or prosthetists). An appropriate neonatal resuscitation team should be in attendance at delivery and assume care of the infant as soon as possible after birth. Ideally, delivery is accomplished at as late a gestational age as is safely possible, since prematurity increases the morbidity and mortality of infants with congenital anomalies, particularly if early surgical correction is required.

The potential impact of the congenital anomaly on fetal monitoring must be taken into consideration, particularly when interpreting the findings. External fetal monitoring is the preferred route. If this is unsatisfactory, internal fetal monitoring in the form of a scalp electrode may be used, providing there are no concerns that the congenital anomaly could interfere with its placement. Expectations regarding the tracing should be in keeping with the type of anomaly. For example, cardiac anomalies may be accompanied by intermittent or sustained arrhythmias despite adequate fetal oxygenation. Similarly, fetuses with anomalies of the central nervous system may not display the usual variability and accelerations that are characteristic of a normal tracing. There should be clear, preestablished, and individualized parameters for fetal monitoring–based intervention, in order to avoid confusion or conflicts amongst the different members of the care team.

Special considerations may arise during planned vaginal deliveries of fetuses with known congenital anomalies. In some situations, intervention is required to facilitate vaginal delivery of the infant. For example, a fetus with megacystis may require vesicocentesis to allow the abdomen to be delivered through the maternal pelvis. The same can be true of a large abdominal or pelvic cyst such as can be found with multicystic dysplastic kidneys or rarely ovarian cysts.

For several reasons, operative delivery in the form of cesarean section before the onset of labor may be entertained, including:

Malpresentation. Noncephalic presentation is more common in fetuses with congenital anomalies, particularly in those with polyhydramnios.

Protection of the Mother. Occasionally, fetal congenital anomalies (e.g., macrocephaly, conjoined twins) place the mother at risk for complications during labor by preventing vaginal delivery, particularly as pregnancy advances. In this scenario, delivery by cesarean section may be indicated.

Protection of the Anomalous Area. Some external congenital anomalies (e.g., omphalocele involving the liver, large vascular sacrococcygeal teratoma) may be at risk of damage during the process of labor and delivery. In this instance, cesarean section may be beneficial. As always, care should be taken to avoid inadvertent laceration of the fetus and undue manipulation of the affected area.

Facilitation of Neonatal Resuscitation. If the fetus has a congenital anomaly that may obstruct the upper airway, a procedure called ex utero intrapartum treatment (EXIT) may be considered, for which cesarean delivery is required.

Minimizing Fetal Distress. In the presence of certain congenital anomalies, the fetus may experience unnecessary or detrimental distress (e.g., arthrogryposis). Delivery by cesarean section could be considered if the process of vaginal delivery is believed likely to cause significant pain to the fetus. This should be balanced by the recognition that cesarean delivery is not entirely atraumatic.

Fetuses with Life-Limiting Conditions

When the diagnosis of a life-limiting fetal condition is made antenatally, parents should be presented with all options from termination to palliation. Examples of such conditions include anencephaly, bilateral renal agenesis, trisomy 18 (T18) or 13 (T13), and thanatophoric dysplasia. They are commonly referred to as lethal, yet none of them fit the actual strict definition as such (Table 33-2). For example, more than 50 percent of babies with T18 or T13 survive for more than a week, up to 20 percent survive for more than a year, and when cardiac surgery is performed, 1-year survival rates as high as 50 percent have been reported.

A great majority of those pregnancies will be terminated or naturally result in an intrauterine fetal demise. However, the high rate of terminations may be partly related to the way counseling is provided. A survey of over 1000 obstetricians in the United Kingdom, Australia, and New Zealand showed that 85 percent of obstetricians regarded T18 as a lethal condition and more than 50 percent of them regarded T18 as incompatible with life. When surveying T18/T13 parents, it appeared that 93 percent had been told by health professionals that their child's condition was "lethal or incompatible with life" and two-thirds of them reported feeling pressured to terminate their pregnancy. In instances where parents of fetuses with T18 chose to continue with the pregnancy, 23 percent of obstetricians would never discuss or offer fetal monitoring in labor and 28 percent of them would never offer a cesarean section for fetal distress. This implies that a personal judgment around the quality of life of a child with severe cognitive impairment influences the clinician's decision to provide treatment.

It is key that health care professionals provide nondirective, unbiased, and value-neutral counseling to parents following prenatal diagnosis of a life-limiting fetal condition. The concept of shared decision making derives from a *patient-centered* view of health care. It focuses on what matters to parents and fundamentally derives from basic ethical principles. Autonomy means respecting the parents' views, wishes, concerns, and accepting that they can best determine these. Evaluating what is best for the fetus or neonate (when the parents are surrogate decision makers) and assessing the impact on the family units' adaptive and coping ability further complicates these difficult decisions. There is a dearth of data as to the frequency of parents choosing active or palliative approaches of care for the neonate,

OTHER ISSUES

TABLE 33-2: PUBLISHED OUTCOME FOR SEVERE CONGENITAL ANOMALIES FREQUENTLY DESCRIBED AS LETHAL[a]

Severe Congenital Anomalies	Prevalence	Probability of Live Birth (in absence of termination)	Median Postnatal Survival	Proportion Surviving >1 week/>1 year	Longest Reported Survivals
Renal agenesis	1.7/10,000	not reported	<24 hours	<5%/<5%	13 months
Anencephaly	10/10,000 pregnancies 1.6/10,000 births	62-72%	<24 hours 55 minutes	0-14%/7%	10 months 2.5 years
Thanatophoric dysplasia	0.4/10,000	not reported	not reported	not reported	5-9 years
Trisomy 18	2.6/10,000	48-51%	14 days	35-65%/14-19%	27-50 years
Trisomy 13	1.2/10,000	46-51%	10 days	45-57%/14-21%	19-27 years
Holoprosencephaly	0.5/10,000	not reported	4-5 months	71%/47%	6-19 years

[a]Using recent population cohort studies where available.

Reproduced with permission from Wilkinson et al, Ethical language and decision-making for prenatally diagnosed lethal malformations, Semin Fetal Neonatal Med. 2014;19(5):306-11.

following the diagnosis of severe congenital malformations in general and in life-limiting fetal conditions in particular. For all we know, there may be an increasing tendency for couples to consider pursuing the pregnancy when the option of palliative care is discussed. Furthermore, offering this palliative approach from the time of diagnosis, throughout pregnancy, at delivery, and beyond is of considerable benefit to the family.

As those pregnancies progress into the third trimester, it is important for the family and the care givers to establish a birth plan. A portion of women carrying fetuses with congenital anomalies will go into spontaneous preterm labor or will end up with premature rupture of the membranes. There is an increased risk of antepartum or intrapartum fetal demise that patients should be made aware of. As difficult as this discussion may be, it is still best to hold it in advance of the patient being admitted to the labor ward and to have it clearly documented in her medical chart. The timing of, conduct, and mode of delivery for these at-risk fetuses must be addressed with the family as well as all members of the health care team. Iatrogenic preterm delivery, whether to preempt an IUFD or to reduce parental distress, carries risks to the mother, including that of a failed induction of labor.

A maternal-focused approach to obstetrical care may mean that it is appropriate to limit the number of antenatal visits and fetal ultrasounds, avoid monitoring in labor, and aim for a vaginal delivery, if this reflects the parents' wishes. In the same spirit, active fetal-oriented obstetrical management, including monitoring or even cesarean section, may also be acceptable and is not necessarily against the best interests of the child. Interventions such as amnioinfusion during labor to reduce the frequency of fetal heart decelerations and assisted second stage to accelerate the birth of the liveborn child, short of performing a cesarean section, represent other "fetal-oriented" options. For some parents, the opportunity to experience as much time as they can with their child, while he or she is still alive, is extremely important. However, whatever the decision, the risks to the mother should never outweigh the benefits to the unborn child, which is why every case should be individualized.

If the fetus survives the process of labor and delivery, newborn care measures such as swaddling, soothers, the use of a warmer and sucrose should be provided. After all, palliative care is not synonymous with "withdrawal" or "withholding" of certain or all treatments. It is about goal-directed care for a patient with a life-limiting condition and their family. Memory-making strategies such as castings, moldings, and hair locks should be adopted in order to support the family. Where available, it may be valuable to involve an experienced palliative care team to do this in the

OTHER ISSUES

best possible way and to offer the opportunity of perinatal hospice care, should the infant survive beyond mom's "hospital" stay. In the absence of such a trained team, the obstetric team should be involved in providing information and comfort to the parents in a timely, compassionate, and sensitive manner.

Fetuses with Unexpected Congenital Anomalies

Due to prenatal ultrasound becoming routine in most countries, it is relatively uncommon to deliver a fetus with an unanticipated major congenital anomaly. Sonographic detection rates for anomalies such as neural tube defects and gastroschisis are approaching 100 percent. In comparison, detection rates are considerably lower for other conditions (e.g., cleft palate). Furthermore, a small number of patients who have not had any prenatal care or ultrasounds may present in labor. It should be remembered that there may be no hint of an abnormality before the birth and the obstetrical care provider needs to be prepared for the possibility of an unanticipated congenital anomaly in every delivery. Upon recognition of an abnormality, the most responsible person (MRP) should inform the parents of the finding/s. Depending on the setting at the delivery, this may be the attending obstetrician, midwife, or pediatrician. In general, the MRP should provide the most relevant and up-to-date information to the parents as soon as it is deemed reasonable to do so. The impact of the abnormality on the health of the infant should be explained clearly and further treatment and investigation offered when appropriate (including karyotype, diagnostic imaging, and genetic examination). Because some congenital anomalies have the potential to be life threatening, it is crucial that emergent conditions be excluded (e.g., ambiguous genitalia secondary to congenital adrenal hyperplasia and electrolyte abnormalities or ductus arteriosus dependent complex heart defects). Once the diagnosis is confirmed, the risk of recurrence should be discussed with the parents, although it may be most appropriate to provide this prepregnancy counseling remote from the acute event of their child's birth.

Fetal Anomalies: Destructive Operations

The purpose of destructive operations is to reduce the size of the head, shoulder girdle, or body of an unborn child or to increase the diameter of the maternal pelvis in order to enable the vaginal delivery of the baby. Although there is little role for them in advanced countries, they may occasionally be required in the developing world. Indeed, the dangers of those destructive procedures to the mother far outweigh the risks of a cesarean section delivery, such that they are almost never performed today. On the rare occasion where they must be done, a thorough examination of the birth canal should be conducted immediately after delivery to ensure that no injury has been caused by the instruments or the sharp edges of the skull bones. We will focus our discussion on the destructive operation specific to congenital anomalies.

Cephalocentesis

The aim of this procedure is to reduce the bulk of the head. It should be reserved for cases of hydrocephalus. The excess cerebrospinal fluid can be drained, even in a live infant, by inserting a large-bore needle (16-18 gauge) through the fontanelle. The size of the head is reduced, and its delivery made possible. The most direct approach is vaginal where the needle is inserted through the dilated cervix and into the cranial cavity via a fontanelle or suture. The sagittal sinus should be avoided. If necessary, the needle can be pushed through one of the cranial bones. When the presentation is breech, drainage of the cerebrospinal fluid can be achieved by spondylectomy or, if possible, by direct entry into the ventricles beneath the occipital plate or behind the ear. Alternatively, a transabdominal approach can be used. In this case, the needle is passed through the abdominal and uterine walls and through the fetal cranial bones into the skull.

Other destructive procedures include decapitation, cleidotomy, and symphysiotomy. The latter two are discussed in Chapter 18 of this book, which covers shoulder dystocia.

SELECTED READING

American College of Obstetrics and Gynecology: Practice Bulletin Number 227: Fetal Growth Restriction. Obstet Gynecol 137:e16-e28, 2021

Breeze AC, Lees CC: Antenatal diagnosis and management of life-limiting conditions. Semin Fetal Neonatal Med 18: 68-75, 2013

Dolk H, Loane M, Garne E: The prevalence of congenital anomalies in Europe. Adv Exp Med Biol 686:349-364, 2010

Drotar D, Baskiewicz A, Irvin N, Kennell J, Klaus M: The adaptation of parents to the birth of an infant with a congenital malformation: a hypothetical model. Pediatrics 56: 710-717, 1975

Heuser CC, Eller AG, Byrne JL: Survey of physicians' approach to severe fetal anomalies. J Med Ethics 38:391-395, 2012

International Society for Ultrasound in Obstetrics and Gynaecology: ISUOG Practice Guideline: diagnosis and management of small-for-gestational-age fetus and fetal growth restriction. Ultrasound Obstet Gynecol 56:298-312, 2020

OTHER ISSUES

Janvier A, Farlow B, Barrington KJ, Bourque CJ, Brazg T, Wilfond B: Building trust and improving communication with parents of children with Trisomy 13 and 18: A mixed-methods study. Palliat Med 34:262-271, 2020

Smale LE: Destructive operations on the fetus. Review of literature and application in 10 cases of neglected dystocia. Am J Obstet Gynecol 119:369-374, 1974

Society for Maternal-Fetal Medicine: SMFM Consult Series #52: Diagnosis and management of fetal growth restriction. Am J Obstet Gynecol 223:B2-B17, 2020

Society of Obstetricians and Gynaecologists of Canada: Clinical practice guideline: Intrauterine growth restriction: screening, diagnosis, and management. J Obstet Gynaecol Can 35:741-748, 2013

Society of Obstetricians and Gynaecologists of Canada: Clinical practice guideline: Magnesium sulphate for fetal neuroprotection. J Obstet Gynaecol Can 41:505-522, 2019

Spinnato JA, Cook VD, Cook CR, Voss DH: Aggressive intrapartum management of lethal fetal anomalies: beyond fetal beneficence. Obstet Gynecol 85:89-92, 1995

Wilkinson D, de Crespigny L, Xafis V: Ethical language and decision-making for prenatally diagnosed lethal malformations. Semin Fetal Neonatal Med 19:306-311, 2014 (Erratum in: Semin Fetal Neonatal Med 20:64, 2015)

CHAPTER 34

Intrapartum Infections

Wesley J. Edwards
Griffith D. Jones

INTRODUCTION

Infections are increasingly recognized as important contributors of maternal, fetal, and neonatal complications. These can be divided into two major categories: ascending genital tract infections and hematogenously spread infections from the mother. Some infections may be entirely asymptomatic and recognized by antenatal screening. For others, the symptoms can vary significantly and it is not infrequent for some of these entities to be subtle or subclinical. As such, a high index of suspicion is required, along with appropriate knowledge of preventive and therapeutic approaches. Diagnostic tools include serologic testing: markers of inflammation in blood and amniotic fluid and culture of blood, amniotic fluid, placenta, and membranes. Pathologic examination of the placenta, cord, and membranes can be helpful retrospectively.

VIRAL INFECTIONS

Human Immunodeficiency Virus

Mother-to-child transmission (MTCT) can occur antenatally, intrapartum, or postpartum through breastfeeding. Most commonly, the infant acquires the infection intrapartum. Without antiretroviral (ARV) therapy, the risk of transmission to the fetus or infant is as high as 25 percent but can decrease to below 2 percent with appropriate management, including antenatal screening, ARV therapy to maximally suppress viral load, and careful selection of the mode of delivery. Labor must be managed in a way to minimize the potential exposure of the fetus to maternal blood. Significant risk factors for MTCT are listed in Table 34-1.

Intrapartum Care

Antiretroviral Therapy

- Canadian guidelines recommend that intrapartum IV zidovudine is offered to all HIV-infected pregnant women, regardless of their antepartum regimen or viral load, to reduce perinatal transmission of HIV (grade III-B recommendation). The UK guidelines suggest offering this only to women with a viral load more than 50 copies/mL

TABLE 34-1: RISK FACTORS FOR MOTHER-TO-CHILD TRANSMISSION OF HIV

High maternal viral load (the amount of HIV RNA in the plasma)
Breastfeeding
Sexually transmitted infections
Chorioamnionitis
Prolonged rupture of the membranes
Young maternal age
History of stillbirth
Vaginal mode of delivery (in the context of high viral load)
Low CD4 count
Advanced maternal HIV disease
Bleeding during labor (episiotomy, perineal laceration, and intrapartum hemorrhage)

- Women who are receiving an antepartum combination ARV drug regimen should continue this regimen on schedule as much as possible during labor and before scheduled cesarean delivery
- Women receiving combination regimens that include zidovudine should receive IV zidovudine during labor while other oral ARV components are continued

Cesarean Delivery

- For women who have either an unknown or a significant viral load (i.e., HIV RNA >50 copies/mL at 34 to 36 weeks) in late pregnancy, delivery by scheduled cesarean delivery is recommended in Canada. This is regardless of the use of antepartum ARV drugs
- It is not clear whether cesarean delivery after ruptured membranes or onset of labor provides benefit in preventing perinatal transmission. Management of women originally scheduled for cesarean delivery who present with ruptured membranes or in labor must be individualized based on duration of rupture, progress of labor, plasma viral load, current ARV regimen, and other clinical factors

Trial of Labor. Women with maximally suppressed viral loads (<50 copies/mL) can be offered a vaginal delivery. However, it is essential to minimize

OTHER ISSUES

the contact with maternal blood or body fluids and secretions during that time. As such, the following is recommended:

- Avoid routine use of fetal scalp electrodes for fetal monitoring
- Avoid artificial rupture of membranes unless clear obstetric indications are present
- Operative delivery with forceps or a vacuum extractor and/or episiotomy should be performed only if there are clear obstetric indications

Postpartum Care

- The infant should be carefully washed before any injections are administered
- Breastfeeding is contraindicated
- Contraceptive counseling is recommended

Herpes Simplex Virus

In Canada, the incidence of type 2 herpes simplex virus (HSV-2) seropositivity in pregnant women varies from 7.1 to 28.1 percent, and the incidence of neonatal HSV is one in 17,000 births. Neonatal HSV is typically acquired during delivery as a result of exposure to genital tract lesions. It is diagnosed based on clinical presentation and cultures of the infant 48 hours after birth. The infant can develop a variety of complications, including long-term neurological sequelae or disseminated disease carrying a 90 percent mortality rate.

It is imperative to recognize and treat maternal infections with HSV for the adequate prevention of neonatal disease. Maternal HSV can be categorized as primary (no antibodies to HSV-1 or -2) or recurrent infections (has antibodies to HSV-1 or -2). The greatest risk of neonatal infection occurs in the context of a primary infection in the third trimester because this does not confer sufficient time for transplacental passage of protective maternal antibodies to the newborn.

Primary Infection

Because primary infection in the third trimester carries a neonatal risk of HSV of 30 to 50 percent, most authorities, including the SOGC, recommend that these women be delivered by cesarean section. Neonatal cultures should then be performed and the infant observed closely.

Recurrent Disease

In these circumstances, maternal antibodies are present that cross the placenta. In this context, women presenting in labor with a genital lesion carry a risk of neonatal disease of less than 5 percent. The absence of such lesions at delivery carries a trivial risk of asymptomatic shedding and calculated risks of neonatal disease of less than two per 10,000. Cultures are not predictive of neonatal disease in these instances.

Therefore, women with recurrent infection presenting at delivery should be examined carefully for the presence of HSV lesions. If lesions are seen in the genital area or even as far as over the thighs or buttocks or if prodromal symptoms are present, Canadian guidelines recommend cesarean delivery. UK guidelines suggest that the neonatal risks of HSV and maternal risks from cesarean section should be discussed and vaginal delivery offered, with the final choice made by the mother. As an "ascending infection," the cesarean section should be performed within 4 hours of ruptured membranes. In addition, scalp sampling and scalp electrodes should be avoided.

BACTERIAL INFECTIONS

Listeriosis

The risk of fetal infection hematogenously spread from the mother is much less common during labor. This is partly related to the physiologic, mechanical, and immunologic barriers provided by the placenta. However, rarely, organisms such as staphylococci, streptococci, or pneumococci may infect the pregnant woman, resulting in a significant degree of maternal bacteremia. This then reaches the placenta and occasionally crosses to the fetus. These patients may present with classical symptoms of maternal fever, tachycardia, malaise, and uterine tenderness. The fetus may show evidence of tachycardia. Prompt treatment with antibiotics should be initiated, and delivery should be planned accordingly (see section "Chorioamnionitis"). Perhaps the most relevant perinatal hematogenous infection is listeriosis. Although rare (12 per 100,000 in pregnancy), this gram-positive bacillus has severe consequences for the fetus and newborn. Maternal listeriosis is associated with increased risks of fetal demise, preterm delivery, neonatal sepsis, meningitis, pneumonia, and death. The perinatal mortality rate varies between 27 and 33 percent.

Listeria monocytogenes has a particular predilection for pregnant women, who are 20 times more likely to become infected compared with the general population. The organism is acquired by the mother through contaminated water and food such as milk, cheese, chicken, coleslaw, undercooked meat, fruits, and vegetables. It can then spread transplacentally to the fetus. Mothers infected with *Listeria* are often asymptomatic or present with nonspecific flu-like symptoms. A high index of suspicion is thus necessary.

The predilection for pregnant women is well illustrated by a 1981 Canadian outbreak, which affected 100 individuals, of whom 34 were pregnant. In this group were nine stillbirths, 23 neonatal infections, and only two live healthy births.

Diagnosis

Confirmation of diagnosis can be done reliably by cultures of amniotic fluid, meconium, membranes, placenta, blood, or spinal fluid. Placental pathologic examination may reveal the presence of acute villitis and of multiple microabscesses.

Because *Listeria* is an intracellular organism and can resemble diphtheroids, pneumococci, or *Hemophilus*, Gram stains are helpful clinically only one-third of the time. Cultures of the vagina or stools are not recommended because women can be normal carriers without being infected. Serologic test of listeriosis are also not recommended. Therefore, if a pregnant woman presents with a clinical scenario suggestive of listeriosis, blood cultures are recommended.

Treatment

The antibiotics recommended for the treatment of listeriosis must be given in high dose to cross the placenta and to penetrate intracellularly. These include ampicillin as a first line and erythromycin as a second line. In women allergic to penicillins, trimethoprim–sulfamethoxazole has been effective. Therapy should continue for 7 to 14 days (Table 34-2).

TABLE 34-2: RECOMMENDED TREATMENT APPROACHES MATERNAL LISTERIOSIS

First line:
• Ampicillin 2 g every 6-8 hours

Second line:
• Erythromycin 4 g/day
• Penicillin-allergic women: trimethoprim–sulfamethoxazole 1-2 tablets every 6 hours

Group B Streptococcus

Group B streptococcus is a gram-positive organism responsible for infections mostly in infants and pregnant women. Maternal colonization of the lower gastrointestinal (GI) and urinary tracts with GBS occurs in 15 to 30 percent of women. As such, this organism is considered to be part of the "normal" flora of the vagina. However, GBS also represents one of the most important causes of neonatal mortality and morbidity, with a case fatality rate that can be as high as 50 percent. Two types of neonatal infection can occur: early onset or late onset. Early-onset disease (EOD) manifests itself in the first 7 days of life and is the result of transmission from mother to fetus. The incidence of this serious disease is reported as 0.3 per 1000 infants.

Risk Factors for Early-Onset Disease

1. Maternal colonization: The most important risk factors for EOD is maternal colonization. A pregnant woman with positive GBS vaginal or rectal culture near term has a 25-fold increased risk of having an infant with EOD. The GI tract serves as the reservoir for GBS, and it is noteworthy that colonization during pregnancy can be transient or persistent. In addition, the extent of colonization also plays a role in disease transmission, with heavy colonization representing an even higher risk to the infant. Finally, the presence of GBS in the urine at any time during pregnancy also carries a much higher risk of EOD
2. Gestational age less than 37 completed weeks
3. Prolonged duration of membrane rupture (12-18 hours)
4. Intrapartum temperature more than 38°C
5. Intraamniotic infection
6. Previous delivery of an infant with invasive GBS disease
7. Young maternal age, black race, and low maternal levels of GBS-specific anticapsular antibody

Prevention

All pregnant women should be offered screening with a rectovaginal swab at around 36 weeks' gestation. The negative predictive value of GBS cultures performed 5 weeks or less before delivery is 95 to 98 percent. However, because of a decrease in negative predictive value, the clinical utility decreases when a prenatal culture is performed more than 5 weeks before delivery.

Intrapartum treatment of all women with a positive GBS culture or unscreened women with risk factors as described in Table 34-3 should be initiated at the onset of labor or rupture of membranes.

OTHER ISSUES

TABLE 34-3: RISK FACTORS REQUIRING ANTIBIOTIC TREATMENT INTRAPARTUM OR AT THE ONSET OF MEMBRANE RUPTURE FOR THE PREVENTION OF GROUP B STREPTOCOCCUS EARLY-ONSET DISEASE

Women with a positive rectovaginal culture at 35 to 37 weeks[a]
Women with a previously affected infant
Women with GBS bacteriuria at any time during pregnancy (regardless of the amount of colony-forming units present)
Women at less than 37 weeks' gestation unless a negative swab has been obtained in the 5 weeks before presentation
Women with intrapartum fever (>38°C)
Women with an unknown GBS status and either known GBS positive status in a prior pregnancy or ruptured membranes at term for greater than 18 hours or intrapartum fever

[a]Guidelines from the American College of Obstetricians and Gynecologists has also added to this list "intrapartum nucleic acid amplification test," a form of rapid testing available in the United States.

GBS, group B streptococcus.

Recommended antibiotics are listed in Table 34-4. Although both ampicillin and penicillin are efficacious against GBS, penicillin has a narrower spectrum and is the antibiotic of choice. In the case of low-risk penicillin allergy, cephazolins are considered appropriate. Otherwise, clindamycin or erythromycin is recommended for those at high risk of anaphylaxis to penicillins.

Chorioamnionitis

Chorioamnionitis is an infection of the chorion and amnion, which can progress to involve the umbilical cord, placenta, and fetus itself. It is characterized

TABLE 34-4: ANTIBIOTIC DOSAGES FOR THE PREVENTION OF EARLY-ONSET DISEASE DUE TO GROUP B STREPTOCOCCUS

Penicillin G 5 million units IV; then 2.5 million every 4 hours
Penicillin-allergic, low risk of anaphylaxis: cefazolin 2 g IV; then 1 g every 8 hours
Penicillin allergic and at risk of anaphylaxis: clindamycin 900 mg IV every 8 hours or erythromycin 500 mg IV every 6 hours
In rare cases, GBS resistance may occur; vancomycin is then the antibiotic of choice

GBS, group B streptococcus; IV, intravenous.

by the infiltration of these membranes by neutrophil polymorphs, which starts at the interface between the decidua and chorion at the level of the os. The most common microorganisms involved include *Ureaplasma* spp., *Mycoplasma* spp., enterococci, streptococci, coliforms, and staphylococci.

Intrapartum risk factors for the development of chorioamnionitis include multiple examinations during labor, prolonged labor, nulliparity, bacterial vaginosis or group B streptococcal (GBS) colonization, meconium, use of internal monitoring, and epidural anesthesia. Finally, alcohol use and cigarette smoking are predisposing factors.

Frequently associated with preterm prelabor rupture of the membranes (PPROM) and preterm labor (PTL), chorioamnionitis is often suspected as playing a causative role in these pathologies. Ascension of microorganisms via the genital tract to the membranes results in the production and release of proinflammatory cytokines and chemokines, which in turn may weaken the membranes and lead to PPROM. In addition, the release of prostaglandins associated with the process of inflammation may induce cervical changes and result in preterm delivery. Inflammation of the amniotic cavity, independent of the presence of positive cultures, is associated with a higher risk of preterm delivery, chorioamnionitis, low APGAR scores, admission to the neonatal intensive care unit, and low birth weight.

In addition, exposure of a fetus to such an environment can lead to the development of an intense inflammatory reaction in the fetal compartment itself. This is referred to as fetal inflammatory response syndrome (FIRS), which is characterized by elevated levels of interleukin-6 (IL-6) in the fetal blood and by the possibility of multiorgan damage, including effects on the hematopoietic system, lungs, brain, heart, kidneys, and adrenal glands. Long-term sequelae for these newborns include bronchopulmonary dysplasia and cerebral palsy. A meta-analysis examining the association between chorioamnionitis and cerebral palsy reported a 140 percent increased risk for fetuses exposed to clinical chorioamnionitis and an 80 percent increased risk for a histologic but asymptomatic chorioamnionitis.

Clinical Presentation

Chorioamnionitis can present with maternal and fetal signs or be subclinical. Maternal fever (one reading of $\geq 39.0°C$ or two readings of $\geq 38.0°C$) is often associated with general malaise and may present with uterine contractions. In addition, the presence of a tender uterus and a foul-smelling discharge help strengthen the diagnosis. Associated with this are maternal and fetal tachycardia (>100 and >160 beats/min, respectively) and a

OTHER ISSUES

nonreassuring tracing. Although these symptoms and signs can raise the possibility of chorioamnionitis, they are neither sensitive nor specific, and as such, an overall evaluation of the risk factors present and the clinical presentation are both important.

Diagnostic Criteria

Laboratory investigations in cases of suspected chorioamnionitis are based on the presence of a maternal response and the presence of inflammation and of an invading microorganism. As such, an evaluation of maternal leukocytosis or a left shift may help the clinician but remain nonspecific, particularly in the context of labor, which may be associated with increases in maternal leukocyte counts because of dehydration or the administration of steroids.

C-reactive protein (CRP), an acute phase reactant, moderately predicts histologic chorioamnionitis. In the presence of maternal fever and tachycardia, a maternal blood culture, although not useful in diagnosing chorioamnionitis itself, may be helpful in certain complex cases for selection of antibiotics.

Finally, the evaluation of amniotic fluid has been the scope of much research in the hope to uncover a specific and sensitive diagnostic strategy. Various rapid testing methodologies have been evaluated, including Gram stain (98% specificity), glucose levels (74% specificity), and white cell count. The need for an amniocentesis has severely limited their use clinically.

Although levels of cytokines (especially IL-6) and MMPs (especially MMP-8) were consistently found to be higher in the amniotic fluid of women with a chorioamnionitis and their sensitivities and specificities were acceptable, they are only currently available in research settings.

Amniotic fluid cultures remain the "gold standard" but the time required for a result is often too long in a clinical setting, where rapid decisions regarding delivery must be made. In addition, recent data are now revealing the presence of unsuspected microorganisms, which would not necessarily be identified on culture. Innovative technologies such as proteomics may assist the clinician in this context in the future.

Management

Supportive Care. Upon diagnosis of chorioamnionitis, supportive measures for both the mother and fetus must be put in place and a plan for delivery initiated. Given the possible maternal risks of sepsis, attention to intravenous (IV) fluids is essential. A Foley catheter may be useful to assess fluid balance. Monitoring of vital signs is crucial, with prompt attention paid to hypotension and tachycardia. Oxygen saturation should be evaluated regularly and maintained at 95 percent and above. Anti-pyretics should be administered to normalize maternal temperature given the association between maternal fever and adverse neonatal out-comes, including encephalopathy. Electronic fetal monitoring should be implemented.

Delivery. The mode of delivery in these cases should be dictated by obstetrical determinants because cesarean delivery has not been shown to improve outcomes for either the mother or the fetus upon initiation of appropriate antibiotic use.

Antibiotics. Parenteral antibiotics must be administered promptly and their choice based on the most commonly found microorganisms. In that context, it is suggested to treat with a combination of ampicillin 2 g IV every 6 hours (or vancomycin 1 g IV every 12 hours for those with allergy to penicillins) and gentamicin 1.5 mg/kg every 8 hours. Although this par-ticular administration of gentamicin is widely used, a once-daily dosage approach (one dose of 5 mg/kg) has been found to be as efficacious in treating the infection.

Finally, if better anaerobic coverage is desired (e.g., if a cesarean section is planned), the addition of clindamycin (900 mg IV every 8 hours) or met-ronidazole (500 mg IV every 8 hours) may be wise.

The duration of treatment generally is limited. In the case of a vagi-nal delivery, antibiotics can usually be discontinued at delivery or after one postpartum dose has been administered. However, in the context of a cesarean delivery, most clinicians continue antibiotics until the patient has been afebrile for a period of 24 hours.

Antibiotic Prophylaxis to Prevent Perinatal Infections

The most important risk factor is delivery by cesarean section. Women delivered by cesarean section are 20 times more likely to suffer a postpartum infection compared with those delivered vaginally. These infections include endomyometritis, wound infection, and infection of the urinary tract, pelvic abscess, septic pelvic thrombophlebitis, pneumonia, and sepsis.

To reduce this risk, a significant number of studies have investigated the use of prophylactic antibiotics before performing a cesarean section. The evidence suggests that there was a significantly decreased risk of endome-tritis and wound infections when prophylactic antibiotics are administered

OTHER ISSUES

TABLE 34-5: SUMMARY OF RECOMMENDATIONS FOR PROPHYLACTIC ANTIBIOTICS

- Women undergoing either an elective or emergency cesarean section should receive antibiotic prophylaxis

- Women with third- or fourth-degree laceration may benefit from antibiotic prophylaxis

- There is no benefit of prophylaxis with antibiotics in cases of manual removal of the placenta and dilatation and curettage or operative vaginal delivery

to women undergoing emergency or elective cesarean sections. These data with others have led to recommendations by SOGC and ACOG that all women delivered by cesarean section should be offered prophylactic antibiotics (Table 34-5). Administration of antibiotics does not reduce the risk of subsequent infections in operative vaginal deliveries, and there are insufficient data to recommend for or against antibiotic prophylaxis in cases of manual removal of the placenta and postpartum dilatation and curettage. However, antibiotics may decrease perineal wound complications after a third- or fourth-degree perineal laceration.

Choice of Antibiotics

Most studies have examined the use of cephalosporins in the context of prophylaxis at cesarean section. With adequate coverage of gram-positive and modest coverage of gram-negative organisms, this class of agents carries a spectrum that is narrow enough to minimize the risk of developing resistance. In women with penicillin allergy, clindamycin or erythromycin has been suggested.

Finally, cefotetan or cefoxitin is recommended for women with third- or fourth-degree perineal tears. Table 34-6 summarizes the SOGC recommendations regarding antibiotic prophylaxis and obstetric procedures.

TABLE 34-6: ANTIBIOTIC PROPHYLAXIS: RECOMMENDATIONS FROM THE SOCIETY OF OBSTETRICIANS AND GYNAECOLOGISTS OF CANADA

1. Emergency or elective cesarean section
- Cefazolin 1-2 g IV 15-60 minutes before skin incision
- Penicillin-allergic women: clindamycin 600 mg IV or erythromycin 500 mg IV

2. Third- or fourth-degree lacerations
- Cefotetan 1 g IV or cefoxitin 1 g IV

IV, intravenous.

Maternal Sepsis

Introduction

Sepsis is a significant cause of maternal morbidity and mortality. The World Health Organization estimates that sepsis accounts for 10 percent of maternal deaths and is the third most common cause of direct maternal deaths globally. As with other causes of maternal mortality, these numbers represent the tip of the iceberg with many more cases resulting in severe maternal morbidity.

The UK Confidential Enquiry into Maternal Deaths and Morbidity (2009-2012) found that delayed recognition and management was a contributing factor in 63 percent of maternal deaths from sepsis. Data from other jurisdictions suggest that missed management opportunities likely contribute to maternal sepsis deaths globally. The physical, social, and opportunity costs associated with mortality from maternal sepsis, combined with the opportunities for prevention, have made the management of maternal sepsis a global priority.

Definitions

The Third International Consensus (Sepsis-3) definition for sepsis is "life threatening organ dysfunction caused by a dysregulated host response to infection." The updated consensus has not included severe sepsis as a discrete entity. Septic shock occurs when sepsis results in persistent hypotension requiring vasopressors to maintain a mean arterial pressure of 65 mm Hg or higher, despite adequate volume resuscitation. The World Health Organization has used similar wording when they defined maternal sepsis as "a life-threatening condition defined as organ dysfunction caused by an infection during pregnancy, delivery, puerperium, or after an abortion."

Organ dysfunction is identified using the sequential organ failure assessment (SOFA) score. An acute change in the SOFA score by 2 or more points consequent to infection is used. Importantly, the SOFA score was designed and validated as a predictor of mortality and not a diagnostic tool or guide for dynamic medical management.

The quick sequential organ failure assessment (qSOFA) was introduced by Sepsis-3 as a simplified version of SOFA. It was introduced as a more practical bedside assessment tool for patients with infection to predict those at high risk of a poor outcome. Only three variables are used: Glasgow Coma Score <15, a respiratory rate >22/minute, and a systolic blood pressure <100 mm Hg. A patient with two of these variables is considered higher risk for poor outcomes.

OTHER ISSUES

Pathophysiology

A detailed description of the pathophysiology of sepsis is beyond the scope of this chapter. It is important to appreciate however that sepsis occurs when local infection spreads beyond its initial site. A complex systemic inflammatory response acts at a molecular, cellular, and multiorgan level. Examples of organ and system dysfunction include altered mental status, hypotension, tachycardia, edema, hypoxemia, oliguria, hyperglycemia, elevated serum lactate, and coagulation abnormalities.

Infectious Causes in Pregnancy

Infectious causes of sepsis can be divided into either obstetric or nonobstetric categories. Obstetric and genital tract causes are more likely to occur in the intrapartum and postpartum period. Nonobstetric causes can occur at any time during pregnancy. Common infectious causes of sepsis can be seen in Table 34-7.

The most common pathogens isolated in maternal sepsis are group A streptococcus, group B streptococcus, and *Escherichia coli*. However, many organisms including gram-negative bacteria and anaerobic bacteria have been reported depending on the primary site of infection. Mixed infections are also possible.

Diagnosis

Sepsis is not a singular disease state, and, despite its prevalence, there is currently no diagnostic test to confirm a diagnosis of sepsis. One needs to rely on clinical signs and symptoms, and laboratory investigations that signify organ dysfunction when there is suspected or confirmed infection.

Early warning systems (EWS) have been used for many years in nonpregnant patients. These systems use standard patient variables such as

TABLE 34-7: COMMON CAUSES OF SEPSIS IN PREGNANCY

Obstetric Causes	• Chorioamnionitis • Septic abortion • Endometritis • Wound infection following cesarean section or perineal laceration • Invasive intervention such as cervical cerclage
Nonobstetric Causes	• Urinary tract infection • Respiratory tract infection • Appendicitis

heart rate, blood pressure, respiratory rate, temperature, urine output, level of consciousness, and oxygen saturation, which are tracked over time. The number of variables that deviate from normal, combined with the degree of abnormality for each variable, trigger the need for a detailed patient assessment and a proportional escalation in management.

Standardized EWS tools were not designed for, or validated for the pregnant population. Physiological changes of normal pregnancy and labor can overlap with those of evolving infection and sepsis. This can lead to diagnostic uncertainty and delayed management. The modified early obstetric warning system (MEOWS) was designed as a tool to overcome these limitations.

The MEOWS has been in widespread use for many years. The 2003-2005 report on the confidential enquiries into maternal deaths in the United Kingdom recommended the routine use of a national obstetric early warning chart for all obstetric patients to assist in the timely recognition, treatment, and referral of women who have, or are developing, critical illness. An example of a MEOWS chart can be seen in Table 34-8. The MEOWS is not intended to replace clinical decision-making. Rather it determines the urgency of assessment, and prompts an escalation of care proportional to the risk of critical illness.

Management of Sepsis

Sepsis is a medical emergency. Speed of symptom recognition, initiation of appropriate investigations, fluid resuscitation, and antimicrobial therapy are the cornerstones of sepsis management. A linear relationship has been found between the risk of mortality and delays in initiation of management, particularly appropriate antimicrobial therapy. Once sepsis has progressed to septic shock, then the hospital mortality is in excess of 40 percent.

The Surviving Sepsis Campaign introduced an update to their sepsis care bundle in 2018. The updated recommendation introduced a 1-hour bundle. Elements of this bundle can be seen in Table 34-9. This update reiterates the high degree of importance placed on prompt and comprehensive initial management. The first step, however, is thinking that sepsis may be a possibility. One cannot wait for confirmation of an infective organism or source before starting management.

Serum Lactate. Lactate is a biproduct of anaerobic metabolism and is produced when there is a switch from using oxygen to using the glycolytic pathway for energy. Raised serum lactate can be used as a surrogate marker for tissue hypoperfusion. In patients with sepsis, a correlation has been found between increasing levels of serum lactate and mortality. Lactate

OTHER ISSUES

TABLE 34-8: MODIFIED EARLY OBSTETRIC WARNING SYSTEM

Physiological Parameter	3	2	1	0	1	2	3
Respiratory Rate	<12			12-20		21-25	>25
Oxygen Saturations	<92	92-95		>95			
Any Supplemental Oxygen		Yes		No			
Temperature	<36			36.1-37.2		37.3-37.7	>37.7
Systolic BP	<90			90-140	141-150	151-160	>160
Diastolic BP				60-90	91-100	101-110	>110
Heart Rate	<50	50-60		61-100	101-110	111-120	>120
Level of Consciousness				A			V, P, or U
Pain (excluding labor)				Normal			Abnormal
Discharge / Lochia				Normal			Abnormal
Proteinurea						+	++ >

TABLE 34-9: 1-HOUR BUNDLE FROM SURVIVING SEPSIS CAMPAIGN

- Measure serum lactate level. Remeasure if initial lactate is >2 mmol/L
- Obtain blood cultures prior to administration of antibiotics
- Administer broad-spectrum antibiotics
- Begin rapid administration of 30 mL/kg crystalloid for hypotension or lactate >4 mmol/L
- Begin vasopressors if patient is hypotensive during or after fluid resuscitation to maintain mean arterial pressure >65 mm Hg

levels can be used to guide fluid resuscitation and, if abnormal, should be remeasured every 2-4 hours.

Obtain Blood Cultures.   Identifying the responsible pathogen is key to guiding appropriate antimicrobial therapy. As soon as infection is considered as a possible cause for organ dysfunction, blood cultures should be obtained. If an obvious source of infection is present, then samples from this site should also be collected. Sterilization of cultured organisms can occur very quickly after the first dose of an antibiotic. Ideally, cultures should be taken before the administration of an antimicrobials. However, given the increase in mortality with delaying antibiotic therapy, administration should not be delayed for blood cultures in patients suspected of sepsis.

Administer Broad-Spectrum Antibiotics.   Empiric broad-spectrum antibiotic administration is the first part of infection source control. Antibiotic choice will depend on the likely source of infection, and likely organisms accounting for geographic variation in bacteria and antibiotic resistance. Hospital, health region or local specialty society guidelines can guide appropriate antibiotic choice. Initial choices should have coverage of aerobic and anaerobic gram-positive and gram-negative bacteria. Broad-spectrum carbapenem (e.g., Meropenem) or a broad-spectrum β-lactam antibiotic with combination beta-lactamase inhibitor (e.g., Piperacillin/tazobactam) are examples of possible initial therapies. Addition of antifungal and antiviral medication should also be considered based on clinical suspicion. Antibiotic coverage can be narrowed when culture and sensitivity results become available.

Fluid Resuscitation.   Intravenous fluid resuscitation should begin immediately if hypotension or evidence of tissue hypoperfusion (serum lactate >2 mmol/L) is present. The Surviving Sepsis Campaign recommend an initial bolus of 30 mL/kg of crystalloid solution to be completed within the first 3 hours. Although this recommendation is not supported by strong evidence, especially in the pregnant population, it allows a starting position while more clinical information is gathered to accurately guide therapy. Fluid responsiveness is variable in septic patients, and pregnancy related conditions or pathology may also make some patients more susceptible to fluid overload. For this reason, a recommendation of 1-2 L of crystalloid has been an alternative recommendation in the pregnant population. Ongoing reassessment of physiological parameters as well as noninvasive or invasive hemodynamic parameters, if available, will assist in guiding further fluid administration.

Administration of Vasopressors. Prolonged hypotension in patients with sepsis increases the risk of mortality. For patients, whose blood pressure is no longer fluid responsive or where further fluid administration is harmful, administration of vasopressor medication is indicated. A norepinephrine infusion is considered the first-line medication with the target mean arterial pressure of >65 mm Hg. This target pressure has not been adequately studied in the pregnant population but should be the initial target until individualized assessment of organ perfusion is possible.

Specific Pregnancy Considerations. Sepsis in pregnancy is associated with an increased risk of preterm delivery and stillbirth. The presence of sepsis in a pregnant patient is not an indication for delivery. Delivery should be for obstetric indications. The exception being sepsis from chorioamnionitis where delivery should be expedited as a means of source control. Multidisciplinary involvement of senior obstetrical staff, anesthesiology, neonatology, and critical care staff is recommended. Obstetrical management should occur concurrently with sepsis management. Corticosteroids are not contraindicated in maternal sepsis and can be used if indicated for fetal lung maturity.

CONCLUSION

Maternal sepsis is a life-threating emergency. The physiological changes of pregnancy can create diagnostic uncertainty. Clinicians must always consider sepsis as a possibility if hemodynamic abnormalities and evidence of organ dysfunction are present. Misdiagnosis and delaying management significantly increase the risk of maternal death. Each hospital should have readily available access to a pathway for diagnosis and management of maternal sepsis. Early detection using a MEOWS, combined with rapid support for organ perfusion and broad-spectrum antibiotics, are integral to reducing the morbidity and mortality from maternal sepsis.

SELECTED READING

Acosta C, Kurinczuk J, Lucas N, et al: Severe maternal sepsis in the UK, 2011-2012 a national case-control study. PLoS Med 11, 2014

American College of Obstetricians and Gynecologists: ACOG Committee Opinion. Intrapartum management of intraamniotic infection. Obstet Gynecol 130:e95-101, 2017

American College of Obstetricians and Gynecologists: ACOG Committee Opinion. Prevention of group B streptococcal early-onset disease in newborns. No. 797. Obstet Gynecol 135:e51-e72, 2020

Bonet M, Pileggi V, Rijken M, et al: Towards a consensus definition of maternal sepsis: results of a systematic review and expert consultation. Reprod Health 14, 2017

Escobar M, Echavarria M, Zambrano M, et al: Maternal Sepsis. AJOG MFM, 2, 2020

Foley E, Clarke E, Beckett VA, et al: Management of genital herpes in pregnancy. BASHH & RCOG. https://www.bashhguidelines.org/media/1060/management-genital-herpes. pdf, 2014

Gilleece Y, Tariq S, Bamford A, et al: British HIV Association guidelines for the management of HIV in pregnancy and postpartum. HIV Medicine 20:s2-85, 2019

Knight M, Tuffnell D, Kenyon S, et al on behalf of MBRRACE-UK: Saving Lives, Improving Mothers' Care - Surveillance of Maternal Deaths in the UK 2011-13 and Lessons Learned to Inform Maternity Care from the UK and Ireland Confidential Enquiries into Maternal Deaths and Morbidity 2009-13. Oxford: National Perinatal Epidemiology Unit, University of Oxford, 2015

Levy M, Evans L, Rhodes A: The surviving sepsis campaign bundle. Intensive Care Med 44:925-928, 2018

Money D, Steben M, Wong T, et al: Guidelines for the management of herpes simplex virus in pregnancy. J Obstet Gynaecol Can 39:e199-205, 2017

Money D, Tulloch K, Boucoiran I, et al: Guidelines for the care of pregnant women living with HIV and interventions to reduce perinatal transmission. J Obstet Gynaecol Can 36:721–734, 2014

Plante L, Pacheco L, Louis J: SMFM Consult Series #47: Sepsis during pregnancy and the puerperium. Society for Maternal-Fetal Medicine, 2019

Singer M, Deutschman C, Seymour C, et al: The Third International Consensus Definitions for Sepsis and Septic Shock (Sepsis-3). JAMA 315:801-810, 2016

van Schalkwyk J, Van Eyk N, Yudin M, et al: Antibiotic prophylaxis in obstetric procedures. J Obstet Gynaecol Can 39:e293-e299, 2017

OTHER ISSUES

CHAPTER 35

Postterm Pregnancy

Laura M. Gaudet

INTRODUCTION

Definition

Postterm refers to a pregnancy that has reached or exceeded 42 weeks' gestation or 294 days from the first day of the last menstrual period (LMP). Confusion often arises when patients are referred to as "postterm" at 41 weeks' gestation. This appears to have evolved as a result of current recommendations for postterm surveillance, which generally begins at 41 weeks' gestation. Maternity care providers should be clear about gestational age when using the phrase "postterm," which in this chapter refers to pregnancies at or beyond 42 weeks unless otherwise specified.

Prevalence

In general, postterm pregnancy occurs in approximately 7 percent of gestations, with up to 1.4 percent of pregnancies reaching at least 301 days (43 weeks). When first- or second-trimester ultrasound is used for pregnancy dating, rates of postterm pregnancy are decreased. In one study, the incidence fell from 12.1 percent using LMP data to 3.4 percent using an ultrasound estimate. Over time, the number of deliveries occurring at 42 weeks has decreased (from 7.1% in 1980 to 2.9% in 1995). This pattern reflects the decision of many women to undergo delivery at 41 weeks of gestation based on recommendations from national organizations.

Risk Factors

There are several recognized risk factors for postterm pregnancy, including primiparity, maternal age >30 years, and history of previous postterm pregnancy (27% recurrence risk with one previous postterm pregnancy and 39% with two prior postterm pregnancies). Genetic predisposition appears to also play a role, as do excess maternal weight and male fetal sex. Women who were themselves born postterm are more likely to go postterm, and the risk of postterm pregnancy is increased with a paternal history of postterm pregnancy. Rarer associations include fetal anencephaly, fetal adrenal insufficiency, and placental sulfatase deficiency. In the absence of ultrasound dating, postterm pregnancy correlates with predictors of inaccurate recall of LMP, including young maternal age, those of nonoptimal prepregnancy weight, and smoking. Menstrual dating is also more inaccurate in people with long or irregular menstrual cycles in which there is substantial variation in timing of ovulation.

Complications of Postterm Pregnancy

The potential for complications in postterm pregnancy has long been recognized. Much effort has been put into identifying and quantifying these risks. Table 35-1 highlights the generally accepted maternal and fetal neonatal risks associated with postterm pregnancy.

Maternal risks are largely related to the fetal overgrowth that frequently accompanies postterm pregnancy. Most postterm babies are larger than term babies, with a rate of macrosomia (birth weight ≥4500 g) of 2.5 to 10 percent for postterm infants compared to 0.8 to 1 percent of term infants. Thus, complications of macrosomia, including dysfunctional labor, shoulder dystocia, and perineal trauma are all more common in prolonged pregnancies. Maternal risks also include increased risks of postpartum hemorrhage and maternal infection. Finally, studies have shown an increase in anxiety for some mothers during postterm pregnancies.

For the neonate, there may be a gradual increase in perinatal morbidity and mortality in the postterm period, although epidemiologic studies reported inconsistent findings. A UK study classified the risk of perinatal death as a function of ongoing pregnancies (as opposed to all births) and found that the risk rose steadily from 0.7 per 1000 at 37 weeks to 5.8 per 1000 at 43 weeks (Fig. 35-1).

This increase in risk is primarily related to three causes: uteroplacental insufficiency, meconium aspiration, and intrauterine infection. Consequently, there is an increase in the risk of low umbilical cord pH levels (neonatal academia), low 5-minute Apgar scores, neonatal encephalopathy, and infant death in the first year of life. Longer-term, children who were born postterm are slightly more likely to be diagnosed with epilepsy

TABLE 35-1: RISKS ASSOCIATED WITH POSTTERM PREGNANCY

Maternal Risks	Fetal, Neonatal, and Childhood Risks
Increased rate of labor induction	Perinatal death
Dysfunctional labor	Meconium aspiration syndrome
Macrosomia-related birth trauma	Macrosomia and related birth trauma
Postpartum hemorrhage	Epilepsy
Infection (e.g., chorioamnionitis)	Cerebral palsy
Anxiety	

OTHER ISSUES

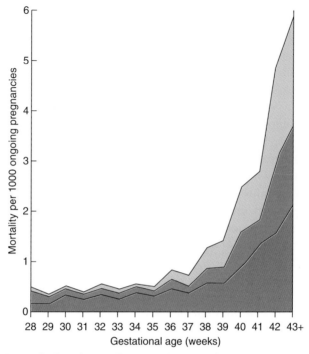

FIGURE 35-1. Perinatal mortality per 1000 ongoing pregnancies. (Reproduced with permission from Hilder L, Costeloe K, Thilaganathan B. Prolonged pregnancy: evaluating gestation-specific risks of fetal and infant mortality. Br J Obstet Gynaecol. 1998;105(2):169-173.)

and cerebral palsy. It is not yet clear whether delivery prior to 42 weeks reduces these risks.

A Cochrane review on induction of labor for improving birth outcomes identified fewer perinatal deaths in women who had labor induced than in those who were followed expectantly. When women at 41 and 42 completed weeks are combined, the relative risk of perinatal death was 0.30 (95% confidence interval [CI], 0.09-0.99) for women who were induced. If deaths caused by congenital anomalies are excluded, there were no deaths in the labor induction group and nine deaths in the expectant management group.

The presence of meconium in the amniotic fluid is often a normal physiologic finding in postterm pregnancy. In the absence of in utero hypoxia, risks to the fetus related to meconium are minimal. Meconium aspiration syndrome (MAS) is thought to result from fetal gasping of meconium-stained amniotic fluid secondary to hypoxia, resulting in a chemical pneumonitis. The Cochrane Database reports a significant decrease in the risk of MAS among fetuses in the induction group compared with the expectant management group (0.29; 95% CI, 0.12-0.68). Labor induction was also associated with a reduction in the prevalence of fetal macrosomia (birthweight greater than 4000 g) in three of the four trials that reported this outcome. Other investigators have reported increased rates of macrosomia-related birth trauma among postterm women who are managed expectantly, including clavicle fracture and Erb's palsy.

Fetal dysmaturity occurs in about 20 percent of postterm pregnancies and refers to a fetus whose weight gain in utero stops after the due date has passed. This is thought to be a variation of placental insufficiency that leads to fetal malnourishment. After birth, the newborns have a distinctive appearance—their arms and legs are long and thin, the skin appears loose and may be dry and/or peeling, scalp hair may be long or thick, and the fingernails and toenails are exceptionally long. Typically, the newborns appear very alert and have a "wide-eyed" appearance. Affected pregnancies are at increased risk of umbilical cord compression from oligohydramnios, meconium aspiration, and short-term neonatal complications such as respiratory depression, symptomatic hypoglycemia, and neonatal seizures.

PREVENTION

Accurate Pregnancy Dating

Ensuring accurate pregnancy dating is the most important factor in reducing the incidence of postterm pregnancy. Traditionally, pregnancies are dated using menstrual history and Naegele's rule. Based on the assumption of a 28-day menstrual cycle with day 14 ovulation, the estimated date of confinement (EDC) is then determined using the following formula: EDC = date of LMP + 1 year – 3 months + 7 days. Most commonly, this is done using handheld pregnancy "wheels" or computer software. In limited-resource setting, this may be the only option. However, maternity care providers must be aware of the limitations of using LMP to determine gestational age. When questioned, many women are uncertain of the first day of their LMP, particularly in the estimated 50 percent of pregnancies that are unplanned. Even when a woman is certain of her menstrual dating, there is marked variation in the follicular phase of the menstrual cycle, making exact timing of ovulation difficult to determine. Furthermore, it has been demonstrated that there is a pattern of "digit preference" in reporting of the LMP.

Research suggests that ultrasound, performed as early as possible in pregnancy, represents a safe and acceptable means of reducing the

OTHER ISSUES

prevalence of postterm pregnancy by up to two thirds. In 2019, the updated UK National Institute for Clinical Excellence guidelines for antenatal care recommend that all pregnancies have their gestational age assigned on the basis of an ultrasound scan, ideally using a either a crown-rump length measured between 10 and 14 weeks or a head circumference measurement at later gestations. Menstrual history is only used to time the scan appointment.

Membrane Sweeping

Sweeping the membranes is a procedure in which a digital cervical assessment is completed with the examining finger advanced between the membranes and the lower uterine segment as far as possible and rotated 360°, thus separating the membranes from the lower uterine segment. It is thought that this elicits endogenous release of prostaglandins that subsequently soften the cervix and potentially augment uterine activity. Some clinicians also advocated stretching of the cervix at the same time.

A 2020 Cochrane Review assessed the effectiveness of membrane sweeping after 38 weeks for the prevention of postterm pregnancy and concluded that it significantly increased the rate of spontaneous labor onset (average risk ratio 1.22, 95% CI 1.08-1.34) and significantly reduced the frequency of induction (relative risk [RR], 0.73, 95% CI 0.56-0.94). In one study, eight women needed to undergo membrane sweeps to avoid one induction of labor. Some evidence suggests that the benefits of membrane sweeping are most marked in the population of nulliparous women with an unfavorable cervix. Commonly reported disadvantages of membrane sweeping include patient pain during the sweep, vaginal bleeding, and irregular contractions following the sweep. Despite this, in one study, 88 percent of women who were questioned in the postnatal period would choose membrane sweeping in the next pregnancy.

MANAGEMENT

Identifying Complicated Pregnancies at Term

At every stage of pregnancy, care providers must make decisions about whether it is safer to continue the pregnancy or to deliver the infant. Before term, the well-being of the premature infant generally precludes delivery unless there is significant risk to the mother or fetus of continuing the pregnancy. Once term is reached, the threshold for delivery in the presence of any maternal or fetal complications falls precipitously because the risks to continuing the pregnancy usually outweigh the risks associated with delivery.

Among postterm pregnancies, the option to manage the pregnancy expectantly may be chosen when complications have been excluded. For this purpose, an ultrasound for fetal growth and well-being along with an assessment of amniotic fluid volume is recommended when the pregnancy reaches 41 weeks. Options for fluid volume assessment include maximum vertical fluid pocket or MVP, in which a largest vertical fluid pocket of less than 2 cm in depth is abnormal, and amniotic fluid index or AFI, in which a result of less than 5 cm is abnormal. If the ultrasound findings are reassuring and the mother is in good health and prefers nonintervention, expectant management may be offered with full discussion of its risks and benefits.

Induction of Labor versus Expectant Management

Despite much investigation and discussion of the ideal management of uncomplicated postterm pregnancies, controversies persist. In a 2020 Cochrane Review, 34 randomized controlled trials reporting on over 21,000 women and infants compared a policy of induction of labor (usually after 41 completed weeks of gestation) with a policy of waiting for labor to start. A policy of induction of labor was clearly associated with fewer perinatal deaths (risk ratio 0.31, 95% CI 0.15-0.64), although absolute rates were low—there were four perinatal deaths in the labor induction group and 25 deaths in the expectant management group. The same review showed a decrease in the risk of neonatal intensive care admission (risk ratio 0.88, 95% CI 0.80-0.96). After excluding contraindications to labor, the American College of Obstetricians and Gynecologists recommends induction of labor be routinely recommended after 42^{+0} weeks and by 42^{+6} weeks of gestation and considered between 41^{+0} weeks and 42^{+0} weeks. A thorough discussion of risks, benefits and alternatives to induction of labor versus expectant management with appropriate surveillance should be conducted. Gestational age, results of antepartum testing, condition of the cervix, and maternal preference should be taken into consideration and a plan formulated (Fig. 35-2).

Surveillance During Expectant Management

If an informed patient declines delivery, expectant management should be provided with appropriate surveillance. There is no consensus on the optimum time to initiate postterm surveillance, nor is there agreement

OTHER ISSUES

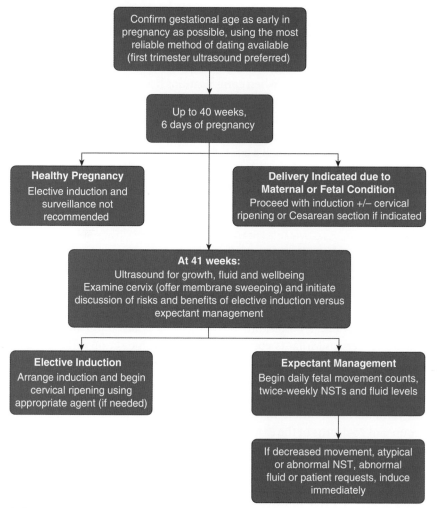

FIGURE 35-2. Algorithm for management of postterm pregnancy. NST, nonstress test; US, ultrasonography.

on the frequency of monitoring. It is reasonable to instruct the woman to perform daily fetal movement counts. Women should perceive six fetal movements in an interval of 2 hours. Failure to meet these criteria should prompt women to contact their maternity care provider or hospital as soon as possible for further antenatal testing. After 41 weeks' gestation, formal surveillance should be offered, such as follow-up ultrasound assessments of amniotic fluid volume and nonstress tests, that, if normal, should both be performed twice weekly until delivery. Throughout this period, the woman and her care provider should be in close contact and have a low threshold to proceed with induction. Nonetheless, expectant management with appropriate surveillance is a reasonable care plan for uncomplicated postterm pregnancies. The small increase in absolute risk of perinatal mortality and maternal and newborn complications of continuing the pregnancy must be weighed against the patient's preference for nonintervention.

CONCLUSIONS

Postterm pregnancy occurs in 2 to 10 percent of pregnancies, depending on definition and determination of postterm pregnancy. Once maternal and fetal complications have been excluded, the patient should be informed of the risks and benefits to induction of labor and expectant management with surveillance. If induction is chosen, cervical ripening is essential for maximizing the chance of vaginal birth. Birth complications should be anticipated and managed appropriately.

SELECTED READING

American College of Obstetricians and Gynecologists: Practice Bulletin No.146. Management of Late-Term and Postterm Pregnancies. Obstet Gynecol 124:390-396, 2014

Finucane EM, Murphy DJ, Biesty LM, Gyte GML, Cotter AM, Ryan AM, Boulvain M, et al: Membrane sweeping for induction of labour (review). Cochrane Database Syst Rev 2, 2020

Galal M, Symonds I, Murray H, Petraglia F, Smith R: Postterm pregnancy. Facts, Views & Vision in ObGyn 4:175-187, 2012

Hannah ME, Hannah WJ, Hellmann J, Hewson S, Milner R, Willan A: Induction of labour compared with serial antenatal monitoring in post-term pregnancy. N Eng J Med 326:1587, 1992

Hilder L, Costeloe K, Thilaganathan B: Prolonged pregnancy: Evaluating gestation-specific risks of fetal and infant mortality. B J Obstet Gynecol 105:196, 1998

Middleton P, Shepherd E, Morris J, Crowther CA, Gomersall JC: Induction of labour at or beyond 37 weeks' gestation. Cochrane Database Syst Rev 7, 2020

Society of Obstetricians and Gynaecologists of Canada: Guidelines for the management of pregnancy at 41+0 to 42+0 weeks. J Obstet Gynaecol Can 39:e164-e174, 2017

Wang M, Fontaine P: Common questions about late-term and postterm pregnancy. Am Fam Physician 90:160-165, 2014

OTHER ISSUES

CHAPTER 36

Obstetric Anesthesia and Analgesia

Catherine Gallant

The practice of obstetric anesthesia began in 1847 when Sir James Young Simpson introduced ether, or "twilight sleep," into obstetric practice for the final stages of labor and delivery. Today obstetric anesthesia has evolved into a complex subspecialty. Although the majority of deliveries are uncomplicated, parturients are presenting with increasingly complex comorbidities because of medical and surgical advances in the treatment of their underlying conditions. For any hospital providing obstetrical care, the availability of qualified personnel and equipment to provide general or neuraxial anesthesia is essential for good obstetric care. Modern regional anesthetic techniques have contributed to maternal and neonatal safety. Persons administering or supervising obstetric anesthesia must be qualified to manage the rare but potentially life-threatening complications of neuraxial anesthesia, which include respiratory failure and cardiovascular collapse, local anesthetic toxicity including seizures, or vomiting and aspiration.

This chapter provides an overview of the physiologic changes seen with pregnancy, describes commonly used methods of labor analgesia, and provides an overview of anesthetics administered during pregnancy for cesarean section and nonobstetric surgery.

PREPARATION FOR PAIN DURING LABOR

The experience of birthing a child is personal and unique to each parturient. Each woman's expectations of labor will influence the birthing experience. The experience of pain during labor is highly variable. In a meta-analysis of 10 studies that looked at the ability to cope with pain during labor, both the presence of individualized support throughout labor and an acceptance of pain during birth were found to be important. Pain management during labor involves more than the timely administration of analgesics. Some women may seek out nonpharmacological therapies to cope with the pain of labor, which may be independent of or complementary to the more traditional forms of labor analgesia. It is important to understand and respect the patient's wishes and beliefs, regardless of culture and background.

The majority of parturients experience moderate to severe pain during labor and delivery, which they describe as being more intense than any other previous pain experience. Women who deliver for the first time describe the pain as more intense than that of subsequent labor. It is reported that the pain is exceeded only by traumatic amputation or causalgia.

The American Society of Anesthesiologists (ASA) states:

There is no other circumstance where it is considered acceptable for an individual to experience untreated severe pain, amenable to safe intervention, while under a physician's care. In the absence of a medical contraindication, maternal request is a sufficient medical indication for pain relief during labor.

Control of pain during labor should begin with prenatal education and counseling. Lack of proper psychological preparation can contribute to the pain experienced with birth. Considerable evidence exists that preparation for childbirth can significantly modify the amount of pain experienced. Continuous support throughout labor is associated with increased satisfaction with the birth experience and less need for analgesia. Satisfaction in childbirth does not result from the absence of pain as many women are willing to experience some pain but do not wish it to overwhelm them. Women may choose to avoid medications or circumstances may limit their access to pharmacological pain relief.

Excessive pain may result in more harm to the fetus than the judicious use of analgesics and anesthetics. The pain and stress of labor contribute to elevated levels of circulating catecholamines, especially epinephrine. Epinephrine has beta-adrenergic tocolytic effects on the myometrium. Effective epidural analgesia reduces plasma epinephrine levels and may shift a dysfunctional to a normal labor pattern.

Elevated plasma catecholamine levels observed during labor may lead to increases in maternal cardiac output and peripheral vascular resistance, as well as decreased uteroplacental perfusion.

Hyperventilation consistently accompanies labor pain. It leads to maternal hypocarbia, which can inhibit ventilatory drive between contractions and result in maternal hypoxemia. Maternal alkalosis shifts the oxygen–hemoglobin curve to the left, thus reducing the offloading of oxygen to the fetus. Maternal alkalosis can cause uteroplacental vasoconstriction and impair oxygen transfer to the fetus. Epidural analgesia has been shown to reduce plasma levels of maternal epinephrine, beta-endorphin, and cortisol, likely by reduced pain and anxiety.

CAUSES OF PAIN DURING LABOR

In the first stage of labor, pain is caused by changes in the lower uterine segment and cervix. It is visceral or cramp-like in nature. Pain impulses are carried by the visceral afferent type C fibers (sympathetic) entering the

OTHER ISSUES

spinal cord from T10 to L1. Pain can be referred to the abdominal wall, lower back, and thighs.

In the late first stage and second stage of labor, pain caused by distension of the vaginal vault and perineal stretching is carried by the pudendal nerve from S2 to S4. Pain is more severe. The parturient experiences rectal pressure and the urge to bear down as the presenting part descends into the pelvic outlet.

During cesarean delivery, additional nociceptive pathways are involved in pain transmission. A T6 or T4 sensory level of anesthesia is required for adequate anesthesia. During surgery, stretching of the skin, manipulation, and dissection intraperitoneally involve visceral pain pathways.

Various factors may influence the degree and intensity of the pain that is experienced with labor and delivery. Some of these are listed in Table 36-1.

MATERNAL PHYSIOLOGY

Profound physiologic changes affecting most maternal organ systems occur during pregnancy, which may affect anesthetic management. A summary of these changes is given in Table 36-2.

TABLE 36-1: FACTORS THAT MAY INFLUENCE THE PAIN OF LABOR AND DELIVERY

The parturient's psychological state
Mental preparation
Family support
Presence of trained support person such as doula
Medical support
Cultural background
Parity
Previous childbirth experiences
Size and presentation of fetus
Size and anatomy of pelvis
Use of medications to augment labor
Duration of labor

TABLE 36-2: THE PHYSIOLOGIC CHANGES OF PREGNANCY

Nervous System			
Variable	**Change**	**Cause**	**Importance**
General Anesthesia	MAC requirements decrease by 25%-40%	CNS effect of progesterone and (or) beta-endorphin	General anesthesia drug requirements are decreased.
Regional anesthesia	LA dose requirements decrease by ~40%	Decrease in size of epidural space caused by engorged epidural veins and (or) hormonal changes	Increased epidural spread of LA may occur, especially if aortocaval compression is not prevented.
Cardiovascular System			
Blood volume (BV)	Total BV ↑ by 35% Plasma BV ↑ by 45% RBCs' BV ↑ by 20%	Hormonal effect	An ↑ of ~1000 mL compensates for the 400-600 mL of blood loss with delivery.
Cardiac output (CO)	↑ by 40% at 10 weeks' gestation Labor↑ CO 45% above prelabor values After delivery, CO ↑ 60% above prelabor values	Increases in CO are in response to increased metabolic demands (stroke volume increases more than heart rate)	Patients with preexisting heart disease may decompensate (e.g., pulmonary edema may occur during labor or after delivery in the patient with significant mitral stenosis).
Peripheral circulation	BP normal or ↓ SVR ↓ by 15% Venous return from legs decreases	SVR decreases to compensate for ↑ in CO, leaving BP normal or ↓	Supine hypotensive syndrome (see text)

(Continued)

OTHER ISSUES

TABLE 36-2: THE PHYSIOLOGIC CHANGES OF PREGNANCY (*Continued*)

Cardiovascular System			
Variable	Change	Cause	Importance
Regional blood flow	Uterus increases blood flow by 500 mL/min	Blood flow in the placenta depends on blood pressure	Placental blood flow cannot ↑ but can ↓ with maternal ↓ BP because of blood loss, aortocaval compression, or catecholamines.
Respiratory System			
Upper airway	Mucosal edema makes the parturient prone to bleeding	Capillary engorgement	Trauma may occur with suctioning and placing nasal or oral airways. Choose a smaller ETT.
Ventilation	Minute ventilation increases by 50% Tidal volume ↑ 40% Respiratory rate ↑ 10%.	Increases in O_2 consumption begin in the first trimester Labor may increase O_2 consumption more than 100%	Normal resting maternal $PaCO_2$ ↓ to ~30 mm Hg in the first trimester. Pain from labor and delivery result in further hyperventilation.
Lung volumes	FRC ↓ 20% No change in VC	By the fifth month, the rising uterus begins to force the diaphragm up	Uptake of inhaled anesthesia occurs faster because of increased minute ventilation with a smaller FRC.
Arterial oxygenation PaO_2	Increased by 10 mm Hg	Caused by hyperventilation	Decreased FRC with increased O_2 consumption results in very rapid decreases in PaO_2 during apnea (e.g., induction of general anesthesia). Pulse oximetry is important.

(Continued)

TABLE 36-2: THE PHYSIOLOGIC CHANGES OF PREGNANCY (*Continued*)

Gastrointestinal System			
Variable	**Change**	**Cause**	**Importance**
Gastric fluid volume	Increased	Enlarged uterus displaces pylorus Gastric emptying delayed	All parturients are considered to have a "full stomach." Pain, anxiety, and drugs (especially narcotics) all slow gastric emptying. Metoclopramide may be useful in reducing volume.
Gastric fluid acidity	Increased	Gastrin secreted by placenta Stimulates H+ secretion	Use of H2-receptor antagonists (ranitidine) and (or) a nonparticulate antacid (Na citrate) is recommended to increase gastric pH.
Gastroesophageal junction	Decreased competence	Enlarging uterus distorts the angle of the junction	Pulmonary aspiration of gastric contents is the major risk of general anesthesia. Placement of an ETT is mandatory in every parturient rendered unconscious by anesthesia.

BP, blood pressure; CNS, central nervous system; ETT, endotracheal tube; FRC, functional residual capacity; LA, local anesthesia; MAC, minimum alveolar concentration; RBC, red blood cell; SVR, systemic vascular resistance; VC, vital capacity.

Physiologic changes of pregnancy alter neuraxial anatomy. There is accentuation of lumbar lordosis, a softer ligamentum flavum and decreased space in the spinal canal due to vascular engorgement of the epidural veins. Physiological changes of pregnancy also cause a more pronounced response to neuraxial induced sympathetic blockade compared to nonpregnant patients. There is higher baseline sympathetic tone and potential for aortocaval compression.

OTHER ISSUES

Twenty to 30 percent less local anesthetic is required for epidural and spinal anesthesia in pregnant patients.

Profound changes in physiology are due to increased concentrations of various hormones, mechanical effects of the gravid uterus, greater metabolic demand, and the hemodynamic changes of the low-pressure placental circulation. Hormonal changes are likely responsible for most of the changes during the first trimester. Mechanical effects are apparent during the second half of gestation as the uterus arises from the pelvis.

Respiratory and Acid Base Changes

Alveolar ventilation inverses by 30 percent or more by mid pregnancy, resulting in chronic respiratory acidosis. Oxygen consumption is increased. Functional residual capacity (FRC) decreases by 20 percent with expansion of the uterus, with resulting decreased oxygen reserve and the possibility of airway closure which may result in hypoxemia. This risk of airway closure is increased with morbid obesity, and supine, Trendelenburg, or lithotomy positions.

Weight gain and engorgement of respiratory tract mucosa increase difficulties with mask ventilation and tracheal intubation. Adjuncts for securing the airway should be readily available when administering general anesthesia at any stage during pregnancy, because the risk of failed intubation is increased.

Cardiovascular Changes

Cardiac output increases up to 50 percent due to increased heart rate and stroke volume. These changes are seen as early as 8 weeks' gestation. The heart increases in size, due to both greater blood volume and increased force of contraction. A grade II systolic ejection murmur is commonly heard at the left sternal border, which is felt to be a benign flow murmur.

Systemic vascular resistance is reduced early in pregnancy, likely secondary to the presence of the low resistance utero-placental vascular bed and maternal vasodilation caused by prostacyclin, estrogen, and progesterone.

Aortocaval Compression

In up to 15 percent of parturients, the gravid uterus may compress the inferior vena cava (IVC) when the parturient lies supine. This may be seen as early as week 20 and increases in frequency in the third trimester. There is an increased risk in parturients with polyhydramnios and in multiple pregnancy because of the increased size of the uterus. This is known as supine hypotensive syndrome.

With IVC compression, there is reduced venous return to the heart. This may lead to signs of shock in the parturient such as maternal hypotension, diaphoresis, nausea, vomiting, and altered mentation. Venous pressure in the lower limbs and uterus increases. Uterine blood flow is not autoregulated but depends on the difference between arterial and venous pressures. There may be a reduction in uterine blood flow, resulting in fetal distress or asphyxia. However, it is important to appreciate that a lack of maternal symptoms does not exclude decreased placental perfusion.

Displacing the uterus to the left during labor with the placement of a right hip wedge helps prevent this phenomenon from occurring. A minimum left lateral tilt of 15° should be used. In women who remain symptomatic, increasing the tilt may be beneficial because individual susceptibility to this syndrome varies.

Changes in Blood Volume

Blood volume expands by 30 to 50 percent by term gestation, with a resultant dilution anemia due to increased plasma volume relative to red blood cell volume. White cell count increases.

Pregnancy is associated with enhanced platelet turnover, clotting, and fibrinolysis. It represents a state of accelerated but compensated intravascular coagulation.

PAIN MANAGEMENT OPTIONS DURING LABOR AND DELIVERY

The wide range of options available for pain relief during labor are summarized in Table 36-3.

Opioid Analgesia

Opioid analgesia includes intravenous (IV) and intramuscular (IM) techniques. Advantages include ease of use and patient acceptance. It is useful for those who prefer less invasive techniques and when regional anesthetics are contraindicated or unavailable.

Although sedatives and tranquilizers have been used in the past, the increasing availability of regional anesthesia has largely replaced their use.

OTHER ISSUES

TABLE 36-3: OPTIONS FOR PAIN MANAGEMENT

Nothing
Psychological support (birthing coach, partner, other family members)
Behavioral modification (Lamaze)
Hypnotherapy (relaxation exercises practiced before presentation to birthing unit)
Education (prenatal classes)
Massage, walking, various birthing positions
Nitrous oxide (Entonox)
Opioid analgesics
Epidural analgesia
Spinal anesthesia
Combined spinal and epidural anesthesia
Local infiltration
Pudendal block
Paracervical block

However, opioids are still used in many cases either as the sole agent for labor analgesia or in early labor as a temporizing measure until regional anesthesia is available. There is a risk of maternal and neonatal depression with their use. All parenteral opioids readily cross the placenta and cause neonatal central nervous system and respiratory depression. The choice of drug, timing of administration, and method of administration must be carefully considered. Side effects common to all opioids include respiratory depression, orthostatic hypotension, delayed gastric emptying, nausea, and vomiting.

Morphine. The dose used is approximately 0.1 mg/kg maternal body weight every 3 to 4 hours. Peak effect is seen 1 to 2 hours after IM injection and 20 minutes after an IV injection, with a duration of action of 4 to 6 hours. The effect on the fetus depends on the time relationship of administration to delivery. If given within 3 hours of delivery, the risk of fetal narcosis is high.

Meperidine. The dose is 1 mg/kg every 3 to 4 hours. Peak effect is 40-50 minutes after an IM injection and 5 to 10 minutes after an IV injection. The duration of action is 3 to 4 hours. Maternal effect is similar to morphine. It is quickly transferred across the placenta, but peak levels are reached in the fetus 2 to 3 hours after administration. Infants born 2 to 3 hours after administration are most susceptible to opioid-induced respiratory depression. Elimination may take 2 to 3 days, and this manifests as lower APGAR scores and impaired neurobehavioral scores for the first 3 days of life. Normeperidine, an active metabolite, may be responsible for these changes.

Nalbuphine. A mixed agonist antagonist, provides good pain relief without respiratory depression and may be a better choice. Doses of 10 to 20 mg IM every 4 to 6 hours usually provide adequate analgesia.

Fentanyl. This is a synthetic opioid. It has been used to provide pain relief in labor, but because of its short duration of action, it must be administered IV, usually through a patient-controlled analgesia (PCA) pump. Remifentanil is an ultra-short-acting synthetic opioid that has been used as an alternative to fentanyl in PCA pumps. Remifentanil has a half-life of 2 minutes and is rapidly metabolized by the fetus, so there should be minimal neonatal depression. Use of remifentanil PCA requires one-to-one nursing because of the risk of maternal hypoventilation Narcotic effects in the newborn are best antagonized with naloxone, 5 to 10 mcg/kg.

Nitrous Oxide

Nitrous oxide is a weak analgesic and amnesic. It is relatively insoluble in blood, so induction and recovery are both rapid. For labor analgesia, it is offered in a 50:50 mixture in oxygen (Entonox) to decrease the chances of maternal hypoxemia. Advantages are ease of use, the safety profile for the mother and infant, rapidity of onset of effect (50 seconds), and widespread availability. It is relatively simple to use because the patient self-administers it using a handheld face mask. To be effective, there must be adequate analgesic concentrations of nitrous oxide present in the blood and the brain at the peak of uterine contractions. This requires maternal cooperation, with deep inhalation as soon as the woman is aware of the onset of a contraction. Some patients may become drowsy. However, this effect is short lived after discontinuation of the agent. Common side effects include dizziness, nausea, dysphoria, and a sense of claustrophobia.

OTHER ISSUES

Accumulation is negligible, and neonatal depression is rare.

Disadvantages are that if it is not administered correctly, peak analgesic effect may be delayed until after the contraction. Studies on its effectiveness have shown mixed results. It may be ineffective in up to half of parturients. Specialized equipment is required for its administration. Efficient scavenging is difficult, resulting in environmental pollution. It is unclear what, if any, the effects of long-term exposure to subanesthetic concentrations of nitrous oxide are.

Epidural Analgesia

Continuous lumbar epidural analgesia is the gold standard of labor analgesia. Its use has increased in the last 10 years with 57.8 percent of Canadian women using this technique during labor. It is the most effective way to block the pain of labor and can provide effective pain relief throughout all stages of labor and delivery.

It involves the injection of a dilute local anesthetic, usually combined with an opioid analgesic, into the lumbar epidural space. The drugs diffuse across the dura into the subarachnoid space, where they act on the spinal nerve roots to provide analgesia. Various combinations of drugs have been used as either intermittent boluses or by continuous infusion.

Placement of an epidural catheter allows analgesia to be maintained until after delivery. If a cesarean delivery is deemed necessary, conversion to epidural anesthesia can be completed rapidly, avoiding the need for general anesthesia in most cases.

Epidural analgesia produces a segmental and sensory nerve block with the onset of pain relief. Blood pressure may normalize because of vasodilatation and may lower in some instances. This may be beneficial in patients with pre-eclampsia. There may be a significant improvement in uteroplacental blood flow, both in healthy patients and those with hypertensive disorders of pregnancy. This is because of a reduction in vascular resistance as long as blood pressure is maintained.

Patient-controlled epidural analgesia (PCEA) has become increasingly popular. A low baseline infusion is given and the patient has the ability to "top up" with bolus doses of the same mixture. Alternatively, there is no background infusion, and the patient gives herself bolus doses on demand only. There is high satisfaction with this method and overall less medication is given than by the conventional infusion technique.

Another alternative to continuous infusion is programmed intermittent epidural bolus (PEIB). The pump will deliver a bolus dose at specific intervals (e.g., 8 mL every 45 minutes). This technique allows for greater spread of local anesthetic in the epidural space when compared to a continuous infusion. It can be used with PCEA. There is better analgesia, enhanced maternal satisfaction, less motor block, and reduced local anesthetic consumption when compared with a continuous infusion.

Contraindications to Epidurals

Absolute contraindications include patient refusal or inability to cooperate, uncorrected coagulopathy, sepsis or infection at the puncture site, uncorrected hypovolemia, and raised intracranial pressure. Any preexisting neurologic disease should be carefully documented before initiation of the epidural.

Technique of Epidural Analgesia

Before the initiation of the epidural, several steps must be taken. The anesthetist must review the patient's obstetric history; review her medical and anesthetic history; and perform a focused physical examination, including the vital signs, airway, heart, lungs, and back. Emergency resuscitation equipment, drugs, and supplies must be readily available. An IV catheter, preferably 18 gauge, should be placed. Many anesthesia providers administer a 500-mL bolus of crystalloid, although the ASA Taskforce on Obstetric Anesthesia has stated that a fixed volume of IV fluid is not required before placement of a labor epidural. With the use of more dilute local anesthetics for epidural analgesia, severe hypotension is rarely seen.

After obtaining informed consent, the patient is either seated or placed in the lateral decubitus position. The lumbar area is prepped with an antiseptic solution. In the authors' institution, 2 percent chlorhexidine in 70 percent isopropyl alcohol is the agent of choice. A sterile drape is placed over the prepped area. In the second or third lumbar interspace, the skin is infiltrated with 1 or 2 percent lidocaine. Either a paramedian or midline technique with a 16- or 17-gauge Tuohy needle is used, using loss of resistance to saline or air. The epidural space is identified, and a 20-gauge polyurethane multiorifice catheter is threaded 3 to 5 cm into the epidural space through the Tuohy needle, which is then withdrawn. The catheter is secured to the mothers' back with an adhesive dressing and tape.

In the past, a test dose of 3 mL of lidocaine 1.5 percent with epinephrine 1:200,000 was injected at this point to rule out intrathecal or intravascular catheter placement. If the dose was injected intravascularly, the patient would experience tinnitus, a metallic taste, and dizziness. Tachycardia would be seen because of the beta-adrenergic effects of the epinephrine. However, because of the wide variations in heart rate that occur with contractions, this effect may be masked. It is recommended that the traditional test dose should be given immediately after a contraction to maximize sensitivity.

The use of a traditional test dose is controversial. Epinephrine may reduce placental blood flow by producing uterine artery constriction. It is relatively contraindicated in cases such as diabetes mellitus or pre-eclampsia, where there may be decreased uteroplacental blood flow. An undesirable side effect of the traditional test dose is that it produces motor block. There may be maternal hypotension caused by block of sympathetic nerves.

Today, the anesthetist may elect to "test" the epidural with a more dilute solution that will be used for infusion. The epidural is loaded with 3- to 5-mL increments of the epidural solution. Examples are 0.0625 to 0.1 percent bupivacaine with fentanyl 2 mcg/mL or 0.08 to 0.125 percent ropivacaine with fentanyl 2 mcg/mL. A total of 15 to 20 mL of these solutions can be used to incrementally load the epidural while watching the vital signs.

Effects on Labor and Delivery

Many studies have attempted to identify factors associated with cesarean delivery. In the past, observational studies have suggested that epidural analgesia, particularly when administered in early labor, is associated with an increased risk of cesarean delivery. Studies are difficult to perform because it is not ethical to assign women to a placebo group with no analgesia. A recent Cochrane Database Systemic Review from 2018 compared epidural analgesia to nonepidural or no analgesia in labor. In trials of singleton, uncomplicated pregnancies conducted since 2005, epidural analgesia does not increase the proportion of women who have an assisted vaginal delivery. It is felt that changes in administration of epidural analgesia such as the use of low dose local anesthetics and opioid account for this.

Historically, multiple observational studies have found that early initiation of epidural analgesia (cervical dilatation 3-5 cm) is associated with a higher risk of cesarean delivery. Randomized controlled trials have not shown this to be true. In 2006, the American College of Obstetricians and Gynecologists (ACOG) rescinded their recommendation to delay epidural placement until mothers were in active labor. Epidurals can be safely placed at any stage of labor, including the second stage.

Studies have attempted to address whether or not neuraxial analgesia prolongs the duration of the first and second stages of labor. Studies are conflicting regarding the effect on the first stage of labor. If it does prolong it, it is to a minor degree. The bulk of evidence suggests that neuraxial analgesia does prolong the second stage of labor to a small degree. However, neonatal outcomes do not appear to be affected.

Risks of Epidural Analgesia

Risks of epidural analgesia and anesthesia should be disclosed to the patient. Studies looking at informed consent have shown that patients want to be informed of significant material risks even if the incidence is low.

Common side effects include pruritus, nausea and vomiting, urinary retention, and fever. There is a failure rate of up to 12 percent in labor epidurals. The risk of postdural puncture headache (PDPH) is quoted at 1 percent, but this incidence is increased with new trainees and is reduced with experience. It is common to have localized pain or backache at the site of skin entry, especially if there are multiple passes with the Tuohy needle. This may last for up to several weeks. There is no evidence to suggest that epidural analgesia causes long-term backache.

Infection at the site of insertion is rare, as is meningitis. It has been reported in the literature. Meticulous sterile technique during insertion and during top ups of the epidural must be observed.

Traumatic injury to a vessel in the epidural space leading to an epidural hematoma is rare. If a patient has back pain or a worrisome neurologic examination, then imaging should be obtained urgently. Surgical decompression should be performed urgently or paralysis may result.

Epidural analgesia rarely causes neurologic complications. In fact, most postpartum neurologic complications are obstetric palsies from nerve compression by the fetal head. Nerves may also be stretched with positioning in labor. A detailed neurological exam and imaging may be required to determine the cause.

Systemic toxicity is related to high plasma levels of local anesthetics and is extremely rare. Most commonly, it is caused by accidental IV injection. Initial signs and symptoms include tinnitus and disorientation and ultimately seizures and cardiovascular collapse. It is more likely to be seen after epidural than after spinal because the doses are higher for epidurals, especially when dosing epidurals for cesarean sections. The risk of toxicity is reduced by dosing incrementally and by aspirating the catheter before injecting.

If signs of central nervous system toxicity occur, the injection should be stopped. Seizures should be treated with benzodiazepines (midazolam 2-5 mg) or barbiturates (thiopental 50-100 mg). The airway should be secured and supplemental oxygen provided.

OTHER ISSUES

If cardiovascular toxicity develops, advanced cardiac life support protocols should be followed. The airway should be secured. When performing chest compressions, the uterus must be displaced leftward after 20 weeks' gestational age so that the major vessels are not compressed by the enlarged uterus. If spontaneous circulation has not returned, the current recommendation is to deliver the baby within 5 minutes after cardiac arrest.

Early administration of lipid emulsion (20% intralipid) is recommended for local anesthetic toxicity. After the airway has been secured, a bolus of 1.5 mL/kg is administered IV over 1 minute followed by an infusion of 0.25 mL/kg/min for at least 10 minutes after return of spontaneous circulation. The bolus may be repeated. Total dose should not exceed 10 mg/kg over 30 minutes.

Failed Blocks

The definition of a failed block is inadequate analgesia or anesthesia after an epidural. Failed blocks may be caused by inadequate dosing of drugs, patient factors, or technical issues related to the placement of the epidural. If inadequate amounts of drugs are injected, then the required spinal segments will not be blocked and analgesia will not be achieved. Scar tissue or other anatomical features in patients may rarely cause epidural failure. Another factor to consider is that the Tuohy needle or the catheter may not be sited within the epidural space. The catheter may migrate after being positioned, either out through an intervertebral foramen or back out through the skin. With multiorifice catheters, one or more of the orifices may not be in the epidural space. The catheter may be positioned more to one side, causing a unilateral block. Ideally, the catheter should be placed 3 to 5 cm within the epidural space to avoid migration of the catheter.

Spinal Anesthesia and Combined Spinal Epidural

Spinal anesthesia is not often used alone for labor analgesia because of the finite duration of action of the agents used. However, it may be combined with epidural analgesia for rapid onset of pain relief. Anesthesia is initiated with a subarachnoid injection of opioid and local anesthetic, then maintained via the epidural catheter. This can be done in several ways. The most popular is with a needle through needle technique, where the Tuohy needle is inserted into the epidural space and then serves as an introducer for the spinal needle. The spinal needle passes though the Tuohy needle and punctures the dura. Small doses of local anesthetic combined with opioids, such as bupivacaine 2 mg and fentanyl 10 to 15 mcg, are injected intrathecally, the spinal needle is removed and the epidural catheter is threaded.

Alternatively, two different interspaces can be utilized, with the epidural placed first then the spinal performed at a lower level sequentially.

The duration of analgesia is about 90 minutes. If the patient has not delivered within that time period, the epidural catheter can be activated. The author starts the epidural infusion immediately rather than waiting for patient request so that there is uninterrupted analgesia. In this situation, the epidural test dose is omitted.

The needle through needle technique does require the use of a long spinal needle, which must protrude 12 to 17 mm beyond the tip of the epidural needle when the two needles are fully engaged. To reduce the risk of PDPH, a small (25 or 27 gauge) noncutting spinal needle is preferred.

The combined spinal–epidural (CSE) technique does result in a greater incidence of fetal bradycardia compared with epidural techniques. The mechanism is believed to be attributable to a transient imbalance in epinephrine compared with norepinephrine levels. Epinephrine has a tocolytic effect and causes uterine relaxation. With rapid onset of analgesia, circulating epinephrine levels drop. This results in a relative increase in uterine tone and may lead to a prolonged tetanic contraction. This is usually short lived and does not result in increased cesarean delivery rates.

With the use of pencil point or atraumatic spinal needles for this technique, the risk of PDPH is not significantly increased.

Dural puncture epidural anesthesia is another technique that is identical to CSE anesthesia other than there is no drug injection intrathecally. The intent is to allow for augmented transfer of epidural injected drugs into the subarachnoid space, which possibly results in faster onset of analgesia.

Postdural Puncture Headache

Headache is one of the most common symptoms seen in the postpartum period. When the dura is breached by a 16-gauge Tuohy needle, a PDPH will develop in up to 88 percent of parturients. The headache is believed to be caused by leakage of cerebrospinal fluid through the rent in the dura, which causes intracranial hypotension. When standing, there is traction on pain-sensitive structures. Cerebral vasodilatation is also believed to play a role. This headache has a strong postural component with relief of symptoms when supine. The International Headache Society has defined PDPH as a bilateral headache that develops within 7 days after lumbar puncture and disappears within 14 days after the lumbar puncture. The headache worsens within 15 minutes of assuming the upright position and disappears or improves within 30 minutes of resuming the recumbent position.

The headache is usually described as occurring in the frontal and/or occipital areas, but may also involve the neck and upper shoulders.

OTHER ISSUES

The usual onset of symptoms is within 48 hours of the dural puncture, but in 25 percent of cases, it presents later than 3 days. Nausea, vomiting, nuchal rigidity, hearing loss, and diplopia may be seen.

This headache can be debilitating and may significantly impair the mother's ability to care for herself and her infant. The natural history is that symptoms will resolve over 10 days, but there have been case reports of persistent headaches for weeks to months. The duration of headache is usually related to the gauge of the needle that breached the dura.

Management of the second stage may affect the incidence of headache after accidental dural puncture. One study of 33 patients who had accidental dural puncture showed that the incidence of headache was 10 percent (1 in 10) in those who went on to have cesarean section compared to 74 percent (17 of 23) in those who pushed.

Many treatments have been proposed for treatment of PDPH including caffeine infusions, ACTH injections, and more recently sphenopalantine ganglion nerve block. However, epidural blood patch remains the definitive treatment for severe headache. Treatment of PDPH usually begins with conservative measures such as bed rest and analgesics. This delay increases the success rate of the blood patch, which has a failure rate of up to 71 percent if performed within the first 24 hours of dural puncture versus a failure rate of 4 percent if performed later than 24 hours after dural puncture. The optimal volume of autologous blood to be injected is believed to be 20 mL. Success rates vary from 75 to 93 percent and a second blood patch may be required in some cases.

Paracervical Block

This method is now rarely used in North America for labor analgesia because there has been a high incidence of complications with its use, specifically fetal asphyxia and poor neonatal outcome, especially with the use of bupivacaine. However, it is an easily performed method of achieving pain relief during the first stage of labor. It is ineffective for the second stage of labor. Its main advantage is that the block can be performed by the obstetrician, and the attendance of an anesthetist is not required. It is more commonly used to provide analgesia for other gynecologic procedures.

The injection is made transvaginally into the posterolateral fornices, thus blocking the sensory pathways at the junction of the uterosacral ligaments with the cervix. The procedure can be carried out in the patient's bed or the delivery table. The block is instituted during the active phase of labor with the cervix at least 3 to 4 cm dilated.

Equipment consists of a 20-gauge needle, 13 to 18 cm long, with a sheath or needle guide of such length that 1.5 cm of the tip of the needle protrudes when it is inserted up to its hub. The needle sheath is guided by the fingers into the vagina and placed in the fornix just lateral to the cervix at a tangent to the presenting part. The needle (with the attached syringe) is introduced through the guide until the point rests against the mucosa. With quick, slight pressure, the needle is pushed through the mucosa to a depth of 6 to 12 mm. Aspiration is performed to guard against direct intravascular injection. If no blood returns, the desired amount of anesthetic agent is used. It is advisable to wait for a few minutes after the injection of one side. Fetal heart auscultation is performed, and if it is normal, the other side is injected. If fetal bradycardia occurs, the procedure should be discontinued. Mepivacaine, lidocaine, and procaine in 1 percent concentrations are effective. Bupivacaine is not recommended because of a high incidence of fetal bradycardia.

Sites of injection vary. Some inject at 3 and 9 o'clock, but others give several injections at 3, 4, 8, and 9 o'clock. In any case, 10 mL is given on each side in single or multiple doses.

Most parturients experience complete or partial relief from pain almost immediately with a duration of about 1 hour. If the cervix is not yet fully dilated, a second block may be required. Other forms of anesthesia are required for the actual delivery.

Transient numbness and paresthesias of one or both lower extremities occur commonly as a result of spread of the local anesthetic to the sciatic nerve or part of the lumbosacral plexus.

Rapid absorption or intravascular injection may cause symptoms of local anesthetic toxicity, including dizziness, anxiety, shaking, and occasional seizures and loss of consciousness. Occasionally, transient hypotension may occur. There is a risk of hematoma formation at the site of injection. There have been case reports of parametritis.

The main concern of paracervical block is the effect on the fetus. Changes in fetal heart rate (FHR) can be seen in up to 30 percent of cases with the majority being fetal bradycardia. In up to 20 percent of the cases when bradycardia is seen, it is sufficient to impair tissue perfusion, with acidosis and neonatal depression the ultimate result.

The etiology of the bradycardia is complex and likely occurs by several pathways:

1. Uterine artery vasoconstriction because of the proximity of the injection, leading to placental hypoperfusion and fetal asphyxia
2. Direct uterine artery injection

3. Direct intramyometrial injection
4. Diffusion of local anesthetic through the uterine arteries and deposition into the intervillous spaces with subsequent fetal uptake and direct fetal cardiotoxicity
5. Direct fetal injection

Changes in FHR are seen more frequently in primigravidas, in those with previous nonreassuring FHR patterns, and in very low birthweight infants (<2500 g). Onset is usually within 2 to 10 minutes after injection and may last 3 to 30 minutes. With prolonged bradycardia, fetal acidosis and neonatal depression may be seen, especially if delivery is within 30 minutes of injection.

Due to the high risk of complications, this technique should be avoided if the fetus is compromised, as in cases of placental insufficiency, prior fetal distress, and prematurity. Use only small doses of dilute local anesthetics. Avoid vasoconstrictors such as epinephrine. Do not perform this block if delivery is anticipated within 30 minutes. If the cervix is dilating rapidly, the chance of aberrant injection is increased, and the block should not be performed. The FHR should be monitored continuously during and after the block.

Do not use this block if there is a known sensitivity to local anesthetics or if there is vaginal bleeding or infection.

Direct Infiltration Anesthesia

The main purpose of perineal infiltration is to permit incision and repair of episiotomy, as well as suturing of lacerations.

1. Xylocaine 1 percent provides a rapid onset of action and profound anesthesia. Total volume of 30 to 50 mL is sufficient for most cases
2. Either the needle is inserted at the posterior fourchette and the injections are made lateral *or* the needle is inserted at a point halfway between the anus and the ischial tuberosity and the injections are made toward the midline
3. Using a 25- to 27-gauge needle, a wheal is made by injecting a small amount of the local anesthetic solution into the skin where the needle is to be inserted
4. The needle is then changed to a 22 or 20 gauge, which is inserted through the wheal. Multiple injections are made into the subcutaneous tissue, muscles, and fascia after aspiration to ensure that the needle is not intravascular
5. Adequate analgesia is achieved within 5 minutes

The technique is simple to perform, with no special anatomic knowledge necessary. The success rate is almost 100 percent. However, complete perineal anesthesia is not achieved because only the infiltrated areas are anesthetized.

Pudendal Nerve Block

The pudendal nerve originates from S2, S3, and S4. It exits the pelvis through the lower part of the greater sciatic foramen, curves around the ischial spine, crosses the sacrospinous ligament close to the attachment to the ischial spine and then reenters the pelvis alongside the internal pudendal artery at the lesser sciatic foramen. At this point, the pudendal nerve breaks up into the inferior hemorrhoidal (rectal) nerve, the perineal nerve, and the dorsal nerve of the clitoris. These nerves are best blocked at the ischial tuberosity. Additional innervation is received from the pudendal branch of the posterior femoral cutaneous nerve, which supplies the posterior labial portion of the perineum. A secondary innervation is provided by the ilioinguinal and genitofemoral nerves. These nerves must be blocked by supplemental infiltration to achieve thorough anesthesia of the anterior portions of the labia majora and mons pubis.

The timing of administration of this block is important to its success. In primigravidas, it is done when the cervix is fully dilated and the presenting part is at station +2. In multiparas, the block is administered at 7- to 8-cm dilatation. Pudendal anesthesia is sufficient for spontaneous delivery or low forceps extractions, breech delivery, and repair of episiotomy and lacerations. It may be combined with local infiltration. Before the widespread availability of epidurals, it was the preferred analgesic technique for delivery. It can be used when contraindications to neuraxial anesthesia exist or when low forceps delivery is required.

Either a transvaginal or transperineal approach may be used. The transvaginal approach is most commonly used.

Transperineal Approach

The local anesthetic is injected around the pudendal nerve through a 15.2 cm needle with a .625 cm spacer. A commonly chosen agent is 1 percent lidocaine. Effective analgesia is achieved within 15 minutes. After an intradermal wheal has been raised, the needle is inserted through the skin midway between the anus and the ischial tuberosity. As the needle is advanced, small amounts of local anesthetic are injected. The index finger of the left hand is inserted into the vagina or rectum to palpate the tuberosity of the

OTHER ISSUES

ischium. The needle is then directed toward the ischial spine. A number of injections are made:

1. Five to 10 mL is injected at the anterolateral aspect of the spine, as well as under the tuberosity, to block the inferior pudendal branch of the posterior cutaneous nerve. At this point, the syringe can be detached from the needle and refilled

2. The needle is then advanced to the medial aspect of the ischial spine, where another 5 to 10 mL is injected to block the branches of the pudendal nerve. Because the pudendal artery and vein run parallel to the nerve, intermittent aspiration to ensure the needle is not intravascular should be performed

3. Another 5 to 10 mL of the solution is injected as the needle is advanced 2.5 cm past the ischial tuberosity into the ischial fossa. This blocks the pudendal nerve in Alcock's canal

4. The point of the needle is advanced posteriorly to the ischial spine. The finger can palpate the sacrospinous ligament, and it guides the needle in this direction until a "popping" sensation indicates that the needle has pierced the ligament. The needle is advanced another 0.5 cm, and 5 to 10 mL of solution is injected at this point to block the pudendal needle before it divided. The needle is withdrawn, and the other side is blocked

5. The final step is to infiltrate the area that lies 1.5 cm lateral and parallel to the labia majorum from the middle of the labium to the mons pubis. This effectively blocks the secondary innervation from the iliohypogastric, ilioinguinal, and genitofemoral nerves. This must be done bilaterally

Transvaginal Approach

A 10- or 20-mL syringe is attached to a 15.2 cm needle with a .625 cm spacer. The left pudendal nerve is blocked first. The index and middle fingers of the left hand are inserted into the vagina, and the ischial spine and sacrospinous ligament are palpated.

Holding the syringe in the right hand, the needle is placed in a specialized pudendal needle sheath, such as an Iowa trumpet with the sharp tip retracted into the sheath. Using the groove formed by the apposition of the index and middle fingers, the needle is inserted into the wall of the vagina toward the tip of the ischial spine. The needle is advanced 1.5 cm into the sacrospinous ligament, and 5 to 10 mL of local anesthetic solution is injected. The needle is then advanced until it "pops" through the sacrospinous ligament, and 5 to 10 mL of local anesthetic is injected with intermittent aspiration to ensure the needle is not intravascular. Supplementary infiltration of the area lateral to the labia majora is carried out as described in the section "Transperineal Approach." The procedure is then repeated on the other side.

CESAREAN SECTION

Cesarean delivery now accounts for approximately one-third of all deliveries in North America. The updated Practice Guidelines for Obstetric Anesthesia from the ASA Task Force on Obstetrical Anesthesia observe that neuraxial techniques (spinal, epidural, and CSE) are associated with improved outcomes for both mother and baby when compared with general anesthesia, especially in the presence of a high body mass index and airway issues. However, the choice of anesthetic should be made in each instance after a careful assessment of patient, medical, anesthetic, and obstetric issues.

Complications related to anesthesia are the sixth leading cause of peripartum maternal mortality in the United States. Most commonly, these deaths result from failures in oxygenation and ventilation and may be seen at extubation as well as induction of anesthesia.

At the authors' institution, most cesarean sections are performed under regional anesthesia. For elective cesarean sections with no contraindication to regional anesthesia, spinal anesthesia is preferred. After establishing IV access with a 16- or 18-gauge IV and with standard monitors in place, the back is prepped with a 2 percent chlorhexidine in 70 percent isopropyl alcohol solution. Using sterile technique, the intrathecal space is identified with an atraumatic 25- to 27-gauge spinal needle. Bupivacaine 9 to 12 mg with 15 mcg of fentanyl and 100 mcg of preservative-free morphine are then injected.

The patient is then placed supine with left uterine displacement. If hypotension and nausea occur, small boluses of phenylephrine 50 to 100 mcg are given, or alternatively an infusion of phenylephrine is started at 40 mcg/min and titrated to effect.

If an epidural is in situ and functioning well, then the catheter is topped up with a combination of 2 percent lidocaine and epinephrine 1:200,000. Twenty mL of this combination, with 50 to 100 mcg of fentanyl, is given in 3- to 5-mL increments through the epidural catheter. Preservative-free morphine given in doses of 2.0 to 2.5 mg provides analgesia for about 18 hours.

When the surgery may be prolonged, a CSE technique is used. General anesthesia is reserved for the emergencies when there is no time to establish a regional block.

At the authors' institution, after the baby is delivered, a bolus of 1 to 3 units of oxytocin is given prior to starting an infusion. Oxytocin (40 units/liter) is started at 75 mL/hr. If there is uterine atony, the rate may be increased. Alternatively, 100 mcg of carbetocin may be injected IV over 1 minute. If atony persists, prostaglandin F2 (PGF2) alpha or Hemabate 250 mcg should be given intramuscularly or intramyometrially. Ergonovine is reserved for resistant uterine atony.

Postoperative analgesia routines include 500 mg of acetaminophen and 400 mg of ibuprofen every 4 hours. This provides excellent analgesia in the majority of patients. Hydromorphone may be added if necessary.

Currently, the author administers prophylactic antibiotics before skin incision in all cesarean sections. Cefazolin is the agent of choice, with clindamycin or vancomycin being the alternate drugs in case of allergy.

NONOBSTETRIC SURGERY DURING PREGNANCY

In 2016, the U.S. Food and Drug Administration issued this warning:

> …repeated or lengthy use of general anesthetic and sedation drugs during surgeries or procedures in children younger than 3 years or in pregnant women during their third trimester may affect the development of their children's brains.

Most procedures which are performed in pregnant women are medically necessary. Alternative anesthetic techniques may not be feasible. Estimates of the frequency of nonobstetric surgery performed during pregnancy range from 0.3 to 2.3 percent. Indications include acute abdominal disease, malignancies, and trauma. The anesthesia provider may have to modify standard anesthesia protocols to accommodate the physiological changes of pregnancy and the presence of the fetus.

Anesthetic considerations in these patients must include any underlying medical conditions, the reason for the surgery, the physiologic effects of the pregnancy, and any potential effects on the fetus.

Surgical diagnosis of an acute abdomen may be made more difficult because of the presence of the gravid uterus. The white blood cell count is normally elevated during pregnancy. Surgical technique and patient positioning must take into account the gravid uterus.

Because surgery is normally avoided during pregnancy, patients who do present are usually more seriously affected. Surgery is generally delayed until the second trimester if at all possible.

Anesthetic management should include a careful assessment of the airway. The supine position should be avoided, especially after 18 to 20 weeks of gestation. The choice of general versus regional anesthesia should be carefully weighed for each case. However, most women require an urgent laparotomy for exploratory surgery and require general anesthesia.

General anesthesia usually consists of rapid-sequence induction with standard agents, tracheal intubation, and maintenance with a volatile agent. Minimum alveolar concentration (MAC) is decreased by up to 40 percent. Drugs with an established safety record in pregnancy should be used rather than newer drugs.

Maternal arterial CO_2 levels should be kept in the normal pregnant range during ventilation (32-34 mm Hg); otherwise, fetal acidosis may result in fetal myocardial depression. Maternal alkalosis may lead to decreased uterine blood flow. Maternal hypotension must be treated aggressively with fluids and vasopressors. Data suggest that phenylephrine is the vasopressor of choice.

Because pregnancy is a hypercoagulable state, there is an increased risk of thromboembolic events postoperatively. The need for anticoagulants should be determined on a case-by-case basis.

SELECTED READING

Anim-Somuah M, Smyth RM, Cyna AM, Cuthbert A: Epidural versus non-epidural or no analgesia for pain management in labour. Cochrane Database Syst Rev 5, 2018

Chestnut DH, Wong CA, Tsen LC, et al: Chestnut's Obstetric Anesthesia: Principles and Practice, 6th ed. Philadelphia: Elsevier, 2019

Practice Guidelines for Obstetric Anesthesia: An updated report by the American Society of Anesthesiologists Task Force on Obstetrical Anesthesia. *Anesthesiology* 124: 270-300, 2016

OTHER ISSUES

CHAPTER 37

Peripartum Imaging

Asma Assiri
Abdalmajed Eisa

ULTRASOUND IN THE MODERN ERA

Advances in medical technologies have allowed us to think out of the box and augment our practical skills with direct visualization using ultrasound, including portable machines. Some use handheld ultrasound probes that can be wirelessly connected to any device with a screen, such as smartphones. Although ultrasound cannot replace clinical assessment, it can improve the quality of care and answer questions that no clinical exam can (e.g., location of the placenta).

The chapter focuses on imaging techniques directly applicable to patients presenting to the labor and delivery unit. This can be collectively referred to as *peripartum ultrasound* (Table 37-1). Regardless of the type of scan, fetal viability should be assessed every time.

The following ultrasound assessments should be within the skill set of most obstetricians practicing in labor and delivery. A key practical point is to always ensure that the probe orientation matches the screen orientation. This ensures "left" and "cranial" are always depicted correctly on the screen. Gently moving your finger on one corner of the probe and observing the screen will confirm this before you start scanning.

Because ultrasound is transmitted poorly through air, the face of the transducer must be coupled to the patient's skin by a fluid medium, such as gel, so that the sound waves may penetrate the skin surface–air interface. Higher ultrasound frequencies are used on vaginal probes, giving finer, more detailed resolution of structures. However, the higher frequency beam can only penetrate a short distance, and therefore the field depth is limited. Lower frequency probes are used transabdominally, giving greater depth and penetration.

In order to reflect real obstetric practice, the images used in this chapter were either obtained using a basic, older-model ultrasound machine (as typically found in most labor and delivery units) or a newer handheld, portable unit.

ANTEPARTUM ULTRASOUND

Fetal Viability

Using real-time ultrasound, fetal cardiac motion can be readily appreciated within the fetal chest. Confirming fetal viability can help avoiding a Cesarean section in some cases of nonviable fetus. By applying color or power Doppler, the movement of blood within the cardiac chambers can

TABLE 37-1: ROLES FOR PERIPARTUM ULTRASOUND

Antepartum Ultrasound	Intrapartum Ultrasound	Postpartum Ultrasound	Other Uses

• Fetal viability
• Fetal number
• Antepartum bleeding (placenta previa, vasa previa, or placenta abruption)
• Biometry
• Amniotic fluid volume
• Preoperative mapping
• Biophysical profile
	• First stage:
	  I. Presentation
	  II. Placenta location
	  III. Breech assessment (type, neck flexion, and EFW)
	• Second stage:
	  I. Head position
	  II. Head station
	  III. Head direction
	  IV. Midline angle
	  V. Subpubic angle
	  VI. Second twin assessment
		• Third stage of labor complications (retained products of conception and PPH)
		• Ultrasound-guided operative procedures (D&C, MROP, and placement of a Bakri balloon)
			• Invasive procedures
			  I. Amnioreduction
			  II. Drainage of abnormal fetal fluid collections
			• Bladder residual volume
			• Local and regional anesthesia
			• Nuchal cord
			• Fetal Dopplers
			• Placental maturity

also be appreciated. An approximate heart rate can be obtained by applying M-mode (motion mode) or pulsed Doppler techniques. Fetal heart rate (FHR) in obstetrics is considered normal between 110 and 160 bpm.

Fetal Number

If the patient had no previous antenatal care, it is very important to rule out multiple gestations. In cases with more than one fetus, knowing the chorionicity and amnionicity is the next step, although it may be difficult to define the former in the second and third trimester, especially if the two placentae are not separated. However, observing a membrane between the fetuses is crucial to rule out a monoamniotic multiple gestation.

Antepartum Bleeding

When a patient presents with antepartum hemorrhage, ultrasound plays an important rule to help to identify the cause of the bleeding, such as placenta previa, placental abruption (Fig. 37-1), vasa previa, or even uterine rupture. The first three clinical situations are covered in more detail in their respective chapters.

Uterine rupture is a rare but a catastrophic situation with high maternal and fetal mortality and morbidity. The diagnosis usually is made through a clinical suspicion in high-risk patients. Using ultrasound, the sonographic features associated with uterine rupture include the presence of the gestational sac and fetus outside the uterus, empty uterus, extra-peritoneal

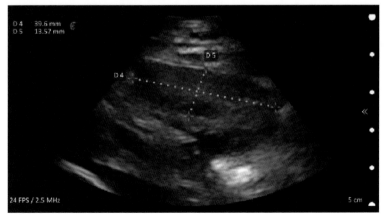

FIGURE 37-1. A subchorionic hematoma seen in a patient presenting with vaginal bleeding. Although this may aid in diagnosis, placenta abruption remains a clinical diagnosis.

hematoma, intrauterine blood, free peritoneal blood, and large uterine mass with gas bubbles.

Biometry

Fetal biometry (biparietal diameter, head circumference, abdominal circumference, and femur length) can be used to give an estimated gestational age, if previously unknown, but it is only accurate to within 3 to 4 weeks in the third trimester.

Biometry can estimate fetal weight, screening for fetal growth restriction when the gestation is known and aiding in neonatal counseling for smaller babies.

When the operator does not feel confident in his or her measurement technique, the unique shape of the cerebellum is readily recognized and its length easily measured (Figs. 37-2A, B). This can provide an approximate estimate of gestation when other options are limited.

Preoperative Mapping

When Cesarean section is being undertaken for a placenta previa with an anterior component, for vasa previa, or for obstructive or lower segment fibroids, mapping can be performed immediately before surgery to help guide the optimal uterine incision site.

Biophysical Profile

Biophysical profile (BPP) is mainly used as antepartum surveillance to assess fetal well-being. It can be used in Obstetric Triage departments but this is not within the scope of this book.

Amniotic Fluid Volume

Assessment of the amniotic fluid volume is principally a component of antenatal fetal assessment in the second and third trimester. It is also a component of the BPP. The simplest quantitative method for amniotic fluid evaluation is the single deepest vertical pocket (SDP). The deepest vertical pocket of fluid that is free from any umbilical cord, or fetal parts is measured. A value less than 2 cm is considered oligohydramnios and a value greater than 8 cm is considered polyhydramnios. It is known that a significant reduction in amniotic fluid volume is associated with an increased

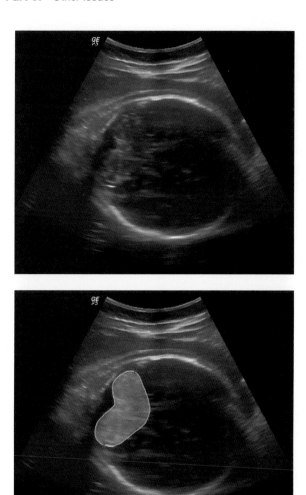

FIGURE 37-2. Fetal cerebellum (highlighted in yellow). Its unique shape and simple measurement allow for an approximate assessment of preterm gestational age.

incidence of nonreassuring FHR patterns and subsequent emergency Cesarean section. However, evidence also suggests that the knowledge that the amniotic fluid volume is low alters obstetric decision-making and results in increased Cesarean sections. For this reason, it has been largely abandoned as an admission screening test in labor and delivery units.

Amnioinfusion is sometimes used to relieve variable decelerations in the presence of oligohydramnios. In this situation, amniotic fluid volume assessments can guide therapy.

INTRAPARTUM ULTRASOUND

First Stage of Labor

Presentation
Probably one of the commonest uses of portable ultrasound in birthing units has been to assess presentation. The position of the head and orientation of the longitudinal axis of the spine should be used.

Cord Presentation
On occasion, the suspicion of a cord presentation will arise either from a vaginal examination or from marked decelerations related to contractions. Transperineal or transvaginal ultrasound, aided by color Doppler, can assist diagnosis (Fig. 37-3).

Abdominal delivery is the only option for an abnormal heart rate. If there is no suspicion of fetal compromise, expectant management can be undertaken provided there is rapid access to emergency Cesarean section because there is an ever-present risk of acute cord prolapse. Cases with intrapartum resolution of the cord presentation as labor progresses have been reported. It is also important to distinguish cord presentation from vasa previa. The latter may be associated with an accessory placental lobe and will usually only have two vessels. Alternatively, there may be a membranous cord insertion into the lateral margin of a low placenta (velamentous cord insertion). In such case, vaginal delivery is not recommended.

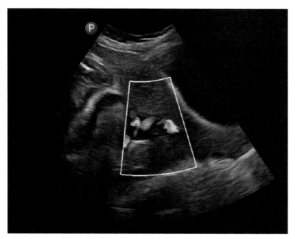

FIGURE 37-3. Cord presentation seen on color Doppler views. Pulsed Doppler can confirm fetal umbilical arterial wave pattern.

Placental Localization

Transabdominal ultrasound can usually exclude previa, but a transvaginal or transperineal approach is required to diagnose it (see Chapter 31). Clinicians should avoid the temptation to search for abruption that may delay proper management because the diagnostic sensitivity of ultrasound is poor. However, moderate and large hematomas can be seen by ultrasound (Fig. 37-1).

Breech Assessment

There has been renewed interest in vaginal breech delivery. Most guidelines recommend knowledge of the type of breech presentation to identify the footling breech at risk of cord complications (Fig. 37-4).

The longitudinal orientation of the cervical spine should be visualized to exclude the hyperextended "star-gazing" position associated with an increased risk of neurologic complications. Finally, attempts at vaginal birth are often tied to certain birthweight ranges. If the breech was previously undiagnosed, some attempt at assessing this using biometry will be necessary.

Second Stage of Labor

Head Position

Occipitoposterior (OP) positions remain a prominent cause of dystocia in labor and operative delivery. Transabdominal ultrasound can reliably

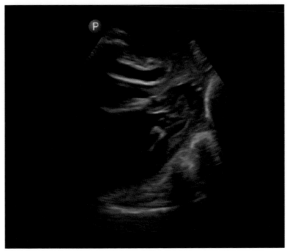

FIGURE 37-4. Translabial ultrasound in sagittal views showing footling breech presentation in a woman presenting in preterm labor.

assess head position using the position of the fetal eyes and the spine in a cross section through the chest (Figs. 37-5A, B). Translabial ultrasound can also be used (Fig. 37-5C).

It has shown that transient OP positions are seen in up to one-third of labors but that the majority rotate to occipitoanterior (OA) even after

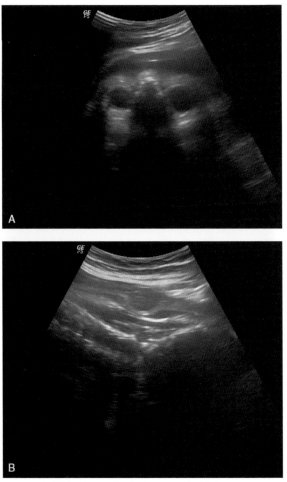

FIGURE 37-5. A. Transabdominal views showing fetal eyes looking straight upward in a direct occipitoposterior (OP) position. **B.** The spine can help when maternal acoustic shadows don't permit visualization of fetal eyes as in this occipitoanterior position. **C.** Transverse views of translabial scan showing the midline falx and the choroid plexi diverting away from the midline toward the back of the occiput, which here shows an OP position. **D.** Asynclitism can be demonstrated using a translabial view in transverse section. **E.** The interrupted red line overlying the falx divides the brain into two equal halves with the yellow lines defining the angle between the falx and the midline pelvis (known as midline angle and can be used as an indicator of birth progress).

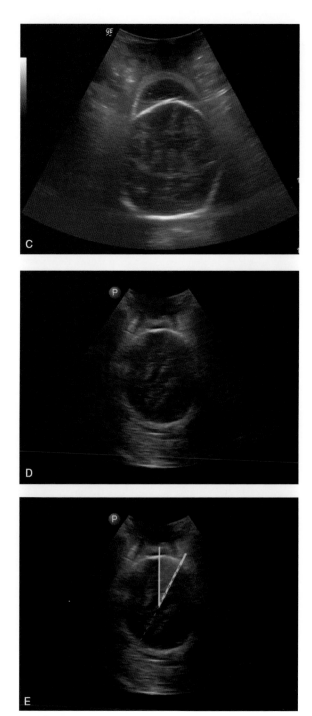

FIGURE 37-5. (*Continued*)

full dilatation. Epidural anesthesia has been shown to reduce this rotation, leading to a higher persistence of posterior positions. Most importantly, ultrasound has shown how inaccurate digital vaginal examination is at assessing head position, with some studies reporting error rates as high as 75 percent. The accuracy of digital assessment was poorest when the head was in a non-OA position or when the station was not below the ischial spines. These are the exact clinical situations that can be associated with difficult instrumental deliveries. Correct placement of the ventouse cup or forcep blades is predicated by an accurate assessment of fetal position.

Another factor to be considered when assessing the head position is synclitism (Figs. 37-5D, E). Asynclitism can complicate operative vaginal deliveries. This can be achieved by ensuring the brain midline (falx) is seen.

Head Station

Several methods have been studied using transperineal ultrasound with either direct measurements using the symphysis pubis as a landmark (angle of progression, progression distance, and head symphysis distance) or indirect method using the fetal head as a landmark (head perineal distance) (Figs. 37-6A, B).

Angle of progression (AoP) is the most studied method with the strongest evidence. It is the angle between the long axis of the pubic bone and a line from the lowest edge of the pubis drawn tangentially to the deepest bony part of the fetal skull. Vaginal delivery was 88 percent with AoP $\geq$110 and 38 percent with AoP <110 in a prolonged first stage of labor. Tutschek et al have developed a table that correlates the AoP and the head station.

Other measurements include: progression distance (PD), head symphysis distance (HSD), and head perineum distance (HPD). References at the end of this chapter provide more details about each technique.

Head Direction

The angle between the longest recognizable axis of the fetal head and the long axis of the pubic symphysis, measured in a midsagittal transperineal view.

Midline Angle

Utilizing the angle of head rotation as an indicator of birth progress. This can be assessed thorough the same view in Fig. 37-5E.

Subpubic Angle

Using 3D techniques.

OTHER ISSUES

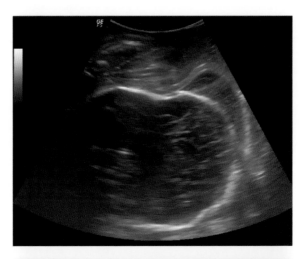

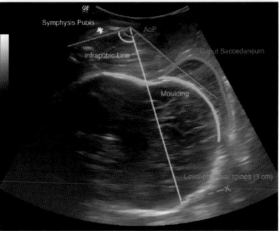

FIGURE 37-6. In a sagittal view of translabial scan, the symphysis pubis (*) is used as the landmark for head station. The yellow "infrapubic line" drops at a 90° angle to the front of the symphysis pubis and represents the "−3" station. Ischial spines (representing "0" station) are therefore 3-cm anterior to the "infrapubic line" (x). Angle of progression (AoP) is represented by the red lines. Molding (green) and caput succedaneum (blue) are seen.

Second Twin Assessment

After delivery of the first twin, the lie of the remaining twin needs to be assessed along with the FHR. These can both be accomplished quickly and efficiently by real-time scanning. Knowing the fetal cardiac position allows prompt and accurate placement of the external monitors' Doppler probe. Alternatively, the heart rate can be monitored by ultrasound, because the relatively rapid descent that will occur will require frequent readjustments of the Doppler probe. If either a breech extraction or internal podalic version is required, the position of the fetal feet can be identified before the procedure is started. Real-time guidance can be provided to the accoucheur during intrauterine manipulation.

POSTPARTUM ULTRASOUND

Third Stage of Labor Complications

The placental bed vessels vasoconstrict after delivery of the fetus, and this precedes placental expulsion. Abnormal placental adherence can be identified if flow persists or postpartum hemorrhage is diagnosed. If the patient hemodynamics status permits, ultrasound can be used to confirm or rule out suspicion of retained products when the delivered placental appears abnormal in shape or missing cotyledons.

Acute uterine inversion can be recognized on ultrasound, which can then guide manual replacement and confirm correct repositioning.

Ultrasound-Guided Operative Procedures

If retained products are seen, guidance can be given to aid the manual removal of retained placenta tissue or performing dilation and curettage (Figs. 37-7A, B).

OTHER USES

Amnioreduction

In the presence of marked polyhydramnios, a gradual reduction in fluid volume can play a part in a stabilizing induction and minimize the risk of acute abruption sometimes seen with a sudden reduction in uterine volume. It also can be used during pregnancy when the patient has symptoms associated with increased abdominal pressure. There is no certain guidelines regarding the amount of fluid should be removed, the use of tocolytic or antibiotics. However, it is been proposed that maximum of 2.5 L of amniotic fluid removed gradually at one time, is reasonable, effective, and with less side effects.

OTHER ISSUES

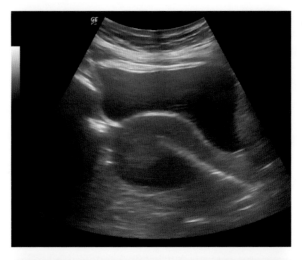

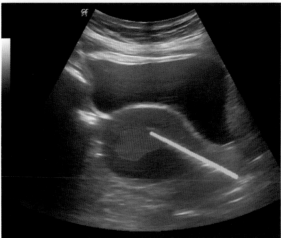

FIGURE 37-7. Retained part of the placenta (highlighted in red) is seen after a full-term vaginal delivery with ultrasound guiding the curette (yellow line). An intrauterine balloon is an effective and safe method to manage PPH due to uterine atony. Balloon placement can be guided by ultrasound, although the inflated balloon is typically pushed down into the lower uterine segment by the dominant fundal myometrium.

Drainage of Abnormal Fetal Fluid Collections

Excessive fluid collections within the fetal head or abdomen can lead to dystocia. After appropriate counseling as to risk, ultrasound-guided drainage can be performed. Bilateral pleural effusions can seriously compromise neonatal respiratory function during delivery. Even a partial drainage in utero can significantly lower the ventilation pressures needed after intubation.

Maternal Bladder Residual Volumes

Bladder dysfunction with retention is common in the immediate postpartum period. It can be related to a transient pelvic nerve apraxia or an epidural effect. The concern is that large-volume retention, if unrecognized, can lead to prolonged difficulties with bladder emptying. The distended bladder can be visualized and the bladder volume measured by ultrasound. This is a noninvasive, pain-free method and can be done by personal without ultrasound training. Indeed, there are now portable ultrasound machines whose sole purpose is to assess bladder volume using built-in software.

Local and Regional Anesthesia

Using probes that allow imaging of the superficial structures, ultrasound guidance can be used to guide epidural or central line placement, especially in patients with high BMI or difficult anatomy. This allows accurate needle placement to the correct depth and reduces the risk of complications. An abdominal block under ultrasound guidance has been used to limit post–Cesarean section pain.

Nuchal Cords

It is not recommended to screen for the presence of a nuchal cord, because it does not appear to improve perinatal outcome, increasing obstetric intervention and maternal anxiety for no benefit.

Fetal Doppler

No intrapartum role has yet been found for arterial Doppler studies. There is a limited data on the usefulness of the intrapartum ductus venosus (DV) Doppler in predicting hypoxia and acidosis in the fetus. However, the technique requires highly skilled operators and high-quality ultrasound machines.

Placental Maturity

A "mature" placenta, as reflected by a Grannum grade III appearance, was originally thought to identify a fetus with lung maturity. This is no longer considered true. It remains contentious as to whether this test has any role in fetal assessment. Certainly, there is considerable interobserver

OTHER ISSUES

variability in assessing grade, with a significant tendency to overcall the more advanced grades.

RADIOGRAPHY

As a diagnostic aid, x-ray has a limited range of uses in modern obstetrics. The use of diagnostic ultrasound has almost eliminated the need for x-ray examination of developing fetuses.

Although not routinely recommended in pregnancy and labor, x-ray can be used when resources are limited. Please refer to earlier editions of this book where more details about this topic have been covered.

SELECTED READING

American College of Obstetrics and Gynecology: Practice Bulletin no. 175. Ultrasound in Pregnancy. Obstet Gynecol 128:e241-e256, 2016

International Society of Ultrasound in Obstetrics and Gynecology Practice Guidelines: Intrapartum Ultrasound. Ultrasound Obstet Gynecol 52:128–139, 2018

Malvasi A: Intrapartum Ultrasonography for Labor Management. Springer, 2021

Molina FS, Nicolaides KH: Ultrasound in labor and delivery. Fetal Diagn Ther 27:261, 2010

The Puerperium

Felipe Moretti

CHAPTER 38

NORMAL ANATOMIC AND PHYSIOLOGIC CHANGES

The puerperium is the period that begins after the delivery of the placenta and lasts until the reproductive organs have returned to approximately their prepregnant condition. The puerperium is usually considered to last 6 weeks.

Shivering

Postpartum shivering is observed in 25 to 50 percent of women after normal delivery. The pathogenesis of postpartum chills is not clear. No treatment is necessary other than supportive care. When shivering is anesthesia related, it can be treated pharmacologically.

Uterine Involution

After the delivery of the placenta and membranes, contractions reduce the size of the uterus so that it can be felt as a hard, globular mass lying just below the umbilicus. Contraction of interlacing myometrial muscle bundles constricts the intramyometrial vessels, impeding blood flow and preventing postpartum hemorrhage. Moreover, large vessels at the placental site thrombose, a secondary hemostatic mechanism for preventing blood loss at this site.

The uterus weighs 1000 to 1200 g immediately after delivery. It rapidly falls to 500 g by 7 days, disappears into the pelvis by 2 weeks, and is back to its nonpregnant weight of 50 to 70 g by 6 weeks. This reduction is the result mainly of a decrease in the size of the myometrial cells rather than of their number.

Involution of the placental site also takes up to 6 weeks. Immediately after delivery, the placental site is elevated, irregular, and friable and is composed of thrombosed vascular sinusoids. These undergo gradual hyalinization. Most of the decidua basalis is shed over a period of weeks and is replaced by regenerating endometrium. Failure of normal involution of the placental site may lead to late postpartum hemorrhage.

Lochia

The basal portion of the decidua remains after delivery of the placenta. The decidua divides in two layers: the superficial layer and the deep layer. The deep layer, which contains some endometrial glands, regenerates new endometrium. Restoration of the endometrial cavity is rapid and is complete in 16 to 21 days. The superficial layer of decidua surrounding the placental site becomes necrotic and is sloughed off during the first 5 to 6 days. This postpartum vaginal discharge, made up of a mixture of blood and necrotic decidua, is called "lochia." It is red for 2 to 3 days (lochia rubra), becomes paler as the bleeding is reduced (lochia serosa), and by 7 days is yellowish-white (lochia alba). The total volume of postpartum lochial secretion is 200 to 500 mL and lasts from 3 to 6 weeks.

Regeneration of the Endometrium

The deeper part of the decidua that contains some endometrial glands remains intact and is a source of a new lining of the uterine cavity. Restoration of the endometrium is rapid; by the seventh day, it resembles the nonpregnant state and is complete by 16 to 21 days.

Cervix

Immediately after delivery, the cervix is floppy and ragged with several small tears and bleeding points that are insignificant. The cervical os closes gradually. It admits two to three fingers for the first 4 to 7 days and by the end of 10 to 14 days is barely dilated.

The glandular hypertrophy and hyperplasia of pregnancy regresses gradually, and this process is complete by about 6 weeks. The squamous epithelium that was lacerated during delivery heals and undergoes rapid re-epithelialization, but not all cervices regain their prepregnant appearance. Persistence of glandular epithelium on the exocervix is described as a cervical ectropion.

Vagina

After delivery, the vagina is a spacious, smooth-walled cavity with poor tone. Gradually, the vascularity and edema decrease, and by 4 weeks, the rugae reappear, although they are less prominent than in nulliparas. The vaginal epithelium appears atrophic for some time (longer in lactating women) but looks normal by 6 to 10 weeks.

Lacerations of the lower vagina and perineum heal gradually. Perineal care is a matter of hygiene. Showers and washing with soap and water are sufficient for most patients. Hot sitz baths reduce perineal tenderness and promote healing of episiotomy and lacerations. The suggestion has been put forward that ice baths, by causing vasoconstriction, reduce edema,

OTHER ISSUES

inflammation, and bleeding. They may also decrease the excitability of nerve endings, relieving muscular irritability and spasm. This may relieve pain more effectively and for a longer period than hot baths. The drawback to this treatment is that the patient has to endure the sensation of cold, burning, and aching until the numbness and analgesia supervene.

Fallopian Tubes

The cells decrease in size and number. Two weeks after delivery, the tubal epithelium is similar to that seen in menopause, with atrophy and decilia-tion. After 6 to 8 weeks, the normal structure has been regained.

Ovaries and Ovulation

The puerperal period is one of relative infertility, especially for women who are lactating. In nonlactating mothers, initial postpartum ovulation can occur within 6 weeks. In women, who exclusively breastfeed without supple-mentation, ovulation is usually reliably delayed by at least 6 months. The incidence of conception in this situation is only 2 percent, but additional con-traception should be considered, depending on individual circumstances.

The occurrence of the first menstruation varies, but most nonlactating women have menstruated by 12 weeks after delivery. The return of men-struation is usually delayed in lactating women. Menses within the first 6 weeks are rarely ovulatory.

Breasts

In the early puerperium, the breasts undergo marked changes. Between the second and fourth day, the breasts become engorged with increased vascularity and areolar pigmentation. There is enlargement of the lobules resulting from an increase in the number and size of the alveoli. At this time, lactation begins, controlled by various hormones. The production of milk occurs spontaneously but is enhanced by suckling. Once lactation is established, the most important stimulus for the continuation of the pro-duction of milk is suckling. A message is sent via the nervous system to the hypothalamus, and there is an increase in the production and release of oxytocin. Oxytocin stimulates the myoepithelial cells of the alveoli of the breasts to contract, causing milk to be transported to, and sometimes through, the nipple. This is the "letdown" reflex.

Some mothers are unable to breastfeed their infants for a variety of rea-sons, including insufficient milk, inverted nipples, diseases of the breast, or the need to take drugs that may be excreted in the milk and effect the baby. Others simply choose not to.

In 60 to 70 percent of women, who do not wish to breastfeed, lactation can be suppressed by the use of a tight bra and the avoidance of stimulation of the nipple. Pharmacologic suppression is no longer advised because of a high incidence of rebound phenomenon.

Cardiovascular System

The cardiac output increases during the first and second stages of labor. It rises even higher immediately after the birth as the reduction in uterine size squeezes an additional amount of fluid into the circulation. After a short interval, the cardiac output decreases to about 40 percent above the prelabor levels and returns to normal after 2 to 3 weeks. The decrease in heart rate is partly responsible for the reduced cardiac output. Changes in blood volume result from loss of blood at delivery and from the mobilization and excretion of extravascular fluid.

Urinary Tract

The dilatation that takes place in the urinary collecting system during pregnancy does not return to normal for more than 6 weeks. The combination of loss of tone, trauma to the bladder during delivery, and anesthesia (especially of the conduction variety) may lead to retention of urine, necessitating catheterization.

Gastrointestinal Tract

Mobility of the intestines, which is decreased during pregnancy, gradually returns to normal. The use of excessive analgesia may delay this process. Laxatives or an enema may be required.

BREASTFEEDING

Advantages

Breastfeeding is convenient, economical, and emotionally satisfying to most women. It also helps to contract the uterus, decreasing maternal blood loss.

OTHER ISSUES

Breast milk is digestible, has the ideal temperature and nutrient composition, and has no bacterial contamination. Colostrum and milk contain immunologic components such as immunoglobulin A (IgA), complement, macrophages, lymphocytes, lactoferrin, lactoperoxidase and lysozymes.

Breastfed infants have decreased incidences of diarrhea, respiratory infections, otitis media, urinary tract infections (UTIs), necrotizing enterocolitis, invasive bacterial infection, and sudden death. Additionally, cognitive development and intelligence may be improved.

Breastfeeding should always be encouraged by care-givers. Mothers and infants who are able to start breast feeding within one to two hours after delivery are more successful than those whose initial interactions are delayed for several hours.

Breastfeeding and COVID-19

Mothers should practice skin-to-skin care and breastfeed while in the hospital with some modifications to usual processes according hospital guidance.

The Public Health Agency of Canada and the World Health Organization (WHO) recommend mother with suspected or confirmed COVID-19 continue to breastfeed. The Centers for Disease Control and Prevention (CDC) recommends mother and health care providers discuss benefits and risks of breastfeeding and come to a shared decision.

Contraindications

Mothers should not breastfeed, or feed expressed milk to their infants diagnosed of Galactosemia, infected with human T-cell lymphotropic virus type I or type II, who are using an illicit street drug such as cocaine, suspected or confirmed Ebola virus disease, and are undergoing treatment for breast cancer.

For HIV, breastfeeding is not recommended in the United States. The Canadian Pediatric Society also recommends avoiding breastfeeding in this group of patients.

In resource-limited settings, such as some parts of Africa, the World Health Organization (WHO) recommends that HIV-infected mothers breastfeed exclusively for the first 6 months of life and continue breastfeeding for at least 12 months, with the addition of complementary foods. These mothers should be given ART to reduce the risk of transmission through breastfeeding.

Mothers with active tuberculosis or varicella should not breastfeed but can feed expressed breast milk to their infants.

Few medications are contraindicated while breastfeeding. The health care providers should weigh the risks and benefits when prescribing a medication to breastfeeding mother. An up-to-date information available on medication and lactation can be found on Drugs and Lactation Database (LactMed).

In women who are not breastfeeding is recommended the use of a tight brassiere and avoidance of breast stimulation as nondrug suppresses. Cabergoline 1 mg per oral single dose during the first day postpartum has shown to be effective for lactation suppression and breast engorgement.

Breast Fever

Puerperal fever from breast engorgement is common and may occur in 13 percent of all women postpartum. Fever can range from 37.8°C to 39°C. Treatment of engorgement consists of firm breast support, analgesics, and applying ice bags. Pumping of the breast or manual expression is recommended.

Mastitis

Infection of the mammary glands is often caused by coagulase-positive *Staphylococcus aureus*. Most frequently, symptoms of a painful erythematous lobule in one quadrant of the breast are noted during the second or third week of the puerperium.

Infection may be limited to the subareolar region but more frequently involves an obstructed lactiferous duct and the surrounding breast parenchyma. If cellulitis is not properly treated, a breast abscess may develop. If the infected breast is too tender to allow suckling, gently pumping until nursing can be resumed is recommended. Apply local heat and provide good support. Penicillins or cephalosporins are the antibiotics of choice. Erythromycin is given to women who are penicillin sensitive. Treatment should be continued for 10 to 14 days.

Breast Abscess

Clinical suspicion occurs when a mass is palpable, or a fever fails to subside after 48 to 72 hours. Pitting edema over the inflamed area and some degree of fluctuation are indicative of abscess formation. If an abscess occurs, it is usually necessary to undertake drainage. Ultrasound-guided needle aspiration followed by antibiotics has an 80 to 90 percent success rate.

ENDOMETRITIS

Postpartum endometritis is essentially an infection of the decidua. It may also extend to the myometrium (called endomyometritis) or involve the parametrium (called parametritis). The route of delivery is the most important single risk factor for puerperium infection. The French Confidential Enquiry on Maternal Deaths cited a nearly 25-fold increased infection-related mortality rate with cesarean section versus vaginal delivery. The incidence of cesarean section has increased rapidly in Europe and in the rest of the world, with some places in Latin America reporting rates of 50 percent.

Antibiotic prophylaxis is widely used to reduce the incidence of puerperium infection after cesarean section, resulting in a two-thirds reduction in endometritis and a decrease in wound infection. In contrast, endometritis is relatively uncommon after vaginal delivery.

Risk Factors for Endometritis

1. Antepartum
   a. Low socioeconomic status
   b. Lack of prenatal care
   c. Anemia
   d. Maternal diabetes mellitus
   e. Obesity
   f. Bacterial colonization of the lower genital tract (e.g., group B streptococcus)
   g. HIV infection
2. Intrapartum
   a. Prolonged membrane rupture
   b. Prolonged labor
   c. Multiple cervical examinations
   d. Intrapartum chorioamnionitis
   e. Intrauterine fetal monitoring
3. During delivery
   a. Cesarean section
   b. Manual removal of the placenta
   c. Operative vaginal delivery
   d. Hemorrhage
   e. Devitalization of tissue from episiotomy and lacerations

Pathogenesis of Endometritis

The cervicovaginal flora may have access to uterine cavity during labor and delivery. It can be facilitated by the risk factors mentioned earlier. The colonization of the decidua may lead to invasive infection of the myometrium and parametrium. The potential for invasive infection is enhanced in cesarean births because of the presence of foreign bodies such as suture material, myometrial necrosis at the suture line, and formation of hematomas or seromas. A wide range of bacteria may be involved, including both aerobes and anaerobes. Broad-spectrum coverage is necessary for treatment.

Clinical Manifestations

The most common symptom is pyrexia. It is considered postpartum fever when the temperature is 38°C or more. After the first 24 hours, two episodes of fever within 10 days postpartum is suggestive of infection. Other symptoms include uterine tenderness, foul lochia, chills, and lower abdominal pain. The uterus may be soft and subinvoluted, which can lead to excessive uterine bleeding.

Other common causes of fever are:

- Surgical site infection (cesarean delivery incision, episiotomy incision, perineal laceration)
- Mastitis or breast abscess
- UTI
- Aspiration pneumonia
- Deep vein thrombosis (DVT) and pulmonary embolism (PE)

Laboratory Studies

Leukocytosis is a normal finding during labor and early puerperium. However, white blood cell counts as high as 20,000/mL can be expected with an infection. Urinalysis should be routinely performed to rule out a UTI. Lochia cultures should be obtained using speculum to allow direct visualization of the cervix. Accurate cultures can be achieved only if specimens obtained transcervically are free from vaginal contamination.

Imaging

Postpartum imaging is often used to rule out any other cause of fever such as pneumonia, DVT, or pulmonary embolus if there is persistent postpartum fever. Patients refractory to 48 to 72 hours of adequate antimicrobial therapy should be imaged, searching for abscesses, retained products of conception, hematomas, and septic pelvic thrombophlebitis. Imaging can also be used to guide therapy, such as abscess drainage.

Treatment

Treatment of mild metritis after vaginal delivery with outpatient oral antibiotics is usually sufficient. For moderate to severe infections, intravenous broad-spectrum antibiotic therapy is recommended. The response of therapy should be monitored clinically and by laboratory testing as needed. Improvement follows in 48 to 72 hours in nearly 90 percent of women treated with one of the several standard regimens. Deterioration or failure of treatment requires a complete reevaluation.

Antimicrobial Regimens

In mild endometritis, outpatient treatment with ampicillin (1 g every 6 hours) has been shown to be effective and should be given up to 2 to 3 days after remission of fever and clinical improvement.

In moderate or severe cases or after cesarean section, intravenous therapy with a broad-spectrum antimicrobial agent regimen, such as clindamycin 900 mg + gentamicin 1.5 mg/kg every 8 hours, should be administered. If sepsis or enterococcal infection is suspected, ampicillin (1 g intravenously every 6 hours) should be added to the regimen.

Alternative Regimens

- Clindamycin + aztreonam (gentamicin substitute with renal insufficiency)
- Cefoxitin + clindamycin or metronidazole
- Ceftriaxone
- Imipenem + cilastatin

WOUND INFECTION

Cesarean Section Incision

When prophylactic antibiotics are given, the incidence of wound infection is usually less than 2 percent. Fever that persists to the fourth or fifth postoperative day suggests a wound infection. Wound infection is characterized by local erythema and tenderness. Spontaneous drainage may occur and is often accompanied by reduction of symptoms and signs.

Treatment

The incision should be opened, encouraging drainage of infected material. Mechanical cleansing of the wound is the mainstay of therapy. The wound can be packed with saline-soaked gauze two to three times per day, which will remove necrotic debris each time the wound is unpacked. The wound can be left open to heal or it can be closed secondarily when granulation tissue has begun to form.

Episiotomy Infection

The incidence is 0.5 to 3 percent, and clinical findings are characterized by local pain. Spontaneous drainage is frequent, and inspection of the episiotomy site shows disruption of the wound and a gaping incision. A necrotic membrane may cover the wound and should be debrided if possible.

Treatment

By opening and cleaning the episiotomy wound, the formation of granulation tissue is promoted. Warm sitz baths may help the debridement process.

URINARY TRACT INFECTION

The incidence of postpartum UTI is approximately 2 to 4 percent. The anatomical proximity of the lower gastrointestinal tract and genital tract exposes the urinary tract to bacteria present in the vicinity. Asymptomatic bacteriuria is found in 2 to 7 percent of women during pregnancy and up to 13 percent postpartum. Catheterization significantly increases the rate of bacteriuria. Operative delivery, epidural anesthesia, and frequent pelvic examinations are also associated with increased risk for a UTI. Moreover, after delivery, the bladder and lower urinary tract remain somewhat hypotonic, and residual urine and reflux result, which provides an excellent environment for infection.

Cystitis

Most UTIs are limited to the bladder. The presenting symptoms are frequency and dysuria. Rarely is there fever or malaise.

OTHER ISSUES

Escherichia coli is the most common organism isolated from infected urine postpartum. In women with persistent or repeated infections, bacteria such as *Proteus, Pseudomonas, Enterobacter,* and *Klebsiella* spp. are often cultured. Treatment consists of antibiotics with specific activity against the causative organism. These drugs include sulfonamides, nitrofurantoin, trimethoprim–sulfamethoxazole, oral cephalosporins, and ampicillin.

Pyelonephritis

Patients who develop pyelonephritis appear unwell. They develop fever, shaking chills with fever spikes, pain in the back and flank, and tenderness in the costovertebral angle. In contrast with cystitis, pyelonephritis requires initial therapy with high doses of intravenous antibiotics such as ampicillin 8 to 12 g/day or a first-generation cephalosporin such as cefazolin 3 to 8 g/day. When the patient has clinical signs of sepsis or a resistant organism, aminoglycoside can be added. The response to therapy may be fast and after resolution of fever, antibiotics should be continued intravenously or orally for a total of 10 days. Urine cultures should be obtained to guide any necessary modification in drugs.

DEEP VENOUS THROMBOSIS AND PULMONARY EMBOLISM

Venous thromboembolism (VTE) complicates between one in 500 and one in 2000 pregnancies and is more common postpartum than antepartum. PE is the leading direct cause of maternal death in the United Kingdom (1.56 of 100,000 maternities) and is the second most cause of maternal death overall (11% of maternal deaths).

The highest incidence of VTE, PE in particular, is during the postpartum period. Cesarean section is a significant risk factor, but women having vaginal deliveries are also at risk, and 55 percent of the postpartum maternal deaths from VTE in the United Kingdom between 1997 and 2005 occurred in women who had delivered vaginally. DVT is more common in the left than the right leg. The risk of VTE is twice as high after cesarean section than vaginal delivery.

Pathogenesis

Pregnancy itself puts all women at higher risk of VTE, with a four- to 10-fold increase compared with an age-matched nonpregnant female population.

Venous stasis, endothelial injury, and a hypercoagulable state (Virchow's triad) are marked in pregnancy and the postpartum period, increasing the risk of thromboembolic events. Major additional risk factors are a previous VTE and/or a documented thrombophilia. A history of thrombosis increases the risk of pregnancy-related VTE to up to 12 percent.

Clinical Manifestations

Clinical diagnosis of DVT and PE is unreliable and is even more inaccurate during pregnancy. DVT can present with leg discomfort, leg swelling, pitting edema, discoloration, and warmth. PE is the most difficult diagnosis. Dyspnea, the most common symptom of PE, occurs in up to 70 percent of normal pregnancies, often stabilizing near term. Usually PE is considered in the differential diagnosis of many clinical presentations, including chest pain, dyspnea, hemoptysis, and unexplained tachycardia.

Thromboprophylaxis

The management strategy for postpartum thromboprophylaxis should be based on assessment of prepregnancy and antenatal risk factors for VTE, modified by intrapartum events, including mode of delivery and any obstetric complications (Table 38-1).

Postpartum Thromboprophylaxis

Thromboprophylaxis involves both nonpharmacologic and pharmacologic measures. Early mobilization after delivery and hydration should be encouraged. Graduated compression stockings and pneumatic compression boots may also be used to achieve improved blood flow and reduce stasis in the femoral and popliteal vessels. Women with known thrombophilia should be considered for heparin prophylaxis for at least 7 days postpartum even if they did not receive antenatal thromboprophylaxis. It can be extended to 6 weeks if there is a family history or other risk factors present. Patients who have an emergency cesarean section should be considered for thromboprophylaxis with heparin for 7 days after delivery. For patients who have an elective cesarean section and have one or more risk factors such as body mass index greater than 30 should also receive thromboprophylaxis for 7 days after delivery. Where resources allow it, low-molecular-weight heparin (LMWH) is appropriate for postpartum thromboprophylaxis (Table 38-2). If women are receiving long-term anticoagulation with warfarin, this can be started when the risk of hemorrhage

OTHER ISSUES

TABLE 38-1: RISK FACTORS FOR VENOUS THROMBOEMBOLISM IN PREGNANCY

Preexisting		
Previous Venous Thromboembolism		
Thrombophilia	Inherited	Antithrombin deficiency
		Protein C deficiency
		Protein S deficiency
		Factor V Leiden
		Prothrombin gene G20210A
	Acquired (antiphospholipid syndrome)	Persistent lupus anticoagulant
		Persistent moderate or high-titer anticardiolipin antibodies
		Persistent moderate or high-titer β2 glycoprotein 1 antibodies
Medical comorbidities	(e.g., inflammatory diseases, nephrotic syndrome, sickle cell disease,[a] IV drug user)	
Age >35 years or parity ≥3		
Obesity (BMI >30 km/m²)		
Smoking		
Gross varicose veins	Symptomatic or above knee or with associated phlebitis, edema, or skin changes)	
Obstetric		
Multiple pregnancy		
Assisted reproductive therapy		
Preeclampsia		
Prolonged labor, midcavity rotational operative delivery		
Cesarean section		
PPH (>1 L) requiring transfusion		

(Continued)

TABLE 38-1: RISK FACTORS FOR VENOUS THROMBOEMBOLISM IN PREGNANCY (*Continued*)

New Onset or Transient
Surgical procedure in pregnancy or puerperium
Hyperemesis, dehydration
Ovarian hyperstimulation syndrome
Admission or immobility (≥3 days bed rest)
Systemic infection (requiring antibiotics or admission to hospital)
Long-distance travel (>4 hours)

BMI, body mass index; IV, intravenous; PPH, postpartum hemorrhage.

[a]Villers MS, Jamison, MG, De Castro LM, James AH: Morbidity associated with sickle cell disease in pregnancy. Am J Obstetr Gynecol 199:125, e1-125, 2008

Reproduced with permission from Reducing the risk of thrombosis and embolism during pregnancy and the puerperium. Green-top Guideline No. 37a. Royal College of Obstetricians and Gynaecologists, 2009.

TABLE 38-2: THROMBOPROPHYLACTIC DOSE FOR ANTENATAL AND POSTNATAL LOW-MOLECULAR-WEIGHT HEPARIN

Weight (kg)	Enoxaparin	Dalteparin	Tinzaparin (75 U/kg/day)
<50	20 mg/day	2500 units/day	3500 units/day
50-90	40 mg/day	5000 units/day	4500 units/day
91-130	60 mg/day[a]	7500 units/day[a]	7000 units/day[a]
131-170	80 mg/day[a]	10000 units/day[a]	9000 units/day[a]
>170	0.6 mg/kg/day[a]	75 units/kg/day[a]	75 units/kg/day[a]
High prophylactic dose	40 mg 12-hourly	5000 units 12 hourly	4500 units 12 hourly for women weighing 50-90 kg

[a]May given in two divided doses.

Reproduced with permission from Reducing the risk of thrombosis and embolism during pregnancy and the puerperium. Green-top Guideline No. 37a. Royal College of Obstetricians and Gynaecologists, 2009.

is low, usually 5 to 7 days after delivery. Heparin and warfarin are safe when breastfeeding.

Contraindications to Anticoagulation

- Active antenatal or postpartum bleeding
- Increase risk of major hemorrhage such as placenta previa
- Bleeding diathesis, such as von Willebrand's disease, hemophilia, or acquired coagulopathy
- Thrombocytopenia
- Acute stroke in the past 4 weeks (ischemic or hemorrhagic)
- Severe renal disease
- Severe liver disease
- Uncontrolled hypertension (systolic blood pressure greater than 200 mm Hg and diastolic blood pressure greater than 120 mm Hg)

SEPTIC PELVIC THROMBOPHLEBITIS

The incidence of septic pelvic thrombophlebitis (SPT) is approximately one in 3000 deliveries (one in 9000 vaginal deliveries and one in 800 cesarean sections). There are two types of SPT: ovarian vein thrombophlebitis (OVT) and deep septic thrombophlebitis (DSPT). The pathogenesis is similar to that of VTE.

Clinical Manifestation

Ovarian vein thrombophlebitis usually presents within 1 week of delivery. Patients appear clinically ill and develop fever and abdominal pain localized to the flank, the back, or the side of the affected vein. Pelvic tenderness may be present.

Patients with DSPT usually present with fever in the early postpartum or postoperative period. They are not usually clinically ill. Fever or chills may be the only symptoms, and patients appear clinically well between spikes. DSPT is frequently diagnosis of exclusion and should be suspected in persistent postpartum fever despite antibiotic therapy.

Diagnosis

SPT is often a diagnosis of exclusion. It should be suspected in the setting of unexplained fever during the week after delivery or persistent postpartum fever despite antibiotic therapy for metritis. Imaging should be obtained to evaluate SPT. CT or MRI can be useful for diagnosis of OVT but not for DSPT.

Treatment

Antibiotic therapy combined with anticoagulation is the most common treatment for this condition. Most patients have already been receiving parenteral antibiotics for endometritis. Options for appropriate antibiotic regimens are shown in Table 38-3.

Anticoagulation is recommended, and unfractionated heparin in an initial bolus of 5000 units followed by continuous infusion of 16 to 18 U/kg can be used. Therapeutic doses of LMWH are also used by many clinicians.

TABLE 38-3: EMPIRIC ANTIBIOTIC THERAPY FOR SEPTIC PELVIC THROMBOPHLEBITIS

Options for empiric gram-negative and anaerobic coverage include:
Monotherapy with a beta-lactam/beta-lactamase inhibitor, such as one of the following:
Ampicillin–sulbactam (3 g every 6 hours)
Piperacillin–tazobactam (4.5 g every 8 hours)
Ticarcillin–clavulanate (3.1 g every 4 hours)
A third-generation cephalosporin such as ceftriaxone (1 g IV every 24 hours) plus metronidazole (500 mg IV every 8 hours)
For patients with beta-lactam intolerance, alternative empiric regimens include:
A fluoroquinolone (e.g., ciprofloxacin 400 mg IV every 12 hours or levofloxacin 500 mg/day IV daily) plus metronidazole (500 mg IV every 8 hours)
Monotherapy with a carbapenem, such as one of the following:
Imipenem (500 mg every 6 hours)
Meropenem (1 g every 8 hours)
Ertapenem (1 g/day)

SELECTED READING

Benson MD, Haney E, Dinsmoor M, Beaumont JL: Shaking rigors in parturients. J Reprod Med 53:685, 2008

Centers for Disease Control and Prevention: Breastfeeding and Special Circumstances. March 2022

Confidential Enquiry into Maternal and Child Health: Saving Mothers' Lives: Reviewing Maternal Deaths to Make Motherhood Safer, 2003-2005. The Seventh Report of the Confidential Enquiries into Maternal Deaths in the United Kingdom. London: CEMACH; 2007

Deneux-Tharaux C, Carmona E, Bouvier-Colle MN, Bréart G: Postpartum maternal mortality and cesarean delivery. Obstet Gynecol 108:541, 2006

Liu S, Liston RM, Joseph KS, et al: Maternal mortality and severe morbidity associated with low-risk planned Caesarean delivery versus planned vaginal delivery at term. CMAJ 176:455, 2007

Marik PE, Plante LA: Venous thromboembolic disease and pregnancy. N Engl J Med 359:2025, 2008

Moore DL, Allen UD: HIV in pregnancy: Identification of intrapartum and perinatal HIV exposures. Paediatr Child Health 24:42-49, 2019

Narvey M: Clinical Practice: Breastfeeding and COVID-19. August 10, 2021. Canadian Paediatric Society, Fetus and Newborn Committee.

Negishi H, Kishida T, Yamada H, Hirayama E, Mikuni M, Fujimoto S: Changes in uterine size after vaginal delivery and cesarean section determined by vaginal sonography in the puerperium. Arch Gynecol Obstet 263:13, 1999

Panel on Treatment of Pregnant Women with HIV Infection and Prevention of Perinatal Transmission: Recommendations for Use of Antiretroviral Drugs in Transmission in the United States. February 2021

Royal College of Obstetricians and Gynaecologists: Reducing the risk of thrombosis and embolism during pregnancy and the puerperium. Green-top Guideline No. 37a. http://www.rcog.org.uk/guidelines, 2009

Smaill FM, Gyte GM: Antibiotic prophylaxis versus no prophylaxis for preventing infection after cesarean section. Cochrane Pregnancy and Childbirth Group. Cochrane Database Syst Rev 2014:CD007482, 2014

Villar J, Valladares E, Wojdyla D, et al: Caesarean delivery rates and pregnancy outcomes: the 2005 WHO global survey on maternal and perinatal health in Latin America. Lancet 367:1819, 2006

Witlin AG, Mercer BM, Sibai BM: Septic pelvic thrombophlebitis or refractory postpartum fever of undetermined etiology. J Matern Fetal Med 5:355, 1996

CHAPTER 39

The Newborn Infant

Nadya Ben Fadel
Sally Mashally

ADAPTATION TO EXTRAUTERINE LIFE

The successful transition from intrauterine to extrauterine life is dependent upon significant physiologic changes that occur at birth. For the transition to be successful, the following changes must occur.

Alveolar Fluid Clearance

During pregnancy, lung growth and development occurs through the accumulation of alveolar fluid. During late gestation and labor, catecholamine and other hormones are increased, resulting into active resorption of fluid from alveoli, which is enhanced further by increased oxygen tension (PaO_2) at birth. A minor mechanism of alveolar fluid clearance is the squeeze of the infant chest wall during vaginal delivery; the thorax is compressed as it traverses the birth canal. This expresses some fluid from the upper airways. Most of what remains is absorbed by the pulmonary capillaries and lymphatics.

Lung Expansion

After birth, the air movement into the lungs expands the alveolar air spaces resulting in stimulation of surfactant release, which reduces alveolar surface tension and prevents alveolar collapse.

Establishment of Regular Breathing and Gas Exchange

The mechanical expansion of the lungs at first breath and the rise in alveolar PO_2 lead to a rapid decrease in pulmonary vascular resistance and an increase in pulmonary blood flow. A number of factors are involved in the initial stimulus to respiration. The most important is the fall in PO_2 and the rise in PCO_2 that follows the cessation of umbilical circulation. Tactile, thermal, and proprioceptive inputs also play significant roles.

Circulatory Changes

Changes in Pressure
Fetal circulation is characterized by relatively high right ventricular and pulmonary artery pressures. These are maintained by elevated pulmonary

arteriolar resistance and by the presence of a large ductus arteriosus. The ductus equalizes pressures between the pulmonary artery and aorta and directs most of the right ventricular output into the systemic circulation. Systemic pressures are decreased by the presence of the umbilical circulation, which acts as a low-pressure shunt.

After clamping the umbilical cord and removal of the placenta and its low vascular resistance, the systemic vascular resistance increases; meanwhile, lung expansion after the first effective breaths results in a drop of pulmonary vascular resistance and pulmonary artery pressure. This will result in elevation of left ventricle pressure above that of the right ventricle.

Closure of Fetal Vascular Channels

Foramen Ovale. The increase in pulmonary venous return to the left atrium leads to a rise in left atrial pressure. As the left atrial pressure increases and the right atrial pressure falls, right-to-left shunting across the foramen ovale decreases. Eventually, the left atrial pressure exceeds the right atrial pressure. This compresses the valve of the foramen ovale and produces functional closure of the interatrial septum. Anatomic closure takes place over a period of months or years.

Ductus Arteriosus. The ductus arteriosus closes functionally over the first 24 to 72 hours of life. This process is related to the rise in arterial oxygen saturation and is mediated by decreased circulating prostaglandins levels.

IMMEDIATE CARE OF THE INFANT IN THE DELIVERY ROOM

Initial Resuscitation

Of all newborn infants, 10 percent will need some assistance to initiate and establish breathing, and around 1 percent will require more extensive resuscitation. Before the actual delivery, it is important to identify infants who may need support for their initial transitioning to extrauterine life. This step helps to minimize any delay in resuscitative measures, thereby improving prognosis and outcome. Some examples of infant groups that may warrant the presence of a neonatal resuscitation team at the time of their birth are shown in Table 39-1.

OTHER ISSUES

TABLE 39-1: RISK FACTORS FOR THE NEED FOR NEONATAL RESUSCITATION

Maternal Conditions	Fetal Conditions	During Delivery
Age (>40 years, <16 years)	Prematurity	Abnormal fetal heart rate
Poor socioeconomic status	Postmaturity	Abnormal presentation
Smoking, drug and/or alcohol abuse	Intrauterine growth restriction	Instrumented delivery
Medical conditions	Macrosomia	Cesarean delivery
Diabetes mellitus, hypertension	Multiple gestations	Chorioamnionitis
Chronic heart, lung diseases, kidney diseases/ urinary tract infections, and blood disorders	Congenital anomalies	Systemic maternal infection
Obstetric conditions	Hydrops	Foul-smelling or meconium-stained amniotic fluid
Prior stillbirth/early neonatal death		Cord prolapse
Prior birth of a high-risk infant		Narcotic administered to mother within 4 hours of birth
Antepartum hemorrhage		
Premature rupture of the membranes		
Serious infection during pregnancy		
Placental anomalies		

To identify newborns needing support rapidly and efficiently during the early neonatal transition, physicians should consider the American Academy of Pediatrics (AAP) guidelines, the most recent version of which was updated in 2020.

If a high-risk delivery is anticipated, individuals skilled in neonatal resuscitation should be present. If time permits, the team should meet with the parents to discuss the anticipated problems, plans for infant care, and address parental concerns to the best of their ability.

The following equipment should be prepared:

- Turned-on radiant warmer
- Opened oxygen source with adequate flow through the tubing
- Suctioning apparatus
- Laryngoscope
- Resuscitation bag and mask with adequate seal and generation of pressure

Upon the birth of any newborn, the following four questions should be asked:

1. Is this a term newborn?
2. Amniotic fluid clear or not?
3. Additional risk factors?
4. Umbilical cord management plan?

If, after considering the above four questions, no concerns are identified. The answer to all questions is yes; then the newborn should be dried, delayed cord clamping after placing skin to skin on the mother, and covered by a dry blanket to avoid heat loss. Such newborns simply need to be monitored for their respiratory pattern and their color.

If concerns are identified, then the newborn needs extra support and should be transferred to a bed equipped with a warmer. During the first 30 seconds, initial steps are done, and resuscitation aims to dry and stimulate the newborn, followed by clearing the airway. Suctioning the mouth is followed by the nose if necessary. Tactile stimulation to facilitate the respiratory effort. The primary assessment of breathing pattern, colour by pulse oximetry and heart rate should follow immediately after the above primary supportive steps have been taken. Heart rate assessment via chest auscultation is the initial preferred method. However, the electrocardiography is more accurate and rapid and should be used to confirm heart rate before the initiation of chest compression for bradycardia. If the newborn does not respond to these measures by establishing a strong cry and a heart rate above 100 bpm, the pediatrician should be paged, and the following sequential steps in resuscitation should be undertaken:

1. A baby who has heart rate below 100 bpm or is apneic needs to be started on positive-pressure ventilation with room air at a rate of 40 to 60 breaths per minute immediately and have the preductal circulation assessed using an oxygen saturation monitor attached to the right hand in conjunction with electrocardiographic (ECG) monitoring. The most sensitive indication of successful resuscitation is an increase in heart rate
2. If a prompt increase in heart rate does not happen, ventilation corrective steps known with the acronym "MRSOPA" should be performed. They include mask readjustment, repositioning airway by ensuring correct head position known as "sniffing position, suctioning mouth and nose, opening the mouth and tilting the jaw forward, increasing the pulse pressure variation (PPV) using increments of 5 to 10 cm H_2O

OTHER ISSUES

to maximum of 40 cm H_2O and using alternative airway as endotracheal intubation or laryngeal mask if the heart rate remains less than 100 bpm despite delivery of effective ventilation

3. At any point during the resuscitation, if newborn initiates strong breathing efforts and maintains a heart rate above 100 bpm, positive-pressure ventilation should be stopped, and free flow oxygen is administered as needed to maintain target preductal oxygen saturation by pulse oximetry monitoring. Consider the use of continuous positive airway pressure (CPAP) regardless of gestational age if labored breathing or persistent cyanosis are present with a heart rate ≥100 bpm. However, cautions should be taken due to increased risk of pneumothorax in term and late preterm infants when using high pressures

4. Chest compressions are indicated if the heart rate less than 60 bpm after 30 seconds of adequate ventilation with supplemental oxygen. Compressions should be delivered to the lower third of the sternum using a depth of approximately one-third of anteroposterior diameter of the chest. Two thumbs technique (both hands encircle the infant's chest with the thumbs on the sternum and the fingers under the infant) is preferred. Compressions and ventilation should be coordinated with a 3:1 ratio of compressions to ventilation. Coordinated chest compressions and ventilations should continue until the spontaneous heart rate is 60 bpm or above

5. If heart rate remains below 60 bpm despite adequate ventilation with 100 percent oxygen and chest compressions, administration of epinephrine, volume expansion, or both is indicated. If intravenous access has not yet been established, a higher dose of epinephrine can be administered via an endotracheal tube. Epinephrine may be repeated every 3 to 5 minutes if the heart rate remains less than 60 bpm. Hypovolemia in neonates is uncommon; hence volume resuscitation should only be considered if the heart rate remains less than 60 bpm despite adequate ventilation. Volume expanders can be normal saline (10 mL/kg over 5 to 10 minutes). O Rh-negative blood is preferred if there is evidence of blood/volume loss

6. Close monitoring should be provided to newborns who required resuscitation because they are at increased risk of deterioration after their vital signs returned to normal

7. In any newborn with an undetectable heart rate after 20 minutes of effective resuscitation, including intubation and the use of epinephrine, consideration should be given to redirection goals of care and discussion with members of the health care team and family discontinuing resuscitation

8. For detailed information on this topic, refer to the American Heart Association Guidelines for Cardiopulmonary Resuscitation and Emergency Cardiovascular Care 2020

Special Considerations

Oxygen and PPV

The AAP 2020 guidelines recommended the initial oxygen concentration for PPV for preterm infants born at less than 35 weeks' gestational age should be 21 to 30 percent, then adjusted to maintain the recommended target saturations. Initial support with CPAP is suggested if the baby has labored spontaneous breathing at an adequate respiratory rate. CPAP pressures of 5 to 8 cm H_2O may be considered. It is important to monitor ongoing respiratory status, because subsequent intubation may be required due to respiratory failure or for the administration of surfactant.

Temperature Control in Preterm Infants

Preterm infants are more prone to hypothermia because of their relatively large body surface area, decreased subcutaneous fat, and inability to produce enough heat. Hypothermia in the immediate period after delivery is associated with higher mortality and morbidities as intraventricular hemorrhage, respiratory distress, hypoglycemia, and pulmonary hemorrhage. The temperature should be maintained between 36.5°C and 37.5°C.

Hypothermia can be prevented by maintaining the delivery room temperature at 24 to 25°C, warm blankets, and removing wet blankets.

Additional interventions have been used to reduce hypothermia including head caps and polyurethane bags wrapped around babies with very low birth weight (<1500 g).

Delayed Cord Clamping

The AAP and the American College of Obstetricians and Gynecologists (ACOG) recommend delayed cord clamping (DCC) for at least 30 to 60 seconds after birth in both vigorous term infants and preterm. Studies have shown better hemodynamic stability in infants who had DCC and better hemoglobin and iron stores.

In preterm babies, DCC is appropriate if the baby is stable and immediate resuscitation is not required. It has been shown to reduce mortality and need for blood transfusion. However, it increases the risk of hyperbilirubinemia in term and preterm infants.

OTHER ISSUES

Antenatal Corticosteroids

Antenatal corticosteroids have been shown to reduce infant mortality in less than 24 weeks and reduce the incidence and severity of respiratory distress syndrome, circulatory instability, intraventricular hemorrhage, and necrotizing enterocolitis.

A single course of corticosteroids is recommended for pregnant women between 24^{+0} weeks and 34^{+6} weeks of gestation who are at risk of preterm delivery within 7 days as per ACOG and Society of Obstetricians and Gynaecologists of Canada (JOGC).

Antenatal corticosteroids should be considered for mothers at gestational age less than 24 weeks at risk of preterm delivery within 7 days based on a family's decision regarding resuscitation. It can also be considered for mothers at gestational age between 34^{+0} weeks and 36^{+6} weeks at risk of preterm birth within 7 days and who have not received a previous course of antenatal corticosteroids.

Magnesium Sulfate for Neuroprotection

Maternal treatment with magnesium sulfate has been shown to improve neurologic outcomes when administered before 30 weeks of gestation. Magnesium sulfate prophylaxis is recommended if the periviable delivery of a potentially viable infant is anticipated per ACOG recommendation.

APGAR Score

The APGAR score is a method of grading newborns; 0, 1, or 2 points are awarded for each of five signs, depending on their presence or absence (Table 39-2). The grading is done at 1 minute after birth and may be

TABLE 39-2: APGAR SCORING OF NEWBORNS

Sign	0 Points	1 Point	2 Points
Heart rate	Absent	Under 100	Over 100
Respiratory effort	Absent	Slow, irregular	Good, crying
Muscle tone	Limp	Flexion of extremities	Active motion
Reflex irritability: response to catheter in nostril	No response	Grimace	Cough or sneeze
Color	Blue-white	Body pink; extremities blue	Completely pink

repeated at 5 minutes. Most children are normal and fall in the 7- to 10-point range. A score of 3 to 6 indicates mild to moderate depression. When the APGAR score is 2 or less, the infant is severely depressed.

The APGAR scoring system has become established as the method by which the condition of babies is assessed immediately after birth. Recent investigations have shown that the APGAR score by itself is not a totally accurate index of the health of the neonate and that the predictive value of the system is limited. Analyses of blood from the umbilical cords of infants from mothers in the high-risk category revealed that many acidotic babies were born in a vigorous condition with high APGAR scores and that numerous infants with low APGAR scores did not have acidosis at birth. The conclusion is that although scoring the infant's condition by the APGAR criteria is important, other tests and examinations are necessary for a full assessment.

POOR POSTNATAL ADAPTATION

Respiratory Distress Syndrome

Respiratory distress syndrome (RDS) results from inadequate production or early inactivation of surfactant. Surfactant molecules form a layer over the interior of the alveoli, effectively reducing surface tension during expiration and preventing collapse. It mainly affects preterm infants, but it can certainly happen at term, especially after a nonlabor cesarean section.

In the immature lung, where surfactant is deficient, progressive alveolar collapse tends to occur with each expiration. Worsening lung compliance increases the work of breathing. Areas of atelectatic alveoli cause intrapulmonary shunting. The result of these changes is increasing respiratory failure and hypoxia. If left untreated, recovery may occur in time as surfactant production increases, or the baby may die in the absence of exhaustion or hypoxia treatment. At autopsy, the lungs are collapsed and airless. Histologically, the bronchioles and alveoli are lined with hyaline membranes composed of fibrin and cellular debris.

Clinical and Laboratory Findings

Evidence of respiratory difficulty immediately or within the first few hours of life is the classical clinical syndrome. There is indrawing of the sternum and lower ribs on inspiration, flaring of the alae nasi, and an audible expiratory grunt. The baby can be cyanotic in room air, but his or her color improves with the administration of oxygen.

The condition may stabilize. More typically, however, there is deterioration over the first 24 to 48 hours. The baby's oxygen requirements increase. As the infant tires, he or she becomes increasingly hypercarbic and begins to have apneic spells. Hypoxia and acidosis may cause a reversion to the fetal circulatory pattern with pulmonary vasoconstriction, a rise in pulmonary artery pressure, and right-to-left shunting through the still patent ductus arteriosus.

Because the signs of respiratory distress are nonspecific, chest x-ray is important for diagnosis. This will show small, poorly aerated lungs with a granular appearance, the result of areas of micro atelectasis. The airways stand out against the opaque lung fields as air bronchograms.

Prevention

Administering antenatal steroids to pregnant women at risk of preterm delivery less than 34 weeks of gestational age has been the main preventive measure.

Treatment

Positive-pressure ventilation is the mainstay of treatment. This can be done using CPAP machines without needing to intubate the newborn or by use of invasive mechanical ventilation. Surfactant therapy should be given to all infants who are still on a considerable amount of oxygen and need to be intubated.

Other therapies are essentially supportive. Oxygen is given as necessary. A neutral thermal environment is provided to minimize oxygen consumption. Blood gases, glucose, calcium, and electrolytes are monitored carefully.

Meconium Aspiration Syndrome

Meconium aspiration syndrome (MAS) is defined as respiratory distress in an infant born through a meconium-stained amniotic fluid (MSAF). Unlike RDS, which is mostly a disease of preterm infants, this condition is usually seen in term or postterm babies. Hallmarks of this syndrome include early onset of respiratory distress in a meconium-stained infant, hypoxia and characteristic radiologic lung appearances caused by chemical irritation, and physical partial or complete obstruction of small airways.

The incidence has declined due to changes in obstetrical care. It is reported to be 0.1 to 0.4 percent of births and approximately 2 to 10 percent of infants born with meconium-stained amniotic fluid.

Pathophysiology

Intrauterine stress may cause in utero passage of meconium into the amniotic fluid. Meconium staining of the amniotic fluid can probably be regarded as a physiologic finding that does not, in itself, indicate the presence of fetal distress. The great majority of infants born with meconium staining are well at birth and have no respiratory problems.

Thick meconium may cause partial or complete block of the airways causes lung collapses and pneumothorax. It can also induce inflammation of the lung leading to chemical pneumonitis. Although meconium is sterile, the mucopolysaccharide component provides an excellent growth medium for microorganisms and results in infection and pneumonia.

Clinical and Laboratory Findings

The infant shows signs of respiratory distress, with grunting, indrawing, and cyanosis in room air. Severe refractory hypoxia may result from the persistence of pulmonary hypertension. Chest x-ray shows the presence of areas of pulmonary collapse as well as areas of hyperinflation. Air leak with pneumothorax or pneumomediastinum is a common complication. The picture is frequently complicated by other signs of perinatal asphyxia, such as seizures and anuria.

Prevention

The most important form of management is prevention. This approach begins with recognition of high-risk pregnancies and maternal factors that may cause uteroplacental insufficiency and subsequent fetal hypoxia during delivery. In the presence of meconium staining, the fetus should be carefully monitored by continuous or periodic fetal heart monitoring to detect early evidence of suspected fetal compromise. In the presence of confirmed compromise, delivery should be accomplished promptly by cesarean section if necessary. Induction of labor should be done to women greater than 41 weeks' gestation, since MAS is higher in postterm infants.

Intrapartum and Delivery Room Management

Resuscitation of infants with meconium-stained amniotic fluid should be guided by the general neonatal resuscitation principles. Routine intubation and endotracheal suctioning of meconium is not recommended as per the American Academy of Pediatrics (AAP) and Canadian Paediatric

OTHER ISSUES

Society (CPS) to avoid delay in providing ventilation and preventing complications of intubation. Endotracheal intubation and tracheal suction may be beneficial when there is evidence of airway obstruction during positive pressure ventilation. Infants with meconium aspiration are at risk of pulmonary hypertension, air leak, and chemical pneumonitis and must be observed closely for signs of respiratory distress.

Treatment of established MAS is mainly supportive and follows the general principles described above for RDS such as maintaining adequate oxygenation and ventilation, and correction of any metabolic abnormality such as hypoglycemia and acidosis, which increase oxygen consumption. Infants with persistent pulmonary hypertension may have to be treated with high-frequency ventilation and inhaled nitric oxide. The CPS position statement recommends that intubated infants with MAS requiring more than 50 percent oxygen should receive surfactant therapy.

Perinatal Asphyxia

Asphyxia results from impairment of fetal blood supply and/or impairment of fetal gas exchange before or during delivery. In mild asphyxia, apnea is the principal clinical manifestation. In severe cases, the neonate presents with an abnormal level of consciousness or seizures, often accompanied by difficulty of breathing and decreased tone and reflexes.

The ACOG executive summary refers to this as *Neonatal Encephalopathy*. It is a general term in which hypoxic-ischemic encephalopathy (HIE) is included. The ACOG consensus states that the insult due to HIE is presumed to be associated with abnormal neonatal signs and contributing events close to labor and delivery that are consistent with an acute hypoxic-ischemic event.

Epidemiology

The incidence of HIE is approximately 1-6 in 1000 live births and higher in resource-limited countries. Moderate-to-severe HIE remains an important cause of mortality, acute neurological injury, and subsequent long-term neurodevelopmental disability despite advances in perinatal care.

The incidence of long-term complications depends on the severity of HIE. As many as 80 percent of infants who survive severe HIE develop serious complications, 10 to 20 percent develop moderate disabilities, and up to 10 percent are healthy. Among the infants who survive moderately severe HIE, 30 to 50 percent may have serious long-term complications, and 10 to 20 percent have minor neurologic morbidities. Infants with mild HIE tend to be free from serious neurological complications.

Diagnostic Criteria for Perinatal Asphyxia

Guidelines from the AAP and ACOG for HIE indicate that all of the following must be present for the designation of perinatal asphyxia severe enough to result in acute neurologic injury:

1. "Sentinel" obstetric event (e.g., uterine rupture, placental abruption) occurring immediately before or during labor
2. Low Apgar scores less than 5 at 5 minutes and 10 minutes
3. Profound metabolic acidosis in fetal umbilical cord arterial blood obtained at delivery (pH <7, base excess [BE] ≥12) in an umbilical artery blood sample
4. Evidence of multiorgan dysfunction (e.g., kidney, lungs, liver, heart, intestines)
5. Early-onset neonatal encephalopathy seen on brain MRI or magnetic resonance spectroscopy consistent with hypoxia-ischemia
6. Exclusion of other causes of neonatal encephalopathy (e.g., congenital anomalies of the central nervous system)
7. Spastic quadriplegic or dyskinetic cerebral palsy

Supportive Management

The initial evaluation should be done to determine the presence and extent of end-organ damage, identify a possible etiology or concomitant condition that requires specific therapy, and obtain a baseline to compare changes in organ function over time. The management of depressed infants is mostly supportive intensive care. Intervention strategies aiming to avoid any further brain injury in these infants include immediate resuscitation of any infant with apnea following NRP guidelines, and maintain adequate oxygenation and ventilation. Cardiovascular support may be required, and inotropic agents may be used to support cardiac function for infants with evidence of myocardial failure. On the first day of life, infants are maintained on intravenous fluids of 10 percent dextrose without additional sodium and potassium at 60 cc/kg per day. This degree of fluid restriction is to avoid the risk of water retention due to acute kidney injury and the potential risk of the syndrome of inappropriate antidiuretic hormone (SIADH).

Therapeutic Hypothermia

The ACOG recommends comprehensive clinical assessment to determine eligibility for therapeutic hypothermia.

OTHER ISSUES

It is the only proven neuroprotective therapy for neonatal encephalopathy, started within the first 6 hours after delivery and continued for 72 hours. It has become the standard of care for infants with moderate-to-severe HIE.

Eligibility Criteria. The AAP recommends starting hypothermia for term and late preterm infants ≥36 weeks' gestation with HIE who are ≤6 hours old and who meet either treatment criteria A or treatment criteria B, and also meet criteria C:

A. Cord pH ≤7.0 or base deficit ≥−16 **OR**
B. pH 7.01 to 7.15 or base deficit −10 to −15.9 on cord gas or blood gas within 1 h **AND** History of an acute perinatal event (such as but not limited to cord prolapse, placental abruption or uterine rupture) and Apgar score ≤5 at 10 minutes or at least 10 minutes of positive-pressure ventilation
C. Evidence of moderate-to-severe encephalopathy demonstrated by the presence of seizures **OR** at least one sign in three or more of the six categories of Sarnat staging

Assessment should be done to depressed infants at birth to determine whether they meet criteria A or B. Infants who fulfill criteria A or B should then undergo a careful neurological examination to decide whether or not they fulfill criteria C. Infants who meet criteria A and C, or B and C, should be offered hypothermia.

Target Temperature. The optimal rectal temperature is 33 to 34°C. Passive cooling (e.g., removing the infant's hat, blanket, and turning off an overhead warmer) should be initiated in community hospitals, following consultation with a receiving neonatologist. Rectal temperature should be monitored every 15 minutes to ensure the infant's temperature does not decrease below 33°C.

Contraindications of Hypothermia

- Major congenital or genetic abnormalities for which no further aggressive treatment is planned.
- Infants with severe intrauterine growth restriction
- Infants with clinically significant coagulopathy and infants with evidence of severe head trauma or intracranial bleeding.

Side Effects of Hypothermia

- Bradycardia (heart rate of 80-100 bpm)
- Hypotension with possible need for inotropes
- Persistent pulmonary hypertension with impaired oxygenation
- Infants with HIE, whether they receive therapeutic hypothermia or not, are more prone to arrhythmias, hypoglycemia, hypokalemia, urinary retention, and coagulopathy

Consequences of Perinatal Asphyxia

The initial physiologic response to perinatal asphyxia is redistribution of blood flow from the nonvital organs (e.g., liver, kidney, intestine, skin, and splanchnic area) to the vital organs (brain, heart). At least one organ dysfunction other than the brain develops in infants with moderate to severe HIE. Systemic effects of perinatal asphyxia may be present even in the absence of encephalopathy. Severe perinatal asphyxia has a profound impact on almost every organ system. Some of the most important of these are as follows.

Central Nervous System. HIE results in extensive neural damage or destruction. The neonatal period may be complicated by an altered state of consciousness, seizures, disturbances of tone and activity, and signs of damage to the brain stem (e.g., apnea, instability of temperature). The rate of mortality is significant, and morbidity occurs in the form of mental retardation, deafness, cortical blindness, and cerebral palsy. However, only 10 percent of cerebral palsy cases are believed to have an intrapartum origin.

Respiratory System. Asphyxia increases the incidence of RDS, probably because of damage to the surfactant producing type 2 alveolar cells and the persistent pulmonary hypertension. Pulmonary hemorrhage may also complicate asphyxia

Cardiovascular System. Profound hypoxia can cause acute myocardial failure and severe hypotension. In such cases, the electrocardiogram will show changes consistent with myocardial ischemia.

Urinary System. Renal function is commonly impaired after severe perinatal asphyxia. Anuria or oliguria result from acute tubular necrosis. Cortical necrosis may also occur. In most cases, the changes are reversible, but occasionally, chronic renal disease results.

OTHER ISSUES

BIRTH INJURIES

Birth injury is defined as an impairment of the neonate's body function or structure due to an adverse event that occurred at birth. Injury may occur during labor, delivery, or after delivery. With advances in obstetric practice, the incidence of birth injuries has significantly decreased. However, they are still considered a major cause of neonatal morbidity.

They range from minor problems to severe injuries that may result in significant neonatal morbidity or mortality. Risk factors include macrosomia, maternal obesity, abnormal fetal presentation, operative vaginal delivery, small maternal stature, maternal pelvic anomalies, and primiparous women.

Soft Tissue Injuries

Bruising and Petechiae
They are usually self-limited and seen in the presenting part of the newborn. Petechia are present at birth, do not progress or are associated with bleeding. Significant bruising is a major risk factor for the development of hyperbilirubinemia requiring close follow-up.

Lacerations
The most common birth injury is associated with cesarian delivery and more commonly on the presenting part of the fetus, typically the scalp and face.

Subcutaneous Fat Necrosis
Uncommon and usually occurs in the first few weeks of life adjacent to a bony structure due to adipose tissue ischemia following a traumatic delivery. It is self-limiting and resolves by 6 to 8 weeks of age. Long-term follow-up is required for the development of hypercalcemia.

Ocular Injuries

Common minor ocular injuries include retinal and subconjunctival hemorrhages and lid edema. They resolve spontaneously without affecting the newborn within 1 to 5 days for the retinal hemorrhage and 1 to 2 weeks for the subconjunctival hemorrhage. They are usually associated with forceps-assisted delivery.

Nasal Septal Dislocation

It occurs due to compression of the nose from the maternal symphysis pubis or sacral promontory during labor. It can present with respiratory distress due to airway obstruction. The examination reveals deviation of the nose to one side with asymmetric nares and flattening of the dislocated side. Manual reduction should be performed by 3 days of age to prevent nasal septal deformity.

Caput Succedaneum

It is an edematous swelling of the scalp above the periosteum and occurs after prolonged engagement of the fetal head in the birth canal or after vacuum extraction. Except for rare, very severe cases, the newborn is usually asymptomatic and resolves within few days with no special intervention is necessary. The differentiating sign of caput secundum is that the superficial edema may pass the suture line and fontanels.

Cephalohematoma

It presents as demarcated with sharp borders swelling that does not cross suture lines as a result of a subperiosteal collection of blood caused by rupture of vessels beneath the periosteum (usually over the parietal or occipital bone). Prolonged vaginal deliveries and the use of forceps are risk factors. It does not cause significant blood loss and rarely expands after delivery. It usually resolves spontaneously over few weeks. Up to 5 percent of affected newborns may have an underlying skull fracture. Rarely, calcification of the hematoma can occur with a subsequent bony swelling that may persist for months, causing significant skull deformities.

Subgaleal Hemorrhage

Occurs when blood accumulates in the loose connective tissue of the subgaleal space as a result of traction on the scalp during delivery. It can be considered the most important type of extracranial bleeding due to a higher mortality rate, which contributes to massive blood loss (20-40% of a neonate's blood volume resulting in a loss of 50 to 100 mL) into the subgaleal space. Usually, it appears as fluctuating edema crossing the suture line and fontanel, which spreads over to the neck and back of the ears as bleeding progresses. Expansion of the swelling due to continued bleeding may occur hours to days after delivery. A newborn physical examination should take place after all attempted vacuum or difficult operative deliveries.

These infants should be observed closely with ongoing monitoring, including frequent vital signs (minimally every hour) and serial measurements of hematocrits and head circumference.

Intracranial Hemorrhages

Intracranial hemorrhages include subdural, subarachnoid, epidural, intraventricular hemorrhages, and less frequently, intracerebral and intracerebellar hemorrhages.

Subdural Hemorrhage

The most common type of intracranial hemorrhage in neonates. Vacuum extraction, forceps or cesarian section increase the risk of subdural hemorrhage. It can be asymptomatic and discovered incidentally or symptomatic presenting with signs of neurologic dysfunction such as irritability, altered tone and level of consciousness and seizures, respiratory depression, and apnea within the first 24 to 48 hours of life that can be managed conservatively without surgical intervention due to the plasticity of the neonatal skull. Rarely, it is associated with increased intracranial pressure necessitating urgent surgical evacuation.

Subarachnoid Hemorrhage

The second most commonly neonatal intracranial hemorrhage. Bleeding occurs into the subarachnoid space, the interval between the arachnoid membrane and pia mater. Small subarachnoid hemorrhages can happen in preterm infants without causing any symptoms. Infants with large subarachnoid hemorrhage present at 24 to 48 hours of life with nonspecific neurologic signs and symptoms such as irritability or seizures, apnea and respiratory depression. The diagnosis is made by CT of the head or, in nonemergent scenarios, MRI of the head.

Epidural Hemorrhage

It occurs as a result of injury to the middle meningeal artery between the dura and inner table of the skull. It is very rare in neonates. It is often accompanied by a linear skull fracture. Infants with epidural hemorrhage can present with nonspecific neurologic symptoms, such as seizures and hypotonia or signs of increased intracranial pressure as bulging fontanelle, changes in vital signs, and level of consciousness in large hemorrhages. It can deteriorate quickly because of the arterial source of bleeding. CT or MRI of the head can help differentiate it from subdural hemorrhage, and the infant should be followed closely with neurosurgery.

Intracerebellar Hemorrhage

Intracerebellar hemorrhage mainly happens in preterm infants. It has been reported in up to 2.5 percent of preterm infants and even higher on autopsy results. The prognosis is guarded.

Intraventricular Hemorrhage

Intraventricular hemorrhage (IVH) is the most concerning of all intracranial hemorrhages. The overall incidence of IVH is estimated at 10 to 20 percent, which has declined during recent decades. This type of hemorrhage is caused by the prominence of germinal matrix vessels, which regress by term. Therefore, most IVHs happen in infants below 32-weeks' gestational age. A screening ultrasound is necessary for the diagnosis. Intraventricular hemorrhage in full-term infants occurs as a consequence of birth injury. In the absence of a clotting disorder or severe asphyxia, most IVH in term infants resolves spontaneously with no long-term sequelae. There are four types of intraventricular hemorrhage, previously named as grades I to IV:

a. Subependymal germinal matrix hemorrhage
b. IVH with no ventricular dilatation
c. IVH with ventricular dilatation
d. IVH associated with intraparenchymal hemorrhage

Infants with IVH accompanied by ventricular dilatation or intraparenchymal bleeding are at risk of developing hydrocephalus and have poor long-term neurodevelopment outcomes.

Bony Injuries

Skull Fracture

Neonatal skull fractures, although uncommon, can happen secondary to a forceful vaginal delivery or a forceps-assisted delivery. Linear skull fractures develop due to pressure upon the soft fetal skull during labor and delivery from maternal structures. Linear skull fractures can be completely asymptomatic except if associated with internal bleeding or injury. Linear skull fractures at the base of the skull can be particularly dangerous, with severe hemorrhage from the underlying venous system. This type of linear fracture is more common in breech deliveries. Uncomplicated linear fractures do not need any intervention. However, in case of hemorrhage or cerebrospinal fluid leak in basal skull fracture, appropriate supportive treatment, including transfusions and antibiotic therapy, should be considered.

Depressed fractures are usually associated with forceps assisted delivery and occur because of inward buckling of the skull bones. It is associated with an increased risk of intracranial bleeding and/or cephalohematoma. Neurosurgical consultation should be done in infants with evidence of an intracranial hemorrhage and if the depression is greater than 1 cm.

Clavicle Fracture

This is the most common bony injury, and risk factors include instrumental delivery, shoulder dystocia, increased maternal age, and increased birth weight. Displaced (complete) fractures are usually diagnosed early because they are more likely to be accompanied by physical findings in the immediate postdelivery time period such as crepitus, edema, lack of movement of the affected extremity, asymmetrical bone contour, and crying with passive motion.

Nondisplaced fractures are commonly asymptomatic and diagnosed late with the formation of a visible or palpable callous. They heal spontaneously with no long-term sequelae. The arm on the affected side can be placed in a long-sleeved garment for comfort.

Humerus Fracture

Humeral fractures are rare. They are associated with shoulder dystocia, macrosomia, cesarean delivery, breech delivery, and low birth weight. They present with decreased movement of the affected arm, decreased Moro reflex, localized swelling, and crepitation. A careful examination should be done to rule out brachial plexus injury because it is a common association with humeral fractures. Usually, no treatment is required other than stabilization against the thorax by an elastic wrap or long-sleeved shirt with the elbow in 90 degrees flexion to prevent rotational deformities. However, they need assessment and follow-up by a pediatric orthopedic surgery team

Femur Fracture

Femur fractures are uncommon, usually spiral, and located in the proximal half of the femur. Risk factors are twin pregnancies, breech presentations, and prematurity. A pop or a snap may be heard in infants delivered by vaginal breech extraction.

Sternomastoid Muscle

A firm, painless swelling may be palpated in the midportion of the sternomastoid muscle at birth or within the first 1 to 2 weeks. It was postulated that this was fibrosis related to a hemorrhage into the muscle after birth trauma.

In the absence of treatment, shortening of the muscle can occur with the production of torticollis and eventual deformation of the skull. A regular program of passive stretching of the involved muscle should avoid this outcome and obviate the need for surgical intervention.

Injury to Peripheral Nerves

Brachial Plexus Palsy

Brachial plexus palsy is uncommon with an incidence of 0.15 percent as per ACOG. The network of nerves is fragile and can be damaged by stretching, which can occur when the head and neck are forced away from the shoulder; such injury might happen during breech delivery when there is difficulty with the arms and in cephalic presentations with shoulder dystocia. Brachial plexus palsy is most commonly unilateral and can be divided into three subtypes.

Erb's Palsy. This accounts for approximately 50 percent of cases involving C5 and C6. The arm hangs limply by the side and is rotated internally. The elbow is extended, but the wrist and fingers' flexion is preserved, giving rise to the so-called "waiter's tip" position. The possibility of phrenic nerve injury (C3, C4, and C5) should be considered, and diaphragmatic paralysis excluded.

Klumpke Paralysis. This involves the C8 and Tl. There is a weakness of the wrist and finger flexors and the small muscles of the hand. A true isolated Klumpke palsy is extremely rare. The term is sometimes loosely applied when there is total brachial plexus palsy. This pattern of injury is much less common than Erb's palsy. The prognosis is worse than in Erb's palsy.

Total Plexus Injury. This involves all brachial nerves, C5 to T1. The newborn will have a flaccid arm with absent reflexes throughout.

Management. Daily physical therapy and observation for evidence of recovery is the main treatment method. Physical therapy aims to prevent contractures starting early in the first week of life. Supportive splints may be used. Several surgical techniques can aid recovery if functional recovery does not ensue within 3 to 9 months. In general, if a physical examination shows incomplete recovery by 3 to 4 weeks, full recovery is unlikely. If there are no signs of improvement by 3 to 6 months, spontaneous recovery is unlikely, and surgical exploration (nerve transfer) can be considered. Otherwise, the damage will most likely be permanent.

Facial Nerve

Injury to the facial nerve usually occurs distal to its emergence from the skull. The result is a weakness of the muscles on the affected side of the face. The characteristic signs are the failure of one side of the mouth to move and the eyelid to close. An oblique application of obstetric forceps may compress the nerve. However, this may occur after spontaneous vaginal delivery. It has been suggested that the lesion might result from pressure on the face from the sacral promontory. Clinical presentation depends on the site of injury. In central paralysis, forehead muscle function remains intact. In peripheral paralysis, the entire side of the face will be affected, and the newborn will have difficulty closing the eye on the affected side.

Treatment is limited to the protection of the eye when it is involved. Methylcellulose eye drops are applied, and the eye should be taped shut to avoid corneal injury.

The prognosis for affected infants is good. There is some return of function in most cases in 2 to 3 weeks and complete recovery by 2 to 3 months.

Injury to the Spinal Cord

Spinal cord injuries in neonates are most commonly secondary to difficult deliveries, especially breech deliveries or those associated with extensive traction during labor. Upper cervical injuries are the most common type. Ligamentous laxity and the lack of muscular support are the main causes of neonates' vulnerability to spinal cord damage without obvious vertebral fractures. However, in any neonate with suspicion of spinal cord injury, vertebral fractures should be ruled out. MRI is the modality of choice.

Clinical Outcome

The clinical outcome may be divided into four groups:

1. Stillbirth or early neonatal death because of lower brain stem injury
2. Respiratory failure leading to death or permanent ventilator dependence
3. Long-term survival with paralysis or weakness of the limbs
4. Survival with minimal neurologic damage. Most of these develop spasticity later and maybe erroneously diagnosed as having cerebral palsy

Management

Management is essentially supportive. There is little evidence that there is a place for neurosurgical intervention in spinal cord injury. Supportive care, including mechanical ventilation and physiotherapy, minimizes disability in less severely affected infants.

Abdominal Injuries

Abdominal injuries are not common and include mainly rupture or subcapsular hemorrhage into the liver, spleen, and adrenal glands.

Hepatic Rupture

The liver is the organ most often injured or lacerated. A subcapsular hematoma may develop, increasing in size until it ruptures into the peritoneal cavity. Infants are at increased risk if they have hepatomegaly (e.g., infants of diabetic mothers), coagulation disorders, or are asphyxiated at birth, preterm or postterm, or delivered breeches.

Splenic Rupture

This accident is less common than injury to the liver. Splenomegaly increases the danger of its occurrence. The clinical presentation is dependent upon the amount of blood loss. Infants may need urgent resuscitation and transfer to a tertiary care center for further management.

PERINATAL MORTALITY

The accurate and timely reporting of live birth and fetal and infant death is the cornerstone of perinatal mortality data. Because reducing fetal and infant mortality is among any nation's health goals, accurate definitions of these events are essential for understanding causes and researching potential solutions.

Perinatal mortality is defined as the sum of intrauterine deaths plus deaths in infants' first 7 days of life, expressed per 1000 total births. The most recent data for Ontario, Canada, showed perinatal mortality of seven per 1000 total births in 2007. This is roughly split equally between stillbirths (fetal deaths) and neonatal mortality.

Stillbirth

Deaths before or during delivery (stillbirths) are most commonly caused by anoxia. These may be associated with:

1. Placental insufficiency in which the placenta is small or its function impaired by infarcts or disease. There is usually evidence of decreased fetal growth, and some of these deaths may be avoidable by careful monitoring and early delivery when indicated

OTHER ISSUES

2. Antepartum hemorrhage, especially abruptio placentae. This accident can occur as an emergency 1 to 2 months before term and may result in immediate fetal death caused by extensive placental separation

3. Umbilical cord problems: Prolapse of the cord carries a high risk of fetal death. Knots or loops in the cord are considered causes of fetal death only when they are very tight, and no other cause can be found

4. Maternal disease, especially diabetes. The risk of sudden unexpected fetal death has been much reduced by improved medical care of pregnant women with diabetes

5. Abnormalities of labor and delivery such as breech presentation and prolonged labor, particularly in underresourced settings

Neonatal Death

Early neonatal deaths are most commonly related to:

1. *Preterm delivery* with its attendant complications, especially RDS and intraventricular hemorrhage. Some infants born at 25 weeks' gestation or less show inadequate lung development to allow for gas exchange

2. *Congenital malformations:* Abnormalities causing early death include extensive lesions of the central nervous system and severe forms of congenital heart disease, especially the hypoplastic left heart syndrome. Pulmonary hypoplasia, incompatible with life, accompanies Potter syndrome and many cases of diaphragmatic hernia

3. *Infection:* Bacterial infections remain a serious problem in the neonatal period. The organism most frequently associated with overwhelming infection in term newborns is group B, beta-hemolytic streptococcus, while in preterm infants, *Escherichia coli* was recently found to be the most common cause of sepsis. Pneumonia or generalized sepsis may result, especially in preterm infants, with a very high mortality rate

4. *Intrapartum asphyxia or trauma:* Deaths from these causes have been reduced because of better fetal monitoring and the more judicious use of cesarean section. However, unexpected complications continue to cause occasional neonatal deaths

SELECTED READING

American Academy of Pediatrics. Committee on Fetus and Newborn; Papile LA, Baley JE, et al: Hypothermia and neonatal encephalopathy. Pediatrics 133:1146-1150, 2014

American College of Obstetricians and Gynecologists: Executive summary: Neonatal encephalopathy and neurologic outcome. Obstet Gynecol 123:896-901, 2014

Demissie K, Rhoads GG, Smulian JC, et al: Operative vaginal delivery and neonatal and infant adverse outcomes: population based retrospective analysis. BMJ 329:24, 2004

Drury PP, Gunn ER, Bennet L, Gunn AJ: Mechanisms of hypothermic neuroprotection. Clin Perinatol 41:161–75, 2014

Ferriero DM: Neonatal brain injury. N Engl J Med 351:1985-1995, 2004

Gluckman PD, Wyatt JS, Azzopardi D, et al: Selective head cooling with mild systemic hypothermia after neonatal encephalopathy: Multicentre randomised trial. Lancet 365:663-670, 2005

Holden R, Morsman DG, Davidek GM, et al: External ocular trauma in instrumental and normal deliveries. Br J Obstet Gynaecol 99:132, 1992

Kilani RA, Wetmore J: Neonatal subgaleal hematoma: presentation and outcome–radiological findings and factors associated with mortality. Am J Perinatol 23:41, 2006

Podoshin L, Gertner R, Fradis M, Berger A: Incidence, and treatment of deviation of nasal septum in newborns. Ear Nose Throat J 70:485, 1991

Smit E, Liu X, Jary S, Cowan F, Thoresen M: Cooling neonates who do not fulfil the standard cooling criteria—short- and long-term outcomes. Acta Paediatr 104: 38-45, 2015

Whitby EH, Griffiths PD, Rutter S, et al: Frequency and natural history of subdural haemorrhages in babies and relation to obstetric factors. Lancet 363:846, 2004

CHAPTER 40

Medical Education and Simulation-Based Training

Adam Garber

If the license to practice meant the completion of 'their' education how sad it would be for the practitioner, how distressing to 'their' patients! More clearly than other the physician should illustrate the truth of Plato's saying that education is a life-long process.

—*William Osler*

Osler W: An address on The Importance of Post-graduate Study. Lancet 156:73-75, 1900

INTRODUCTION

Ongoing education and team training are paramount to the provision of safe obstetrical care. The burden of evidence pointing toward this continues to grow (Satin, 2018). The paradigm of "see one, do one, teach one" has given way to deliberate practice in simulated and native contexts.

This chapter aims to provide practical information that may facilitate departmental educational mandates. For this purpose, the chapter includes four sections: fundamental aspects of educational theory, curriculum design, team training and simulation-based education, and current and future directions in education.

FUNDAMENTAL ASPECTS OF EDUCATIONAL THEORY

This section describes three theoretical lenses that can serve to inform medical education and team development.

Andragogy—Adult Learning

As learners progress from children to adults, they bring with them a growing set of skills, experiences, and values. Although there is overlap, andragogy—"the art and science of helping adults learn"—possesses some distinct assumptions and principles from those of pedagogy (Knowles, 1984). Malcolm Knowles identified assumptions and principles of adult learning that can be used to inform curricular initiatives. Such initiatives acknowledge, build on, or even challenge learner's existing knowledge and skills (Mukhulalati and Taylor, 2019).

Principles of andragogy serve to guide the creation of educational interventions for adult learners in several ways (Knowles, Kauffman):

- The learning environment should be safe and empower learners to express themselves
- Curriculum should be learner-centered, and learners should be involved in curriculum planning
- Learners should help in assessing their own learning needs, create their own objectives, and identify resources/strategies that will assist in accomplishing these objectives
- Teachers should support learners in carrying out their devised plans to accomplish their learning objectives
- Learners should reflect on their experience and evaluate their own learning

Experiential Learning—Learning by Doing

Experiential learning emphasizes the importance of actual experience in the process of education. Kolb's experiential learning cycle describes four stages in an ongoing cycle of learning (see Fig. 40-1). This "begins" with a concrete experience that could take place in a real clinical environment or in a simulated context. The learners then go through a process of reflection that leads to forming new ideas or modifying existing ones. Learners then actively test these new ideas, which leads to new experiences and the cycle starts over.

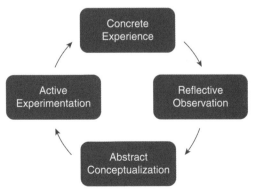

FIGURE 40-1. Kolb—Learning styles and experiential learning cycle. (Modified from Kolb DA (1984). Experiential learning: experience as the source of learning and development. Englewood Cliffs, NJ: Prentice Hall.)

OTHER ISSUES

For example, learners participate in a simulated case of managing a patient with postpartum hemorrhage—a concrete experience. They then undergo a debrief where they reflect on the experience—an opportunity for reflective observation. They decide that they may need to change their tone of voice when leading the scenarios so that others will feel more comfortable speaking up around them—an abstract conceptualization. They then practice their new tone of voice in the next simulated case—active experimentation. This leads to new experiences and the cycle continues.

Kolb's experiential learning cycle forms a major theoretical underpinning for workplace-based and simulation-based education (discussed later in this chapter).

Situated Learning—Learning in a Social Context

The situated learning model posits that learning occurs through interactions within specific contexts and communities and recognizes the socialization processes that occur in health professions education. This model serves as a lens through which to examine the learning environment. Apprenticeship, for example, is conceived as taking place within a whole community, whereby learners are provided with support commensurate with their level of training and are given more independence as they achieve competence with a particular task.

The situated learning model also highlights the relevance of the informal curriculum, the curriculum that runs parallel to the formal curriculum. This includes the "hidden curriculum"—an area of increasing inquiry found in the implicit lessons learned from the procedures, policies, and practice habits of communities and institutions that reflect their values (Hafferty and Franks, 1994). For example, if learners are assessed only through multiple choice examinations, learners may internalize the notion that other aspects or professional practice such as health advocacy and collaboration are less important. The hidden curriculum is not inherently negative or positive but rather an important element of institutional insight.

CURRICULUM DESIGN

"If we teach today's students as we taught yesterday's, we rob them of tomorrow."

—*John Dewey*

This section addresses the concept of curriculum and describes its design using a particular model—Kern's six-step model. However, many other models of both curriculum design and instructional design exist. These are practical models that can be used by educators to create and implement curriculum.

Curriculum and Instructional Design

A curriculum document is a living document that lays out an educational plan. It includes the following components (Grant, 2013):

- Tells the learner what the content will be, how it will be organized, how learning will be assessed, and how learners will be supported
- Guides the teacher on how to facilitate learning by delivering content and supporting the learner
- Outlines to the educators and the institution the ways in which the curriculum will be evaluated for ongoing improvement
- Takes into account not only clinical content but also local context, professional values, and social accountability
- Evolves in accordance with its evaluation

In developing a curriculum, both curriculum and instructional design, are relevant (Grant, 2013). While somewhat overlapping constructs, curriculum design focuses more on the content: what is being taught, in what order, and—to some extent—how the material can be taught. Instructional design focuses on creating efficient and engaging learning experiences for individuals and teams.

Kern's Six-Step Framework for Curriculum Design

It is useful to follow a structure when creating a curriculum. This ensures a systematic approach that is more likely to be focused, feasible, complete, considerate of existing resources, and socially accountable. Kern's six-step framework provides such a structure (Fig. 40-2).

Needs Assessment
The development of a new curriculum begins by identifying a gap through a needs assessment process. This identification of a need for a new curriculum may come from many sources including: (1) a change in unit protocols; (2) the implementation of a novel technology; (3) case reviews of

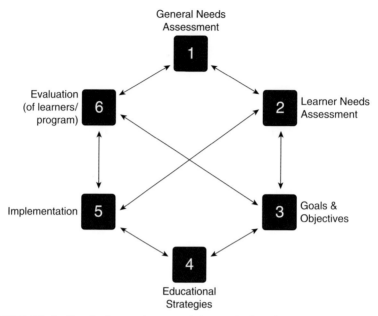

FIGURE 40-2. Kern's six-step framework for curriculum design. (Kern, Thomas, and Hughes, 1998).

quality improvement findings; (4) team-based, interprofessional, and multidisciplinary challenges; and (5) new or changing practice guidelines.

Learner Needs Assessment

A targeted needs assessment considers the needs and characteristics of the learners and the contexts in which they work. Since adult learners are motivated and self-directed, they can actively contribute to this needs assessment.

Goals and Objectives

The overarching aims of the curriculum should be stated. It can be helpful to utilize an organizing framework such as the CanMEDS framework from the Royal College of Physicians and Surgeons of Canada (Frank et al., 2015).

Learning objectives describe what a learner should be able to do after completing a learning activity. Helpful tips for constructing well-written learning objectives include (Chatterjee and Corral, 2017):

1. The **KSA** Pneumonic—A learning objective outlines the **K**nowledge, **S**kills, and/or **A**ttitude to be gained by the learning activity
2. The **SMART** Pnemonic—A learning objective ought to be **S**pecific, **M**easurable, **A**ttainable, **R**elevant, and **T**ime-bound
3. Blooms' Taxonomy—Bloom described six cognitive domains in a hierarchy (remember, understand, apply, analyze, evaluate, create) and attached action verbs to each cognitive domain. This table helps the writer incorporate the relevant action verbs into the learning objective

Educational Modalities

Upon completing the learning objectives, the educational modalities of the curriculum must be set. This component describes both the core content and how the content will be delivered. A range of educational modalities exist, such as didactic lectures, flipped classroom approaches, problem-based learning, E-learning, simulation, and workplace-based learning. Choosing the most appropriate educational tools requires the consideration of available resources (time, equipment, and personnel) and of learner characteristics. The benefits and drawbacks of a given modality must also be considered.

Implementation

The implementation section of a curriculum moves beyond which educational modalities will be utilized. It answers the "who, what, when, and where" questions.

Assessment and Evaluation

A given curriculum must make clear its approach to assessment of the learners and evaluation of the curriculum. Assessment refers to the judgment of a learner's or team's performance. Evaluation refers to the judgment of the curriculum and educational program Assessment, broadly speaking, can be understood as *formative* or *summative*. Formative assessments refer to assessments that are not used to make decisions about progression through a training program and instead are only for the sake of learning itself. Summative assessments are, in addition to their contribution to learning, used to make judgments that contribute to decisions regarding progression through a training program. The intention of an assessment—formative or summative—should be explicitly articulated in a curriculum document.

Miller's Prism of Clinical Competence (Fig. 40-3) helps explicate the hierarchy of assessments most used in health professions education.

OTHER ISSUES

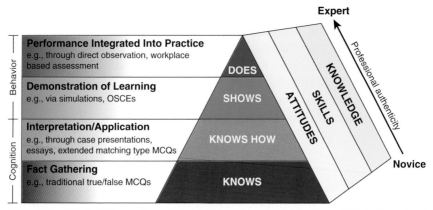

FIGURE 40-3. Miller's Pyramid of Clinical Competence. (From Miller's Pyramid of Clinical Competence by R. Mehay and R. Burns In The Essential Handbook for GP Training and Education by R. Mehay (Ed.). Copyright © 2009 by CRC Press. Reproduced by permission of Taylor & Francis Group.)

Workplace-based assessment resides at the top of the pyramid as this assesses the clinician's actual practice while multiple choice questions reside at the bottom of the pyramid because they reflect pure factual knowledge possessed by the clinician.

Through both informal means and formal means such as questionnaires and focus groups, among others, a curriculum must be evaluated and iterated. This evaluation data forms a portion of the ongoing needs assessment and can contribute to ongoing curricular improvements.

INTERPROFESSIONAL EDUCATION AND SIMULATION-BASED EDUCATION

Providing intrapartum care is a complex task. The birthing unit is reliably unreliable, and crises are sure to occur. When they do happen, it is rarely the action of a single individual that influences a patient outcome but rather the cumulative response of the interprofessional team. Given that health care is delivered in teams, it follows that a component of training should also be team-based. For this reason, interprofessional education and simulation are increasingly understood to be essential to improving patient safety and quality of care.

Interprofessional Education

Interprofessional education (IPE) is the deliberate practice of bringing together different professions to participate in a specific educational task such as case-based learning or simulation. In addition to learning alongside individuals of other professions, IPE is unique in that a primary focus is to learn from and about each other's professional practice in order to come to a deeper understanding of team members' contributions to care and, in so doing, gain competence as a team (Freeth, 2013).

There is good and growing evidence that well-designed interprofessional education improves patient outcomes, patient-centred communication, and team functioning. Paramount to any IPE effort is the involvement of the relevant professions in the design and implementation of an educational activity. For example, in training teams to manage a critically ill preeclamptic patient, it is essential to involve obstetrical, nursing, anesthesia, and perhaps internal medicine in the design of the learning activity such as the creation of a case for review or the creation of a simulation scenario.

Simulation-based Education

Simulation is a broad reaching term referring to any learning activity that mimics an authentic component of clinical experience to give individuals or teams an opportunity to practice or demonstrate a particular task and its accompanying skill set. Simulation is not inherently an expensive, resource intensive activity—although it can be. Simulation does not require a comprehensive simulation center, nor does it require elaborate costly manikins. Just like other educational modalities, once the intended learning outcome is defined, a simulation activity can be designed to achieve this outcome in as simple and inexpensive a way as possible.

The use of simulation dates back at least as far as the 18th century when Madam Coudray created "Le Machine," a part-task trainer, to teach midwives and surgeons about labor and birth.

A range of simulators exist that aid in obstetrical education. Five common types of simulators include part-task trainers, integrated simulators, virtual reality simulators, simulated patients, and hybrid simulators.

Part-task Trainers include objects that provide the opportunity to practice specific tasks, such as a birthing pelvis or a synthetic arm for venipuncture. Common objects can be used for this purpose as well. For example, an orange can also be considered a part-task trainer when used to practice punch biopsies of the skin. The *PROMPT* pelvis is an example

OTHER ISSUES

of a birthing pelvis part-task trainer that, when coupled with a training program, has been shown to decrease the sequelae of shoulder dystocia at participating centers in the United Kingdom and elsewhere (Draycott et al. 2008).

Integrated simulators or *High Fidelity Manikins* such as *SimMom* are manikins connected to a computer. Their physiologic output such as their palpable pulses or breathing can be adjusted. Their vital signs are typically displayed on an electronic monitor. These outputs can be adjusted by instructors in real time according to the actions of those participating in the simulation.

Virtual reality simulators allow the learner to interact with a specific clinical environment through images seen on a screen or, more recently, a three-dimensional headset. Some virtual simulators possess haptic systems that provide the tactile component of a clinical skill that the learner experiences while interacting with the virtual reality-based simulation.

Simulated patients are people trained to simulate patients, portray their particular clinical presentations, and respond in real time to the actions of the participants.

Hybrid simulators combine the use of a simulated patient and a part-task trainer. They therefore allow learners to interact with a patient while practicing a technical skill. For example, when simulating a shoulder dystocia, the use of a birthing pelvis placed between the legs of a simulated patient allows learners to practice communicating with the patient in a critical moment while also performing the shoulder dystocia maneuvers on a birthing pelvis. Hybrid simulators have a particular value in the effort to create low-cost, realistic obstetrical simulation scenarios.

Realism

High Fidelity simulators became synonymous with expensive, physically real-appearing manikins. Diekmann et al. advanced the understanding of "fidelity" or "realism" by parsing out the concept of realism in physical, semantical, and phenomenological domains. Rudolph et al. further reframed these concepts as Physical, Conceptual, and Emotional Realism (Rudolph et al., 2007). The careful consideration of these domains is vital to achieving the learning objectives of the simulation scenario:

Physical realism refers to the look and feel of the simulator used in the scenario. If the aim of the simulation is to develop specific technical skills, physical realism may be most important.

Conceptual realism refers to the ability of the simulator to respond to "if-then" relationships in a clinically realistic way. For example, if a learner gives a blood pressure lowering medication then the blood pressure should go down. The blood pressure could be displayed on a monitor connected to a manikin, a tablet next to a simulated patient, written on a piece of paper or a whiteboard, or even called out by the simulation instructor. As long as the blood pressure goes down and this is somehow communicated, the conceptual realism of the scenario is upheld.

Emotional realism refers to the affective experience when engaging in a simulation scenario. The emotional tone of the scenario should consider the level of the learner and the objectives of the scenario. For example, when teaching the steps of a cesarean section to a junior learner, it may be harmful to simulate an anxious patient voice speaking nervously across the drapes. In contrast, when training an interprofessional team to respond to an eclamptic seizure, having an anxious partner in the room for the team to manage may increase the emotional experience of realism for the participants.

Considering the different domains of realism is critical to designing a practical, cost-effective scenario that will engage participants and lead them toward achieving the learning objectives of the scenario.

Crisis Resource Management

The concept of "Crisis Resource Management" (CRM) was adapted by David Gaba from "Crew Resource Management" born out of the aviation industry to teach teams how to manage crises using simulation drills. CRM skills are nontechnical skills such as leadership, followership, resource management, situational awareness, and communication. Like technical skills and clinical expertise, CRM is a skill set that requires practice and honing.

Prebriefing and Debriefing

Prebriefing the learners on the upcoming simulation activity helps to create psychological safety that is paramount to a constructive learning experience. This is an opportunity to orient the learners to the space and the equipment, emphasize the aim of the activity, encourage the "suspension of disbelief," and normalize the debriefing process.

Debriefing refers to a period of deliberate facilitated reflection on performance following a simulation scenario. Debriefing is critical to translating the simulated experience into meaningful learning. Whether facilitated by an expert debriefer or a structured written guide, there is value to the debriefing process. There are several models for debriefing. Eppich and Cheng created an integrated framework for debriefing—the PEARLS

OTHER ISSUES

framework—that is commonly employed. It emphasizes a learner-centred approach to debriefing and moves through four phases: reactions, summary, analysis, and wrap-up (Eppich and Cheng, 2015).

In Situ Simulation

Simulations can take place in a number of settings depending on the objectives of the simulation and the availability of resources. In situ simulation takes place in the native clinical context. For example, a simulated postpartum hemorrhage would take place on the birthing unit in a birthing room and the participants in the simulation would be the on-call team that is working at that time.

Depending on unit acuity, in situ simulation may pose some logistical challenges given the need to provide concurrent clinical care. However, it allows for the actual clinical team to work through relevant challenges to care on site. In so doing, in situ simulation can serve to audit clinical practices and identify latent safety threats that may be specific to the local context. This is in addition to the teamwork and CRM skills that can be practiced.

With the onset of the COVID-19 pandemic, obstetrical units had to rapidly change longstanding practices and evaluate the feasibility of novel protocols. At our center and others, in situ simulations and walkthroughs were utilized to integrate practice and policy, create novel protocols, and adapt existing systems, ushering in a new way in which simulation can be utilized to create and disseminate changes to systems of clinical practice.

CURRENT AND FUTURE DIRECTIONS

This section highlights the growing emphasis on competency-based medical education and patient engagement in education.

Competency-based Medical Education

Competence, most simply stated, is the ability to complete a particular task. Postgraduate programs are increasingly following a Competency Based Framework in which learning objectives take the form of entrustable professional activities (EPAs) and milestones (Frank et al. 2015). Entrustable professional activities describe the authentic tasks of a discipline. They are observable and can be delegated to the learner.

The Royal College of Physicians and Surgeons of Canada (RCPSC) has mapped EPAs and CanMEDS milestones within Obstetrics and Gynecology postgraduate across stages of training. For example, "Performing a Cesarean Section with a Skilled Assistant" is an EPA in the "Foundations of Discipline" stage of training. The task can then be assessed using an entrustment scale. This is an intuitive scale for the clinician teacher because the notion of "entrustability" represents a judgment that the supervisor is frequently making for a given trainee, at a given stage of training, completing a certain task. The scale employed by the RCPSC uses a 5-point rating system, including: 1 ("I had to do"), 2 ("I had to talk them through"), 3 ("I needed to prompt"), 4 ("I needed to be there just in case"), and 5 ("I did not need to be there"). A higher rating reflects a higher level of entrustability.

Overall, competency-based medical education tries to emphasize the value of a growth mindset when approaching learning—one in which supervisors serve as coaches to facilitate the growth of their learners.

Patient Engagement in Education

Patient engagement, in general, has been a new value of institutions in their effort toward improving quality and safety. In particular, the involvement of patients in the creation and evaluation of learning activities is a trend that is gaining momentum.

Collaborating with patients can be beneficial in a number of ways. First, such a collaboration helps to ensure a level of social accountability when designing an educational program or activity. Second, it can help protect against bias and stereotyping when constructing cases and simulation scenarios. Third, such collaboration provides authenticity when training simulated patients. Moreover, engaging patients grounds the educational event by making the link between the clinical team, the disease process, and the patient for whom they care.

CONCLUSION

Sound educational practices are a fundamental component of ensuring safe maternal and newborn care. This chapter aimed to provide some foundational educational theory alongside commonly utilized practical

OTHER ISSUES

frameworks for curriculum and simulation design. Maternal and newborn care is provided by teams. It behooves us then to create educational programs that train the whole team and not only the individual. These training experiences—simulated or otherwise—can be efficient, inexpensive, and still lead to important skill building, while also promoting a culture of interprofessional excellence.

APPENDIX A: SIMULATION SCENARIO—A WORKED EXAMPLE

The following is an example of the way that a simulated case of postpartum hemorrhage can be designed and implemented.

Title: Management of Postpartum Hemorrhage

Needs Assessment: The quality assurance team identified a gap in patient care after reviewing cases of postpartum hemorrhage. The team found delayed intervention, and a lack of closed loop communication during clinical management. They suggested an in situ simulation to train medical teams on postpartum hemorrhage management.

Participants: May include all or some of the following professional roles— Obstetrician, Midwife, Family Physician, Nurse, Anesthesiologist

Location: In situ simulation in an unoccupied birthing room on the birthing unit

Objectives for the Simulation:

1. Integrate key aspects of crisis resource management such as leadership, followership, situational awareness, and closed loop communication while managing postpartum hemorrhage as an interprofessional team.
2. Initiate early medical management of postpartum hemorrhage utilizing the unit's postpartum hemorrhage protocol and kit.
3. System Objective: Identify latent safety threats on the unit during this in situ simulation.

Required Personnel and Equipment:

1. Facilitator(s)—to prebrief the participants, run the simulation scenario, and debrief the participants.
2. Simulated patient—wearing gown and pants with red fabric taped or sewn to simulate postpartum bleeding. Can use mannequin and simulated bleeding if available.
3. Local birthing room supplies—might include blood pressure cuff, oxygen saturation, IV cannula, crystalloid fluid, syringes with labels for postpartum hemorrhage medications, and postpartum hemorrhage checklist/kit if available. Bakri balloon if available.

Vignette: The scenario begins with the facilitator (acting as the off-going nurse) providing the following as handover to the participant nurse.

"This is *Rosa Bledsoe*. She is a 28-year-old primigravid who underwent spontaneous vaginal birth following a 30-hour labor and a 4-hour second stage of labor. She is healthy with no medical history and no allergies. She is now 20 minutes postpartum and has begun to experience more heavy bleeding. Thank you for taking over."

Flow: (can write this out or use a chart or story board to outline scenario flow)

Timeline	Patient Status	Trigger Action by the Learner or Simulator Causing the state to Change	Expected Nurse Actions	Expected Midwife or Obstetrician Actions	Facilitator Actions
Baseline	HR 120 bpm BP 90/50		Participant nurse enters room and requests handover from off-going nurse		Provide handover to participant nurse and "leaves room"
0–5 mins	HR 120 bpm BP 90/50 Simulated patient might say: "I don't feel so good...." "I'm so dizzy"	Uterus noted to be atonic on exam	Initiates uterine massage Calls for help—OB/Midwife Provides handover to OB/Midwife	Receives handover from nurse Requests 2nd IV & Bolus of IV Fluid Request blood work Initiates medical uterotonic therapy	Announce change in vital signs if monitor not available Announce atonic uterus when nurse initiates uterine massage
5–10 mins	BP: 80/50 HR: 130 SPO2: 97% RR: 20 Simulated patient is more confused: "I'm scared. What is happening?"	Continued uterine atony as announced by the facilitator	Inserts 2nd IV, Provides boluses Gives the ordered medications Utilizes closed loop communication	Considers other causes (tissue/trauma/thrombin) Orders blood products Orders 2nd and 3rd uterotonic agents Provides ongoing uterine massage Consider Bakri balloon/laparotomy	Announces vital sign change or changes the display on the monitor Announces ongoing uterine atony and ongoing bleeding
10–12 mins	BP 100/65 HR: 110 Simulated patient: "I'm feeling a bit better"	Uterine tone improves	May initiate huddle or disposition conversation	Initiates huddle or disposition conversation	Announces improved uterine tone and change in vital signs
12 mins	END SCENARIO				

Debriefing: Key phases (per PEARLS debriefing framework):

Reactions: How did that feel?

Summary: Can someone summarize the case to make sure that we are all on the same page?

Analysis: What went well? What could have gone better? What about our system (e.g., room, equipment, etc.) can be changed to make things safer?

Wrap up: What will you take away from this case out into real clinical practice?

Evaluations: Collect feedback from participants on the simulation itself for ongoing improvement of the simulation. Compile any identified latent safety threats and provide these to leadership and relevant stakeholders so that changes can be made to improve unit safety.

SELECTED READING

Chatterjee D, Corral J: How to write well-defined learning objectives. J Educ Perioper Med 19:E610, 2017

Eppich W, Cheng A: Promoting Excellence and Reflective Learning in Simulation (PEARLS): development and rationale for a blended approach to health care simulation debriefing. Simul Healthc 10:106-115, 2015

Draycott TJ, Crofts JF, Ash JP, Wilson LV, Yard E, Sibanda T, et al: Improving neonatal outcome through practical shoulder dystocia training. Obstet Gynecol 112:14-20, 2008

Frank JR, Snell L, Sherbino J: CanMEDS 2015 Physician Competency Framework. The Royal College of Physicians and Surgeons of Canada, Ottawa. http://canmeds.royalcollege.ca/uploads/en/framework/CanMEDS%202015%20Framework_EN_ Reduced.pdf, 2015

Freeth, D: Interprofessional education. In: Swanwick T (ed.), Understanding Medical Education. John Wiley & Sons, Ltd: 2013

Grant, J: Principles of curriculum design. In: Swanwick T (ed.), Understanding Medical Education. John Wiley & Sons, Ltd: 2013

Hafferty FW, Franks R: The hidden curriculum, ethics teaching, and the structure of medical education. Acad Med 69:861-871, 1994

Knowles, Malcolm S: Andragogy in Action. San Francisco: Jossey-Bass, 1984

Kolb DA: Experiential Learning: Experience as the Source of Learning and Development. Englewood Cliffs, NJ: Prentice Hall: 1984

Rudolph JW, Simon R, Raemer DB: Which reality matters? Questions on the path to high engagement in healthcare simulation. Simul Healthc 2:161-163, 2017

Satin AJ: Simulation in obstetrics. Obstet Gynecol 132:199-209, 2018

OTHER ISSUES

CHAPTER 41

Patient Safety and Quality Assurance in Obstetrics

Megan M. Gomes

WHY SHOULD PHYSICIANS CARE ABOUT PATIENT SAFETY AND HEALTH CARE QUALITY?

Patient safety is a global concern and landmark publications and reports have highlighted the extent of concerns present in health care systems. The Institute of Medicine (IOM) released the ground-breaking report "To Err is Human: Building a Safer Health System," which estimates that between 44,000 and 98,000 hospital deaths per year are due to medical error. The Canadian Adverse Events Study reported a 7.5 percent incidence rate of adverse events in Canadian hospitals. Among the adverse events reported, 36.9 percent were judged to be preventable and 20.8 percent resulted in a patient death. It is estimated that one in 10 patients in high-income countries are harmed while receiving care in a hospital setting. Patient safety incidents also represent a significant financial burden on the health care system across the world.

Health care providers and institutions must make an ongoing commitment to patient safety by shifting the culture to focus on patient safety and incorporating patient safety education at all levels of medical training. The creation and implementation of reliable patient safety incident reporting systems should reduce patient safety incidents, provide learning opportunities for the health care team, and improve the quality of patient care in a sustainable fashion.

Definitions

Patient safety is defined as the freedom from potential or unnecessary harm for a patient related to the delivery of health care. Patient safety aims to reduce the risk of patient harm that occurs during health care provision and utilizes best practices demonstrated to lead to optimal patient outcome. The key component of patient safety is continuous improvement guided by learning from adverse events and errors.

The World Health Organization (WHO) Conceptual Framework for the International Classification for Patient Safety was developed to provide patient safety terminology that can be utilized globally.

Patient Safety Incident. An event or circumstance which could have resulted, or did result, in unnecessary harm to a patient. A patient safety incident (PSI) can be classified as a reportable circumstance, near miss, no harm incident, or harmful incident.

Reportable Circumstance. A situation in which there was significant potential for harm, but no incident occurred (e.g., a busy labor and delivery unit remaining grossly understaffed for an entire shift, or bringing a vacuum to an operative vaginal delivery only to discover it does not work although it was not needed).

Near Miss. An incident which did not reach the patient (e.g., an antibiotic being connected to the wrong patient's intravenous line, but the error was detected prior to starting the infusion).

No Harm Incident. An event reached a patient but no discernable harm resulted (e.g., an antibiotic was infused into a patient's intravenous line, but it was not needed).

Harmful Incident. An incident that results in harm to a patient (e.g., the wrong antibiotics were infused into a patient and they were allergic to the medication and the patient experienced and anaphylactic reaction). This replaces the term *adverse event*.

Patient Safety Education

The health care environment has changed: patient populations are becoming more medically complex, new technologies are used, patients are more informed, and health care systems are more complex with an increasing number of interdisciplinary team members responsible for the care of an individual patient. Transforming the way in which we practice medicine and educate our trainees requires a team effort including medical students, residents, staff physicians, department heads, nurses, and allied health professionals. The team approach incorporates a diverse set of knowledge and skills that will provide continuous improvement in patient safety and education in this area.

Effective communication among all members of the health care team is critical to providing safe obstetrical care. Health care team communication issues have been reported in 70 percent of obstetrical sentinel events and have been identified as one of the top three leading root causes of reported sentinel events. Team training and increased awareness of the importance of communication between members of the health care team are key. A robust patient safety program requires teamwork and communication training. The Agency for Healthcare Research and Quality and Department of Defence jointly developed TeamSTEPPS (Team Strategies and Tools to Enhance Performance and Patient Safety). TeamSTEPPS is an example of

OTHER ISSUES

an evidence based teamwork system training program to improve institutional collaboration and communication involving patient safety, and involves tools and concepts applicable to all health care providers.

Awareness of the importance of physician training and participation in quality and patient safety is rapidly growing. The incorporation of patient safety and health care quality into core medical education curriculums will pave the way to necessary change that will integrate patient safety into the daily practice of health care providers. New international standards have been set by organizations such as the Royal College of Physicians and Surgeons of Canada and the Accreditation Council for Graduate Medical Education that include quality concepts in the curriculum. Current leaders and practicing physicians also require education in the importance of patient safety and training in order to incorporate health care quality and patient safety into their daily practice.

The patient safety and health care quality curriculum must extend beyond the classroom into the hospital wards and outpatient clinics. A powerful way to educate health care trainees is through their daily work environment and through clinically relevant experiences. Health care professionals must strive to continually improve the care that they provide and the system in which they work in order to integrate patient safety and health care quality into medical training in the clinical setting.

Patient Safety Culture

A culture of safety is fundamental in the effort to reduce error. A culture of patient safety is defined as "the incorporation of safe thinking and practise into clinical medicine." A safe culture includes the development of systems for reporting and data collection, a reduction in the predisposition of placing blame on individuals, and a focus on systemic latencies. A "Just Culture" is also an essential component to promoting a safety culture. A just culture recognizes that competent medical professionals make errors and that errors are inevitable, especially in the context of delivery of health care given its complexity. Just culture recognizes the responsibility of all health care workers to follow safe practices and to avoid reckless behaviours. Reckless behavior is an action that puts a patient at risk of significant harm and shows a conscious disregard of risk. A just culture will investigate patient safety incidents fairly and openly. One key component of creating a culture that supports patient safety is developing an atmosphere where health care providers feel safe in reporting PSI, are encouraged to report PSI, are motivated to identify systemic problems and collaborate to create change.

A dedicated Quality Assurance (QA) Committee is recommended to facilitate effective and sustainable change. Leadership is required to advocate for allocation of financial and human resources to achieve the recommendations developed by the QA team. A forum for dissemination of knowledge and policy change that reaches all levels of the health care team is required. Regular departmental maternal and morbidity rounds and educational rounds on various topics in patient safety is required. In addition, frequent memos, a department quality newsletter, and email communications are recommended to provide continuous updates and education on patient safety.

Patient Safety Reporting System and Quality Assurance Committee

A fundamental shift in the way health care providers perceive patient safety incidents is imperative. The prevailing culture of blame is a prominent source of safety issues in the health care system. The IOM report highlights the fact that patient harm due to medical error is not the result of health care professionals themselves but rather due to the entire health care system. The health care profession must shift the focus of simply placing blame on individuals toward scrutinizing the system in which we work. Every member of the health care team must acquire the skill set to recognize the potential of systemic errors. Health care must be delivered in an environment that encourages patient safety incident reporting.

Health care providers at all levels have a duty to actively participate in the process of change. Leaders in the field need to educate health care providers that patient safety incidents can be used as an opportunity to improve the system as opposed to placing blame. When health care professionals are educated on the importance of reporting PSIs and the subsequent system wide change that is generated from patient safety reports there will be a shift in the way providers perceive PSI reporting.

The key principle of patient safety is continuous improvement guided by knowledge acquired from patient safety incidents and medical errors. Effective patient safety initiatives require a mechanism to report patient safety incidents, a Quality Committee to analyze the incident reports and provide recommendations, and infrastructure to implement the recommendations generated to develop subsequent policy change thereby decreasing the likelihood of recurrence. Health care institutions require a commitment to allocate financial resources toward a safety incident reporting system and the personnel required to support and analyze the system.

OTHER ISSUES

Institutions require a formal system to report patient safety incidents in order to analyze and learn from patient safety incidents. The Ottawa Hospital (TOH) incorporated a formalized system of reporting patient safety incidents in 2009, called the Safety Learning System (SLS). The SLS is a voluntary electronic patient safety reporting system that can be completed by any member of the health care team. The SLS system is available on all hospital computers and through remote access with hospital identification log in. The SLS system classifies events in four separate categories including: patient safety incident, employee incident report, security incident, or privacy incident. Additional prompts and drop-down menus appear that trigger reporting of additional mandatory details including incident date, location, associated service, affected patient, and other parties involved. A mandatory text box is included to allow a brief description to include all relevant details surrounding the incident, the outcome, and what was done in response. Indications for completion of an SLS report were developed by the QA Committee and are outlined in Table 41-1.

Each individual SLS report completed in the Obstetrics department is reviewed following the algorithm outlined in Figure 41-1. Each SLS entry is reviewed by a core reviewer, for example the clinical care leader or clinical manager, to determine if the incident requires review at prescreen, can be addressed independently, or if the report can be closed without further review. All SLS reports submitted by a health care team member are reviewed, and pertinent details of the case and follow-up action items are included in the SLS report prior to closing the report. The SLS report is graded on an ordinal scale with regards to the severity (Table 41-2) and likelihood of recurrence (Table 41-3) and recommendations are provided. If a critical patient safety incident is identified by the core reviewer as outlined in Table 41-4, the SLS report is escalated to the Corporate Quality Department at our Institution for a more detailed review.

The core reviewer generates the SLS case list to be reviewed by a smaller group of the Quality Assurance (QA) Committee members at monthly prescreen meetings. The QA Committee prescreen meeting is led by the Director of Quality and Patient Safety, a physician with an area of expertise in patient safety, and is comprised of a multidisciplinary group of health care providers, including labor and delivery and postpartum clinical managers, labor and delivery and postpartum nurse educators, physicians from obstetrics and maternal fetal medicine, a patient relations representative, and a quality coordinator. The prescreen group reviews all SLS cases deemed required for further investigation by the core reviewer. Each SLS case is reviewed and a decision is made to analyze the case at the prescreen meeting with recommendations, grading of incident severity, and

TABLE 41-1: MEDICAL INDICATORS FOR SAFETY LEARNING SYSTEM (SLS) REPORTING (BIRTHING UNIT AND MOTHER BABY UNIT)

MATERNAL INDICATORS FOR REPORTING		
SLS Entry Required	**Strongly Consider SLS Entry**	
Adverse Drug Reaction/ Medication Error	Death or serious disability associated with labor and delivery*	Anesthesia related complications*	Chorioamnionitis w/ wadverse outcome/Sepsis	Code 333
Cardio-Respiratory Arrest	Hemorrhage requiring transfusion/Code Bleed Obstetrics	DVT/PE/Other embolus	Failed Forceps/ Vacuum w/ adverse outcome	Placental abruption
Hysterectomy-unplanned	Injury during surgery*	4th degree tear	Placenta previa/ accreta w/ adverse outcome	Other serious incidents
Seizures	Severe medical illness/ Admission to ICU*	Unplanned transfer to OR	Unattended delivery	Hypertensive emergency
Uterine rupture	Retained foreign body	Post-partum readmission		

(Continued)

TABLE 41-1: MEDICAL INDICATORS FOR SAFETY LEARNING SYSTEM (SLS) REPORTING (BIRTHING UNIT AND MOTHER BABY UNIT) (Continued)

FETAL INDICATORS FOR REPORTING				
SLS Entry Required		**Strongly Consider SLS Entry**		
Abduction or discharge to wrong person	Transfer to CHEO for cooling	Apgar <5 at 5 minutes	Base Excess > than –12.5	Code 222
Birth Trauma	Neonatal Intrapartum Death*	Cord Prolapse	Neonatal loss	Other serious incidents
Unexpected admission to SCN/NICU due to poor gases/APGARS/anomalies*	Unexpected Neonatal Death*	Shoulder dystocia with suspected injury	Late or Term Stillbirth**	
Cord pH <7	Seizures/Significant neurologic event/Abnormal MRI	Unexpected congenital anomalies		

SYSTEM/ENVIRONMENT INDICATORS FOR REPORTING
Communication
Documentation (Records/Results)
Equipment/Resources
Human Resources
Protocol Deviations
No system issues identified

*Does not result primarily from the patients underlying medical condition or from a known risk inherent in providing the treatment

**Late stillbirth: occurs between 28–36 completed weeks of pregnancy.

**Term stillbirth: occurs between 37 or more complete weeks of pregnancy.

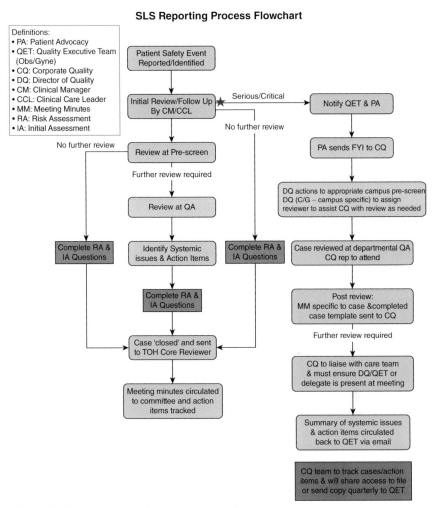

SLS Reporting Process Flowchart

Definitions:
• PA: Patient Advocacy
• QET: Quality Executive Team (Obs/Gyne)
• CQ: Corporate Quality
• DQ: Director of Quality
• CM: Clinical Manager
• CCL: Clinical Care Leader
• MM: Meeting Minutes
• RA: Risk Assessment
• IA: Initial Assessment

Patient Safety Event Reported/Identified

Initial Review/Follow Up By CM/CCL → Serious/Critical → Notify QET & PA

No further review

PA sends FYI to CQ

No further review

Review at Pre-screen

Further review required

Review at QA

DQ actions to appropriate campus pre-screen DQ (C/G – campus specific) to assign reviewer to assist CQ with review as needed

Complete RA & IA Questions

Identify Systemic issues & Action Items

Complete RA & IA Questions

Case reviewed at departmental QA CQ rep to attend

Complete RA & IA Questions

Post review: MM specific to case &completed case template sent to CQ

Further review required

Case 'closed' and sent to TOH Core Reviewer

CQ to liaise with care team & must ensure DQ/QET or delegate is present at meeting

Meeting minutes circulated to committee and action items tracked

Summary of systemic issues & action items circulated back to QET via email

CQ team to track cases/action items & will share access to file or send copy quarterly to QET

FIGURE 41-1. SLS reporting process flowchart.

OTHER ISSUES

likelihood of recurrence and closing the SLS event, or the case is selected for a more detailed review at the monthly QA committee meeting.

An active multidisciplinary QA committee is an essential component to the analysis and review of SLS reports and generation of recommendations. The QA Committee is comprised of a larger multidisciplinary team including physicians from Obstetrics, Maternal Fetal Medicine, Neonatology, Obstetrics Anesthesiologists, nursing, patient advocacy representative and the quality coordinator and is led by the Director of Quality and Patient Safety. Each SLS case is presented using a standard QA Case Review

TABLE 41-2: SLS SEVERITY OF INCIDENT

Severity of the Incident	Patient Safety	Critical	Incident leading to death or loss of limb/organ.
		Serious	Major injury resulting in irreversible damage.
		Moderate	Moderate injury requiring treatment. Increased length of hospital stay.
		Minor	Minor injury requiring minimal treatment.
		No Harm	No harm or minimal injury requiring no treatment.

TABLE 41-3: SLS LIKELIHOOD OF RECURRENCE

	Term	Definition
Likelihood of Reoccurrence	High	Expected to reoccur
	Medium	Might reoccur
	Low	Not expected to reoccur
	Rare	Should never reoccur

TABLE 41-4: LISTS OF INCIDENTS THAT MUST BE REPORTED FOR SERIOUS INCIDENT REVIEW

- Maternal mortality or serious disability associated with labor and delivery
- Neonatal intrapartum death that does not result primarily from the patient's underlying medical conditions or from a known risk inherent in providing the treatment
- Unexpected neonatal death that does not result primarily from the patient's underlying medical conditions or from a known risk inherent in providing the treatment
- Neonatal transfer to CHEO for head cooling due to asphyxia
- Patient death or serious disability associated with a medication error (i.e., death involving a narcotic)
- Patient transferred back to ICU within 48 hours
- Infant abducted or discharged to wrong person
- Outside the above criteria, any incident deemed critical or serious as decided by interdisciplinary team

QA Case Review Template	
MRN: SLS:	Date:
1. **Case Summary** - brief summary of pertinent history and details.	**2 min**
2. **Case Analysis (What was the primary reason for a QA review?)** • What happened? • What normally happens? • What does the procedure require?	**3 min**

3. **Discussion**
• Why did it happen?
• Did you identify any system issues in this case?
  ➤ Communication
  ➤ Equipment/Resources
  ➤ Human Resources
  ➤ Protocol Deviations
  ➤ Documentation
  ➤ No systemic issues identified
• How was TOH managing the risk at the time of the incident?
	5 min

4. **Action Items** • Do you have any recommendations that would improve patient care?	**5 min**

FIGURE 41-2. Standard QA case review template.

Template (Fig. 41-2) in order to provide consistency of case analysis. All pertinent details regarding the case are reviewed and a complete risk assessment of the case is performed by the committee. Because all SLS cases reviewed at QA have been prescreened and identified for review, the goal is to develop action items to prevent future occurrences of similar events. An update on the progress of the generated action items are reviewed at the next QA committee meeting. After review at QA, the case is closed and sent to TOH's core review quality and patient safety department, which is comprised of a large hospital-wide multidisciplinary group (Fig. 41-1). Each case reviewed at QA is considered for presentation at department maternal morbidity and mortality rounds.

The quality committee recommendations and reminders are disseminated in a quarterly department quality newsletter, at monthly divisional and department meetings, the department quality Share Point site, and via email communication to ensure regular department-wide dissemination.

OTHER ISSUES

Conclusion

As the medical field advances at a rapid pace, the health care system must adapt in order to continue to provide high-quality care to patients. Landmark publications and reports alerted the medical profession and patients of the major issues in patient safety and health care quality present in our current health care system. In order to improve patient outcomes and provide safe quality care, health care providers require education on the core concepts of patient safety and health care quality and learn to integrate the patient safety culture into our daily clinical practice. Communication and team collaboration is required to optimize and promote patient safety principles. Institutions require a reliable patient safety incident reporting system with a dedicated patient safety team to analyze and generate recommendations to improve the quality of care provided.

SELECTED READING

Agency for Healthcare Research and Quality: TeamSTEPPS™: national implementation. https://www.ahrq.gov/teamstepps/index.html, 2021

American College of Obstetricians and Gynecologists: Patient safety in obstetrics and gynecology. ACOG Committee Opinion No. 447. Obstet Gynecol 114:1424-1427, 2009

Asch DA, Nicholson S, Srinivas S, Herrin J, Epstein AJ: Evaluating obstetrical residency programs using patient outcomes. JAMA 302:1277-1283, 2009

Baker R, Norton P, Flintoft V, Blais R, Brown A, Cox J, Tamblyn R: The Canadian Adverse Events Study: The incidence of adverse events among hospital patients in Canada. CMAJ 170, 1678-1686, 2004

Brennan T, Leape L, Laird N, Hebert L, Localio R, Lawthers A, Newhouse J, et al: Harvard Medical Practice Study I. Incidence of adverse events and negligence in hospitalized patients: Results of the Harvard Medical Practice Study I. 1991. Qual Safety Health Care 13: 145-151; discussion 151-152, 2014

Committee on Quality of Health Care in America; Institute of Medicine: Crossing the Quality Chasm: A New Health System for the 21st Century. Washington, DC: National Academies Press, 2001

Kohn L, Corrigan J, Donaldson, M: To Err Is Human: Building a Safer Health System. Washington, DC: National Academies Press, 2000

Mann S, Pratt S: Team approach to care in labour and delivery. Clin Obstet Gynecol 51: 666-679, 2008

Panagioti M, Khan K, Keers RN, Abuzour A, Phipps D, Kontopantelis E, Bower P, et al: Prevalence, Severity, and nature of preventable patient harm across medical care settings: Systematic review and meta-analysis. BMJ 366:l4185-l4185, 2019

Patow CA, Karpovich K, Riesenberg LA, Jaeger J, Rosenfeld JC, Wittenbreer M, Padmore JS: Residents' engagement in quality improvement: A systematic review of the literature. Acad Med 84:1757-1764, 2009

Pettker CM, Thung SF, Raab CA, Donohue KP, Copel JA, Lockwood CJ, Funai EF: A comprehensive obstetrics patient safety program improves safety climate and culture. Am J Obstet Gynecol 204:216.e1-216.e6, 2011

Singer SJ, Gaba DM, Geppert JJ, Sinaiko AD, Howard SK, Park KC. The culture of safety: Results of an organization-wide survey in 15 California hospitals. Qual Saf Health Care 12:112-118, 2003

Singh R, Naughton B, Taylor JS, Koenigsberg MR, Anderson DR, McCausland LL, Wahler RG, et al: A comprehensive collaborative patient safety residency curriculum to address the ACGME core competencies. Med Educ, 39:1195-1204, 2005

Slawomirski L, Auraaen A, Klazinga N. The Economics of Patient Safety: Strengthening a Value-Based Approach to Reducing Patient Harm at National Level. Paris: OECD; 2017

Stevens DP, Kirkland KB: The role for clinician educators in implementing healthcare improvement. J Gen Intern Med, 25:S639-643, 2010

The Joint Commission: Sentinel Event Data Root Causes by Event Type 2004-2013

The Joint Commission: Sentinel event alert, Issue 30. http://www.jointcommission.org/assets/1/18/SEA_30.PDF, 2021

Walton M, Woodward H, Van Staalduinen S, et al: The WHO patient safety curriculum guide for medical schools. BMJ Quality & Safety 19:542-546, 2010

Wong R: Teaching Quality Improvement in Residency Education (pp. 1–102). Royal College of Physicians and Surgeons of Canada. http://www.royalcollege.ca/rcsite/documents/cbd/teaching-quality-improvement-in-residency-education-e.pdf, 2015

World Health Organization: The Conceptual Framework for the International Classification for Patient Safety. World Health Organization: Geneva, 2009.

OTHER ISSUES

Note: Page numbers followed by *f* and *t* refer to figures and tables respectively.